Lippincott's Review Series

Mental Health and Psychiatric Nursing

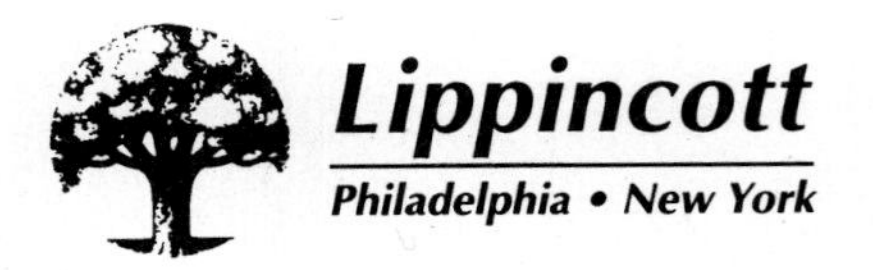
Lippincott
Philadelphia • New York

Lippincott's Review Series

SECOND EDITION

Mental Health and Psychiatric Nursing

Ann Isaacs, RN, CS, MSN
Associate Professor
Luzerne County Community College
Nanticoke, Pennsylvania

Acquisitions Editor: **Susan Glover, RN, MSN**
Sponsoring Editor: **Deedie McMahon**
Project Editor: **Sandra Cherrey Scheinin**
Production Manager: **Helen Ewan**
Design Coordinator: **Doug Smock**
Indexer: **Sandy Nickerson**

2nd Edition

Library of Congress Cataloging in Publications Data

Isaacs, Ann.
Mental health and psychiatric nursing.—2nd ed. / Ann Isaacs.
p. cm.—(Lippincott's review series)
Rev. ed. of: Mental health and psychiatric nursing. © 1992.
Includes bibliographical references and index.
ISBN 0-397-55215-7
1. Psychiatric nursing—Examinations, questions, etc. I. Title.
II. Series.
[DNLM: 1. Mental Health—examination questions. 2. Psychiatric Nursing—examination questions. WY 18.2 I74m 1996]
RC440.L57 1996
610.73'68'076—dc20
DNLM/DLC
for Library of Congress 95-41442
CIP

The material contained in this volume was submitted as previously unpublished material, except in the instances in which credit has been given to the source from which some of the illustrative material was derived.

Any procedure or practice described in this book should be applied by the health-care practitioner under appropriate supervision in accordance with professional standards of care used with regard to the unique circumstances that apply in each practice situation. Care has been taken to confirm the accuracy of information presented and to describe generally accepted practices. However, the authors, editors, and publisher cannot accept any responsibility for errors or omissions or for any consequences from application of the information in this book and make no warranty, express or implied, with respect to the contents of the book.

The authors and publisher have exerted every effort to ensure that drug selection and dosage set forth in this text are in accordance with current recommendations and practice at the time of publication. However, in view of ongoing research, changes in government regulations, and the constant flow of information relating to drug therapy and drug reactions, the reader is urged to check the package insert for each drug for any change in indications and dosage and for added warnings and precautions. This is particularly important when the recommended agent is a new or infrequently employed drug.

Materials appearing in this book prepared by individuals as part of their official duties as U.S. Government employees are not covered by the above-mentioned copyright.

9 8 7 6 5 4 3 2 1

REVIEWERS

Barbara K. Boyer, RN, BSN
Director of Nursing Education
Mental Health Institute
Independence, Iowa

Penny S. Brooke, RN, MS, JD
Assistant Dean
University of Utah College of Nursing
Salt Lake City, Utah

Edward J. Edwards, RN, EdD, CHES
Assistant Professor
Indiana University of Pennsylvania
Indiana, Pennsylvania

INTRODUCTION

Lippincott's Review Series is designed to help you in your study of the key subject areas in nursing. The series consists of six books, one in each core nursing subject area:

Medical-Surgical Nursing
Pediatric Nursing
Maternal-Newborn Nursing
Mental Health and Psychiatric Nursing
Pathophysiology
Fluids and Electrolytes

Each book contains a comprehensive outline content review, chapter study questions and answer keys with rationales for correct and incorrect responses, and a comprehensive examination and answer key with rationales for correct and incorrect responses.

Lippincott's Review Series was planned and developed in response to your requests for outline review books that address each major subject area and also contain a self-test mechanism. These books meet the need for comprehensive subject review books that will also assist you in identifying your strong and weak areas of knowledge. Each book is a complete source for review and self-assessment of a single core subject—all six together provide an excellent comprehensive review of entry-level nursing.

Each book is all-inclusive of the content addressed in major textbooks. The content outline review uses a consistent nursing process format throughout and addresses nursing care for well and ill clients. Also included are necessary additional concepts such as growth and development, nutrition, pharmacology, and body structures, functions, and pathophysiology. Special features of each book are Key Concepts and Nursing Alerts, which are identified by distinctive icons. Key Concepts are basic facts the nurse needs to know to perform his or her job with ease and efficiency. Nursing Alerts are fundamental guidelines the nurse can follow to ensure safe and effective care.

You can use the books in this series in several different ways. Overall, you can use them as subject reviews to augment general study throughout your basic nursing program and as a review to prepare for the National Council Licensure Examination (NCLEX-RN). How you use each book depends on your individual needs and preferences, and on whether you review each chapter systematically or concentrate only on those chapters whose subject areas are particularly problematic or challenging.

You may instead choose to use the comprehensive examination as a self-assessment opportunity to evaluate your knowledge base before you review the content outline. Likewise, you can use the study questions for pre- or post-testing after study, followed by the comprehensive examination as a means of evaluating your knowledge and competencies of an entire subject area.

Regardless of how you use the books, one of the strengths of the series is the self-assessment opportunity it offers in addition to guidance in studying and reviewing content. The chapter study questions and comprehensive examination questions have been carefully developed to cover all topics in the outline review. Most important, each question is categorized according to the components of the National Council of State Boards of Nursing Licensing Examination (NCLEX).

- Cognitive Level: Knowledge, Comprehension, Application, or Analysis
- Client Need: Safe, Effective Care Environment (Safe care); Physiological Integrity (Physiologic); Psychosocial Integrity (Psychosocial); and Health Promotion and Maintenance (Health Promotion)
- Phase of the Nursing Process: Assessment, Analysis (Dx), Planning, Implementation, Evaluation

For those questions not related to a client need or to a phase of the nursing process, NA (not applicable) will be used, as in questions that test knowledge of a basic science.

Unlike the NCLEX examination that tests the cumulative knowledge needed for safe practice by an entry-level nurse, these practice tests systematically evaluate the knowledge base that serves as the building block for the entire nursing educational process. In this way, you can prepare for the NCLEX examination throughout your course of study. Good study habits throughout your educational program are not only the best way to ensure ongoing success, but also will prove the most beneficial way to prepare for the licensing examination.

Keep in mind that these books are not intended to replace formal learning. They cannot substitute for textbook reading, discussion with instructors, or class attendance. Every effort has been made to provide accurate and current information, but class attendance and interaction with an instructor will provide invaluable information not found in books. Used correctly, these books will help you increase understanding, improve comprehension, evaluate strengths and weaknesses in areas of knowledge, increase productive study time, and, as a result, help you improve your grades.

MONEY BACK GUARANTEE—Lippincott's Review Series will help you study more effectively during coursework throughout your educational program, and help you prepare for quizzes and tests, including the NCLEX exam. If you buy and use any of the six volumes in Lippincott's Review Series and fail the NCLEX exam, simply send us verification of your exam results and your copy of the review book to the address below. We will promptly send you a check for our suggested list price.

Lippincott's Review Series
Marketing Department
Lippincott-Raven Publishers
227 East Washington Square
Philadelphia, PA 19106-3780

CONTENTS

Lippincott's Review Series

Mental Health and Psychiatric Nursing

Professional Role and Practice of Mental Health and Psychiatric Nursing

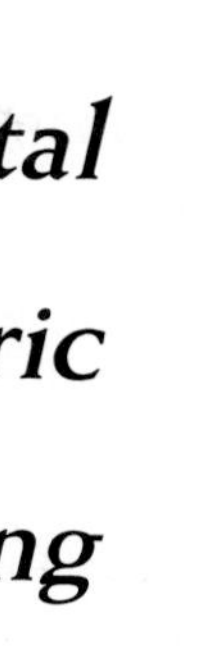

I. Overview

A. Evolution

1. Among her many accomplishments, Florence Nightingale (1850s) noted that client care must involve psychologic and social, as well as physiologic, aspects.
2. In the 1880s, Linda Richards promoted better care for psychiatric clients and directed the first school for mental health and psychiatric nursing.

3. Working as Assistant Superintendent of Nurses at the psychiatric clinic of The Johns Hopkins Hospital, Harriet Baily wrote the first psychiatric nursing textbook, *Nursing Mental Diseases*, in 1920.
4. In 1937, the National League for Nursing (NLN) recommended that mental health and psychiatric nursing be included in nursing school curricula. The NLN also assumed responsibility for standardizing and accrediting psychiatric nursing education.
5. In 1948, Esther Lucille Brown wrote a report, "Nursing for the Future," in which she recommended incorporating psychiatric nursing into the basic schools of nursing.
6. **Hildegard Peplau's 1958 book *Interpersonal Relations in Nursing* presented the first major framework for psychiatric nursing practice and also emphasized the interpersonal nature of nursing and the use of psychodynamic principles in nursing practice.**
7. In 1958, the American Nurses Association (ANA) established the Conference Group on Psychiatric Nursing, now known as the Council on Psychiatric and Mental Health Nursing Practice.
8. **In 1973, the ANA published the first standards of mental health and psychiatric nursing practice; these standards were revised in 1982 and in 1994.**

B. Nursing roles and functions

1. The nurse uses the nursing process in providing direct care to clients and families.
   a. **Promotes self-care and independence**
   b. **Assists with problem solving to facilitate activities of daily living**
   c. **Communicates in a therapeutic manner**
   d. **Establishes effective interpersonal relationships**
   e. **Helps the client examine problem behaviors and test alternatives**
   f. **Teaches health measures and provides information about specific disorders and recommended treatments**
   g. **Administers, monitors, and informs the client about prescribed medications and other treatments**
   h. **Ensures a safe environment**
2. **The nurse establishes and maintains a therapeutic milieu.**
   a. Views interactions with the client as having potential to enhance self-esteem and improve coping
   b. Participates in team approach to treatment
   c. Promotes client responsibility for treatment and self-governance

d. Reinforces policies and procedures established to govern inappropriate behavior

3. The nurse coordinates diverse aspects of client care.

4. The nurse acts as client and family advocate.

a. Teaches about rights and responsibilities of clients
b. Shares information about self-help and support groups
c. Makes appropriate referrals to community resources

5. The nurse works as a member of the interdisciplinary team in planning, implementing, and evaluating client care.

6. The nurse promotes primary prevention measures.

a. Teaches principles of mental health
b. Teaches stress management; promotes life and/or coping skills
c. Encourages effective family communication and function
d. Participates in community-oriented programs related to mental health

C. Practice settings

1. Acute care inpatient settings
   a. General community hospitals
   b. Medical centers
   c. State facilities
   d. Veterans' facilities
2. Crisis care settings
   a. Walk-in clinics
   b. Outpatient services
   c. Crisis hot line units
3. Community mental health centers
4. Private organizations (HMOs, private practices, groups)
5. Ongoing care for clients with chronic mental illness
   a. Halfway houses
   b. Clinics
   c. Structured work programs and sheltered workshops
6. Partial hospitalization programs
7. Prisons

D. Levels of care

1. Primary preventive care involves altering causative or risk factors to impede a developing illness. Primary prevention encompasses:

a. Client and family teaching
b. Stress reduction
c. Psychosocial support
d. Substance abuse avoidance and other preventive measures

2. **Secondary preventive care focuses on reducing or minimizing the effects of mental illness. Aspects include:**
   a. Screening
   b. Crisis intervention
   c. Suicide prevention
   d. Short-term counseling
   e. Emergency nursing care and short-term hospitalization

3. **Tertiary preventive care involves minimizing long-term residual effects of illness. Examples include:**
   a. Rehabilitation programs
   b. Vocational training
   c. Aftercare support
   d. Partial hospitalization options

E. Levels of practice

1. **Basic level: Psychiatric-mental health registered nurse**
   a. Education: baccalaureate degree in nursing
   b. Certification: formal process validating nurse's clinical competence; RN,C
   c. Practice: staff nurse in variety of inpatient and community settings

2. **Advanced level: psychiatric-mental health advanced practice registered nurse (APRN)**
   a. Education: master's degree in psychiatric-mental health nursing as a clinical specialist
   b. Certification: formal process validating competence in advanced clinical nursing skills; RN, CS
   c. Practice: structured and unstructured settings in primary care and community; independent practice as psychotherapist

F. Standards of practice

1. The ANA's Council on Psychiatric and Mental Health Nursing developed the first widely accepted standard of practice in 1973 (revised in 1982 and 1994).
2. In 1994, a collaborative effort of members of the Coalition of Psychiatric Nursing Organizations, under the leadership of the Executive Committee of the ANA's Council on Psychiatric and Mental Health Nursing, revised these standards of practice, which are divided into two general areas:
   a. Standards of care: "pertain to professional nursing activities that are demonstrated by the nurse through the nursing process" (ANA, 1994, p. 25).
   b. Standards of professional performance: "describe a competent level of behavior in the professional role, including

activities related to quality of care, performance appraisal, education, collegiality, ethics, collaboration, research, and resource utilization" (ANA, 1994, p. 34).

II. Therapeutic nurse-client relationships

A. Elements

1. Goal-directed and purposeful interaction involves:
   a. Establishing a contract for the time, place, and focus of nurse-client meetings
   b. Planning conditions for termination at the onset of and throughout the relationship

2. **Roles and responsibilities should be clearly defined; the nurse is the professional helper and facilitator, and the client's needs and problems are the focus of the relationship.**
3. Confidentiality is maintained by:
   a. Sharing information only with professional staff who have a need to know
   b. Informing the client of all information to be shared beforehand
   c. Obtaining the client's written permission to share information with any others outside of the healthcare team
4. Therapeutic behaviors by the nurse include:
   a. Self-awareness of thoughts, feelings, behaviors
   b. Clarification of personal values
   c. Empathic listening
   d. Effective communication
   e. Realistic goal setting
   f. Collaborative work with clients
   g. Responsible and ethical practice

B. Phases

1. **The orientation (assessment and analysis) phase involves:**
   a. **Developing trust and open communication**
   b. Assessing the client's reason for seeking help or hospitalization
   c. Establishing mutually agreed-upon goals
   d. Developing a therapeutic contract (see Display 1-1)
   e. Formulating nursing diagnoses

2. **The working (planning and implementing) phase involves:**
   a. **Planning outcomes and related interventions to assist client to meet goals**
   b. Facilitating expression of thoughts and feelings
   c. Exploring problems
   d. Encouraging constructive coping measures

DISPLAY 1-1.
Essential Elements of a Therapeutic Nurse-Client Contract

- Nurse and client know each other's names.
- Client understands the nurse's role.
- Responsibilities of nurse and client are defined.
- Goals of the relationship are clarified.
- Meeting places and times are established.
- Conditions for termination are outlined.
- Confidentiality is discussed and ensured.

e. Practicing and evaluating more adaptive behaviors
f. Working through resistance behavior

3. **The termination (evaluation) phase involves:**
   a. **Evaluating therapeutic outcomes**
   b. **Expressing feelings about termination**
   c. Observing for regressive behavior
   d. Evaluating the nurse-client relationship

C. Therapeutic (facilitative) communication

1. Structural elements of communication include:
   a. Sender: originator of the message
   b. Message: information transmitted
   c. Receiver: recipient of the message
   d. Feedback (sometimes referred to as "feedback loop"): response of the receiver to the message
   e. Context: setting in which communication takes place
2. Nonverbal communication techniques include:
   a. Kinetics: body movements such as gestures, facial expressions, and other mannerisms
   b. Proxemics: the space between communicators (eg, intimate space, up to 18 in; personal space, 18 in to 4 ft; social-consultative space, 9 to 12 ft; and public space, more than 12 ft apart)
   c. Touch
   d. Silence
   e. Paralanguage: voice quality or how message is delivered
3. Variables influencing communication include:
   a. Perception: one's viewpoint about the situation
   b. Values: one's beliefs about what is desirable
   c. Cultural background: distinctive, learned ways of life (eg, language, customs)
   d. Roles: social or professional functions (eg, parent, nurse, student)
4. Aims of therapeutic communication include:
   a. Initiating a professional, helpful relationship

b. Building trust
c. Maintaining a helping relationship over time
d. Providing emotional support

5. Essential elements for therapeutic communication include:
a. An unconditionally positive regard for the client
b. Empathy (see Table 1-1)
c. Genuineness
d. Warmth and respect
e. Immediacy
f. Purposefulness

6. Therapeutic communication approaches include:
a. Offering self: being available to listen to the client
b. Asking open-ended questions: neutral questions that encourage the client to express concerns
c. Providing opening remarks: general statements based on assessment of the client
d. Restating: repeating to the client the main content of the communication
e. Reflecting: questions and feelings are directed back to the client
f. Focusing: asking goal-directed questions to help the client focus on a specific content area
g. Encouraging elaboration: helping the client to describe more fully the concerns or problems under discussion
h. Seeking clarification: helping the client put into words unclear thoughts or ideas

TABLE 1-1.
Comparing Empathic and Nonempathic Nursing Behaviors

EMPATHIC BEHAVIORS	NONEMPATHIC BEHAVIORS
▸ Focusing on the client's feelings	▸ Ignoring the client's feelings
▸ Asking open-ended questions	▸ Asking closed-ended questions
▸ Using a warm vocal tone	▸ Using a flat vocal tone
▸ Conveying a nonjudgmental attitude	▸ Conveying a judgmental attitude
▸ Maintaining eye contact	▸ Looking away
▸ Nodding the head periodically	▸ Nodding too much
▸ Smiling periodically	▸ Picking at clothing
▸ Making smooth gestures	▸ Maintaining facial inexpressiveness
▸ Opening arms	▸ Laughing too much
▸ Leaning forward slightly	▸ Making jerky, stabbing gestures
▸ Appearing comfortable	▸ Crossing arms
▸ Synchronizing movements with those of the client	▸ Leaning away
	▸ Looking uncomfortable
	▸ Not synchronizing movements with those of the client

i. Giving information: sharing with the client information that is relevant to healthcare and well-being
j. Examining alternatives: helping the client explore options in light of his or her needs and the resources available
k. Using silence: allowing periodic pauses in communication to give the nurse and client time to think about what has taken place
l. Summarizing: highlighting the important points of a communication by condensing what has been said or observed

III. Legal and ethical issues

A. Levels of hospital admission

1. In informal admission:
   a. Admission is initiated by the client.
   b. The client retains his or her civil rights.
   c. The client is free to leave at any time.
2. In voluntary admission:
   a. Admission is initiated by the client, a family member, or another on the client's behalf.
   b. The client signs a formal agreement for hospitalization.
   c. The client retains all his or her civil rights.
   d. A written request must be submitted before discharge in order for the client to leave.
3. In involuntary admission (or commitment):
   a. Admission is ordered by the court or an administrative panel. Involuntary admission involves a specific legal process governed by state law.

   b. **The client has been judged dangerous to himself or herself, dangerous to others, or in need of treatment.**
   c. The client may or may not retain his or her civil rights (depending on specific state legislation).
   d. The client can be hospitalized against his or her will and must be formally discharged in order to leave.
   e. Involuntary commitment may be on an emergency basis (3 to 10 days on average) or a temporary basis (generally 60 to 180 days).

B. Client rights

1. **Most psychiatric inpatient units have adopted a Patient's Bill of Rights based on one issued by the American Hospital Association in 1975 and the Mental Health Systems Act of 1980.**
2. These rights include the following:
   a. The right to treatment provided by the least restrictive means

b. The right to communicate with people outside the hospital by telephone or written communication
c. The right to keep clothing and personal effects
d. The right to religious freedom, employment, education
e. The right to make purchases, manage property
f. The right to habeas corpus
g. The right to independent psychiatric evaluation and periodic review of status
h. The right to civil service status
i. The right to retain licenses (eg, driver's, professional)
j. The right to sue or be sued and to have legal representation
k. The right not to be subjected to unnecessary mechanical restraints
l. The right to privacy
m. The right to informed consent

C. Competency

1. Definition: Competency is related to the capacity to understand the consequences of one's decision.
2. A psychiatric client is competent unless judged otherwise by a court of law.
   a. Competent clients have the right to consent to and/or refuse treatment.
   b. Clients judged incompetent by court procedure will have a legal guardian appointed. Consents for treatment will then be given by legal guardian.

D. Restraints

1. Pharmacologic drugs given to inhibit a specific behavior
2. Physical: any manual or mechanical device, material, or equipment that will inhibit free movement
3. Legislation governing use of restraints is specified by state laws as well as federal legislation.
   a. Restraints are to be used only to ensure the physical safety of the client or other clients.
   b. Restraints are to be used only upon written order by physician specifying duration and circumstances under which they are to be used.

E. Ethical issues

1. When can a client refuse hospitalization, therapy, or medications?
2. When should a client's movement or privileges be restricted?
3. When should confidential information be shared?
4. When should the nurse intervene to prevent the client from harming self or others?

F. Legal and ethical responsibilities
1. **Comply with the law.**
2. **Uphold clients' rights.**
3. **Practice within scope of a specific state's nurse practice act.**
4. **Maintain practice standards of the profession.**
5. **Clarify personal and professional values.**
6. **Act as an advocate for the mental health needs and rights of clients, families, and the community.**

IV. Cultural issues

A. Concepts
1. Through the process of *enculturation,* values and beliefs are learned.
2. One's sense of belonging to particular cultural group is called *ethnicity.*
3. Members of specific cultural groups share similar patterns of behavior, values, and beliefs.
4. Values and beliefs about health, illness, mental disorders, and acceptable treatments may differ among diverse cultural groups.

B. Culturally diverse nursing care includes consideration of the following (Giger and Davidhizer, 1991):

1. **Communication, both verbal and nonverbal**
2. **Space, especially personal space in particular cultures**
3. **Social organization, including particular culture's defined family group**
4. **Concepts of time, including orientation to present and future**
5. **Environmental control, including special cultural health practices**
6. **Biologic variations among different groups**

C. Guidelines for relating to clients from diverse cultures (Giger and Dividhizer, 1991)
1. Respect particular cultural group.
2. Assess and analyze personal beliefs regarding different cultures.
3. Plan care based on client's communicated needs and cultural background.
4. Modify communication approaches to particular culture.
5. Use validation as an important therapeutic technique.
6. Use an interpreter if client speaks another language.

Bibliography

American Nurses Association (1994). *A statement on psychiatric-mental health clinical nursing practice and standards of psychiatric-mental health clinical nursing practice.* Washington, DC: American Nurses Publishing.

Giger, J., & Davidhizar, R. E. (1991). *Transcultural nursing*. St. Louis: Mosby-Year Book.

Townsend, M. C. (1993). *Psychiatric-mental health nursing: Concepts of care*. Philadelphia: F. A. Davis.

Varcarolis, E. (1994). *Foundations of psychiatric-mental health nursing* (2nd ed.). Philadelphia: W. B. Saunders.

Wilson, H., & Kneisl, C. (1992). *Psychiatric nursing* (4th ed.). Menlo Park, CA: Addison-Wesley.

STUDY QUESTIONS

1. Of the following descriptions of roles assumed by nurses, which one is unique to the mental health and psychiatric nurse?
   a. provides direct client care, including administering medications and treatments and promoting self-care
   b. strives to assist client to communicate and relate to others more effectively
   c. coordinates diverse aspects of care by working with other members of the healthcare team
   d. serves as an advocate on behalf of clients and their families
2. All but one of the following statements about a therapeutic nurse-client relationship are true. Which one is not true?
   a. The relationship considers social needs of both participants.
   b. The relationship is focused on the client's needs and problems.
   c. The relationship is directed toward specific goals.
   d. The relationship has clearly defined parameters.
3. Getting acquainted and developing trust and open communication characterize which phase of the nurse-client relationship?
   a. orientation
   b. working
   c. termination
   d. evaluation
4. The overall purpose of therapeutic communication is to
   a. analyze the client's problems
   b. facilitate and maintain a relationship that is helpful to the client
   c. provide emotional support during difficult times
   d. ensure that the client will remain cooperative
5. Whether or not to administer medications to a psychotic client who refuses them because he or she believes they are poison is an example of which legal/ethical issue?
   a. maintaining role parameters of the nurse-client relationship
   b. using authority in the nurse-client relationship
   c. exhibiting unconditional positive regard
   d. encountering a conflict of interest over client's rights
6. In the communication process, feedback refers to
   a. response of the receiver to the sender
   b. originator of a message
   c. setting in which communication takes place
   d. information transmitted
7. Which of the following would be an inappropriate topic to raise during the orientation phase of the nurse-client relationship?
   a. the client's perception of the reason for hospitalization
   b. clarification of the roles of nurse and client
   c. conditions for termination of the relationship
   d. exploration of the client's inadequate coping mechanisms
8. A newly admitted client says, "I just don't know if I should be here. What will my family think?" Using the approach of reflection, the nurse may respond most appropriately with which of the following statements?
   a. "It's hard to be here; you're concerned about your family's reaction."
   b. "What your family thinks isn't important. It's you that we're concerned about."
   c. "It sounds like your family doesn't understand you."
   d. "You can't always please your family, can you?"
9. The psychiatric nurse is caring for a

domineering client who resembles the nurse's own rather harsh and demanding mother. At the end of the interaction, the nurse seeks out a colleague with whom feelings are explored about the client. This action by the nurse indicates
  a. inability to cope effectively
  b. the presence of dependency needs
  c. appropriate self-awareness
  d. the need for psychotherapy

10. After having one conversation with a female nurse, a young male client asks the nurse for her phone number, stating that he would like to date her. Which of the following responses would be most appropriate?
  a. "I'm sorry, but I'm married and not interested in dating."
  b. "It's against hospital policy for me to date clients."
  c. "This is a professional relationship, and we need to stay clear on that."
  d. "I may consider dating you once you have fully recovered."

11. The nurse and client are in the working phase of their relationship. During the interaction, the client has been talking about some important problems and revealing a lot about himself. Now he falls silent. The best initial nursing action would be to
  a. encourage the client to continue talking
  b. remain silent with the client, staying attentive
  c. ask the client a nonthreatening question
  d. terminate the interaction

12. A client was admitted for acute psychosis, manifested by auditory hallucinations and withdrawal. The client refuses to take antipsychotic medications, saying "They make my head feel fuzzy." The staff observes the client becoming more psychotic without the medications and meets to discuss the problem of noncompliance. Which of the following statements made during the discussion reflects consideration for the ethics involved in solving this problem?
  a. "The client needs the medications to prevent worsening the psychosis. We can give an injectable form and use restraints while giving it."
  b. "Because the client needs the medication, we can secretly put a liquid form of it into the orange juice."
  c. "This client has the right to be psychotic. Let's consider a transfer to a unit where the client can be as psychotic as desired."
  d. This client has the right to refuse medications. Let's explore other options to deal with this behavior.

13. Which of the following suggestions made by staff members reflects the best potential solution to the problem of client noncompliance?
  a. Have client's family meet with the staff to decide whether or not the client should be forced to take medications.
  b. Have client's psychiatrist and primary nurse explore options with the client about taking medications.
  c. Consider discharge because the client does not qualify for commitment proceedings.
  d. Take away privileges until the client complies with the treatment program.

14. A client hospitalized under a voluntary admission wants to call a lawyer about a personal matter involving a lawsuit with a neighbor. Which of the following nursing actions would be appropriate in this case?
  a. Allow the phone call without seeking further information.
  b. Ask the client detailed questions about the lawsuit.
  c. Allow the phone call only after the client explains what the matter is about.
  d. Call the lawyer to announce the hospitalization of the client.

15. The ANA Standards of Practice for the

nurse who is prepared at the basic level include

a. using the nursing process as a guide for client care
b. being accountable to a psychiatrist for client care
c. conducting clinical research
d. practicing as a psychotherapist

ANSWER KEY

1. ***Correct response: b***
Psychiatric nursing is an interpersonal process aimed at promoting effective communication and interpersonal relationships. Primary work in the interpersonal area is unique to psychiatric nursing.
a, c, and d. These responsibilities apply to all areas of nursing.
Knowledge/Safe care/Implementation

2. ***Correct response: a***
The therapeutic relationship differs from a social one because it is based on the needs of the client, is goal directed, and has clear boundaries. It is a professional relationship, with the nurse functioning as a therapeutic agent.
b, c, and d. All of these statements regarding a therapeutic relationship are true.
Knowledge/Safe care/Planning

3. ***Correct response: a***
During the orientation phase, the introductory and assessment phase of the nurse-client relationship, a primary task is to establish trust and open communication so that the nurse and client can begin to work together.
b and c. Working and termination both are later phases in the nurse-client relationship.
d. Evaluation is a task in the termination phase.
Knowledge/Psychosocial/Assessment

4. ***Correct response: b***
The aim of therapeutic communication is to foster a helping relationship so that the client can develop more effective communication and coping behaviors.
a, c, and d. None of these tasks reflects the overall aim of therapeutic communication.
Knowledge/Safe care/Planning

5. ***Correct response: d***
Power over clients forms the basis for a conflict of interest. The problem of administering medications to a psychotic client who the staff believes needs them is a common ethical problem in psychiatric care.
a, b, and c. None of these responses specifies the ethics involved in this scenario.
Comprehension/Safe care/Implementation

6. ***Correct response: a***
This question is based on the structural model of communication, which has five components: sender, message, receiver, feedback, and context. Feedback refers to the response (verbal or nonverbal) of the receiver to the sender.
b, c, and d. These are definitions of sender, context, and message, respectively.
Knowledge/Safe care/Implementation

7. ***Correct response: d***
The orientation phase focuses on developing trust, open communication, and a working contract. Exploring coping mechanisms can be carried out only after a trusting relationship is established; thus, it is an inappropriate intervention for the orientation phase.
a, b, and c. These are all appropriate interventions during the orientation phase.
Knowledge/Psychosocial/Assessment

8. ***Correct response: a***
This is a reflective response in which the nurse indicates an awareness of what the client is experiencing. Reflection indicates understanding, empathy, and respect for the client's feelings.
b. This statement devalues what the client feels by negating what he or she has just said.
c. This statement diverts the conversation from the client's perspective and feelings.
d. This statement is inappropriate because it provides false reassurance.
Application/Psychosocial/Implementation

9. ***Correct response: c***

Self-awareness is a crucial ingredient in therapeutic intervention. Analyzing and sharing perceptions about self in relation to a client help the nurse work through countertransference feelings, which could adversely affect the therapeutic process.

a and b. Seeking peer consultation when countertransference occurs does not indicate inability to cope or underlying dependence.

d. Seeking out peer assistance indicates the ability to work through one's own issues. However, the nurse who often experiences very strong feelings in relation to clients may need psychotherapy.

Application/Safe care/Implementation

10. ***Correct response: c***

At the beginning of a nurse-client relationship, it is wise to clarify the parameters of the relationship.

a and b. These responses avoid the issue of defining the nurse-client relationship.

d. This is an unprofessional response. Because the client is most likely testing the nurse, this response may be very frightening to him. Promising to date a client also could create various problems for the nurse in the future.

Application/Safe care/Implementation

11. ***Correct response: b***

Silence allows the client to think and gain insight into what has been discussed. The nurse should allow the silence and convey interest and support.

a, c, and d. These actions would not be therapeutic in the working phase of a relationship.

Application/Psychosocial/Implementation

12. ***Correct response: d***

The client's right to refuse treatment is a complex issue. Staff must weigh the rights of the client with professional judgment; careful review of all the options will help the staff make a thoughtful decision.

a and b. Enacting these suggestions would violate the client's rights.

c. This represents a way of avoiding the legal and ethical dilemma by moving the client elsewhere.

Application/Safe care/Implementation

13. ***Correct response: b***

One way to deal with medication refusal is to help explore such options as lowering the dosage, changing the medication, or attempting to treat the psychosis without medication. Taking the client's viewpoint seriously by not forcing the medications shows respect for the client and the client's rights.

a. This could violate the client's rights to confidentiality.

c. This action avoids dealing with the medication issue.

d. This action would be punitive.

Application/Safe care/Implementation

14. ***Correct response: a***

One of the client's civil rights is to manage personal affairs—to make phone calls, send letters, and so forth.

b and c. These responses indicate that the nurse is too intrusive in the client's personal affairs.

d. This represents a clear violation of the client's right to privacy.

Application/Safe care/Implementation

15. ***Correct response: a***

The standards clearly state that practice is to be guided by the nursing process.

b. This response is incorrect, because the ANA standards are focused on independent nursing functions.

c and d. These responses are incorrect because conducting research and doing psychotherapy require a minimum of a master's degree preparation.

Knowledge/Safe care/Assessment

2

Conceptual Frameworks for Psychiatric Care

I. Overview

A. Description

1. Conceptual frameworks provide a theoretical view of humanity, developmental processes, behavior, and mental health and illness.

2. Such models organize knowledge in a systematic manner.
3. The assumptions of conceptual frameworks can be tested through research.

4. **Currently there is no single universally accepted model used in psychiatric care.**

B. Purpose of conceptual models

1. **Guide data collection**
2. **Provide reasons and explanations for assessed behaviors**
3. **Guide development of plan of care**
4. **Provide rationale for selecting interventions**
5. **Determine evaluation criteria for outcome measurement**
6. Facilitate research

C. Predominant conceptual models in psychiatric care

1. Psychodynamic
2. Behavioral
3. Interpersonal
4. Cognitive
5. Humanistic (existential)
6. Psychobiologic

II. Psychodynamic framework (focus on intrapsychic process)

A. Concepts (Freud's theory)

1. Levels of awareness

   a. **Conscious: those experiences within individual's awareness**
   b. **Preconscious: those experiences that may be recalled to awareness**
   c. **Unconscious: those experiences (memories, feelings, thoughts, wishes) that are not available to conscious awareness**

2. Personality structure

   a. **Id: most primitive part; instincts and impulses; operates via primary-process thought and pleasure principle**
   b. **Ego: reality-based; the "I" component; validates and tests reality; operates via secondary-process thought; balances impulses from id and demands from superego**
   c. **Superego: moral principle or conscience; culturally acquired values, beliefs, standards of behavior**

3. Psychic determinism
   a. Belief that all human behavior has meaning, although meaning may be on unconscious level
   b. Search for meaning and/or cause of events

4. Psychodynamics
   a. Psychic energy (cathexis): force required for mental functioning; arises from drives
   b. Instincts (drives): inborn psychologic representations or wishes; include self-preservation and preservation of species, life and death

   c. **Anxiety: response to unconscious conflict or threat to ego**
   d. **Defense mechanisms: mental mechanisms (largely unconscious) that operate in protecting ego against anxiety (see Table 2-1)**
5. Developmental concepts (see Table 2-2)

B. Psychodynamic view of mental illness

1. **Symptoms are caused by internal conflicts.**

TABLE 2-1.
Applied Defense Mechanisms

DEFENSE MECHANISMS	CLINICAL EXAMPLE
▸ Repression (exclusion of unpleasant, or unwanted experiences, emotions, or ideas from conscious awareness)	▸ An accident victim remembers nothing about the accident.
▸ Projection (attributing to another person one's own feelings, wishes that are unacceptable to self)	▸ A frightened client lashes out at the nurse, saying the nurse doesn't know what is going on.
▸ Reaction formation (adoption of behavior or feelings that are exactly opposite one's true emotions)	▸ A client is angry about the care received but behaves in an ingratiating manner.
▸ Displacement (transferring emotions associated with a particular person/event to another person/object/situation that is not as threatening)	▸ A client who is angry with the physician becomes verbally abusive to the nurses.
▸ Identification (adopting the thinking or behavioral patterns of another)	▸ A teenager hospitalized for diabetes wants to become a nurse as a result of the experience.
▸ Denial (refusal to believe or accept unpleasant reality)	▸ A client who drinks alcohol every day and cannot stop fails to acknowledge having a problem.
▸ Isolation (separation of emotions from precipi tating event or situation)	▸ A rape victim talks about the rape experience without showing any emotion.
▸ Intellectualization (use of thinking to avoid experiencing emotions that are unpleasant)	▸ A father talks with his child about what love should be like but fails to demonstrate love toward the child.
▸ Rationalization (justifying one's behavior by presenting reasons that sound logical)	▸ A client being treated for a drug addiction claims an inability to stop taking drugs because of a "bad marriage."
▸ Sublimation (substituting constructive and socially acceptable behavior for strong impulses not acceptable in their original form)	▸ A mother who lost a child in a drunk-driving accident joins an organization that works to educate the public about the dangers of drunk driving.

TABLE 2-2.
Comparing Cardinal Developmental Concepts

DEVELOPMENTAL STAGE	FREUD'S PSYCHOSEXUAL DEVELOPMENT	ERIKSON'S DEVELOPMENTAL STAGES OF MAN
Infancy	Oral stage—gratification of basic oral needs	*Trust vs mistrust*—basic needs fulfillment, trust in mothering one
Toddler	Anal stage—toilet training, social controls	*Autonomy vs shame and doubt*—sense of self-control and independence
Preschool	Phallic stage—sexual identity established	*Initiative vs. guilt*—assertiveness and dependability increase
School age	Latency stage—relationships with same sex, peers	*Industry vs inferiority*—self-confidence via cooperation, competition
Adolescence	Genital stage—relationships with opposite sex, satisfying work	*Identity vs identity diffusion*—sense of self
Young adult		*Intimacy vs isolation*—intimate relationship with another
Middle adult		*Generativity vs stagnation*—contribute to other's well-being
Older adult		Integrity vs. despair—satisfaction with one's life achievements

2. Defenses are fixed at an early developmental stage.

3. **Unresolved conflicts from early childhood cause vulnerability to similar adult situations.**
4. This framework is applied mainly to nonpsychotic conditions.

C. Treatment from a psychodynamic framework

1. **Insight-oriented focus is on interpersonal conflicts, anxiety, defenses, and sexual and aggressive drives.**
2. Unresolved, repressed conflicts are brought to the conscious level by various techniques, such as:
   a. Free association
   b. Dream analysis
   c. Transference analysis (analysis of client's feelings about therapist)
   d. Emotional catharsis (uncovering and reliving traumatic events)
3. Improvement occurs when early conflicts become conscious and are examined and resolved.

D. Application to nursing

1. **Assessment data are collected on client anxiety and use of defense mechanisms.**

2. **Psychodynamic theory can be used to understand and interpret client behavior.**
3. **Psychodynamic approach provides developmental perspective on client behavior.**
4. **Concepts of transference and countertransference are useful in analyzing the nurse-client relationship.**

III. Behavioral framework

A. Concepts

1. Behaviorists focus on identified behaviors.
2. General beliefs about human behavior

   a. **People learn to be who they are by environmental shaping.**
   b. **Behavior can be observed, described, and recorded.**
   c. **Behavior is subject to reward or punishment.**
   d. Experiment can determine which environmental aspects affect behavior.
   e. Behavior can be changed (modified) if the environment is changed.
3. Classical conditioning (Pavlov's theory)
   a. Conditional response: pairing of stimulus with response
   b. Acquisition: gain of learned behavioral response
   c. Extinction: loss of learned behavioral response
4. Operant conditioning (Skinner's theory)
   a. Positive reinforcer: reward will help continue behavior
   b. Negative reinforcer: removing of undesirable consequences will help continue behavior
   c. Positive punishment: aversive consequences will decrease particular behavior
   d. Negative punishment: withdrawal of reward will decrease particular behavior

B. Behavioral view of mental illness

1. **Maladaptive behaviors are learned through classical and operant conditioning; they continue because they are rewarding to the individual.**
2. **Maladaptive behaviors can be changed, without developing insight into underlying causation, by altering the environment.**
3. This framework is commonly applied to phobias, other anxiety disorders, alcoholism, and behavioral problems.

C. Treatment from a behavioral framework

1. Emphasis is on identified symptoms rather than causes.
2. Treatment includes using various behavior modification techniques, such as:

a. Modeling: new behavior learned by imitating specific behaviors of another (either therapist or other persons)
b. Operant conditioning: use of token-economy approach; tradable tokens (rewards) provided for desirable behaviors

c. **Systematic desensitization: gradually confronting a stimulus that evokes anxiety**
d. Aversive therapy: unpleasant consequences result from undesirable behavior
e. Biofeedback: training techniques used to control various physiologic responses
f. Relaxation techniques: training techniques used to counteract anxiety symptoms
g. Assertiveness training: training techniques used to overcome passivity or aggression in interpersonal situations

D. Application to nursing

1. Behavioral principles applied in inpatient psychiatric care include:
   a. Limit-setting techniques based on behavioral principles
   b. Token reward systems to reinforce desirable client behavior
   c. Privileges, such as phone use and off-unit movement, used as reinforcers

2. **Nurse and client collaborate in identifying target behavior needing change.**
3. **Client practices new behaviors with nurse's help.**
4. Nurse uses behavioral principles in teaching client, families, and others.

IV. Interpersonal framework

A. Concepts (Sullivan's theory)

1. Interpersonal therapists focus on interaction of person and environment.

2. **Personality develops through interaction with significant others.**
3. **Child internalizes approval or disapproval of significant others.**
4. Self-system (self-concept) organized as follows:
   a. "Good-me," developed in response to behaviors receiving approval, leads to good feelings about self.
   b. "Bad-me," developed in response to behaviors receiving disapproval, leads to anxiety states.
   c. "Not-me," developed in response to behaviors generating extreme anxiety. These behaviors are then denied as being part of self.

5. Individuals are more similar than different in basic needs, development, and behavior.

6. **Anxiety is an interpersonal phenomena, and occurs when relationships are uncomfortable.**
7. Individuals have two basic needs:
   a. Satisfaction (biologic needs)
   b. Security (emotional and social needs)
8. Framework identifies developmental stages (similar to Freud and Erikson).

B. Interpersonal view of mental illness

1. **Mental illness is defined as inappropriate interpersonal relationships.**
2. **The cause of mental illness is related to past relationships, inappropriate communication, and current crisis.**

C. Treatment from an interpersonal framework

1. Focus is on anxiety and its cause.
2. Therapist is participant-observer in relationship with client.
3. Client is encouraged to verbalize feelings.
4. Problematic relationships of client modified with therapist's help.

D. Application to nursing

1. **Hildegarde Peplau, renowned nurse theorist, developed the interpersonal theory of nursing using Sullivan's ideas.**
2. **Nursing care focuses on the nurse-client relationship, the vehicle through which the client becomes healthy.**
3. Nurses counsel clients by developing a therapeutic relationship.
4. Counseling performed by nurses tends to focus on "here-and-now" interpersonal concerns.
5. Anxiety intervention is an important nursing role (see Chap. 3).
6. Nurses assist psychiatric clients with effective problem solving related to interpersonal issues.
7. Nurses use the nurse-client relationship as a corrective interpersonal experience for clients.

V. Cognitive framework

A. Concepts

1. Focuses on thinking; through maturation, individuals form thoughts about themselves and their world.

2. **Learned thoughts become the basis for emotions and behavior.**
3. **The amount of perceived control over situations affects behavior.**
   a. Internal locus of control: individual believes in own power to affect outcome of situation

b. External locus of control: individual believes self is controlled by powerful outside forces

B. Cognitive view of mental illness

1. **Individual's distorted thinking is the basis for mental illness.**
2. Thought processes that are identified as misperceptions include:
   a. Arbitrary inference: holding beliefs in absence of supporting evidence
   b. Selective abstraction: concentrating on a single detail while ignoring others
   c. Overgeneralization: making global assumptions based on an isolated incident
   d. Magnification: greatly exaggerating a situation
   e. Minimization: belittling personal ability, action, or response
   f. Dichotomous thinking: "all or nothing" patterns of thought

C. Treatment from a cognitive framework

1. Therapist examines client's thought patterns to promote understanding of individual.

2. **Therapist assists client to develop awareness of faulty thinking.**
3. **Client is encouraged to practice alternative thought patterns that are healthier.**
4. Includes several styles of treatment such as:
   a. Rational-emotive therapy (Albert Ellis): Therapist actively disputes irrational client beliefs.
   b. Gestalt therapy (Fritz Perls): Therapist promotes client self-awareness and increased self-responsibility for meeting needs.
   c. Beck's cognitive therapy (Aaron Beck): Therapist teaches client to identify and correct dysfunctional thoughts of self, world, and future.

D. Application to nursing

1. **Nurses assess client's thought patterns.**
2. **Nurses participate in cognitive restructuring as part of team approach.**
3. **Nursing intervention encourages client responsibility for meeting needs and fosters positive client self-image.**
4. **Problem solving and exploring alternatives are approaches used by nurses working with clients.**

VI. Humanistic (existential) framework

A. Concepts

1. **Focus is on here and now.**
2. Unique self is unifying theme.
3. Value development and personal choice guide behavior.
4. Human nature is positive and growth oriented.
5. Existence is search for meaning and authenticity.
6. Human needs are organized in hierarchy of relative order (Maslow's theory) as follows:
   a. Physiologic needs
   b. Safety and security needs
   c. Love and belonging
   d. Self-esteem and esteem for others
   e. Self-actualization

B. Humanistic view of mental illness

1. Mental illness is the failure to fully develop one's potential.
2. Lack of self-awareness and unmet needs interfere with relationships and feelings of security.
3. The fundamental human anxiety is fear of death, which leads to existential anxiety (concern over meaning of one's life).

C. Treatment from a humanistic framework

1. Client-centered therapy (Rogers)
   a. Psychotherapy fosters process of learning to be free, becoming one's self.
   b. Therapist is genuine and without facade when in relationship with client.
   c. Change occurs when therapist conveys acceptance, respect, and genuine empathy for client.
2. Existential therapy
   a. Therapy focuses on life issues of death, freedom, helplessness, loss, isolation, aloneness, and anxiety.
   b. Through psychotherapy, client discovers own meaning of existence.

D. Application to nursing

1. **Humanism establishes theoretical framework for caring component of nursing.**
2. **Nurse-client relationship is based on positive regard, respect, and empathy.**
3. **Before working with psychiatric clients, the nurse assesses own self-concept and self-actualization needs.**
4. **Nursing interventions are designed to enhance client self-esteem following assessment of client self-concept.**

5. **Through reflective listening and empathic responses, the nurse helps client gain self-understanding.**
6. **Nurse advocates client freedom to choose alternatives.**

VII. Psychobiologic framework

A. Concepts

1. Focus is on mental illness as a biophysical impairment.
2. Human behavior is influenced by genetics, biochemical alterations, and function of brain and central nervous system.

3. **The stress response is a neuroendocrine response.**

B. Psychobiologic view of mental illness

1. Mental illness is a disorder of the body.
2. Physiologic, social, and environmental factors cause or predispose one to mental illness.
3. Mental illness can be classified according to criteria put forth by the American Psychiatric Association in *Diagnostic and Statistical Manual of Mental Disorders,* 4th edition (DSM-IV).
4. Relationships between psychobiology and certain mental illnesses have been researched.
   a. Hypotheses related to dopamine (neurotransmitter), monoamine oxidase (brain enzyme), and transmethylation (transfer of molecules from one compound to another) have all been implicated in schizophrenia.
   b. Abnormalities of neurotransmitters (serotonin, epinephrine, and norepinephrine) have been associated with mood disorders of depression and mania.
   c. Endocrine dysfunction (thyroid and adrenal cortex) can contribute to depression and/or manic behaviors.
   d. Relative deficiency of acetylcholine (neurotransmitter) may be associated with Alzheimer's disease.
5. Genetic research has identified genetic markers for some mental illnesses (Huntington's chorea, bipolar disorders in Amish families, familial Alzheimer's disease).
6. Alteration in natural biorhythms have been implicated in mood disorders and abnormal sleep patterns.

C. Treatment from a psychobiologic framework

1. Diagnostic tools, such as brain scanning and imaging techniques, and laboratory data are used to help establish diagnoses as well as evaluate treatment.
2. Somatic therapies (pharmacology, electroconvulsive therapy, and light therapy) are methods of treatment.
3. Psychotherapy may be used in conjunction with somatic therapies.

D. Application to nursing

1. **Client assessment includes physiologic as well as emotional and behavioral aspects of mental illness.**
2. **Administering psychotropic medications, monitoring side effects, and evaluating client responses are nursing responsibilities.**
3. **Teaching clients and families about symptom recognition, medications, treatments, and relapse prevention is a nursing role.**
4. Nurses prepared at the master's level (advanced practice RNs) may conduct psychotherapy and may have prescriptive authority (depending on the individual state's nurse practice act).

Bibliography

Abraham, I., et al. (1992). Integrating the bio into the biopsychosocial: Understanding and treating biological phenomena in psychiatric-mental health nursing. *Archives of Psychiatric Nursing, VI*(5), 295–305.

Carson, R., et al. (1988). *Abnormal psychology and modern life* (8th ed.). Glenview, IL: Scott, Foresman and Co.

Murray, R. B., & Huelskoetter, M. M. (1991). *Psychiatric-mental health nursing: Giving emotional care* (3rd ed.). East Norwalk, CT: Appleton and Lange.

Townsend, M. C. (1993). *Psychiatric mental health nursing: Concepts of care.* Philadelphia: F. A. Davis.

Townsend, M. C. (1994). *Nursing diagnoses in psychiatric nursing* (3rd ed.). Philadelphia: F. A. Davis.

Varcarolis, E. (1994). *Foundations of psychiatric-mental health nursing* (2nd ed.). Philadelphia: W. B. Saunders.

Wilson, H., & Kneisl, C. (1992). *Psychiatric nursing* (4th ed.). Menlo Park, CA: Addison-Wesley.

STUDY QUESTIONS

1. As a consistent aspect of the care environment, the staff meets weekly to discuss the diagnoses and the treatment protocols of newly admitted clients. Which framework for psychiatric care does this approach represent?
   - **a.** psychobiologic
   - **b.** psychodynamic
   - **c.** behavioral
   - **d.** cognitive
2. The client's problems and behaviors are interpreted in terms of anxiety and repressed conflicts. Which framework for psychiatric care does this approach represent?
   - **a.** psychobiologic
   - **b.** psychodynamic
   - **c.** behavioral
   - **d.** cognitive
3. A client newly diagnosed with cancer fails to talk about or acknowledge the diagnosis, acting as if nothing is wrong. Which defense mechanism is this client using?
   - **a.** projection
   - **b.** identification
   - **c.** rationalization
   - **d.** denial
4. In planning a client's care, the nursing staff identifies privileges (eg, use of telephone, participation in recreational activities) to be used as rewards for desirable behavior. These privileges serve as a (an)
   - **a.** extinction
   - **b.** response
   - **c.** operant
   - **d.** reinforcer
5. The *Diagnostic and Statistical Manual of Mental Disorders,* 4th edition (DSM IV) mainly provides
   - **a.** treatment protocols for mental disorders
   - **b.** epidemiologic information about mental disorders
   - **c.** classification and diagnostic criteria for mental disorders
   - **d.** rates of severity of mental disorders according to statistical information
6. Listening carefully as the client talks about choices and responsibilities in life reflects which framework for psychiatric care?
   - **a.** psychobiologic
   - **b.** humanistic
   - **c.** behavioral
   - **d.** cognitive
7. During assessment, a client says to the nurse, "I don't know what to do. My marriage is terrible, and I just got fired from my job." Of the responses below, which one is client-centered?
   - **a.** "Your thoughts are negative right now and this keeps you from making decisions."
   - **b.** "Things in your life are not working well right now and you feel unsure about what to do."
   - **c.** "Have you considered marriage counseling? Many people find that helpful."
   - **d.** "Other people have difficulties too. Have you shared these feelings with others?"
8. The primary nurse encourages a client to record ongoing thoughts in a daily diary. The nurse then reviews the diary with the client to identify thought patterns that appear to contribute to feelings of depression and anxiety. This nursing intervention is based on which framework for psychiatric care?
   - **a.** psychobiologic
   - **b.** psychodynamic
   - **c.** behavioral
   - **d.** cognitive
9. Based on Maslow's theory, which human need must be met first before the others can be considered?
   - **a.** security and safety
   - **b.** love and acceptance
   - **c.** beauty and philosophy
   - **d.** recognition and competence
10. A male client with a diagnosis of mental

retardation is admitted to a unit for clients with unsocialized, aggressive behavior. Even though he has the capabilities, he refuses to bathe, eat with utensils, or participate in structured activities. He carries a teddy bear with him at all times and screams relentlessly if a staff member tries to take the bear away from him. He looks forward to his parents' weekly visits, and he has made some friends on the unit. A plan of care based on behavioral principles is designed for this client. What would a behaviorist be likely to say about this client's unsocialized, aggressive behavior?

a. It has been reinforced so that it continues.
b. It needs to be punished so that it stops.
c. It is too extreme to be modified.
d. It is untreatable because the client is retarded.

11. Using careful observation, staff members list the problematic behaviors of the client in question 10. The list identifies the situations in which the behaviors occur, how long they last, and what happens immediately before and after the behaviors. This procedure is used to

a. enable the client to gain insight into certain behaviors
b. define behaviors that are targeted for change
c. develop a method for desensitizing the client
d. eventually confront the client with the inappropriate behavior

12. Based on the information given in question 10, which reinforcer would best modify this client's behavior?

a. structured activities
b. time with friends
c. the teddy bear
d. visits from parents

13. A 5-year-old girl wants to spend extra time with her "daddy." According to Freud's developmental theory, she is exhibiting

a. latency phase
b. oedipal conflict
c. oral needs
d. anal patterns

14. Which part of the personality houses primitive drives and operates on the pleasure principle?

a. id
b. ego
c. superego
d. alter ego

15. A person released from prison for selling narcotics has been rehabilitated and now works for an agency that educates young people on the dangers of drug use. This person's current behavior reflects which of the following defense mechanisms?

a. displacement
b. identification
c. denial
d. sublimation

ANSWER KEY

1. ***Correct response: a***
The psychobiologic framework is based on the disease model. Syndromes are diagnosed and treatment plans are based on what is currently known about the condition and its treatment.
b, c, and d. These responses refer to other frameworks for psychiatric practice.
Comprehension/Safe care/Planning

2. ***Correct response: b***
Psychodynamic interpretations are based on the idea that repressed conflicts and drives, when not worked through at previous developmental levels, create anxiety. When anxiety is great enough, symptoms of mental disorder occur.
a, c, and d. These responses refer to other frameworks for psychiatric care.
Comprehension/Safe care/Assessment

3. ***Correct response: d***
Failure to acknowledge a problem can be a form of denial. This commonly happens in the earlier stages of a serious diagnosis and occurs so that the ego will not be overwhelmed with anxiety.
a, b, and c. These are other defense mechanisms.
Comprehension/Psychosocial/Assessment

4. ***Correct response: d***
A reinforcer increases the likelihood that a behavior will reoccur. In this instance, the staff wants to increase desirable behaviors by using privileges to reward them.
a. Extinction refers to withholding reinforcement so that the behaviors decrease.
b. Response refers to a behavior directly resulting from a stimulus.
c. Operant refers to a specific behavior.
Comprehension/Psychosocial/Planning

5. ***Correct response: c***
The DSM-IV is used by the four core disciplines in psychiatry to diagnose mental disorders both nationally and internationally.
a and d. This information is not provided in DSM-IV.
b. This is only partially true; some epidemiologic information is provided by the DSM-IV, but it is scant.
Knowledge/Health promotion/Assessment

6. ***Correct response: b***
The humanistic framework focuses on individual choice and responsibility. The focus of psychiatric care from this framework is client-centered. From the humanistic perspective, the nurse waits for the client to introduce particular concerns
a, c, and d. These responses refer to other frameworks.
Comprehension/Psychosocial/Implementation

7. ***Correct response: b***
Client-centered responses are based on active-listening techniques. In this example, the nurse reflects what the client was heard saying. Client-centered responses help the client attain greater self-understanding.
a. This response is incorrect because the nurse focuses on the client's cognitive processes.
c and d. These responses are incorrect because the nurse ignores the client's feelings by suggesting that the client discuss them with someone else.
Application/Psychosocial/Implementation

8. ***Correct response: d***
The cognitive approach is based on the idea that thoughts influence behavior and feelings. In this example, the client must first identify recurrent thought processes that cause ongoing depression and anxiety. Cognitive approaches are especially effective with depressed clients.

a. This refers to care based on a psychobiologic framework, which focuses on identifying and medically treating the chemical imbalance causing the symptoms.

b. Care based on a psychodynamic framework would focus on helping the client gain insight into the past conflicts and the current problems that are causing anxiety and depression.

c. Care based on a behavioral framework would focus on identifying and changing environmental reinforcers that allow symptoms to persist.

Application/Psychosocial/Implementation

9. ***Correct response: a***

After food and water, security and safety are necessary before a person can strive to meet higher needs. Physiologic needs take precedence over psychologic and spiritual needs.

b, c, and d. These all are higher needs on Maslow's hierarchy.

Knowledge/Physiologic/Assessment

10. ***Correct response: a***

Stimuli in the environment are keeping the client's behavior in place. For example, if no one bothers the client when he is aggressive, or no demands are placed on him because he is uncooperative, leaving him alone serves as a reinforcement because he does not have to comply.

b. Punishment is a simplistic and possibly harmful approach to the problem. Punishment should be used only as a last resort in a behavioral approach.

c and d. Extreme behaviors in retarded persons have been successfully treated with behavioral treatment programs.

Analysis/Psychosocial/Assessment

11. ***Correct response: b***

Before behavioral strategies are implemented, the target behaviors—those needing to be changed—must be clearly identified.

a. This is not the behaviorist's primary purpose for documenting the client's behaviors. Insight is not a goal of behavioral intervention. In addition, this client does not have the capacity for insight.

c. Desensitization is not the treatment of choice in this case. Desensitization procedures involve a gradual exposure to an anxiety-producing stimuli after the client has learned relaxation techniques.

d. This approach is not based on behavioral principles.

Analysis/Safe care/Assessment

12. ***Correct response: c***

The fact that the client screams relentlessly when the teddy bear is taken from him shows that this is a very important source of gratification for him. The client becomes aggressive when the teddy bear is removed. He could be told that he must be cooperative for specified amounts of time without the teddy bear. When he complies with this demand, the teddy bear is given to him as a reward. The amounts of time can be gradually lengthened and other rewards can be introduced.

a. At this time, this client does not want to participate in structured activities. He has yet to be cooperative in basic activities of daily living.

b and d. These items are not as important or as immediate to this client and therefore would not be adequate reinforcers.

Analysis/Psychosocial/Planning

13. ***Correct response: b***

According to Freud's theory of psychosexual development, girls experience sexual feelings toward their fathers (and boys toward their mothers) between ages 3 and 5. Oedipal conflict refers to having feelings of attachment for the parent of the opposite sex and feelings of envy and aggression toward the parent of the same sex.

a. According to Freud, the latency phase occurs in the school-age child when focus is on development of same-sex (buddy) relationships.

c. Oral needs are the primary focus of Freud's first stage of psychosexual development (infancy).

d. Anal patterns, according to Freud, are established during the anal developmental phase during toilet training.

Comprehension/Psychosocial/Assessment

14. ***Correct response: a***

In psychoanalytic theory, id refers to that part of the personality that contains primitive drives.

b. The ego deals with reality and mediates conflicts between primitive wishes (id) and internalized standards of conduct (superego).

c. The superego is associated with values, ethics, and conscience.

d. Alter ego is not considered part of the basic personality structure.

Knowledge/Psychosocial/NA

15. ***Correct response: d***

Sublimation is a defense in which socially unacceptable drives are converted into socially acceptable avenues.

a, b, and c. These are other defense mechanisms.

Comprehension/Psychosocial/Assessment

3 Stress, Anxiety, and Anxiety-Related Disorders

I. Overview of stress

A. Definition

1. **Demands on a person that require coping or adapting**
2. **Stimulus or situation that produces distress**
3. Syndrome consisting of nonspecifically induced responses in the body called general adaptation syndrome (Selye's theory)
   a. Alarm reaction: Body defenses are mobilized as the sympa-

thetic nervous system and the endocrine system react to stress by activating large amounts of adrenaline and cortisone (for "fight or flight," see Table 3-1 and Fig. 3-1).

b. Stage of resistance: Adaptive responses attempt to limit damage from stressor.

c. Stage of exhaustion: This can occur if body's attempt to adapt fails.

4. Relationship between person and environment that is assessed by person as exceeding resources and endangering well-being

B. Concepts

1. **Source of stress (stressor) can be internal processes (physical/chemical, developmental, emotional/cognitive) or external life events.**
2. Stress can motivate and challenge person as well as tax coping resources.
3. Stress is more evident during periods of transition and change.

TABLE 3-1.
Components of the Fight or Flight Response

BODY PART OR SYSTEM	ADAPTATION TO STRESS
Hypothalamus	Sympathetic nervous system (SNS) stimulated
SNS	Adrenal medulla stimulated
Adrenal medulla	Epinephrine and norepinephrine released
Eyes	Pupils dilated
Lacrimal glands	Tear secretion increased
Respiratory system	Bronchioles and pulmonary blood vessels dilated Respiratory rate increased
Cardiovascular system	Force of cardiac contraction increased Cardiac output increased Heart rate raised Blood pressure elevated
Gastrointestinal system	Gastric motility (stomach and intestines) decreased Secretions decreased Sphincters contracted
Liver	Glycogenolysis (glucose breakdown) and gluconeogenesis (glucose manufactured from other body substances) increased Glycogen synthesis decreased
Urinary tract	Ureter motility increased Bladder muscle contracted Bladder sphincter relaxed
Sweat glands	Secretion increased
Fat cells	Lipolysis initiated

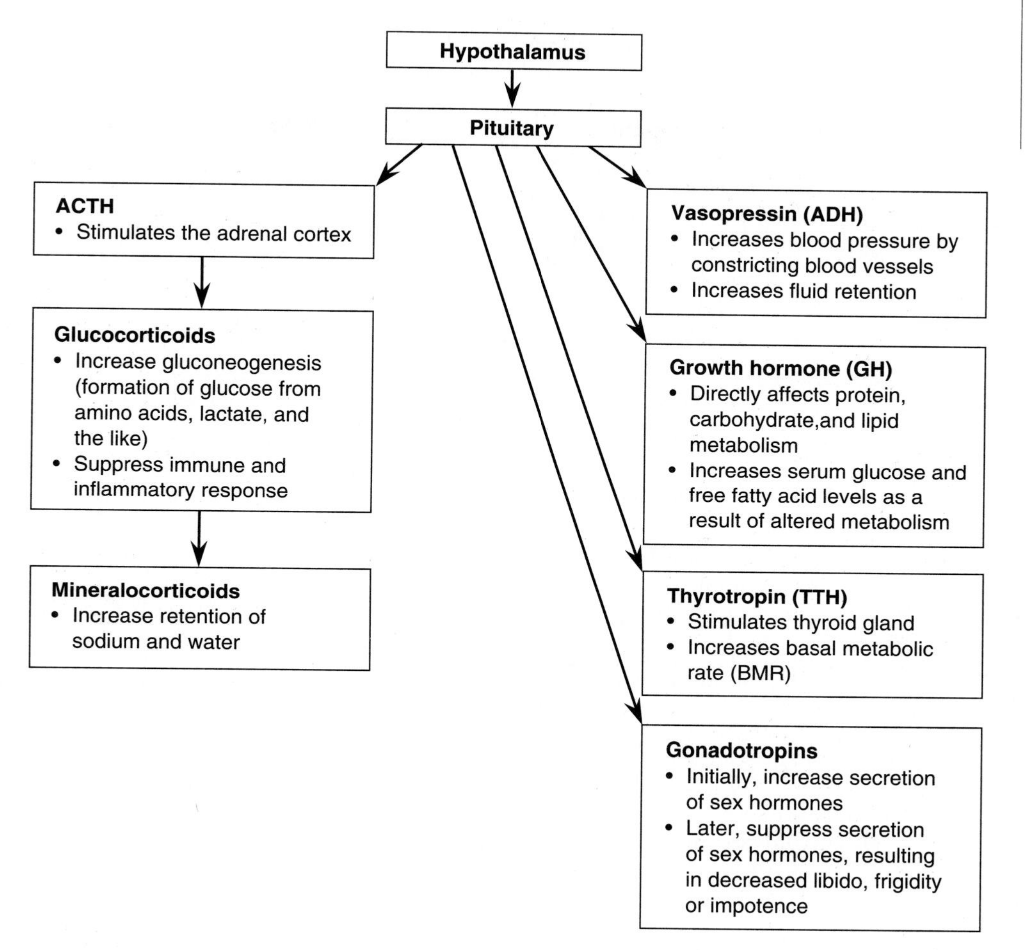

FIGURE 3-1.
Components of sustained-stress response. When a continuing fight-or-flight response becomes a sustained-stress response, the whole body is affected. The hypothalamus stimulates the pituitary gland, which in turn directs the release of various hormones, including adrenocorticotropin (ACTH), which stimulates the adrenal cortex: vasopressin (antidiuretic hormone, also called ADH); growth hormone (GH or somatotropin); thyrotropin (TTH); and gonadotropins.

4. Individual vulnerability to stress depends on predisposing factors that can be biologic, psychologic, or sociocultural.
   a. Biologic factors: genetics, nutritional status, general health
   b. Psychologic factors: intelligence, verbal skills, morale, personality, past experiences, self-concept, motivation, psychologic defenses, locus of control
   c. Sociocultural factors: age, gender, education, income, occupation, social position, cultural background, religious upbringing and beliefs, socialization experiences, level of relatedness to others

5. In 1967, Holmes and Rahe developed a numerical scale ranking both positive and negative life events as sources of stress.

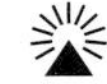

6. **The greater the number of stressful life events, the more likely the person is to develop physical illness or coping deficit.**
7. Axis IV in the *Diagnostic and Statistical Manual of Mental Disorders,* 4th edition (DSM-IV) rates the severity of psychosocial stressors as part of the multiaxial system of diagnosing of mental illnesses.
8. Response to stress depends on many factors, including but not limited to:
   a. Individual's perceived meaning of stressor (could be viewed as harmful, threatening, or challenging)
   b. Coping resources available to individual, such as personal abilities and skills, level of physical well-being, social supports, economic assets, and positive beliefs about self

II. Nursing process in stress

A. Assessment

1. Note physiologic manifestations of stress reflecting fight-or-flight response (Table 3-1).
2. Note psychosocial manifestations including, but not limited to:
   a. Client statements indicating subjective feeling of stress
   b. Decreased interest in usual activities of daily living
   c. Decreased quality and/or quantity of interpersonal relationships

B. Analysis and nursing diagnoses

1. Analyze internal and external stressors affecting client.
2. Establish individualized nursing diagnoses such as:
   a. Ineffective Individual Coping
   b. Altered Role Performance
   c. Impaired Adjustment
   d. Diversional Activity Deficit
   e. Altered Health Maintenance
   f. Altered Nutrition: Less [More] than body requirements
   g. Sleep Pattern Disturbance
   h. Caregiver Role Strain

C. Planning outcomes

1. Work with client in setting realistic goals.
2. Establish desired outcome criteria.
   a. Assist client to identify resources within self for coping.
   b. Encourage demonstration of behavioral and lifestyle changes needed to cope with and/or resolve stressors.

D. Nursing implementations

1. Help client identify stressors.

2. Teach client to monitor:
    a. Physical responses to stress, including increased heart rate, increased respiratory rate, increased sweating, and changes in appetite, sleep, and sexual interest
    b. Psychosocial responses to stress, including subjective feelings of tension, increased level of agitation, decreased frustration tolerance; changes in relationship patterns (overly dependent or exaggerated independence)
3. Encourage use of coping strategies for stress reduction (see Display 3-1).
4. Teach or refer the client to a reputable stress management program.

E. Evaluation

1. Client uses various resources to cope with stress.
2. Client reports successful elimination, reduction, or management of precipitating stressors.

III. Overview of anxiety

A. Definitions

1. **Feeling of apprehension, uneasiness, uncertainty, or dread resulting from real or perceived threat whose actual source is unknown or unrecognized**
2. **Subjective emotional response to stress**
3. State of uneasiness or discomfort experienced to varying degrees

B. Concepts

1. Anxiety is a universal experience.

2. **By increasing alertness and ability, anxiety provides energy that can be constructive.**

DISPLAY 3-1.
Coping Strategies for Stress Reduction

Among various strategies a client may use to deal with stress and anxiety are the following:
Seeking out a supportive person
Striving for self-discipline and perseverance
Ventilating strong emotions
Thinking through options and using problem-solving techniques
Performing physical activities and exercise to release energy
Engaging in activities that induce relaxation, such as:

- Listening to music
- Taking warm showers or baths
- Meditating
- Performing imagery or visualization exercises
- Using progressive muscle relaxation techniques

3. **On the other hand, anxiety can be destructive, producing physical and behavioral symptoms.**
4. Anxiety occurs in degrees (Fig. 3-2). Anxiety affects the ability to deal with stress, to learn, and to focus on a perceptual field.
5. Anxiety is not directly observable but can be assessed from behavior and communicated expressions of feelings by the client.
6. Anxiety is communicated in an interpersonal situation.
7. Anxiety is different from fear.
   a. Fear is a reaction to a known or specific danger.
   b. Response to fear is appropriate to the situation.
8. Various etiologic factors lead to anxiety:
   a. Threats to biologic integrity (eg, illness, physical trauma, impending surgery)
   b. Threats to self-concept, self-esteem (eg, losses, role changes, relationship changes, changes in environment or socioeconomic status)
9. Individual vulnerability to anxiety is related to various factors:
   a. Age

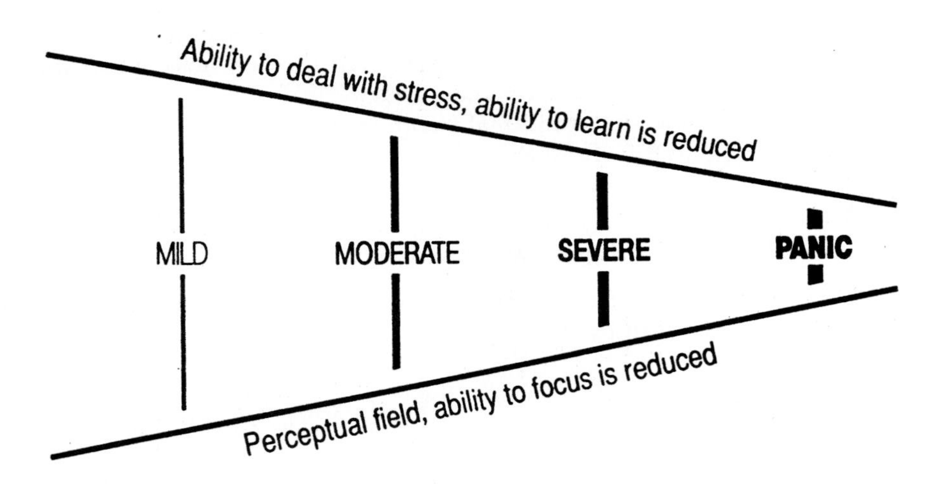

Mild: Increased alertness, enhanced learning ability, enhanced stress management, maximized problem-solving.
Moderate: Ability to focus on central concerns, but more difficulty staying attentive and being able to learn; selective inattention; problem-solving possible with assistance; relaxation techniques helpful.
Severe: Inability to focus or problem-solve, sympathetic nervous system activated; needs structured activities and large muscle activities.
Panic: Complete inability to focus, disintegrated ability to cope; environmental stimuli should be decreased, direction and structure should be provided.

FIGURE 3-2.
Degrees of anxiety and their effects.

b. Health status
c. Genetic predisposition
d. Past experiences with coping
e. Presence or absence of support systems
f. Number of stressors
g. Developmental maturity

IV. Nursing process in anxiety

A. Assessment

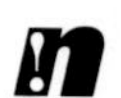

1. **Note any physiologic manifestations of anxiety involving fight or flight response (see Table 3-1).**
2. Note common cognitive responses to anxiety:
   a. Narrowed perceptual field
   b. Difficulty concentrating
   c. Difficulty with decision making
3. Note common behavioral responses to anxiety:
   a. Irritability
   b. Anger
   c. Withdrawal
   d. Restlessness and pacing
   e. Crying
   f. Complaints of dizziness, nervousness, tension
   g. Sleep disturbances

B. Analysis and nursing diagnoses

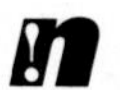

1. **Analyze client's anxiety level as mild, moderate, severe, or panicky (see Fig. 3-2).**
2. **Analyze client's use of coping strategies (see Display 3-1).**
3. Analyze client's use of defense mechanisms (see Chap. 2, Table 2-1).
4. Establish individualized client diagnoses such as:
   a. Anxiety
   b. Altered Thought Processes
   c. Sensory/Perceptual Alterations (Olfactory)
   d. Impaired Verbal Communication
   e. Ineffective Individual Coping
   f. Ineffective Denial
   g. Risk for Violence: Self-directed or directed at others
   h. Sleep Pattern Disturbance

C. Planning outcomes

1. Work with client in setting realistic goals.
2. Establish desired outcome criteria.
   a. Recognize presence of anxiety symptoms, and identify sources of anxiety.
   b. Use effective coping strategies for anxiety reduction.

D. Nursing implementations

1. For the client with moderate anxiety levels:

   a. **Teach about precipitating stressors, coping strategies, and adaptive responses.**
   b. **Use problem-solving process to help client recognize onset of own anxiety, stressors, and coping abilities.**
   c. Promote use of relaxation techniques.
2. For the client with severe or panic level of anxiety:
   a. Establish a supportive, trusting relationship.
   b. **Stay with and attempt to calm the client.**
   c. **Keep demands at a level the client can handle.**
   d. Do not confront the client about defense mechanisms.
   e. Limit environmental stimuli.

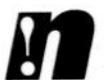

   f. **Convey calmness and give reassurance.**
   g. Encourage the client to engage in physical activity to release energy.
   h. Administer prescribed tranquilizers in a timely manner.
3. General implementations for the client who is anxious:
   a. Encourage client to limit smoking and caffeine intake.
   b. Promote sleep with comfort measures (warm bath, music, back rub, quiet presence of significant other).
   c. Protect from impulsive acts with one-to-one supervision.
   d. Provide client with telephone numbers for emergency or crisis situations (hotline clinics, mental health centers).
   e. Facilitate expression of feelings by listening actively, showing respect, and expressing empathy.

E. Evaluation

1. Client recognizes and verbalizes feelings of anxiety.
2. Client identifies stressors causing anxiety.
3. Client reports reduction in anxiety, and/or increased ability to cope.
4. Client demonstrates appropriate methods to handle anxiety.

V. Anxiety-related disorders

A. Common characteristics

1. Manifestation of anxiety symptoms, both physical and behavioral
2. Avoidance behaviors, occurring when individual attempts to cope with symptoms
3. Associated factors
   a. Biologic vulnerability related to autonomic nervous system overactivity, imbalance of neurotransmitter (serotonin, GABA, norepinephrine) levels
   b. Problem with self-esteem, self-concept
   c. Tendency toward external locus of control beliefs

d. Decreased stress tolerance, decreased coping measures, increased use of defense mechanisms
e. Relationships characterized by excessive dependence on others or avoidance of others

B. Panic disorder

1. **Description (according to DSM-IV diagnostic criteria): recurrent, unexpected attacks followed by at least 1 month of persistent concern about having another attack, worry about the possible implications or consequences of the attack or a significant behavioral change related to the attack**
2. Characteristics
   a. Feelings of "going crazy" or having heart attack
   b. Physiologic symptoms of fight or flight
   c. Personality disorganization, decreased perceptual field
   d. Anticipatory anxiety leading to avoidance of anxiety-provoking situations
3. Management
   a. Pharmacotherapy with antianxiety agents, antidepressants, beta blockers
   b. Behavioral therapy with relaxation training, biofeedback, response prevention
   c. Cognitive restructuring (questioning evidence, examining alternatives, reframing)

C. Generalized anxiety disorder

1. **Description: pervasive, persistent anxiety of at least 6 months duration**
2. Characteristics
   a. Chronic, persistent feelings of apprehension not associated with specific cause
   b. Restlessness or feeling keyed up or on edge
   c. Chronic feelings of inadequacy, difficulty with decision making
   d. Difficulty concentrating or mind going blank
   e. Sleep disturbances
3. Treatment modalities—similar to those used with panic disorder (see above)

D. Obsessive-compulsive disorder

1. Description

   a. **Obsession is a persistent idea or impulse that cannot be eliminated from conscious awareness (eg, aggressive obsessions, contamination obsessions).**
   b. **Compulsion is an uncontrollable, persistent urge to perform an act repetitively or ritualistically (eg, repeti-**

tive hand washing, excessive cleaning behaviors, checking things, counting things).

2. Characteristics
   a. Commonly, obsessions and compulsions occur together.
   b. Behaviors interfere with activities of daily living.

   c. **Individual is aware of the unrealistic, intrusive, and inappropriate nature of obsessions and compulsions (described as ego-dystonic).**
   d. Attempting to resist obsessive-compulsive behaviors causes individual to experience increased anxiety.
   e. Primary gain of obsessive-compulsive behavior is anxiety relief.
3. Management
   a. Pharmacotherapy with antidepressant agents including clomipramine (Anafranil) and sertraline (Zoloft)
   b. Behavioral therapy
   c. Psychotherapy

E. Phobic disorder

1. **Description: irrational fear of specific object, activity, or situation**
2. Characteristics
   a. Irrational fear is accompanied by persistent avoidance of object that elicits phobic response.

   b. **Individual recognizes fear is irrational and inappropriate (ego-dystonic disorder) but feels powerless to control it.**
   c. Simple phobia: fear of specific things (eg, elevators, heights, insects, airplanes)
   d. Social phobia: fear of potentially embarrassing social situations

   e. **Agoraphobia (with or without panic): fear of being in public place from which escape might be difficult or help unavailable**
3. Management
   a. Pharmacotherapy with antianxiety agents, antidepressants, beta blockers
   b. Behavioral therapy with systematic desensitization
   c. Cognitive restructuring
   d. Psychotherapy

F. Post-traumatic stress disorder

1. **Description: recurrently experienced thoughts and feelings associated with severe, specific trauma (eg, combat experiences, rape, serious accident, severe deprivation, torture)**

2. Characteristics
   a. Can be acute or delayed; can become chronic
   b. Includes symptoms such as exaggerated startle response, sleep disorders, guilt (survivor's guilt), nightmares and flashbacks, anger with numbing of other emotions
   c. Alcohol and drugs commonly used to self-treat and relieve symptoms
3. Management

   a. **Pharmacotherapy used cautiously because of potential abuse or dependency**
   b. Behavioral therapy with relaxation training
   c. Support group therapy or self-help groups

G. Dissociative disorders

1. Description: includes a group of five disorders characterized by disturbance in identity, memory, and consciousness
2. Characteristics
   a. The client uses defense mechanism of dissociation or isolation, an unconscious mechanism that serves to detach emotional significance from uncomfortable, unacceptable, or traumatic situations.
   b. These disorders are uncommon, subtle, and usually encountered in nonpsychiatric settings.
   c. These disorders include such behaviors as altered thinking, time disturbance, feeling of loss of control, and fluctuation of emotional expression.
3. Types
   a. Multiple personality disorder (MPD): existence of two or more distinct personalities within one person; usually results from severe abuse in early childhood
   b. Psychogenic fugue: sudden, unexpected flight with an inability to recall areas from one's past
   c. Psychogenic amnesia: sudden inability to recall important personal information
   d. Depersonalization disorder: alteration in self-perception in which one's own reality is temporarily lost or changed
   e. Dissociative disorder not otherwise specified: doesn't fit diagnostic criteria for other disorders
4. Management
   a. Psychodynamic psychotherapy (preferred method)
   b. Behavioral approaches
   c. Pharmacotherapy as appropriate for symptoms of anxiety and/or depression

VI. Nursing process in anxiety-related disorders

A. Assessment

1. Note physiologic manifestations of anxiety involving fight or

flight response (see Table 3-1) as well as special individual physical symptoms.

2. **Note client's specific cognitive, behavioral responses that are congruent or incongruent with established DSM-IV anxiety disorder diagnostic criteria.**
3. Review client's past history of anxiety-related problems.
4. Review client's current internal and external stressors.

5. **Discuss with client his or her own perception of current problem.**

B. Analysis and nursing diagnoses

1. Analyze client's anxiety level (see Fig. 3-2).
2. Analyze client's use of coping strategies (see Display 3-1).
3. Analyze client's use of defense measures (see Chap. 2, Table 2-1).
4. Establish individualized nursing diagnoses (see list of possible nursing diagnoses under anxiety).

C. Planning outcomes

1. Work with client in setting realistic goals.
2. Establish desired outcome criteria for intervention; for example:
   a. Client identifies anxiety responses.
   b. Client identifies possible sources of anxiety in current life situation.
   c. Client knows and uses various coping measures for anxiety reduction.
   d. Client uses resources and/or outside help when anxiety responses escalate.
   e. Client reports reduction in anxiety responses and increased confidence in ability to cope.

D. Nursing implementations

1. For the client with generalized anxiety disorder and or panic disorder, see implementations for anxiety.
2. For the client with obsessive-compulsive disorder:

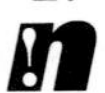

   a. **Convey acceptance of client despite ritualistic behaviors.**
   b. **Allow client time to preform rituals (anxiety will increase if the client cannot perform compulsive behaviors).**
   c. Encourage limit setting on ritualistic behaviors as part of established treatment plan.
   d. Use active listening to encourage client to verbalize feelings (best time for interaction is after client completes ritualistic behavior).

e. Direct need to conduct rituals into more socially useful behaviors (eg, cleaning up after meals, folding laundry).
f. Explore with client the purposes that the behavior fulfills.
g. Teach relaxation techniques and other coping measures to handle anxiety.
h. Teach information about medications used as part of treatment plan.

3. For the client with phobias:
   a. **Do not force contact with phobic object or situation.**
   b. Use selected implementations related to anxiety.
   c. Help client describe feelings prior to response to phobic object.
   d. Encourage client to practice relaxation techniques and other coping measures to handle anxiety.
   e. Participate as member of treatment team in established program for systematic desensitization.
4. For the client with post-traumatic stress disorder:
   a. Use selected implementations related to anxiety.
   b. **Validate with client that traumatic event was indeed highly stressful.**
   c. **Help client verbalize all aspects of traumatic event, including own feelings.**
   d. Encourage use of self-help or support group for follow up.
   e. Teach relaxation techniques and other coping measures to reduce anxiety.
   f. Refer to AA (Alcoholics Anonymous) or NA (Narcotics Anonymous) if drug or alcohol abuse is a problem.
5. For the client with a dissociative disorder:
   a. **Develop a trusting relationship and provide support during times of depersonalization, amnesia, emergence of new personalities.**
   b. Encourage disclosure and discussion of feelings in relation to painful or traumatic experiences.
   c. Facilitate exploration of alternative coping mechanisms.
   d. Help identify sources of conflicts.
   e. Support commitment to insight-oriented therapy with an experienced therapist.

E. Evaluation

1. Client identifies own anxiety responses.
2. Client identifies stressors in current life situation related to anxiety responses.
3. Client uses adaptive coping measures rather than symptomatic behaviors.
4. Client identifies and cooperates in continued treatment plan.

Bibliography

American Psychiatric Association (1994). *Diagnostic and statistical manual of mental disorders (DSM-IV)* (4th ed.). Washington, DC: American Psychiatric Association.

Antai-Otong, D., & Kongable, G. (1995). *Psychiatric nursing, biological and behavioral concepts.* Philadelphia: W. B. Saunders.

Gary, F., & Kavanagh, C. (1991). *Psychiatric mental health nursing.* Philadelphia: J. B. Lippincott.

Rawlins, R., & Heacock, P. (1993). *Clinical manual of psychiatric nursing* (2nd ed.). St. Louis: Mosby-Year Book.

Shives, L. (1994). *Basic concepts of psychiatric-mental health nursing* (3rd ed.). Philadelphia: J. B. Lippincott.

Stuart, G., and Sundeen, S. (1995). *Principles and practices of psychiatric nursing* (5th ed.). St. Louis: Mosby-Year Book.

Townsend, M. C. (1993). *Psychiatric mental health nursing: Concepts of care.* Philadelphia: F. A. Davis.

Varcarolis, E. (1994). *Foundations of psychiatric mental health nursing* (2nd ed.). Philadelphia: W. B. Saunders.

Wilson, H., & Kneisl, C. (1992). *Psychiatric nursing* (4th ed.). Menlo Park, CA: Addison-Wesley.

STUDY QUESTIONS

1. Which of the following statements best describes Selye's general adaptation syndrome?
- **a.** When stress occurs, the body goes through predictable responses no matter what the stressors are.
- **b.** When stress occurs, the body's defenses become depleted as they are used.
- **c.** When stress occurs, the body reacts adversely regardless of the stressors.
- **d.** When stress occurs, the body becomes less able to deal with subsequent stress.

2. When assessing an anxious client, the nurse should recognize that a person deals most effectively with stress when at what anxiety level?
- **a.** mild
- **b.** moderate
- **c.** severe
- **d.** panic

3. Recurring thoughts and behavioral rituals are characteristic of which of the following anxiety disorders?
- **a.** generalized anxiety disorders
- **b.** phobias
- **c.** obsessive-compulsive disorder
- **d.** dissociative disorder

4. When assessing a client for recent stressful life events, the nurse should recognize that these refer to changes experienced by the client that are both
- **a.** undesirable and harmful
- **b.** desirable and growth promoting
- **c.** positive and negative
- **d.** unwanted and unhealthy

5. Which of the following nursing approaches would be most therapeutic in assisting a client to cope with stressful life events?
- **a.** Encourage the client to complain about the stresses experienced.
- **b.** Help the client to refocus only on the positive aspects of stress.
- **c.** Avoid thinking about potential future life changes.
- **d.** Develop ability and patience to deal with life changes.

6. The nurse is teaching a recently diagnosed diabetic client how to take prescribed insulin. The client is having difficulty concentrating on what the nurse says. His respirations are becoming shallow and more rapid, and he is beginning to fidget, crossing and uncrossing his legs frequently and picking at his cuticles. His blood sugar level is within normal range. What degree of anxiety is the client most likely experiencing?
- **a.** mild
- **b.** moderate
- **c.** severe
- **d.** panic

7. Which initial nursing intervention would be most appropriate for the client in question 6?
- **a.** Stop the insulin lesson for awhile, and ask the client how things are going.
- **b.** State that learning about insulin need not be complicated if the client will just relax.
- **c.** Instruct the client to pay closer attention to what is being taught because it is vital to health.
- **d.** Leave that client alone for awhile so that he can become more relaxed.

8. After three diabetes teaching sessions, the nurse evaluates that the client is not progressing well regarding diabetic self-care. For the client to learn, what needs to happen first?
- **a.** The client needs to develop more self-trust.
- **b.** The client needs to practice more often.
- **c.** The client needs to experience less anxiety.
- **d.** The client needs to take control of the illness.

9. A newly admitted client stays up all night scrubbing the toilet and washbasin and washing her hands over and

over. She is constantly bothered by recurrent, intrusive thoughts. Based on this information, the nurse could assume that the client suffers from
   a. hypochondriasis
   b. conversion disorder
   c. psychogenic fugue
   d. obsessive-compulsive disorder

10. When implementing nursing care, the nurse should keep in mind that when a client diagnosed with obsessive-compulsive behavior experiences anxiety increases, ritualistic behaviors likely will
   a. increase
   b. stay the same
   c. decrease
   d. not be related to anxiety

11. A client has been on the psychiatric unit for 3 days for treatment of obsessive-compulsive scrubbing and cleaning behaviors. The client reports feeling more comfortable and at ease on the unit. In light of this change, which nursing intervention could be initiated with regard to ritualistic behaviors?
   a. Allow the client to engage in ritualistic behaviors as much as desired.
   b. Help the client think about ways to limit the ritualistic behaviors.
   c. Focus on the ritualistic behaviors every time they occur.
   d. Strictly limit the ritualistic behaviors.

12. Which nursing action should be taken first for a client exhibiting a higher than usual level of preoperative anxiety?
   a. Ask the client about his or her perceptions and feelings in relation to the upcoming surgery.
   b. Call to inform the surgeon about the client's anxiety.
   c. Ask the client's family to stay with the client for support.
   d. Teach the client what he or she needs to know about the upcoming surgery.

13. The most appropriate nursing intervention for the client with a phobic disorder would include
   a. Confront client with phobic object.
   b. Ignore client's anxiety.
   c. Assess client's response to phobic object.
   d. Teach use of relaxation techniques.

14. Which of the following clients would be most vulnerable to experiencing post-traumatic stress disorder?
   a. husband who has recently lost his wife to cancer
   b. child who fails a grade in school
   c. college student who experienced date rape
   d. wife of a chronic alcoholic

15. Which of the following would be an appropriate outcome for the client with a dissociative disorder?
   a. Client will deal with uncomfortable emotions on a conscious level.
   b. Client will modify stress by use of relaxation techniques
   c. Client will identify own anxiety responses.
   d. Client will utilize problem-solving strategies.

ANSWER KEY

1. ***Correct response: a***
Selye found that no matter what kinds of stressors were applied to rats (chemical, physical, or psychologic), their bodies responded with the same types of physiologic changes (alarm reaction).

b. Stress is not necessarily an adverse response; it may be viewed as challenging by the individual.

c. The body constantly adapts to stress.

d. Only when stress is overwhelming does the body wear down (stage of exhaustion).

Comprehension/Physiologic/Assessment

2. ***Correct response: a***
With mild anxiety, the person feels more alert and is able to focus on the problem at hand.

b. Although the person can still focus and pay attention, with moderate anxiety concentration is reduced.

c and d. Coping is impaired when anxiety is at severe or panic levels.

Knowledge/Health promotion/Assessment

3. ***Correct response: c***
Obsessive-compulsive disorder is characterized by unwanted repetitive thoughts and behaviors. The thoughts are intrusive and the behaviors tend to be concerned with cleanliness, checking, and other rituals.

a, c, and d. These are other disorders related to anxiety.

Knowledge/Psychosocial/Analysis

4. ***Correct response: c***
The concept of stressful life events is based on the research of Holmes and Rahe, who found that both positive and negative changes result in stress.

a, c, and d. None of these responses represents a complete answer to the question asked.

Knowledge/Psychosocial/Assessment

5. ***Correct response: d***
It takes both ability and patience to adjust to life changes. The greater one's coping skills, the more effectively one can deal with life stresses.

a, b, and c. These responses are incorrect; the client needs to look at both positive and negative aspects of change and also to anticipate potential future changes.

Application/Health promotion/Implementation

6. ***Correct response: b***
Moderate anxiety, manifested by restlessness and inability to concentrate, inhibits the learning process.

a, c, and d. These levels of anxiety have manifestations different from those presented in the scenario.

Comprehension/Physiologic/Assessment

7. ***Correct response: a***
Because the client's anxiety is increasing, the nurse should stop and assess what is happening. Asking the client an open-ended question and conveying interest may reduce anxiety and also elicit information on how the client is dealing with the illness of diabetes. It is important for the nurse to recognize that diabetes constitutes a major life change and is therefore a stress-producing diagnosis.

b, c, and d. Through these responses, the nurse avoids having the client express his concerns.

Analysis/Psychosocial/Implementation

8. ***Correct response: c***
The client's anxiety must be reduced because it is interfering with learning.

a, c, and d. Although all of these goals are desirable, they cannot be accomplished until the client's anxiety is reduced.

Application/Safe care/Analysis (Dx)

9. ***Correct response: d***
Obsessive-compulsive disorder is characterized by unwanted recurring thoughts and repetitive, ritualistic behaviors.
a, b, and c. These responses describe other anxiety-related disorders.
Comprehension/Psychosocial/ Analysis (Dx)

10. ***Correct response: a***
Obsessive-compulsive behavior is thought to be an abnormal manifestation of anxiety. If anxiety increases, the client's ritualistic behaviors will probably increase because they serve to alleviate anxiety.
b, c, and d. These responses would not be expected in obsessive-compulsive disorder.
Analysis/Psychosocial/Implementation

11. ***Correct response: b***
Because compulsive behaviors are used to control anxiety, it is helpful if the client thinks of ways to limit them. This way the client stays in control and takes responsibility for the behaviors.
a. In this case, the client may continually engage in ritualistic behaviors. While this may be allowed during initial hospitalization, after a trusting relationship has developed, the client should be encouraged to modify behavior.
c. Focusing on the behaviors will reinforce them.
d. This would greatly increase the client's anxiety, probably leading to additional scrubbing.
Application/Psychosocial/Implementation

12. ***Correct response: a***
The nurse should attempt to assess and reduce the client's anxiety by listening, offering support, and correcting any distortions about the upcoming surgery.
b, c, and d. These interventions could be implemented after talking with the client.
Application/Safe care/Implementation

13. ***Correct response: d***
Relaxation techniques provide the client with a method to cope with anxiety. When anxiety is reduced, phobic behavior will be reduced.
a. This will increase client anxiety and is inappropriate.
b. Anxiety is an uncomfortable emotion that necessitates nursing intervention.
c. This should be done as part of the assessment phase of the nursing process.
Application/Psychosocial/Implementation

14. ***Correct response: c***
Date rape is severe trauma which could serve as a precipitating event causing post-traumatic stress.
a, b, and d. These situations are all stressful but are not considered severely traumatic events.
Comprehension/Psychosocial/ Analysis (Dx)

15. ***Correct response: a***
Dissociative disorders occur when traumatic events are beyond the recall of the person. Bringing the feelings associated with these events into conscious awareness and coping with these feelings will decrease need for dissociation.
b, c, and d. These would be general outcomes for other anxiety-related disorders and, although helpful, are not specific for a client with a dissociative disorder.
Application/Psychosocial/Planning

4 The Mind-Body Continuum: Common Disorders

I. Overview

A. Concepts

1. **Holistic theory does not separate disorders of mind and body; rather, it views illness as a complex mixture of emotional and physical elements.**
2. Mind-body disorders have common components, including:
   a. Physiologic changes and symptoms that are actual or perceived by individual as actual (as in somatoform disorders).

b. Psychologic distress either preceding, accompanying, or following body changes and symptoms.

3. **Treatment of mind-body disorders includes a multidisciplinary approach with medical-surgical specialists as well as specialists from various psychiatric disciplines.**

B. Etiology

1. Stress is perceived differently, depending on individual and specific context.

2. **Stress comes in many forms—psychologic, physiologic, and sociocultural—and is a causative factor in all illness.**
3. Stress is thought to result from multiple causes.

II. Psychophysiologic disorders

A. Concepts

1. **Psychophysiologic disorders include a variety of disorders in which psychologic elements significantly contribute to chemical, physiologic, or structural alterations.**
2. Psychologic factors may precipitate or exacerbate symptoms of general medical conditions by eliciting stress-related physiologic responses.

3. **DSM-IV includes a diagnostic category called "psychologic factors affecting medical condition."**
   a. Essential feature is that these factors adversely affect medical condition.
   b. These factors can be inferred by close temporal association between factors and medical condition.

B. Types

1. Cardiovascular: hypertension, angina pectoris, acute myocardial infarction, migraine headaches
2. Respiratory: asthma, hyperventilation
3. Gastrointestinal: peptic ulcer disease, irritable bowel syndrome, ulcerative colitis, regional enteritis (Crohn's disease)
4. Neuromuscular-skeletal: rheumatoid arthritis, Raynaud's disease, temporomandibular joint (TMJ) pain, back pain.
5. Endocrine: diabetes mellitus, thyroid disorders, premenstrual syndrome (PMS)
6. Integumentary: psoriasis, urticaria, eczema
7. Immune system: allergic disorders, cancer, autoimmune disorders

C. Etiology

1. **Psychologic and environmental factors play an important role in initiation, maintenance, or exacerbation of specific disease process.**

2. Various theories that have been proposed include:
    a. Psychoanalytical: Individual dissociates unacceptable feelings about self and others and then displaces them onto body symptoms.
    b. Behavioral: Illness results from failed attempt to cope with stressful life events.
    c. Psychobiologic: Certain genetic vulnerability coupled with stress triggers illness.
    d. Sociocultural: Competitive lifestyles in urban areas among individuals in higher socioeconomic groups lead to stress-related illnesses.

D. Management

1. Medical disorder is treated in accord with the protocol for the specific medical-surgical condition.

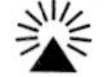

2. **Nonmedical interventions are directed at reducing stress and increasing client control over symptoms.**
    a. Stress management
    b. Biofeedback with relaxation training: electrodes monitor heart rate, muscle tone, and brain waves; individual learns to relax and consciously control physiologic response to stress

III. Somatoform disorders

A. Concepts

1. **Somatoform disorders are a group of disorders characterized by complaints of physical symptoms that cannot be explained by known physical mechanisms.**
2. **Individual experiences a loss or change in physical function.**
3. **Symptoms are not under voluntary control of the individual.**
4. Disorders are characterized by primary gain (anxiety relief) and secondary gains (special attention, relief from responsibilities).
5. Ego syntonic disorders are congruent with individual's view of self.
6. Significant impairment occurs in social or occupational functioning.

B. Types

1. Somatization disorder: history of multiple physical complaints without organic basis, occurring before age 30 and persisting several years
2. Hypochondriasis: unrealistic fear of having serious illness; individual's interpretation of body symptoms is without organic basis
3. Body dysmorphic disorder: preoccupation with imagined physical defect in normal-appearing person; if the individual has a defect, expressed concern is excessive

4. Pain disorder: chronic pain in one or more anatomic sites; a medical condition, if present, plays minor role in accounting for pain
5. Conversion disorder: loss or change of physical function suggesting:
   a. Neurologic disorder (blindness, deafness, loss of tactile sense or pain)
   b. Involuntary motor function disorder (aphasia, impaired coordination, paralysis, seizure)

C. Etiology

1. Psychoanalytic theory: Conflict finds expression by displacement of anxiety onto physical symptoms.

2. **Behavioral theory: Child learns from parents to express anxiety through somatization; secondary gains reinforce symptoms.**
3. Sociocultural factors
   a. Incidence is higher among individuals from lower socioeconomic groups, in rural areas, or with limited education.
   b. Some cultures and religious groups view direct expression of emotions as unacceptable; therefore somatic symptoms are common in these cultures.

D. Management

1. **Aims to recognize and prevent iatrogenic or treatment-induced harm**
2. **Tries to establish long-term relationship with specific healthcare provider to keep client from seeking multiple providers with multiple recommendations for testing and treatment**
3. Psychotherapy
   a. Psychoanalytic therapy assists client to become conscious of repressed conflict.
   b. Behavioral therapy uses exposure and response prevention.
   c. Family therapy teaches the family ways to minimize secondary gains and cope with predictable problems.

IV. Human sexuality and sexual disorders

A. Concepts

1. **Human sexuality includes a sense of maleness or femaleness (gender identity) as well as a desire for contact, warmth, tenderness, and love.**
2. **Sexual health includes integration of somatic, intellectual, and social aspects of sexual being.**
3. Sexual expression is influenced by:
   a. Cultural, ethnic, religious views

b. Age, health status, physical attributes
c. Environment, personal choice as result of personality development

4. Normal sexual behavior is a sexual act between consenting adults, lacking force, performed in a private setting in the absence of unwilling observers.

B. Types of sexual disorders

1. **Paraphilias: unusual or bizarre sexual acts or imagery used to achieve sexual excitement**
   a. May be preference for use of nonhuman objects
   b. Activity with humans may involve real or simulated suffering
   c. Specific paraphilias: fetishism, transvestism, zoophilia, pedophilia, exhibitionism, voyeurism, sexual masochism, sexual sadism

2. **Sexual dysfunctions: psychologically induced inability to be sexually active due to inhibitions, impaired communication between partners, or psychophysiologic changes**
   a. Sexual desire disorders
   b. Sexual arousal disorders
   c. Orgasmic disorders
   d. Sexual pain disorders
   e. Sexual dysfunction due to general medical condition

3. **Gender identity disturbance: sense of discomfort and inappropriateness about one's anatomic sex and the wish to be of the other sex**

C. Etiology

1. Paraphilias
   a. Biologic factors: studies implicate organic factors such as destruction of parts of limbic system, temporal lobe disorders, abnormal levels of androgens; studies inconclusive at this time
   b. Psychoanalytic theory: failure to resolve oedipal conflict, identification with parent of opposite sex or selection of inappropriate object for libidinal cathexis

   c. **Transactional model of stress adaptation: multiple factors, including genetics, past learning, and existing physiologic, psychologic, and sociologic factors**
2. Sexual dysfunctions

   a. **Biologic factors: altered levels of testosterone and serum prolactin; various medications such as antihypertensives, antipsychotics, antidepressants, anxiolytics, and anticonvulsants**

b. Psychosocial factors: associated with hypoactive sexual desire and orgasm disorders; strongly negative emotions become associated with sexual activity

3. Gender identity disorders
   a. Biologic factors currently proposed are inconclusive.

   b. **Psychosocial factors: influence of social learning on gender development in childhood; disturbances are thought to be related to parental dynamics encouraging identity with nongender-based sex role**

D. Management

1. **Specialized training in sex therapy is advocated for professionals treating sexual disorders. American Association of Sex Educators, Counselors and Therapists (AASECT) provides training for certification.**
2. Treatment is based on research by noted sexologists including Masters and Johnson and Helen Singer Kaplan.
3. Treatment includes extensive evaluation of specific problem and relationship dynamics coupled with education and supportive psychotherapy.

V. Eating disorders

A. Concepts

1. **Characterized by severe disturbances in eating behavior**
   a. Morbid fear of becoming fat
   b. Intense preoccupation with weight and dieting
   c. Inaccurate body image
   d. Self-esteem dependent on thinness
2. Other psychopathology may be present, including
   a. Mood disorders (depression)
   b. Personality disorders
   c. Substance abuse (especially with bulimia nervosa)

B. Types

1. **Anorexia nervosa: characterized by refusal to maintain minimally normal body weight**
   a. **Less than 85% normal weight for age and height**
   b. **Although underweight, intense fear of becoming fat**
   c. **Body image disturbance (undue influence of weight or body shape on self-evaluation)**
   d. **Strenuous exercising and peculiar food-handling patterns**
   e. **Lack of sense of competence in any area besides weight control**
   f. **Physical symptoms: absence of menses exceeding 3 months; lanugo growth; hypothyroid-like state; brady-**

cardia and decreased blood pressure; hypokalemia; hypocalcemia leading to osteoporosis

2. **Bulimia nervosa: repeated episodes of binge eating followed by purging behaviors**
   a. Binge eating: consuming enormous quantities of food in discrete time period; emotional events trigger binge
   b. Purging: compensatory behaviors to prevent weight gain, including self-induced vomiting or misuse of laxatives, diuretics, enemas, or other medications.
   c. Fasting or excessive exercise
   d. **Binges leading to feelings of loss of control, guilt, humiliation and self-loathing**
   e. **Physical symptoms: fluid volume deficit, hoarseness and esophagitis, dental erosion from vomiting, enlarged parotid glands, hypokalemia, cardiac arrhythmias**

C. Etiology

1. Psychoanalytic theory: disturbed mother-infant relationships leading to vulnerability in child
   a. Separation: individuation conflicts
   b. Distorted body image with misperception of internal needs
   c. Control of anxiety dependent on control of body and biologic needs
2. Biologic theory: inconclusive; difficult to determine whether physiochemical changes precede, accompany, or follow behavioral problems
3. Sociocultural theory: body-image ideal oriented around thinness; peer pressure factors also important, self-perception powerfully influenced by peer identity in adolescence
   a. 95% of clients female
   b. Age at onset between 13 and 20 years
4. **Family theory: symptoms of eating disorder allow family to avoid dealing with spousal conflict.**
   a. Family members are enmeshed, lacking clear-cut boundaries among parents and children; leads to overinvolvement in child's life.
   b. High value placed on perfectionism; child attempts to meet high standards.
   c. Eating disorder becomes form of rebellion; child gains sense of control through this behavior.

D. Management

1. **Multidisciplinary approach (medicine, psychiatry, psychology, nutrition, nursing) with the priority being to treat physical symptoms first and initiate a refeeding program.**

a. Behavioral therapy: uses contracts to reinforce appropriate eating and prevent harmful behaviors
b. Family therapy: assists families to decrease controlling behaviors and client to increase self-responsibility

2. Somatic treatment
a. Tricyclic antidepressants (for anorexia nervosa)
b. Monoamine oxidase inhibitor (MAOI) antidepressants (for bulimia nervosa)
c. Antihistamine with serotonin antagonist effect; cyproheptadine (Periactin) to stimulate weight gain and treat depression

VI. Nursing process in mind-body disorders

A. Assessment

1. Note objective and subjective symptoms related to specific client diagnosis asserted in diagnostic criteria in DSM-IV.

2. Evaluate cognitive, physiologic, and behavioral responses of individual client.

3. Review client's past history and current internal and external stressors.
a. Discuss client perception of problem.
b. Identify client's self-concept and body image.
c. Identify any secondary gains from physical symptoms.

B. Analysis and nursing diagnoses

1. Determine client's anxiety level, use of coping measures and/or defense mechanisms (see Chap. 3 for determination of anxiety level and coping measures).

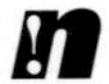

2. Determine meaning of physical symptoms to individual client.

3. Differentiate management priorities for physical and psychologic symptoms.

4. Analyze client insight related to physical symptoms and psychologic problems.

5. Establish individualized nursing diagnoses for client with a psychophysiologic disorder, for example:
a. Pain
b. Ineffective Individual Coping
c. Anxiety
d. Fear
e. Sensory/Perceptual Alteration
f. Risk for Activity Intolerance

6. Establish individualized nursing diagnoses for client with a somatoform disorder, for example:
a. Ineffective Individual Coping
b. Impaired Social Interaction

c. Self Esteem Disturbance
d. Self Care Deficit
e. Ineffective Family Coping: Disabling

7. Establish individualized nursing diagnoses for client with a sexual disorder, for example:
   a. Altered Sexuality Patterns
   b. Sexual Dysfunction
   c. Knowledge Deficit
8. Establish individualized nursing diagnoses for client with an eating disorder, for example:
   a. Altered Nutrition: Less than body requirements
   b. Altered Thought Processes
   c. Social Isolation
   d. Ineffective Individual Coping
   e. Ineffective Family Coping: Disabling
   f. Self Esteem Disturbance
   g. Powerlessness

C. Planning outcomes

1. Work with client in setting realistic goals.
2. Establish desired outcome criteria for client with psychophysiologic disorder, for example:

   a. **Demonstrate ability to cope with physical illness by using stress management and adopting healthy lifestyle.**
   b. Identify specific stressors related to physical illness.
3. Establish desired outcome criteria for client with sexual disorder, for example:

   a. **Identify relationship of stressors and decreased sexual functioning.**
   b. **Express desire to change variant sexual behavior.**
   c. Communicate with partner about sexual matters without discomfort.
   d. Express satisfaction with own sexuality pattern.
4. Establish desired outcome criteria for client with somatoform disorder, for example:

   a. **Express anxiety and conflict verbally rather than with physical symptoms.**
   b. **Reduce and/or eliminate behavior that is demanding or manipulative in relationships with others.**
5. Establish desired outcome criteria for client with an eating disorder, for example:

   a. **Achieve normal or near-normal weight for age and height.**

b. **Replace maladaptive eating behaviors with coping behaviors when anxious.**
c. Identify positive self-concept and realistic body image.
d. State feelings of control in areas of life other than eating.
e. Family establishes open communication and maintains generational boundaries.

D. Nursing implementations

1. For the client with a psychophysiologic disorder:

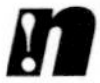

a. **Encourage client to identify and use positive coping measures to handle physical illness.**
b. Help client identify and use support systems.
c. Refer client to specific self-help support group.
d. Teach relaxation training.

2. For the client with a somatoform disorder:

a. Establish trusting relationship.

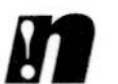

b. **Report and assess new physical complaint, because organic disease is also a possibility in this client.**
c. **Decrease reinforcement and secondary gains derived from physical symptoms.**
d. **Avoid fostering dependency needs, and encourage independent behaviors.**
e. Maintain focus on feelings and/or difficulties in living rather than on somatic symptoms.
f. Set limits on manipulative behavior in matter-of-fact manner.
g. Teach client alternative ways to perform activities if "physical disability" interferes.
h. Help client identify and use positive means to meet emotional needs.

3. For the client with a sexual disorder:

a. Develop supportive relationship with client.
b. Educate client regarding normal sexual behavior and family planning issues.
c. Correct misconceptions regarding sexuality.
d. Review medications prescribed for client and identify side effects related to sexual functioning.
e. Refer to qualified counselor for sex therapy.

4. For the client with an eating disorder:

a. Reinforce dietitian's prescription for caloric intake to accomplish realistic weight gain of 2 to 3 lb weekly.

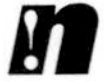

b. **Reinforce treatment plan that establishes privileges and restrictions based on compliance.**
c. **Decrease emphasis on foods and eating.**
d. **Weigh client daily upon rising and after first void.**

e. **Remain with client during meal and for first hour after meal.**
f. **Establish a trusting relationship.**
g. Encourage client to verbalize role within family and discuss issues of dependence/independence.
h. Promote client feeling of control by participation in treatment and independent decision making.
i. Assist family to redefine roles and establish open communication.

E. Evaluation

1. Client identifies relationship between specific stressors and physiologic symptoms.
2. Client verbalizes anxiety about specific problems rather than expressing anxiety with physical symptoms.
3. Client expresses satisfaction with self-concept, body image, and relationships with others.
4. Client uses stress-management techniques and follows health-promoting lifestyle.
5. Client assumes responsibility for self and expresses sense of internal locus of control.
6. Client identifies and cooperates in continued treatment plan.

Bibliography

American Psychiatric Association (1994). *Diagnostic and statistical manual of mental disorders (DSM-IV)* (4th ed.). Washington, DC: American Psychiatric Association.

Gary, F., & Kavanagh, C. (1991). *Psychiatric mental health nursing.* Philadelphia: J. B. Lippincott.

Rawlins, R., & Heacock, P. (1993). *Clinical manual of psychiatric nursing* (2nd ed.). St. Louis: Mosby-Year Book.

Shives, L. (1994). *Basic concepts of psychiatric-mental health nursing* (3rd ed.). Philadelphia: J. B. Lippincott.

Townsend, M. C. (1993). *Psychiatric mental health nursing: Concepts of care.* Philadelphia: F. A. Davis.

Varcarolis, E. (1994). *Foundations of psychiatric mental health nursing* (2nd ed.). Philadelphia: W. B. Saunders.

Wilson, H., & Kneisl, C. (1992). *Psychiatric nursing* (4th ed.). Menlo Park, CA: Addison-Wesley.

STUDY QUESTIONS

1. Psychophysiologic disorders have which of the following in common?
   a. psychologic factors that adversely affect chemical and physiologic processes
   b. physical symptoms that cannot be explained by known physical mechanisms
   c. failed attempts to cope with stressful life events
   d. stress, which causes specific physiologic disease processes

2. A client with benign essential hypertension has been referred for biofeedback training. The nurse would evaluate this training as effective if which of the following occurs?
   a. Client states that stress level is under control.
   b. Client's blood pressure can be maintained on decreased amount of antihypertensive medication.
   c. Client can confront feared object without anxiety.
   d. Client can follow recommended diet and medication plan.

3. A client is preoccupied with numerous bodily complaints even after careful diagnostic work reveals no physiologic problems. Which of the following nursing approaches would be therapeutic for this client?
   a. Listen to the client's complaints carefully and ask the client about them frequently.
   b. Acknowledge that the complaints are real to the client and refocus the client on other concerns.
   c. Challenge the physical complaints by confronting the client with the normal diagnostic findings.
   d. Ignore the client's complaints but have the client write a list of them.

4. A client had a myocardial infarction 3 years ago. Since this time the client has become convinced that another heart attack will occur. The client has severely restricted normal activities despite the physician's advice to resume a normal lifestyle. The nursing diagnosis most applicable to this client would be
   a. Ineffective Individual Coping
   b. Pain
   c. Self Esteem Disturbance
   d. Sensory/Perceptual Alteration

5. A client is taking Mellaril, a drug known to interfere with sexual arousal by inhibiting erectile function. When teaching the client about the drug's side effects, the nurse should provide which of the following information?
   a. Tell the client to expect an erectile problem as a side effect.
   b. Explain that the client's sexual desire likely will decrease.
   c. Do not mention sexual side effects to prevent anxiety from causing an erectile problem.
   d. Explain that the client should report any changes in sexual functioning so medication adjustments can be considered.

6. The nurse is working with a client with a transsexual disorder. The client recently started living as a member of the opposite sex. An unexpected outcome criteria for this nurse-client relationship would be
   a. The client will explore reactions and feelings about living in another gender role.
   b. The client will discuss feelings about the reactions experienced from others.
   c. The client will identify support persons who may be helpful during the change from one sex role to the other.
   d. The client will set the date for sex-change surgery.

7. A teenager has been hospitalized on an eating disorders unit for treatment of anorexia nervosa. The nurse would know that this disorder is characterized by

a. nervous habits related to eating certain foods
b. binge eating in small time periods
c. refusal to maintain minimally normal body weight
d. weight loss of more than 15 lb in 6 months

8. The nurse needs to assess a client with anorexia nervosa for the common physical manifestations of this disorder. Signs and symptoms include which of the following?
a. excessive sweating, polyphagia, polydipsia
b. intolerance to cold, decreased blood pressure, bradycardia
c. intolerance to heat, diarrhea, tachycardia
d. dental caries, nausea, hypercalcemia

9. The psychoanalytic theory regarding etiology of anorexia nervosa includes which of the following concepts?
a. achievement of secondary gain through control of eating
b. conflict between mother and child over separation and individualization
c. family dynamics that lead to enmeshment of members
d. incorporation of body image ideal of thinness

10. Nursing intervention for a client with an eating disorder includes staying with the client for 1 hour after meals. The rationale for this intervention is
a. Assess for and prevent purging behaviors.
b. Develop a trusting nurse-client relationship.
c. Maintain focus on importance of nutrition.
d. Reinforce idea that nurse is in control.

11. The initial treatment priority for a client hospitalized for an eating disorder is
a. Determine current body image.
b. Identify family interaction patterns.
c. Initiate refeeding program.
d. Promote client's feeling of independence.

12. The nurse evaluates treatment as successful if a client with a somatoform disorder
a. practices self-medication rather than change healthcare providers
b. recognizes that physical symptoms increase his or her anxiety level
c. researches treatment protocols for various illnesses
d. verbalizes anxiety directly rather than displaces it

13. The nurse has been asked to develop a sex education program for high school students. Which of the following would be an unimportant consideration in conducting this type of health teaching?
a. The nurse understands that her or his own values include intercourse only with marriage.
b. Group discussion may reveal that some students believe sexual activity is appropriate or expected at their age.
c. Negative consequences of sexual activity should be emphasized to prevent sexual promiscuity.
d. Exploring students' values regarding sexual behavior helps them determine appropriate and inappropriate sexual behaviors.

ANSWER KEY

1. ***Correct response: a***
Stress-related physiologic responses may precipitate or exacerbate symptoms of general medical symptoms. Other factors (genetic, physiochemical, environmental) are also related to psychophysiologic disease processes.
b. This defines a somatoform disorder.
c. This explains the behavioral view of psychophysiologic disease.
d. The relationship between stress and disease is a complex one; a cause and effect relationship has not been established.
Knowledge/Psychosocial/NA

2. ***Correct response: b***
Successful use of biofeedback enables the client to modify physiologic responses to stress, including blood pressure. Decreased need for an antihypertensive medication is an objective measurement of effectiveness.
a. Although this is an outcome of stress management, it is not specifically related to biofeedback.
c. This describes systematic desensitization.
d. This would be a successful outcome of the medical treatment program.
Application/Physiologic/Evaluation

3. ***Correct response: b***
After physical factors are ruled out, somatic complaints are thought to be expressions of anxiety. The complaints are real to the client, but the nurse should not focus on them. Prompting the client to talk about other concerns will encourage expression of anxiety and dependency needs.
a. Focusing on somatic symptoms will reinforce them.
c. Confronting the client in this matter shows lack of sensitivity to the unconscious nature of the problem and will increase client anxiety.
d. Through this action the nurse merely avoids the problem.
Application/Safe care/Implementation

4. ***Correct response: a***
Anxiety over physical health has led to avoidance of activity that would permit the client to live normally. This in an ineffective coping measure.
b and d. There is no evidence that this client has experienced either of these problems.
c. Although the client's self-esteem may be affected in this situation, there is no evidence that this is a primary problem.
Application/Health promotion/Analysis

5. ***Correct response: d***
Clients have a right to information about drug side effects. Clients often discontinue medication to avoid or correct sexual side effects and are less likely to do that if health professionals offer assistance with sexual issues. Clients generally will not raise sexual issues unless health professionals give permission by raising the issue first.
a. This response promotes the expectation of a sexual problem, which can create performance anxiety and lead to erectile failure.
b. Impaired sexual desire most likely would be secondary to the erectile dysfunction.
c. This response does not promote discussion of this sensitive issue. More likely, it reflects the nurse's avoidance of uncomfortable feelings.
Application/Psychosocial/Implementation

6. ***Correct response: d***
Unless the nurse is a certified sex therapist, this would be an unexpected outcome from nursing care of this client.
a, b, and c. These are areas which need to be explored by the client.

The nurse can facilitate exploration by using therapeutic listening skills.

Application/Psychosocial/Evaluation

7. ***Correct response: c***

The chief characteristic of anorexia nervosa is refusal to maintain minimally normal body weight. Weight less than 85% of the normal for age and height is a significant criterion for this diagnosis.

a. This is not a typical symptom of anorexia nervosa. The client with anorexia will restrict eating. The client may omit or severely limit intake of food perceived to be "fattening."

b. This is characteristic of bulimia nervosa.

d. Although weight loss is significant, unless client's weight loss results in less than 85% of the normal it is not significant for this diagnosis.

Knowledge/Physiologic/Assessment

8. ***Correct response: b***

These symptoms are similar to a hypothyroid-like state that is a consequence of anorexia nervosa.

a. These symptoms are unrelated to anorexia nervosa.

c. These symptoms are similar to a hyperthyroid-like state.

d. Dental caries may occur with self-induced vomiting but nausea is not usually present. Hypocalcemia rather than hypercalcemia would be more characteristic.

Knowledge/Physiologic/Assessment

9. ***Correct response: b***

According to psychoanalytic theory, early mother-child dynamics lead to difficulty with the child establishing a sense of separateness from the mother—along with difficulty recognizing normal body cues and needs. Control of eating becomes the one area in which the child establishes a sense of independence.

a. This is the behavioral view of anorexia nervosa.

c. Family theory deals with the issue of lack of generational boundaries.

d. The sociocultural view of anorexia nervosa identifies thinness as being a culturally determined ideal.

Analysis/Psychosocial/NA

10. ***Correct response: a***

The client may experience increased anxiety during treatment which may lead to resumption of behaviors designed to prevent weight gain, such as vomiting or excessive exercise.

b. This is an ongoing part of nursing intervention.

c. Although nutrition counseling is part of treatment, it is not an appropriate rationale for remaining with the client for 1 hour after eating.

d. This would be inappropriate because the treatment focus is on encouraging the client's independent behavior.

Application/Safe care/Intervention

11. ***Correct response: c***

The physical need to reestablish near-normal weight takes priority because of the physiologic, life-threatening consequences of anorexia nervosa.

a, b, d. These are all appropriate but not of highest priority in initial treatment.

Analysis/Physiologic/Intervention

12. ***Correct response: d***

The client with a somatoform disorder unconsciously displaces anxiety with physical symptoms. The ability to recognize and verbalize anxious feelings directly rather than displacing them is a criterion of treatment success.

a and c. These behaviors are indicative of a somatoform problem.

b. Anxiety is decreased by physical symptoms via primary gain in the client with a somatoform disorder. The statement does not reflect a measure of treatment success; rather it suggests a symptom of the disorder.

Knowledge/Health promotion/ Evaluation

13. ***Correct response: c***

No evidence indicates that sex education promotes promiscuity. Adolescents may respond negatively if negative consequences are introduced as threats.

a. The nurse's values need to be clearly identified and efforts made to avoid imposing the values on others during teaching.

b. It is important for clients or students to explore and understand their own values and beliefs about sexuality.

d. In addition to a need for exploration, students need guidance in determining appropriate sexual behaviors.

Application/Health promotion/Planning

Personality Disorders

5

I. Overview

A. Concepts

1. According to diagnostic criteria posed in DSM-IV, a personality disorder is "an enduring pattern of inner experience and behavior that deviates markedly from expectations of the individual's culture, is pervasive and inflexible, has an onset in adolescence or early adulthood, is stable over time, and leads to distress or impairment."

2. **Personality disorder is nonpsychotic illness characterized by maladaptive behavior, which the person uses to fulfill his or her needs.**
3. General characteristics of personality disorders include:

   a. **Troubled relationships, impaired communication**
   b. **Inflexible behavior, use of rigid defense mechanisms**
   c. **Poor stress tolerance, poor coping mechanisms**
   d. **Intact ego that may be defective in controlling impulsive, acting-out behavior**
   e. **Lack of self-responsibility (external locus of control)**
   f. **Denial of maladaptive behaviors, rarely seeks psychiatric help**
   g. **Remains in mainstream of society, despite social or occupational problems**

4. Personality disorders are coded on Axis II of the multiaxial diagnostic system used by the American Psychiatric Association.

B. Types

1. Eccentric personality disorders: individuals typically seem odd or eccentric
   a. Paranoid personality disorder: pattern of distrust and suspiciousness; others' motives are interpreted as threatening to self
   b. Schizoid personality disorder: pattern of detachment from social relationships
   c. Schizotypal personality disorder: acute discomfort in close relationships; cognitive or perceptual distortions; eccentric behaviors
2. Dramatic-erratic personality disorder: difficulty feeling concern or empathy for others

   a. **Antisocial personality disorder: characterized by pattern of disregard for and violation of the rights of others; before age 18 this may involve conduct problems and/ or criminal behavior**
   b. **Borderline personality disorder: characterized by patterns of instability in relationships, self-image, and mood; also characterized by impulsive behavior**
   c. Histrionic personality disorder: characterized by excessive emotionality and attention-seeking behaviors that are dramatic and egocentric
   d. Narcissistic personality disorder: characterized by grandiosity and need for constant admiration from others
3. Anxious or fearful personality disorders
   a. Avoidant personality disorder: characterized by social inhibition, feelings of inadequacy, and sensitivity to potential rejection or criticism
   b. Dependent personality disorder: characterized by submissive and clinging behavior related to excessive need to be cared for by others
   c. Obsessive-compulsive personality disorder: characterized by preoccupation with orderliness, perfectionism, and the need to be in control of situations, objects, and people (see also Chap. 3)

C. Etiology

1. Biologic theory: predisposition related to genetics or neurologic deficits; in antisocial disorder, some evidence of reduced inhibitory anxiety levels
2. Psychoanalytic theory (most research directed to borderline personality disorder)
   a. Failure to work through separation-individuation process;

child unable to separate from mother without significant fear and anxiety

b. Mother perceived by child as both strongly nurturing and hateful and punishing at unpredictable times

3. Behavioral theory
    a. Antisocial personality disorder: proposes that child learns socially undesirable behavior from parents who reward acting-out behavior in child by giving in rather than setting limits
    b. Borderline personality disorder: emphasizes that child is rewarded for clinging, dependent behaviors
4. Sociocultural theory: directed toward antisocial personality disorder, in which deviant behavior may be fostered in an impoverished environment
5. Family theory
    a. Antisocial personality disorder: significant parental deprivation during first 5 years of child's life; chaotic home environment with inconsistent, impulsive parents
    b. Borderline personality disorder: unstable family system leading to unstable personality development

D. Management

1. **Difficult because individual with personality disorder may lack motivation for any change; treatment may be long-term**
2. Psychoanalytic therapy: focuses on restructuring personality
3. Behavior therapy: focuses on individual learning more adaptive behavior
4. Biologic therapy: focuses on prescribed psychotropic medications to relieve specific clinical symptoms such as depression, paranoid thinking, or aggression

II. Nursing process in personality disorders

A. Assessment

1. Assessment findings include cognitive, emotional, and behavioral responses in all clients.
2. Individual with paranoid personality disorder:

    a. **Appears suspicious and mistrustful of others**
    b. **Uses projection as defense mechanism**
3. Individual with schizoid or schizotypal disorder:

    a. **Withdraws socially; emotionally aloof**
    b. **Displays odd mannerisms, speech, behaviors**
    c. **Shows little interest in having sexual experiences with another person**
    d. **Responds with indifference to approval from or criticism by others**

4. Individual with borderline personality disorder:

a. **Has unstable mood and impulsive behavior**
b. **Commonly practices self-mutilation**
c. **Has intense fear of being alone**
d. **Has poor self-concept**
e. **Expresses contradictory ideas or feelings of others, usually views others as all good or all bad (splitting)**
f. Manipulates others

5. Individual with histrionic personality disorder:
a. Has dramatic behavior with exaggerated emotions
b. Displays temper tantrums
c. Exhibits flamboyance; overtones of sexuality
d. Lacks commitment in relationships

6. Individual with narcissistic personality disorder:
a. Incorporates grandiose thinking; exaggerated sense of self-importance
b. Has attention-seeking behaviors
c. Rationalizes failures

7. Individual with antisocial personality disorder:
a. **Behaves in manipulative and controlling manner**
b. **Acts extroverted; has superficial and charming manner**
c. **Lacks concern for rights of others**
d. **Has impaired conscience; lying, cheating, possible criminal behavior**
e. **Desires immediate pleasure and gratification**
f. **Lacks commitment and intimacy in relationship**

8. Individual with avoidant personality disorder:
a. Responds with hypersensitivity to others' reactions and criticisms
b. Fears rejection and failure
c. Desires attention but withdraws socially
d. Fears being alone

9. Individual with dependent personality disorder:
a. Lacks self-confidence and self-esteem
b. Lacks independence and decisiveness
c. Clings in relationship
d. Devalues any personal abilities

10. Individual with obsessive-compulsive personality disorder:
a. **Strives for organization and order**
b. **Is controlling and demanding in relationships**
c. **Strives for perfection; pays great attention to detail**
d. **Forms rigid, moralistic, and judgmental opinions of others**
e. **Conveys indirect expression of anger**

B. Analysis and nursing diagnoses

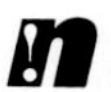

1. **Nurse must analyze own feelings and reactions to specific client with a personality disorder. Nurse should seek peer and/or treatment team direction when own feelings interfere with therapeutic performance.**
2. Analyze individual client's predominant manner of relating to others.
   a. Withdrawn and suspicious (eccentric personality disorder)
   b. Manipulative and controlling (dramatic-erratic disorders)
   c. Dependent (anxious or fearful disorder)

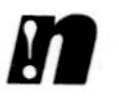

3. **Determine client's level of self-esteem, recognizing that poor self-esteem is present despite apparent egocentricity.**
4. Establish individualized nursing diagnoses. (See Table 5-1 for common nursing diagnoses with specific personality disorders.)

C. Planning outcomes

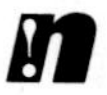

1. **Work with client in setting realistic goals.**
2. Establish desired outcome criteria for clients with an eccentric personality disorder, for example:
   a. Client will verbalize comfort in relating one-to-one with nurse.
   b. Client will participate in group situations with peer group.
   c. Client will control or reduce unusual mannerisms.

TABLE 5-1.
Personality Disorders and Nursing Diagnosis

DIAGNOSTIC CATEGORY	SPECIFIC PERSONALITY DISORDERS	NURSING DIAGNOSES
Eccentric	Paranoid Schizoid/Schizotypal	Impaired Social Interaction Altered Thought Processes Ineffective Individual Coping
Dramatic-Erratic	Borderline Histrionic Narcissistic Antisocial	Anxiety Self Esteem Disturbance Personal Identity Disturbance Ineffective Individual Coping Risk for Self Mutilation Risk for Violence Defensive Coping
Anxious-Fearful	Avoidant Dependent Obsessive-Compulsive	Decisional Conflict Ineffective Individual Coping Social Isolation Self Esteem Disturbance Anxiety

   d. Client will refrain from sharing bizarre or paranoid ideas with others.
3. Establish desired outcome criteria for clients with a dramatic-erratic personality disorder, for example:
   a. Client will control impulsive behaviors.
   b. Client will refrain from self-destructive behaviors.
   c. Client will verbalize anxiety and angry feelings rather than act out.
   d. Client will decrease manipulative behavior and express needs in a direct manner.
   e. Client will respect rights and needs of others.
   f. Client will adhere to rules and regulations in structured environments and relationships.
4. Establish desired outcome criteria for clients with an anxious or fearful personality disorder, for example:
   a. Client will identify positive self statements.
   b. Client will interact with peers in social situations.
   c. Client will manage anxiety when daily living situations are not under individual control.
   d. Client will make decisions in an independent manner.

D. Nursing implementations

1. For the client with an eccentric personality disorder:
   a. **Adopt objective, matter-of-fact manner in interaction with client.**
   b. **Maintain clear, consistent verbal and nonverbal communication.**
   c. Provide daily structure for activities of daily living.
   d. **Maintain focus on reality and reality-based topics.**
   e. Help client identify feelings that are implied.
   f. **Gradually involve client in group situations, providing support when necessary.**
2. For the client with a dramatic-erratic personality disorder:
   a. **Prevent harm by observing client frequently and developing no-harm contract with client.**
   b. **Take a concerned, matter-of fact attitude in interactions with the client.**
   c. Give immediate feedback when confronting inappropriate or manipulative behavior.
   d. Help client examine the consequences of appropriate and inappropriate behavior.
   e. Act as role model for appropriate expression of feelings and negative emotions.
   f. **Avoid rescuing or rejecting client.**

g. **Set limits, reinforce consequences of manipulative behavior or disregard for rights of others.**
h. Give positive feedback for goal achievement and independent behavior.
i. Explore client's feelings regarding rejection, being alone, fear of abandonment.
j. Use problem-solving approach to help client explore changes necessary.
k. Encourage follow-up treatment.

3. For the client with an anxious or fearful personality disorder:

a. **Establish caring, consistent therapeutic relationship.**
b. Establish clear expectations for responsible behavior.
c. Expect client to make decisions.
d. **Teach client how to be assertive or refer to training program.**
e. Encourage client to identify positive attributes.
f. Provide positive feedback when client interacts in social situations.
g. Teach client to use stress-management and relaxation techniques to cope with anxiety.

E. Evaluation

1. Client maintains behavior that is appropriate in social situations.
2. Client expresses satisfaction with self-concept and relationships with others.
3. Client avoids behaviors that are manipulative or exploitative of others.
4. Client expresses angry feelings verbally rather than acts out on self and/or others.
5. Client respects rights and needs of others.
6. Client tolerates areas of imperfection in life without undue anxiety.

7. **Client identifies need for follow-up treatment and agrees to cooperate with appropriate referrals.**

Bibliography

American Psychiatric Association (1994). *Diagnostic and statistical manual of mental disorders (DSM-IV)* (4th ed.). Washington, DC: American Psychiatric Association.

Gary, F., & Kavanagh, C. (1991). *Psychiatric mental health nursing.* Philadelphia: J. B. Lippincott.

Rawlins, R., & Heacock, P. (1993). *Clinical manual of psychiatric nursing* (2nd ed.). St. Louis: Mosby-Year Book.

Shives, L. (1994). *Basic concepts of psychiatric-mental health nursing.* (3rd ed.). Philadelphia: J. B. Lippincott.

Townsend, M. C. (1993). *Psychiatric mental health nursing: Concepts of care.* Philadelphia: F. A. Davis.

Varcarolis, E. (1994). *Foundations of psychiatric mental health nursing* (2nd ed.). Philadelphia: W. B. Saunders.

Wilson, H., & Kneisl, C. (1992). *Psychiatric nursing* (4th ed.). Menlo Park, CA: Addison-Wesley.

STUDY QUESTIONS

1. A client with a dependent personality disorder has been submissive to a spouse's wishes and has taken direction for their lives from the spouse for 25 years. Recently, the spouse died. The nurse would expect the client to experience which of the following responses?
   a. relief, following grief, to begin living life independently
   b. increase in dependent and passive symptoms
   c. take-charge and decisive attitude during this crisis period
   d. paranoia about relationships

2. Which of the following is characteristic of a client with histrionic personality disorder?
   a. very focused on detail
   b. limited expression of emotion
   c. dramatic, always "on stage"
   d. disregard for social norms

3. A client has been diagnosed with schizoid personality disorder. Which of the following behaviors would the nurse probably not observe during assessment?
   a. social detachment
   b. limited emotional expression
   c. odd ideas and mannerisms
   d. actions designed to obtain the nurse's approval

4. A client is an anxious personality type. The client lacks confidence, seems to reject others in relationships before others can reject the client, and sometimes has difficulty accomplishing work assignments because of a fear of failure. Which of the following nursing diagnoses would be most appropriate for this client?
   a. Self Esteem Disturbance
   b. Altered Thought Processes
   c. Self Care Deficit
   d. Risk for Violence: Self-directed

5. Which of the following statements regarding persons with personality disorders is true?
   a. They typically maintain themselves in a marginal manner in society.
   b. They often become psychotic when their illness becomes more acute.
   c. They commonly seek psychotherapy.
   d. With therapy, prognosis for recovery is good.

6. A woman describes herself as a "very religious person" with strong opinions on "what is right and what is wrong." She is quite judgmental regarding others' beliefs and lifestyles. Which of the following principles could support evaluation of the client's behavior as typical of a personality disorder?
   a. Religious fanatics almost always have personality disorders.
   b. Inflexible behavior and use of rigid defense mechanisms is characteristic.
   c. Strong belief systems raise doubts about mental stability.
   d. Judgmental behavior, including self-insight, is typical of personality disorders.

7. A man rents a room from a landlady to whom he is attentive and charming. Sometimes he is late with the rent, but according to the landlady, he always has a good reason and "he is such a nice person" that the landlady is not persistent in collecting from him. One day she loans him money to help him "meet expenses for his ailing mother." The next day, the landlady is surprised to find the tenant and his things gone—with no explanation and no forwarding address. The tenant may well have which of the following personality disorders?
   a. Obsessive-compulsive disorder
   b. Paranoid disorder
   c. Avoidant disorder
   d. Antisocial disorder

8. A person who is perfectionistic, very particular about following rules, and fo-

cused on details is dedicated to work and is effective in producing work. However this person always insists on doing things a certain way. Analysis of the person's rigidity likely would reveal
   a. fear of loss of control
   b. fear of rejection
   c. fear of goal achievement
   d. fear of attention

9. A client has a history of conflict-filled relationships. Despite an expressed desire for friends the client acts in ways that alienate people who befriend her. Which of the following would be an important nursing intervention for this client?
   a. Help the client find friends who are kind and extra caring.
   b. Establish a therapeutic relationship in which role-modeling and role-playing may occur.
   c. Realize that the client cannot change, and accept the client as is.
   d. Point out the client's difficulties in relationships and suggest areas for improvement.

10. A client has a history of problems with people and jobs. This client, who is inflexible, opinionated, and defensive, complains to the nurse that "people are so hard to get along with; if only they weren't so stupid and lazy, things would go much more smoothly." Why is this behavior fairly typical of a person with a personality disorder?
   a. Personality disorders are most common in people with relationship problems.
   b. Lack of insight and blaming others are characteristic behaviors in personality disorders.
   c. Loud, opinionated behavior is typical in personality disorders.
   d. Rationalization and identification are major coping measures in personality disorders.

11. Persons with antisocial personality disorders come to the attention of social agencies more frequently than do persons with other personality disorders because
   a. They are charming and sincere in relationships.
   b. They are more likely to seek therapy.
   c. They are often engaged in criminal activity.
   d. They are most likely to become psychotic and be hospitalized.

12. A person has a schizotypal personality disorder manifested by limited social skills, bizarre thoughts and mannerisms, and inability to hold a job. Having few relatives or friends who can help, this person lives on the streets with other homeless persons. Tonight, the police bring the person to the emergency department, explaining that the client was wandering and complaining of feeling sick. Nursing assessment reveals a high fever and a badly infected leg. After dealing with the infection, a priority nursing diagnosis would be
   a. Altered Role Performance
   b. Diversional Activity Deficit
   c. Risk for Violence: Self-directed
   d. Ineffective Individual Coping

13. An individual thinks people talk about him behind his back and are out to get his job. He is hypersensitive to criticism, and often believes his actions are misjudged. He is mistrustful and jealous in relationships. Which of the following coping measures is this individual exhibiting in his paranoid behavior patterns?
   a. projection
   b. introjection
   c. displacement
   d. sublimation

14. Some clients with personality disorders are defensive and emotionally labile and may become suddenly and explosively angry. When interacting with such a client, the nurse should
   a. Point out how angry the client is becoming and confront the angry behavior.

b. Use gentle and caring touch to calm the client.
c. Tell the client to calm down and stop using derogatory language.
d. Take a calm, quiet, nonconfrontational approach; do not argue.

15. Which of the following is the best definition of personality disorder?
a. a false belief that resists modification
b. a mental state in which the person's ability to perceive reality is impaired
c. an inflexible behavior pattern that causes problems in functioning and relationships
d. a mental disorder involving psychotic disturbances in thought association and affect

16. A woman who is very self-involved believes she is entitled to special privileges in her community. As she puts it, "After all, my family has lived here for over 100 years." She seems preoccupied with issues of societal position and wealth. She treats others somewhat like servants and is insensitive to their needs or reactions. Which of the following personality disorders most likely would apply to this individual?
a. narcissistic disorder
b. histrionic disorder
c. antisocial disorder
d. avoidance disorder

ANSWER KEY

1. ***Correct response: b***
Stress increases symptoms in personality disorders.
a and c. These indicate a change in an ingrained personality pattern.
d. This is another personality disorder behavior.
Application/Psychosocial/Assessment

2. ***Correct response: c***
The histrionic personality is dramatic, reactive, and attention-seeking.
a. This describes obsessive-compulsive personality disorder.
b. This describes paranoid and schizoid personality disorder.
d. This describes antisocial personality disorder.
Knowledge/Psychosocial/Assessment

3. ***Correct response: d***
A client with a schizoid personality disorder is detached, aloof, and socially isolated. This individual has no interest in seeking approval of another and would not seek the nurse's approval.
a, b, and c. These behaviors are characteristic of a schizoid personality disorder and would be expected.
Knowledge/Psychosocial/Assessment

4. ***Correct response: a***
The anxious-fearful personality has problems with insecurity and esteem. These characteristics would therefore meet criteria for a self-esteem disturbance.
b and c. These persons do not have major thought disturbances or self-care problems.
d. There are no data to support potential suicide.
Application/Safe care/Analysis (Dx)

5. ***Correct response: a***
Persons with personality disorders typically are marginally functional despite inflexible personality patterns and social and occupational problems.
b. These persons are not usually psychotic.
c. These persons typically do not seek treatment.
d. These persons commonly have poor prognoses because they usually lack insight and are unwilling to seek therapy.
Comprehension/Psychosocial/Assessment

6. ***Correct response: b***
Individuals with a personality disorder have inflexible behavior patterns and rigid defense mechanisms. They are not likely to change over time.
a. Religious fanatics may be motivated by other psychodynamics (eg, psychotic states).
c. Strong belief systems do not necessarily mean mental instability. A mentally healthy person may have belief systems that are strong and that govern conduct.
d. Individuals with a personality disorder usually lack insight.
Application/Psychosocial/Analysis (Dx)

7. ***Correct response: d***
This behavior is typical of the person with antisocial personality who exploits others in relationships.
a, b, and c. Clients with these personality disorders typically do not behave in criminal ways.
Analysis/Psychosocial/Analysis (Dx)

8. ***Correct response: a***
Persons with obsessive-compulsive personality disorder fear loss of control.
b, c, and d. These features are more characteristic of other personality disorders.
Application/Psychosocial/Analysis (Dx)

9. ***Correct response: b***
Starting with a therapeutic, one-to-one relationship is important in attempting to modify this client's behavior.
a. This would be inappropriate since

these friends could then be easily manipulated.

c. This response negates an individual's potential for growth and improvement.

d. After a nurse-client relationship is established, this intervention may be appropriate.

Analysis/Safe care/Implementation

10. ***Correct response: b***
Lack of self-insight is a major characteristic of individuals with personality disorders.

a and d. These are incorrect statements.

c. This is not typical of all personality disorders, but may be true of dramatic-erratic types.

Analysis/Psychosocial/Analysis (Dx)

11. ***Correct response: c***
Persons with antisocial personality disorder lack social accountability and moral values and may engage in criminal activities.

a. Although this may seem true, superficially, they are not sincere. This response would also not increase frequency of contact with social agencies.

b and d. These are incorrect statements because individuals with a personality disorder are not likely to seek treatment, nor are they likely to become psychotic.

Comprehension/Psychosocial/Analysis (Dx)

12. ***Correct response: d***
Ineffective coping is well supported by the data.

a, b, and c. These are not well supported, nor very pertinent.

Application/Safe care/Analysis (Dx)

13. ***Correct response: a***
A major defense mechanism in paranoid behavior is projection of one's own fears, emotions, or desires onto others.

b, c, and d. These are not pertinent defenses.

Application/Psychosocial/Analysis (Dx)

14. ***Correct response: d***
An important intervention with angry behavior is a calm, nonconfrontational, nonargumentative manner.

a, b, and c. These approaches could exacerbate anger and trigger explosive behavior.

Analysis/Safe care/Planning

15. ***Correct response: c***
The important characteristics of personality disorder include inflexible behavior and difficulty in functioning and relationships.

a, c, and d. These responses describe delusion, psychosis, and schizophrenia, respectively.

Comprehension/Psychosocial/NA

16. ***Correct response: a***
This individual's behavior is self-absorbed and "entitled" and supports narcissistic behavior.

b, c, and d. None of these disorders is supported by this client's behavior patterns.

Application/Psychosocial/Analysis (Dx)

Mood Disorders and Suicidal Behavior

6

I. Overview

A. Concepts

1. **Mood disorders include a group of disorders that involve disturbance in emotion, cognition, and behavior.**
2. **Mood disorders can occur on a continuum ranging from extreme depression to extreme hyperactivity (mania) (see Fig. 6-1).**
3. Ranges in emotion are part of the human condition and occur frequently in everyday life. When emotional responses are exaggerated, prolonged, or interfere with normal functioning, a mood disorder may exist.

4. **Grief is considered a normal response to a loss, such as death of a significant other, divorce, illness or hospitalization, decrease in self-esteem, and loss of personal possessions.**
   a. Acute grieving can occur up to 3 months after a significant loss.
   b. Resolution of grief is characterized by the grieving person's ability to remember, comfortably and realistically, both the pleasures and disappointments associated with the loss.
   c. Grief resolution can take up to 3 years.
   d. Maladaptive grief response can lead to a mood disorder.

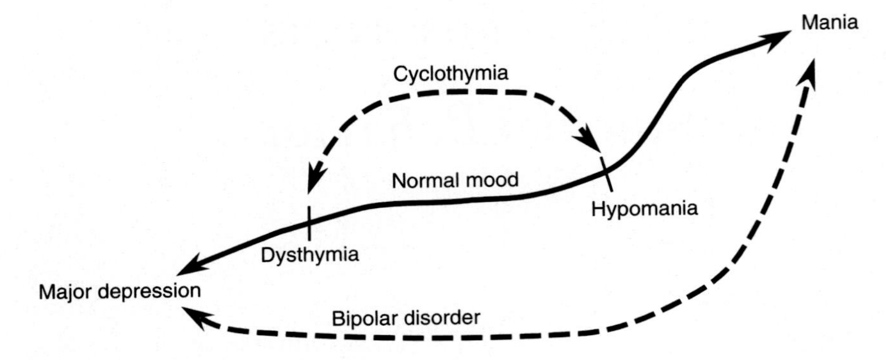

FIGURE 6-1.
Relationships among mood disorders. Characterized by mood swings from elation to despair, mood disorders are related by their episodic and changing nature. Bipolar disorders consist of one or more manic episodes or one or more depressive episodes. Cyclothymia consists of both hypomanic (elevated or irritable) and dysthymic (chronically sad or depressed) mood swings. Situated between the extreme moods, is a normal mood.

The response may be delayed, inhibited, prolonged, or exaggerated.

e. Loss of self-esteem in the grieving person is not characteristic of normal grieving. This may indicate a mood disorder.

5. Depression is an emotional state manifested by:
   a. Sadness
   b. Discouragement
   c. Decreased self-esteem
   d. Helplessness
   e. Increased risk of suicide

6. Mania is an emotional state manifested by:
   a. Elevated mood
   b. High optimism
   c. Increased energy
   d. Exaggerated sense of self-esteem

7. **Mania can be viewed as a reaction formation to underlying depression. Mania or hypomania occur in bipolar disorders.**

8. **Suicidal behavior involves thoughts of taking one's own life.**
   a. Suicidal threat: A suicidal intent is usually accompanied by behavior changes; the threat includes a plan and means to execute the plan.
   b. Suicidal gesture: This self-destructive act does not cause serious injury; it may be followed by a more serious attempt, however.
   c. Suicidal attempt: This self-destructive act has a potential outcome of death.

9. Common risk factors associated with mood disorders and suicidal behavior appear in Table 6-1.

B. Types

1. Depressive disorders

a. **Major depression: characterized by one or more major depressive episodes (at least 2 weeks of depressed mood or loss of interest in activities, accompanied by at least four additional symptoms of depression) (Table 6-2)**

b. **Dysthymia: characterized by 2 years of depressed mood for more days than not; accompanying symptoms not as severe as in major depression**

2. Bipolar disorders

a. **Bipolar I: one or more manic episodes or mixed episodes, usually accompanied by major depressive episode**

b. **Bipolar II: one or more major depressive episodes accompanied by at least one hypomanic episode**

c. **Cyclothymia: at least 2 years of several periods of hypomanic symptoms not as severe as those in manic episode;**

TABLE 6-1.
Common Risk Factors Associated with Mood Disorders and Suicidal Behaviors

RISK FACTOR	MOOD DISORDERS	SUICIDAL BEHAVIOR
Sex	Depression: twice as likely in women as men (2:1) Bipolar: more likely in women than men (1.2:1)	Increased risk in men
Age	Higher in young women and older men	Risk increases with age (but adolescents make more attempts)
Marital status	Higher in married women and single men Lower in married men	Risk lower among married men and women
Family history	Higher risk among first-degree relatives	Higher risk among family members of suicide victims
Precipitators (recent life events)	Birth in family within 6 months Loss of significant other Job problems Separation or divorce Physical illness	Increases with Solitariness (living alone) Unemployment Recent loss Recent surgery or childbirth Social disgrace
Other	Seasonal pattern: depression higher in fall/winter	High risk with alcohol and drug abuse Increased risk in those with mood or thought disorders

TABLE 6-2.
Common Negative Cognitions

NEGATIVE COGNITION	DESCRIPTION	EXAMPLE
Overgeneralization	Believing that everything will go wrong because of a single negative occurrence; the act of blowing things out of proportion. Key words include "never" and "always."	After scoring a low grade in algebra, a student says, "I will never learn this stuff."
All-or-nothing thinking	Viewing everything in extremes—either black or white, with no middle ground	John takes pictures at his friend's wedding. All but three of the pictures are perfect. John is dissatisfied because all the pictures are not perfect and considers himself to be a failure at photography.
Should statements	Using "should," "shouldn't," "must," and "ought to" statements to estabish standards for self and others. Should statements in general lead to frustration. Those directed toward oneself lead to guilt; those directed at others lead to anger and resentment.	John (from previous example) says to himself, "I should have done all of them right."
Labeling	Applying negatively loaded labels to oneself or others	After the student in the previous example was unable to comprehend the 300 pages of her nursing text, she said, "I'm an idiot."
Mind reading	Jumping to conclusions regarding another person's reactions without checking those reactions with the other person	Pat is having an enjoyable lunch with a friend, but the friend looks dejected. Pat asks what the problem is. After coaxing, the friend says, "I know you think that I'm a bad person."
Fortune telling	Being absolutely convinced that things will not turn out right, no matter what the evidence to the contrary	Ellen has received several letters of commendation from her boss, but when it's time to apply for a promotion, she states, "I'd better not apply; my boss will never give me a promotion, I only perform mediocre work."

or periods of depressive symptoms not as severe as those in major depression

3. Seasonal affective disorder (SAD) is currently not classified as a diagnostic category in DSM-IV. However, it is listed as a seasonal pattern specifier when applied to major depression or bipolar disorder.
   a. SAD occurs in fall and winter months and is associated with loss of sunlight.
   b. Common symptoms include loss of energy; hypersomnia; overeating with carbohydrate craving; weight gain.

C. Etiology

1. **Psychobiologic theory: Various biochemical and genetic factors are related to mood disorders.**
    a. Neurotransmitter (norepinephrine, serotonin, dopamine) alterations
    b. Genetic factors: familial tendency, some evidence of chromosomal link in bipolar disorder
    c. Neuroendocrine factors: increased cortisol levels, decreased thyroid levels
    d. Electrolyte imbalances: increased intracellular sodium and calcium
    e. Disturbances in normal circadian rhythms
    f. Medications: some medications associated with mood disorders include anxiolytics, antipsychotics (neuroleptics), antihypertensives, anticonvulsants, calcium channel blockers, steroids.

1. **Psychoanalytic theory (Freud): anger turned inward**
    a. Ambivalent relationship with loved object predisposes to internalization of negative feelings because of fear of rejection or loss.
    b. Loss of loved object is associated with anger and aggression that is turned inward on self leading to negative self feelings.

3. **Cognitive theory (Beck): Child develops negative cognitions leading to negative cognitive triad (see Table 6-2).**
    a. Negative feelings about self: perception of self as unattractive, deprived, defeated, incompetent
    b. Negative feelings about world: perception of outside environment as demanding and unyielding
    c. Negative feelings about future: viewed as hopeless, negative, involving failure

4. **Behavioral-learning theory (Seligman): learned helplessness theory**
    a. Passivity and failure to assert are rewarded by environment.
    b. Lack of positive reinforcement leads to low rate of behavioral output and feelings of unhappiness.
5. Family theory: Dysfunctional family patterns lead to child feeling increased stress to achieve unrealistic parental expectations.

6. **Transactional model: Mood disorders occur due to interaction of various biochemical, genetic, experiential, and behavioral factors.**

D. Management

1. Depressive disorders
    a. Psychotherapy

b. Somatic therapies: antidepressants and/or electroconvulsive therapy (ECT); see Chapter 15
c. Light therapy with broad-spectrum fluorescent lamps (for SAD)
d. Self-help support groups: National Depressive and Manic Depressive Association (NDMDA); Depressives Anonymous; Recovery, Inc.

2. Bipolar disorders
   a. Psychotherapy
   b. Somatic therapy with lithium carbonate, anticonvulsant medications, calcium channel blockers (see Chapter 15)
   c. Self-help support groups (see Section D.1.d)
   d. Family therapy
3. Suicidal behavior
   a. Inpatient psychiatric hospitalization
   b. Crisis intervention
   c. Treatment of associated disorders (ie, depression, addiction, etc.)

II. Nursing process in mood disorders

A. Assessment

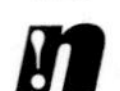

1. **Note characteristic physiologic, cognitive, emotional, and behavioral responses of individual with a mood disorder (see Table 6-3).**
2. **Assess the lethality of the client's suicidal behavior.**
   a. Establish client intent (seeking relief from stress, revenge against significant other).
   b. Evaluate suicidal plan: does client have organized plan and the means to carry out plan?
   c. Explore mental state: identify presence of any thought disorder, level of anxiety, mood.
   d. Review support systems: establish availability of significant others.
   e. Review current stressors affecting client.

B. Analysis and nursing diagnoses

1. Analyze individual client's predominant mood, level of anxiety, degree of self-esteem, severity of symptoms.

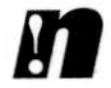

2. **Determine client's risk of suicide, understanding that clients with mood disorders are at increased risk. Suicide is most likely when client is going into or coming out of depression.**
3. Analyze current stressors affecting client, recognizing that recent loss, chronic illness, surgery, childbirth, loss of financial security, and disgrace in community will increase risk of suicide.
4. Establish individualized nursing diagnoses for client with a depressive disorder, for example:

TABLE 6-3.
Comparison of Assessment Data in Mood Disorders

CHARACTERISTICS	DEPRESSIVE DISORDERS	BIPOLAR (MANIC) DISORDERS
Physiologic responses	Altered appetite (increased or decreased)	Reduced appetite due to hyperactivity
	Altered sleep patterns (hypersomnia or insomnia)	Little sleep due to excess energy (insomnia)
	Constipation due to dietary factors, lack of exercise	Constipation possibly from inattention to need for BM
	Fatigue	Boundless energy leading to physical exhaustion.
	Somatic complaints	Physiologic responses ignored
	Restless and undirected activity	Undirected hyperactivity
Cognitive responses	Indecisiveness	Impaired judgment
	Reduced concentration and attention span	Reduced concentration and attention span, distractible, flight of ideas
	Rumination (constant preoccupation with same thoughts), somatic delusions, poverty of thought	Grandiose beliefs and delusions, tangential thinking
Emotional responses	Sadness and despondency	Euphoria, elation
	Anger, agitation, resentfulness	Anger, irritability, rage
	Guilt and worthlessness	Lack of guilt, narcissism
	Hopelessness and helplessness	Exaggerated sense of ability
	Apathy	Emotional lability
Behavioral responses	Poor personal hygiene	Poor personal hygiene
	Psychomotor retardation	Psychomotor agitation
	Decreased motivation	Impulsiveness, lack of inhibition
	Anhedonia	Hypersexuality, increase in high risk sexual behavior
	Frequent complaints and demands	Manipulative, domineering
	Lack of spontaneity	Inappropriate singing, dancing, joking

a. Ineffective Individual Coping
b. Altered Nutrition: Less [More] than body requirements
c. Self Care Deficit: Hygiene, Grooming, Feeding
d. Self Esteem Disturbance
e. Sleep Pattern Disturbance
f. Social Isolation
g. Impaired Verbal Communication
h. Risk for Violence: Self-directed
i. Dysfunctional Grieving
j. Powerlessness
k. Altered Thought Process

5. Establish individualized nursing diagnoses for client with bipolar disorder, for example:

a. Ineffective Individual Coping
b. Risk for Injury

c. Nutrition Altered: Less than body requirements
d. Self Care Deficit: Hygiene, Grooming, Feeding
e. Sleep Pattern Disturbance
f. Altered Thought Processes
g. Impaired Social Interaction
h. Risk for Violence: Self-directed or directed at others

6. Establish individualized nursing diagnoses for client with suicidal behavior, for example:

a. Risk for Violence: Self-directed
b. Risk for Self-Mutilation
c. Ineffective Individual Coping
d. Dysfunctional Grieving
e. Powerlessness
f. Ineffective Family Coping: Compromised

C. Planning outcomes

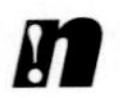

1. Work with client in setting realistic goals.

2. Establish desired outcome criteria for clients with a depressive disorder:

a. Client will eat normal, nutritious meals three times a day to prevent weight loss. (Client will choose foods high in bulk.)
b. Client will reestablish sleep pattern, including at least 6 hours of uninterrupted sleep nightly.
c. Client will report increased energy level and decreased fatigue.
d. Client will verbalize feelings directly during treatment.
e. Client will independently maintain appropriate hygiene practices.
f. Client will verbalize positive self statements.
g. Client will not harm self.
h. Client will report increased feelings of hope for the future.
i. Client will no longer idealize or obsess over lost object.
j. Client will identify aspects of self-control over current life situation.

3. Establish desired outcome criteria for clients with a bipolar disorder:

a. Client will not harm self or others.
b. Client will eat well-balanced diet—snacking to prevent weight loss—and maintain nutritional status.
c. Client will reestablish sleep pattern including, at least 6 hours of sleep nightly.
d. Client will maintain appropriate hygiene practices.
e. Client will report thoughts are not racing.
f. Client will speak without evidence of flight of ideas.
g. Client will report decreased feelings of anger and irritability
h. Client will complete one task at a time.

i. Client will verbalize feelings directly during treatment.
j. Client will interact in social situation without demonstrating impatience or anger with others.
k. Client will accept responsibility for own behaviors.

4. Establish desired outcome criteria for clients with suicidal behavior:
   a. Client will agree to no-self-harm contract.
   b. Client will report feelings of wanting to harm self to staff in timely manner.
   c. Client will verbalize feelings directly during treatment.
   d. Client will state concrete ways to problem solve areas of concern in current life situation.
   e. Client will report increased feelings of hope for the future.
   f. Client will report increased sense of control over life situation.
   g. Client will identify support systems prior to discharge.

D. Nursing implementations

1. For the client with a depressive disorder:
   a. **Facilitate adequate nutrition. Provide smaller or larger portions. Consider client's food preferences. Stay with client during meals.**
   b. Assist with hygiene and grooming as needed.
   c. Accept client, avoiding any action that could be interpreted as criticism.
   d. **Assess the lethality of suicidal behavior and implement appropriate suicide precautions.**
   e. **Avoid excess cheerfulness, sympathy, or superficiality.**
   f. Assist client in developing daily schedule that includes activity and rest.
   g. Promote sleep with daily exercise and activities, as well as bedtime relaxation interventions (eg, quiet time, back rubs, music).
   h. Have brief, therapeutic interactions with client.
   i. Do not force conversation, but encourage participation in social interaction and activity.
   j. Assist client to identify feelings and reduce negative cognitions (see Table 6-2).
   k. Encourage success in achieving goals by structuring simple, manageable tasks.
   l. Question or express doubt about negative self-statements.
   m. Administer antidepressants as prescribed.
   n. Teach client about medication, including action, side effects, dosage, reportable problems.
2. For the client with a bipolar disorder:

a. **Promote adequate nutrition (eg, offer the client high-calorie foods that can be eaten on the run; stay with the client during meals).**
b. **Reduce stimulation throughout the day, especially before bedtime.**
c. Promote rest periods; enhance relaxation (eg, reduce noise, promote quiet time).
d. Assist with self-care as necessary.
e. Promote bowel regularity through adequate dietary roughage, adequate fluid intake, and establishment of a regular schedule for defecation.
f. **Take a matter-of-fact, consistent approach in describing acceptable behavior and realistic limits.**
g. Provide the client with simple tasks that focus attention and yield successful completion.
h. **Assist the client to think through the consequences of behavior in an attempt to control behavior.**
i. **Provide a safe environment and monitor client to prevent accidents and injury.**
j. Administer lithium carbonate (Eskalith) or other medications as prescribed.
k. Teach client about medication, including action, side effects, dosage, reportable problems.

3. For the client with suicidal behavior:

a. **Evaluate client's degree of suicidal risk, noting warning signs, intent to harm self, concreteness of plan, and available resources. Note: Asking the client about suicide does not increase the risk.**
b. Identify any high-risk factors.
c. Determine the degree of client resources and support systems.
d. **Take warning signs seriously.**
e. **Remove dangerous and potentially lethal materials or objects when possible.**
f. **Place the client in a safe, protective environment and monitor closely and consistently. If necessary, mobilize support.**
g. Establish a firm but supportive relationship.
h. Encourage the client to talk about stressors; feelings of pain, anger, and anguish; and suicide plans.
i. Listen empathically.
j. Communicate your presence and desire to protect the client from harming himself or herself.

k. Be aware that suicide risk increases as depression begins to improve (the client has new energy available to carry out intent).
l. Reinforce the client's desire to resolve problems, to live.
m. **Assist the client with problem-solving; break problems down to more manageable parts.**
n. Teach family members about warning signs and encourage them to provide support.
o. Refer the client for outpatient treatment.

E. Evaluation

1. Client maintains weight at level appropriate for age and height.
2. Client does not harm self.
3. Client expresses absence of thoughts of self-harm.
4. Client voices positive self statements.
5. Client expresses hope for future.
6. Client identifies plans for solving current problems.
7. Client exhibits normal sleep patterns, allowing for adequate energy during day.
8. Client expresses satisfaction with improved social interaction.
9. Client demonstrates clear thinking patterns, with no evidence of delusions or flight of ideas.
10. Client maintains hygiene and participates in normal activities of daily living.

Bibliography

American Psychiatric Association (1994). *Diagnostic and statistical manual of mental disorders (DSM-IV)* (4th ed.). Washington, DC: American Psychiatric Association.

Gary, F., & Kavanagh, C. (1991). *Psychiatric mental health nursing.* Philadelphia: J. B. Lippincott.

Rawlins, R., & Heacock, P. (1993). *Clinical manual of psychiatric nursing* (2nd ed.). St. Louis: Mosby-Year Book.

Shives, L. (1994). *Basic concepts of psychiatric-mental health nursing* (3rd ed.). Philadelphia: J. B. Lippincott.

Townsend, M. C. (1993). *Psychiatric mental health nursing: Concepts of care.* Philadelphia: F. A. Davis.

Varcarolis, E. (1994). *Foundations of psychiatric mental health nursing* (2nd ed.). Philadelphia. W. B. Saunders.

Wilson, H. S., & Kneisl, C. R. (1992). *Psychiatric nursing* (4th ed.). Menlo Park, CA: Addison-Wesley.

STUDY QUESTIONS

1. In what ways are bipolar disorder and major depression alike?
   - a. Both are disturbances in thinking.
   - b. Both have strong genetic underpinnings.
   - c. Both are mood disorders.
   - d. Both are equally common in men and women.
2. Which model of depression addresses the issues of negative ideas about self, world, and the future?
   - a. psychoanalytic model
   - b. cognitive model
   - c. learned helplessness model
   - d. transactional model
3. Bipolar disorder is characterized by
   - a. a series of recurrent depressive episodes
   - b. two depressive episodes
   - c. manic episodes that may be followed by a depressive episode
   - d. a depressive episode followed by dysthymia
4. A student client regrets not doing well in English class because of scoring only a "B" on a term paper. The client thought the paper should have earned an "A." Which negative cognitions is this client demonstrating?
   - a. mind-reading and overgeneralization
   - b. overgeneralization and fortune telling
   - c. labeling and all-or-nothing thinking
   - d. all-or-nothing thinking and should statements
5. A client displaying manic behavior likely would exhibit which of the following combinations of symptoms?
   - a. excessive spending, poverty of ideas, impulsiveness, and exultation
   - b. hypersexuality, apathy, poor insight, and irritability
   - c. low tolerance for frustration, lack of inhibition, pressured speech, and social isolation
   - d. labile affect, flight of ideas, clang association, and impaired judgment
6. A client with bipolar disorder, manic type, is hyperactive and has not slept in 4 days. Which of the following nursing interventions would be most appropriate for this client?
   - a. encouraging the physician to prescribe restraints
   - b. reducing distractions and encouraging brief rest periods
   - c. observing the client in hopes that hyperactivity will subside soon
   - d. isolating the client in a room until he or she calms down
7. A client with manic behavior is creating considerable chaos on the psychiatric unit with dominating and manipulative behavior. Which of the following nursing interventions would be most appropriate to deal with this behavior?
   - a. Provide the client with alternative behaviors after treatment team discussion.
   - b. Tell the client that this behavior is unacceptable.
   - c. Work with the treatment team to establish unit controls.
   - d. Establish specific limits on the client's behavior.
8. Which of the following information given by a client indicates that the client is at imminent risk for suicide?
   - a. at least a 2-year history of feeling depressed more days than not
   - b. the recent loss of a love relationship
   - c. reference to feeling loss of energy and appetite
   - d. reference to suicide as possible solution to problems
9. Recognizing the dynamics of suicide, the nurse may initiate which of the following actions most appropriately for a suicidal client?
   - a. Let client spend time alone to reflect on suicidal attempt.

b. Encourage client to verbalize feelings and pain.
c. Stimulate client's interest in activities.
d. Avoid the topic of suicide.

10. A client tells the nurse that her boyfriend ended their relationship and that she would "rather be dead than live without him." Keeping these data in mind, the nurse would establish which of the following outcome criteria for intervention?
a. The client will find another boyfriend.
b. The client will recognize that she was too dependent on her boyfriend.
c. The client will develop adaptive skills.
d. The client will state she feels okay being alive.

11. A husband and wife come to the outpatient clinic. The wife states that she is concerned about her husband because she never knows what to expect of him; he's sometimes happy and sometimes sad. Sometimes he displays self-confidence; at other times he is extremely down on himself. Which of the following assessment data should the nurse gather first?
a. the husband's specific symptoms, their impact on the family and their duration
b. the quality of the couple's marital relationship
c. specific history regarding psychopathology in the husband's family
d. the husband's academic achievements and work history

12. A client has been diagnosed as having a depressive disorder. Which of the following data would the nurse explore as a priority?
a. engagement in high-risk behaviors
b. giving away valued possessions
c. guilt, decreased self-esteem
d. talkativeness, pressured speech

13. The nurse plans to help the client to increase social interaction. Which of the following nursing implementations are most appropriate?
a. Accompany the client to social activities, encouraging participation.
b. Allow client to decide when social interaction is appropriate.
c. Develop daily schedule of activity and rest for client.
d. Question and express doubt about negative self-statements.

14. A client is being admitted to a psychiatric unit for treatment of a depressive disorder. During the nurse's admission assessment, the client expresses feelings of decreased motivation and lack of energy. To add to the complaint the client has insomnia, no appetite, and has sustained a 10-lb weight loss in the past month. The nurse's priority nursing diagnosis for this client would be
a. Altered Nutrition: Less than body requirements
b. Impaired Social Interaction
c. Ineffective Individual Coping
d. Self Care Deficit: Hygiene, Grooming

ANSWER KEY

1. ***Correct response: c***
Both bipolar disorder and major depression involve disturbances in mood and affect.
a. This describes schizophrenia.
b. Genetic research has generated inconclusive evidence, even though genetic factors tend to be stronger for bipolar disorder than for major depression.
d. Major depression is more common in women; bipolar disorders affect both sexes about equally.
Knowledge/Psychosocial/Assessment

2. ***Correct response: b***
The cognitive model describes depression as resulting from negative cognition.
a. The psychoanalytic model attributes depression to the internalization of anger.
c. The learned helplessness model links loss of control with helplessness and depression.
d. The transactional model examines the interaction of biochemical, experiential, and behavioral factors.
Knowledge/Psychosocial/Assessment

3. ***Correct response: c***
To be categorized as a bipolar disorder, the disturbance must include at least one manic episode.
a, b, and d. These describe depressive disorders.
Knowledge/Psychosocial/Assessment

4. ***Correct response: d***
This client is viewing achievement in terms of an "A" being the only passing grade, with any other grade considered a failure (all-or-nothing thinking). The client also has established that an "A" is the standard by which achievement should be evaluated (should statements).
a, b, and c. These negative cognitions do not apply to this situation.
Application/Psychosocial/Assessment

5. ***Correct response: d***
Symptoms of manic behavior include all those listed in response *d* as well as those listed in responses *a, b,* and *c*—except poverty of ideas, apathy, and social isolation, which are typically seen in depressive disorders.
Comprehension/Psychosocial/Assessment

6. ***Correct response: b***
The nurse needs to promote an environment conducive to rest and relaxation (ie, reducing noise level, dimming light, providing a warm bath).
a. This represents a misuse of restraints.
c. Providing no intervention would be inappropriate in this case.
d. This constitutes misuse of isolation.
Application/Safe care/Implementation

7. ***Correct response: a***
The nurse provides alternative behaviors for the unacceptable ones exhibited by the client in assisting the client to develop self-control. Ideally, the treatment team will have discussed alternative behaviors to be reinforced.
b. This intervention is inappropriate because the client is told only what is unacceptable and is not given any alternatives.
c. This intervention is inappropriate because the treatment team's objective for the client is increased self-control.
d. This response is incorrect because the nurse must work with the treatment team. Additionally, this response does not discuss alternative positive behaviors.
Application/Safe care/Implementation

8. ***Correct response: d***
Suicidal thoughts are a specific warning sign of an imminent risk for suicide. Suicidal thoughts need to be taken seriously by the nurse. Further assessment as to suicidal intent is necessary.

a. This indicates a dysthymic disorder.
b. This is a risk factor for depression or suicidal behavior but is not necessarily related to an imminent risk for suicide.
c. These are symptoms of depression.
Knowledge/Safe care/Assessment

9. ***Correct response: b***
This approach gives the client an opportunity to recognize and label painful feelings and to begin developing strategies for effective coping.
a. This approach does not consider that suicidal persons generally feel hopeless and helpless and cannot ask for help.
c and d. These approaches avoid dealing with the issue of suicide, which may communicate the nurse's disinterest and reinforce the client's feelings of hopelessness. It is a myth that discussing suicide will provoke a suicide attempt.
Application/Safe care/Implementation

10. ***Correct response: d***
The immediate focus is on keeping the client alive.
a. This is an inappropriate plan for a therapeutic relationship.
b and c. Although these may be appropriate expected outcomes for treatment, they are not the most immediate focus.
Comprehension/Safe care/Planning

11. ***Correct response: a***
To perform an adequate assessment, the nurse needs thorough and accurate information about the client's symptoms.
b, c, and d. Although this information is necessary, none of it is essential at this point in the assessment.
Application/Psychosocial/Assessment

12. ***Correct response: b***
Giving away possessions is an indicator of suicidal risk. Suicide assessment and prevention would take priority in client situations.
a and d. These are characteristics of bipolar disorders.
c. Although this data is significant in relation to depressive disorders, the nurse would first assess suicide risk in this client.
Knowledge/Safe care/Assessment

13. ***Correct response: a***
Client should be expected to attend any unit social activities but should not be forced to interact. The nurse accompanying the client should provide support and encourage participation.
b. The client who is depressed may not feel that social interaction is desirable. Isolation and withdrawal accompany depression.
c and d. These implementations are appropriate for other problems of depression and are not directed to the goal of increasing social interaction.
Application/Psychosocial/Planning

14. ***Correct response: a***
The client has subjectively expressed a loss of appetite and objectively has lost 10 lb in the past month. The priority nursing diagnosis would be directed to this problem.
b, c, and d. These may all be appropriate nursing diagnoses for a client with depression. Currently the nurse has not collected sufficient assessment data to establish these diagnoses for this client.
Application/Safe care/Analysis (Dx)

Schizophrenic Disorders

I. Overview

A. Definition

1. **A group of psychotic reactions characterized by basic disturbance in relationships and inability to think and communicate clearly**
2. Disturbances in thought processes, perception, and affect resulting in severe deterioration of social and occupational functioning
3. A group of related psychotic disorders that involve difficulties in reality testing and relating
4. According to DSM-IV diagnostic criteria, disturbance that lasts for at least 6 months and includes at least 1 month of active phase symptoms that may involve two or more of the following:
   a. Delusions
   b. Hallucinations
   c. Disorganized speech
   d. Grossly disorganized or catatonic behavior
   e. Negative symptoms such as affective flattening, alogia (poverty of speech), and avolition (inability to persist in goal-directed activities)

B. Concepts

1. **Schizophrenia is more of a syndrome than one disease entity. It can involve any of several combinations of symptoms and reactions.**

2. **Onset of symptoms usually occurs in late adolescence or early adulthood.**
3. **The course of schizophrenia is variable. Onset can be gradual or sudden; remissions may occur; some clients recover completely; some clients have a chronic, unremitting disorder.**
4. The acute phase typically involves psychotic symptoms whereas the chronic phase may involve persistent social and role impairments.

5. **Symptoms of schizophrenia can be characterized by Bleuler's "four As'":**
   a. Autism—withdrawal from interaction with real external environment and retreat into internal fantasy world. Autism leads to confusion about what is generated from inside self and what is stimulus from external environment (Table 7-1).
   b. Affective disturbance—feeling state that is inappropriate to the situation. Affect may be flat or blunted or opposite of what would be expected in a given situation.

TABLE 7-1.
Autistic Disturbances in Schizophrenia

DISTURBANCE	EXAMPLE
Primary process thinking	Ego judgments of time and place possible and impossible are not considered. Rather the individual has dream-like or id thinking.
Concrete thinking	Individual has difficulty with abstract thought, and instead interprets another's communication literally. Can be tested by asking person to interpret a common proverb.
Loss of ego boundaries	Individual loses the sense of body wholeness, leading to difficulty distinguishing between self and not self.
Depersonalization or derealization	Individual feels that the self has been fundamentally changed or altered.
Hallucinations	False sense perceptions, usually occurring as a response to anxiety-provoking stimuli. Any of the five senses may be involved, however, auditory hallucinations are most common in schizophrenia.
Illusions	Misinterpretation of actual environmental stimuli.
Delusions (fixed false beliefs)	Delusions of reference—everything that occurs in external environment has direct reference to one's self. Delusions of persecution—people or institutions are plotting against one or are attacking one's self. Delusions of external influences—one is controlled by others or outside forces. Somatic delusions—involve beliefs about appearance or functioning of one's body. Grandiose delusions—inflated self-worth, power, knowledge, or identity.

c. Associative disturbance—also called *loose associations*—lack of a logical relationship between thoughts and ideas that renders speech and thought inexact, vague, diffuse, and unfocused (Table 7-2)
d. Ambivalence—conflicting or opposite emotions occurring at the same time and leading to inability to make decisions or choices because of simultaneous conflicting feelings (ie, love or hate, happy or sad)

6. **The psychotic thinking and communicative patterns in clients with a schizophrenic disorder indicate severe impairment in perception of reality or a disturbance in ego function.**
   a. Results of reality testing indicate that the individual does not perceive any abnormality and lacks insight about problems.
   b. Individual lacks firm sense of identity and has poor sense of self-esteem.
7. The interpersonal relationships of an individual with schizophrenic disorder are characterized by:
   a. Withdrawal from interactions (ego protection)
   b. Fear of interactions (reflects poor sense of identity)
   c. Basic feeling of rejection
8. Type I schizophrenia (also called *reactive schizophrenia*) is characterized by "positive" (excessive or distorted) symptoms, such as hallucinations, delusions, and thought disorders.
9. *Type II schizophrenia* (also called *process schizophrenia*) is characterized by "negative" (diminished or lost) symptoms, such as flat affect, poverty of speech (alogia), and loss of motivation (avolition).

TABLE 7-2.
Associative Disturbances in Schizophrenia

DISTURBANCE	EXAMPLE
Neologism	Making up new words (eg, potlmp, lemopty)
Word salad	Words seemingly connected in a sentence; however, they do not make up any coherent thought (eg, "The blue isn't silly eating upwards time.")
Illogical or paralogical thinking	Syllogistic thinking that defies logic, such as: "Blessed Mary is a virgin." "I am a virgin." "I am the Blessed Mary."
Echolalia	Senseless repetition of another's words
Echopraxia	Senseless copying of another's behavior or action
Clang association	Words that rhyme are put together without regard to coherent thought (eg, "The sky and pie, for my or dye").

10. The schizophrenic disorders are considered serious mental disorders and, as such, are stigmatized in society. This creates additional burden for client and the family.
11. The chronic nature of these disorders can lead to serious socioeconomic problems for the individual and/or family.
12. An estimated one third of the homeless persons in society are thought to have a schizophrenic disorder.

C. Types

1. Paranoid schizophrenia

   a. **Essential features: systematized delusions or auditory hallucinations (see Table 7-1)**
   b. Individual may be suspicious, argumentative, hostile and aggressive.
   c. Less regressive behavior, less social impairment and better prognosis than other types
2. Disorganized schizophrenia
   a. **Essential features: disorganized speech and behaviors, along with flat and/or inappropriate affect; associative disturbances common (see Table 7-2)**
   b. Individual may have odd mannerisms, exhibit extreme social withdrawal, and neglect hygiene and appearance.
   c. Onset usually occurs before age 25 and course may be chronic.
   d. Behavior is regressive with poor social interaction and poor reality contact.
3. Catatonic schizophrenia
   a. **Essential features: marked psychomotor disturbance that may involve immobility or excessive activity**
   b. Individual may exhibit inactivity, negativism, and waxy flexibility (abnormal posturing). This is called *catatonic stupor.*
   c. Catatonic excitement involves extreme agitation and may be accompanied by echolalia and echopraxia (see Table 7-2).
4. Undifferentiated schizophrenia
   a. **Essential features: varying symptoms including delusions, hallucinations, incoherent speech, and disorganized behaviors**
   b. This classification is used when criteria for other types are not met.
5. Residual schizophrenia
   a. **Essential feature: current absence of acute symptoms but history of past episodes**
   b. Negative symptoms, such as marked social isolation, withdrawal, and impaired role functioning, may be present.

D. Etiology

1. **Exact cause of schizophrenia remains unclear. General consensus is that these disorders result from various combinations of genetic predisposition, biochemical dysfunction, other physiologic disturbances, and psychosocial stress.**
2. Genetic theory: no reliable genetic marker yet discovered; statistical analysis reveals the following:
   a. Incidence in general population is about 1%.
   b. Children having two parents with the disorder have 35% to 45% incidence.
   c. Full siblings of person with schizophrenic disorder have 9% to 12% incidence.
   d. High incidence (9%–35%) in both twins if one has schizophrenic disorder, even when each twin is reared by different parents in different locations.
   e. No increased incidence in children adopted into families with a history of schizophrenia.
3. Psychobiologic theory
   a. Biochemical (the dopamine hypothesis): Excessive dopamine present in the brain suggests that schizophrenia is related to excess production or lack of enzyme responsible for dopamine breakdown.
   b. EEG analysis: some alpha rhythm disturbance apparent in some persons with schizophrenic disorder
   c. Enlarged ventricles: found in some persons with schizophrenic disorders
4. Psychoanalytic theory: Maladaptation in earliest development phase leads to undeveloped ego.
5. Interpersonal theory: Sullivan described parent-child relationships characterized by intense anxiety as leading to later development of schizophrenia.
6. Behavioral theory: Psychotic behavior is learned as result of reinforcement failures; child does not receive reinforcement for appropriate behaviors.
7. Communication theory: Double-bind communication (contradictory messages or cues given by the same person at the same time) leads to child misperceiving meaning of communication in external environment.
8. Family theory: Faulty family development and interaction leads to responses in child that are abnormal but adaptive to that particular family system. Some generalizations about families who have a member with a schizophrenic disorder include:
   a. Too much cohesion (enmeshment) combined with negative emotional tone

b. Unclear generational boundaries with possibility of role reversals between parents and children
c. Closed family system which discourages interaction with outside environment; world perceived as hostile place, fostering mistrust
d. Lack of differentiation of self among succeeding generations of a given family system

E. Management

1. **Psychobiologic regimen: use of antipsychotic (neuroleptic) medications combined with supportive relationship with therapist. Inpatient psychiatric hospitalization common during acute phase.**
2. Individual psychotherapy: reality oriented, aimed at increasing client's trust in another and decreasing anxiety levels; may be long-term due to difficulty in establishing trust
3. Behavioral therapy: aims to decrease inappropriate behaviors associated with schizophrenic disorders; training in social skills by role playing and by reinforcement of acceptable behavior
4. Group therapy: usually occurring on outpatient basis and most successful when combined with drug therapy; difficult in individual experiencing acute disorder
5. Family therapy: focuses on supporting family system, preventing relapse, promoting problem solving and stress management for family members, and educating the family about the illness, treatments, etc.

II. Nursing process in schizophrenic disorders

A. Assessment

1. Review client's history for precipitating stressors, which may include:
   a. Genetic-biologic vulnerability
   b. Difficult family relationships
   c. Stressful life events

2. **Assess for characteristic behavioral responses of the client with a schizophrenic disorder.**
   a. Impaired hygiene, inability to perform activities of daily living (ADLs)
   b. Peculiar mannerisms, posturing
   c. Withdrawal from social interactions
   d. Suspiciousness, hostility
   e. Difficulty making decisions or choices (ambivalence)
   f. Increased or decreased psychomotor activity

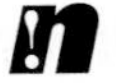

3. **Assess for characteristic cognitive responses of the client with a schizophrenic disorder (see Table 7-1).**

a. Poor attention span
b. Preoccupation with internal stimuli (hallucinations, delusions)
c. Primary process thinking
d. Associative looseness (see Table 7-2)
e. Confused ego boundaries, depersonalization
f. Lack of insight into behavior

4. Note characteristic affective responses of individual with a schizophrenic disorder.
a. Flat or inappropriate
b. Negative
c. Unfocused generalized anxiety

B. Analysis and nursing diagnoses

1. Analyze individual's degree of impaired reality.
a. Determine level of anxiety (see Chap. 3).
b. Determine extent of relationship impairment.
c. Determine degree of autistic disturbances (see Table 7-1) and associative disturbances (see Table 7-2).

2. Analyze client's potential for acting-out behavior.

3. Establish individualized nursing diagnoses for the client with a schizophrenic disorder, including, but not limited to the following:
a. Social Isolation
b. Impaired Verbal Communication
c. Altered Thought Processes
d. Sensory/Perceptual Alterations
e. Self Care Deficit
f. Decisional Conflict
g. Ineffective Individual Coping
h. Noncompliance
i. Self Esteem Disturbance
j. Personal Identity Disturbance
k. Ineffective Family Coping: Disabling
l. Risk for Violence: Self-directed or directed at others

C. Planning outcomes

1. Work with the client in setting realistic goals. (Initially may have to establish goals that are limited depending on client's assessed degree of impairment.)

2. Establish desired outcome criteria for client with schizophrenic disorder. The client will:
a. Demonstrate decreased anxiety level
b. Interact on one-to-one basis with nurse or treatment team member

   c. Maintain personal hygiene and activities of daily living
   d. Decrease or refrain from behaviors that are considered bizarre or inappropriate
   e. Differentiate between thoughts and feelings that are from inside self and those that are from external environment
   f. Increase appropriate social interaction
   g. Identify positive self statements
   h. Cooperate with established treatment plan and agree to follow up with outpatient care
3. Establish desired outcome criteria for families with a member having a schizophrenic disorder. Family members will:
   a. Express feelings about individual needs and problems
   b. Identify anxiety-producing situations and specific coping strategies

D. Nursing implementations

1. For the client who is withdrawn and isolated:
   a. Use self in therapeutic manner.
   b. **Initiate planned, short, frequent and undemanding interactions.**
   c. Plan simple one-on-one activities.
   d. **Maintain consistency and honesty in interactions.**
   e. Gradually encourage client to interact with peers in nonthreatening situations.
2. For the client exhibiting regressive or unusual behaviors:
   a. **Assume matter-of-fact approach to bizarre behaviors (do not reinforce).**
   b. **Treat client as an adult, despite regression.**
   c. Monitor client's eating patterns, encourage and assist when necessary.
   d. **Assist with hygiene and grooming, doing only what client is unable to do.**
   e. **Be cautious with use of touch; this may be perceived as threatening to client with poor ego boundaries.**
   f. Establish routine schedule of activities of daily living.
   g. Give simple choices of two items for client who is ambivalent.
3. For the client who manifests unclear communication patterns:
   a. **Maintain own communication in clear, unambiguous manner.**
   b. Maintain own communication as verbally and nonverbally congruent.

   c. **Clarify any ambiguous or unclear meanings related to client's communication (see Display 7-1).**
   d. Use therapeutic communication techniques (see Chap. 2).
4. For the client who is highly suspicious and hostile:
   a. Establish professional relationship (being overly friendly may be threatening).
   b. **Use touch cautiously; the client may perceive touch as threatening.**
   c. Allow client as much control and autonomy as possible within limits of therapeutic setting.
   d. Work on establishing trust through short interactions that communicate interest and respect.
   e. Explain any treatments, medications, laboratory tests, etc., before initiating.
   f. **Avoid focusing on or reinforcing suspicious thoughts or delusions.**
   g. Identify and respond to emotional needs underlying suspicious thoughts or delusions (see Display 7-2).
   h. **Intervene when client shows signs of increased anxiety levels and of potential acting-out behavior.**
5. For the client who experiences hallucinations and/or delusions:
   a. **Avoid reinforcing hallucinations and/or delusions by discussing them while they are occurring.**
   b. **Point out that you do not share client's perception (eg, "I don't hear the voices you say you hear."), but validate that you believe the hallucination is real to the client.**
   c. Do not argue with the client about hallucinations or delusions.
   d. Respond to the feelings communicated during hallucinatory or delusional experiences (eg, "You seem frightened.").

DISPLAY 7-1.
Making Connections: Clarifying Communications

Client: "The skirts in the sky are flying high and I'm not going with them."
Nurse: "You are trying to tell me something, but I don't understand what it is. Can you tell me in a different way?"
Client: (pointing to a nurse walking briskly down the hall) "They're all in a hurry. . . ."
Nurse: You're telling me that the nurses are very busy and that you feel left out? . . ."
Client: Yes, I need help with my bath. . . ."
Interpretation: In this example, the client uses highly symbolic language in trying to communicate. The nurse indicates that she does not understand what is being said. When the client tries again, the nurse thinks she understands and checks out what she hears with the client. The client then confirms the message.

DISPLAY 7-2.
Making Connections: Responding to Suspicious Thoughts or Delusions

Client: (furtively standing by the nurse's station, looking at the tape recorder on the desk): "That tape recorder is used to record my thoughts. people here are against me."
Nurse: "It doesn't seem to me that this is so. The night nurse uses this tape recorder to make the evening report. I believe that you're safe here."
Client: "I don't feel safe here. Can I stay by the desk while you are here? . . .
Nurse: "Yes; I'll be here for 5 more minutes until lunch trays come. Here's a newspaper for you to read. . . .
Client: "I'll stay here and read the paper."
Interpretation: In this example, the client misinterprets the environment by drawing an unwarranted conclusion about the tape recorder kept at the nurses' station. The nurse responds by presenting reality to the patient in a matter-of-fact manner. Similarly the nurse responds to the underlying meaning of the client's communication by saying that the client is safe here and can remain close by. Then, the nurse refocuses the client on another environmental object, the newspaper.

e. Redirect and focus client on structured activity or reality-based task.
f. Move client to quieter, less stimulating environment.
g. Wait until client is not experiencing hallucinations or delusions before initiating a teaching session about them.
h. Explain that hallucinations or delusions are symptoms of psychiatric disorders.
i. Point out that anxiety or increased stimuli from environment may stimulate hallucinations.
j. Help client control hallucinations by focusing on reality and by taking prescribed medications.
k. If hallucinations persist, help client learn to ignore them and act in appropriate manner despite hallucinations.

6. For the client exhibiting agitated behavior and potential for violence:
   a. **Observe for early cues of agitation; intervene before client begins acting out.**
   b. Provide safe, quiet environment; decrease stimuli when client becomes agitated.
   c. **Avoid retaliating when client is verbally hostile; use quiet, calm tone of voice.**
   d. Offer medications as needed (prn) to agitated client.
   e. Isolate client from general milieu if agitation increases.
   f. Set limits on unacceptable behavior and consistently follow protocol for intervention.
   g. Follow institutional protocol for responding to client with acting-out behavior.
   h. Ensure that enough staff members are available when attempting to subdue violent client.

i. If restraints are necessary, apply them in a safe and non-punitive manner.
j. For a client in restraints, follow protocol and provide safe care.

7. For the family of the client with a schizophrenic disorder:
   a. Encourage each member to discuss feelings and needs.
   b. Assist family members to define basic rules in regard to respecting one another's privacy and living together.
   c. Encourage interaction for each family member with a wider social environment.
   d. Encourage family member to become involved in support groups.
   e. Assist members to identify anxiety-producing situations and plan specific coping strategies.

E. Evaluation

1. Client identifies internal feelings of anxiety and uses learned coping measures to decrease anxiety.
2. Client independently maintains personal hygiene.
3. Client follows routine schedule for ADLs.
4. Client demonstrates appropriate behavior in social situations.
5. Client communicates without evidence of loose, dissociated thinking.
6. Client differentiates between thoughts and feelings that are stimulated from within self and those that are stimulated from the external environment.
7. Client exhibits decreased or controlled magical thinking, delusions, hallucinations, and illusions.
8. Client demonstrates improved social interaction with others.
9. Client displays affect that is appropriate to a given feeling, thought, or situation.
10. Client exhibits decreased suspiciousness, negativity, and anger.
11. Client identifies positive aspects of self.
12. Family members use effective coping strategies to handle anxiety-producing situations.
13. Client participates in treatment plan and follow-up care.

Bibliography

American Psychiatric Association (1994). *Diagnostic and statistical manual of mental disorders (DSM-IV)* (4th ed.). Washington, DC: American Psychiatric Association.

Gary, F., & Kavanagh, C. (1991). *Psychiatric mental health nursing*. Philadelphia: J. B. Lippincott.

Rawlins, R., & Heacock, P. (1993). *Clinical manual of psychiatric nursing* (2nd ed.). St. Louis: Mosby-Year Book.

Shives, L. (1994). *Basic concepts of psychiatric-mental health nursing* (3rd ed.). Philadelphia: J. B. Lippincott.

Stuart, G., & Sundeen, S. (1995). *Principles and practice of psychiatric nursing* (5th ed.). St. Louis: Mosby-Year Book.

Townsend, M. C. (1993). *Psychiatric mental health nursing: Concepts of care.* Philadelphia: F. A. Davis.

Varcarolis, E. (1994). *Foundations of psychiatric mental health nursing* (2nd ed.). Philadelphia: W. B. Saunders.

Wilson, H., & Kneisl, C. (1992). *Psychiatric nursing* (4th ed.). Menlo Park, CA: Addison-Wesley.

STUDY QUESTIONS

1. Which type of schizophrenia is characterized by deteriorated behavior and extreme social withdrawal?
   a. disorganized
   b. catatonic
   c. paranoid
   d. undifferentiated
2. Which of the following statements regarding genetic transmission of schizophrenia is true?
   a. No evidence exists suggesting genetic transmission of schizophrenia.
   b. The incidence of schizophrenia is the same in all families, regardless of family history of schizophrenia.
   c. Twin and adoption studies indicate that the vulnerability for schizophrenia may be inherited.
   d. Conclusive evidence indicates that a specific gene transmits schizophrenia.
3. A client has been newly diagnosed with paranoid schizophrenia. When planning care, which expected changes in the client's perceptions should the nurse keep in mind?
   a. The client will believe that he or she is not functioning normally and will constantly ask for help.
   b. Often, the client will misinterpret environmental stimuli.
   c. The client will notice no changes in self or the environment.
   d. The client will act in a socially appropriate manner.
4. Which of the following nursing actions would be indicated for the client with a paranoid disorder?
   a. spending a great deal of time with the client
   b. establishing a nondemanding relationship with the client
   c. encouraging the client to become involved in group rather than individual activities
   d. leaving the client alone until the client initiates a relationship
5. A client believes that medicines are dangerous and does not want to take them. Which of the following actions should the nurse take first?
   a. Hand the client the medications with firm instructions to take them.
   b. Ask why the client thinks the medicines are dangerous.
   c. Ask the client if an injection would be preferable.
   d. Withhold the medications until the client is less suspicious.
6. A 20-year-old single woman is admitted to the psychiatric unit because, as her mother states, "She is behaving more and more strangely. She stays in her bedroom. She does not bathe or get dressed. She eats with her hands instead of utensils, and she answers her sisters and brothers by mumbling and laughing." Her mother further reports that the client always has been "sensitive and immature" and "a loner." Based on these assessment data, which nursing diagnosis would be of primary importance for this client?
   a. Risk for Violence: Self-directed
   b. Dysfunctional Grieving
   c. Anxiety
   d. Social Isolation
7. In a 20-year-old client newly diagnosed with schizophrenia, which of the following statements regarding age of onset is correct?
   a. Age of onset is typical for schizophrenia.
   b. Age of onset is later than usual for schizophrenia.
   c. Age of onset is earlier than usual for schizophrenia.
   d. Age of onset follows no predictable pattern in schizophrenia.
8. When planning a schizophrenic client's care, the nurse should recognize that withdrawn behavior provides a way for the client to

   a. avoid developing mature relationships
   b. handle altered thoughts and perceptions
   c. remain preoccupied with bizarre delusions
   d. prevent family members from interfering

9. An appropriate nursing strategy to deal with a client's withdrawal would be
   a. Do not attempt to establish a relationship.
   b. Make group interactions the main focus of therapy.
   c. Hold in-depth, one-to-one counseling sessions.
   d. Keep interactions short, frequent, and nondemanding.

10. When evaluating care for a client with schizophrenia, the nurse should keep in mind which of the following points?
   a. Frequent reassessment is needed and is based on the client's response to treatment.
   b. The family need not be included in the care because the client is an adult.
   c. The client is too ill to learn about his or her illness.
   d. Relapse is not an issue for a client with schizophrenia.

11. A 27-year-old client with paranoid schizophrenia has been on the unit for several days. The client, who remains aloof and suspicious, performs outstanding self-care and grooming. The family reports that the client lives at home and holds a clerical job in a nearby general hospital. The client periodically looks intently at the ceiling while tugging at the ear tilted upward toward the ceiling. In assessing this behavior, the nurse should consider that the client
   a. has peculiar mannerisms
   b. may be hearing voices
   c. is avoiding the nurse
   d. is daydreaming

12. One afternoon, a client with paranoid schizophrenia becomes upset, reporting that an item of clothing is missing. Which of the following actions should the nurse take first?
   a. Tell the client that theft is common in hospitals.
   b. Report to the staff that the item is missing.
   c. Suggest that the client be more careful with belongings.
   d. Ask where the client looked for the clothing.

13. While talking with the nurse, a male client states that the FBI is monitoring and recording his every movement and that microphones have been planted in the unit walls for this purpose. Which of the following nursing actions would be most therapeutic in response to this revelation?
   a. Confront the delusional material directly by telling the client that this simply is not so.
   b. Tell the client that this must seem frightening to him but that you believe he is safe here.
   c. Tell the client to wait and talk about these beliefs in his one-to-one counseling sessions.
   d. Isolate the client when he begins to talk about these beliefs.

14. Which of the following behaviors recorded in a client's chart could indicate a potential for violence?
   a. increased agitation and hostility; hallucinations
   b. withdrawal to room; quiet and brooding manner
   c. talking about discharge; calling family members often
   d. assisting with unit clean-up; talking to other clients

15. After treatment, a client with paranoid schizophrenia improves and appears ready to return to work as an assistant in the medical records department of a neighborhood hospital. During discharge planning, the staff evaluates several living arrangements for the client.

Which of the following placements most likely would be beneficial?

a. home—living with family and sharing a bedroom with a teenage sibling

b. a rented room on the same street where family members live

c. a large halfway house in the center of the city in which family members live

d. a state institution about an hour's drive away from family members

ANSWER KEY

1. *Correct response: a*
Disorganized schizophrenia is the more insidious type of schizophrenia. The client's behavior, thinking, and communication regress and become disorganized.
b, c, and d. These types of schizophrenia have different characteristics.
Knowledge/Psychosocial/Assessment

2. *Correct response: c*
Research indicates that various factors apparently contribute to schizophrenia, one of which is genetic vulnerability.
a. Studies show a genetic pattern to the disease.
b. The incidence of schizophrenia is higher in persons whose immediate family has a history of schizophrenia.
d. Such specific evidence has not yet been found.
Knowledge/Physiologic/Analysis (Dx)

3. *Correct response: b*
Clients with paranoid symptoms believe that something is wrong or dangerous in others or in the environment and act accordingly.
a. Most clients with a psychotic illness lack self-insight into changes.
c. The client does notice that things are changing, and as a result, the client's behavior also changes. However, the client usually misinterprets the changes.
d. Socially inappropriate behavior commonly results from misinterpretation of the environment.
Application/Psychosocial/Planning

4. *Correct response: b*
Too much friendliness, intensity, and warmth may be threatening to a paranoid client. It is best to keep interactions short and to maintain a professional distance.
a. This approach would be too intense.
c. A paranoid client does better in individual activities until a sense of trust has developed.
d. This would cause the nurse to avoid the client, an undesirable approach.
Application/Safe care/Implementation

5. *Correct response: a*
It is best to take a matter-of-fact, firm attitude when trying to get a paranoid client to take medications. A nurse's apparent uncertainty will add to the client's insecurity and fear.
b. The nurse already knows that the client believes that medicines are dangerous; this response would only reinforce these beliefs.
c. This action may add to the client feeling more threatened.
d. Withholding medications prescribed to relieve paranoia will likely exacerbate and intensify paranoid thoughts and feelings.
Application/Safe care/Implementation

6. *Correct response: d*
The client manifests social withdrawal, which is related to the general behavioral deterioration and inappropriate affect typical of disorganized schizophrenia.
a, b, and c. These nursing diagnoses are more often associated with other psychiatric conditions and are not implied in the data given about the client.
Comprehension/Psychosocial/Analysis (Dx)

7. *Correct response: a*
The primary age of onset for schizophrenia is late adolescence through young adulthood (ages 17 to 27). Paranoid schizophrenia may sometimes have a later onset.
b, c, and d. These responses are all incorrect.
Knowledge/Health promotion/Assessment

8. ***Correct response: b***
Withdrawal represents a way for the client to defend against the confusion engendered by overwhelming sensory stimuli that cannot be processed normally.

a and c. These are secondary effects of withdrawal.

d. The scenario does not present sufficient information to warrant this conclusion.

Comprehension/Psychosocial/Planning

9. ***Correct response: d***
The nurse must proceed slowly, building trust gradually with a client who is withdrawn and initiating contact by showing interest in the client's daily activities, hygiene, and so forth.

a. This approach suggests ignoring the client, which would be inappropriate.

b and c. These approaches are potentially overwhelming to the client who is withdrawn.

Application/Safe care/Implementation

10. ***Correct response: a***
Because clients respond to treatment in different ways, the nurse must constantly evaluate the client and the client's potentials. Premorbid adjustment is another factor to consider.

b. Most clients with schizophrenia go home, and the family should be involved and supported.

c. The client can learn certain things about the illness if information is given gradually and in easy-to-understand terms.

d. Relapse is common in schizophrenia.

Application/Psychosocial/Evaluation

11. ***Correct response: b***
Clients with paranoid schizophrenia often hear voices; this behavior would indicate that this might be true for the client.

a. A mannerism is usually an involuntary, repetitive movement.

c and d. These are less specific responses.

Application/Psychosocial/Assessment

12. ***Correct response: d***
By staying calm and asking the client this question, the nurse is communicating the ordinary nature of this type of event. A suspicious client often jumps to unwarranted conclusions; perhaps the client did not look carefully for the item before reporting it missing.

a. This response would tend to add to any unsafe feelings the client has.

b. This should not be done until after looking for the item.

c. This is a moralistic, judgmental response.

Analysis/Psychosocial/Implementation

13. ***Correct response: b***
The nurse must realize that these perceptions are very real to the client. Acknowledging the client's feelings provides support; explaining how the nurse sees the situation in a different way provides reality orientation.

a. The direct approach will not work with this client and may decrease trust.

c. This approach will reinforce the delusion.

d. Isolation will increase anxiety. Distraction with a radio or activities would be a better approach.

Application/Psychosocial/Implementation

14. ***Correct response: a***
Indicators of a possible violent episode include increased motor activity, frightening or threatening delusions or hallucinations, and verbal hostility.

b. These are not generally indicators of escalating violence.

c and d. These behaviors are associated with clinical improvement.

Application/Safe care/Assessment

15. ***Correct response: b***
Because the client has a tendency toward aloofness and suspicion, yet is

fairly functional, the best placement would be independent but near family members for social support.

a. Both the client with paranoid schizophrenia and the client's adolescent sibling would benefit from having their own private rooms.

c and d. Both of these choices involve living with a group of people, which is not desirable for the client who has a tendency to be distrustful of others.

Application/Psychosocial/Planning

Substance-Related Disorders

8

I. Overview

A. Definitions

1. Substances: alcohol, medications (prescription and over-the-counter), drugs of abuse (illicit drugs)
2. **Substance abuse: misuse of a substance with significant and recurrent adverse consequences related to repeated use**
3. **Substance dependence: cluster of cognitive, behavioral, and physiologic symptoms indicating continued use of substance despite significant life problems related to that use. Characteristics of substance dependence include:**
   a. Tolerance: need for greatly increased amounts of substance to obtain desired effect
   b. Withdrawal: behavioral, physiologic, and cognitive symptoms occurring when blood or tissue concentrations of substance abruptly decline
   c. Compulsive drug taking behavior

B. Concepts

1. Substance abuse differs from substance dependence in the following ways:
   a. Substance abuse does not include phenomena of tolerance, withdrawal, or pattern of compulsive use.
   b. Substance abuse is more likely in individuals who have only recently started taking the substance.

2. **The most commonly abused substance is alcohol.**
   a. Alcohol abuse ranks as the fourth major health problem in the United States.
   b. Approximately 14% of adults in the United States have had alcohol dependence at some time in their lives.
   c. More than 3 million teenagers are problem drinkers.
3. About one in five nurses is a substance abuser.
   a. Narcotic addiction in nurses is 30 to 100 times greater than in the general population.
   b. Some states have mandatory reporting laws requiring observers to report substance-abusing nurses to state boards of nursing.
   c. In 1982, the American Nurses Association (ANA) adopted a national resolution to provide assistance to impaired nurses.
4. An estimated 4 million people in the United States are cocaine addicts.

5. **Substance abuse is a family problem. About half of all families in the United States have problems with substances. Families of substance abusers may develop common patterns of behavior.**
   a. Codependent behavior: nonsubstance abuser (usually spouse) manifests overfunctioning behavior in attempt to feel good about self by fulfilling needs of others
   b. Children of substance abuser: may adopt various roles, such as family caretaker or family scapegoat, in attempt to compensate
6. Common personality traits are associated with substance abusers.
   a. Dominant and critical behavior toward others (masks self-doubt and passivity)
   b. Personal insecurity, decreased self-esteem
   c. Rebellious attitude toward authority
   d. Difficulty with intimate relationships, tendency toward narcissism
   e. Use of defense mechanisms including denial, rationalization, and projection
7. Polysubstance abuse involves concurrent abuse of two or more

substances (eg, heroin and cocaine, marijuana and cocaine, alcohol and barbiturates).

C. Etiology

1. **Exact cause of substance abuse remains unclear. Genetic factors, biochemical factors, environment, and interpersonal factors, as well as cultural attitudes about substances and their use, may all be implicated.**
2. Biologic theory
    a. Genetic factors: Incidence of alcohol abuse in children of alcoholics is four times greater than in the general population.
    b. Biochemical factors: Research indicates alcoholics may be able to metabolize alcohol more efficiently than nonalcoholics.
3. Sociocultural theory
    a. Hopelessness and defeat of living conditions (eg, poverty and related problems) leading to use of substances for relief
    b. Peer pressure, especially during adolescence when individual is most vulnerable to pressure from peer group
    c. Easy availability of substances combined with attitude that substance use is viable method of stress relief
    d. Societal ambivalence about use of substances, partially validating message that medicine solves problems
4. Family theory: implicates dysfunctional family system, especially characterized by enmeshed families in which children feel increased dependency and turn to substances for pseudo-separation (rebellion)
5. Behavioral theory: Substance use is a response to stressful stimuli; use is reinforced because substances effectively provide temporary relief of anxiety.
6. Psychoanalytic theory: Maladaptation in early stage of development leads to oral fixation in dependent personality. Relief from guilt and shame is sought by taking substances.

D. Management

1. **Detoxification followed by residential or outpatient rehabilitation programs.**
    a. **Withdraw safely from substance(s) abused in controlled environment.**
    b. **Introduce individual with substance abuse to total lifestyle change necessary for drug abstinence.**
2. **Self-help 12-step programs designed to help members achieve and maintain sobriety one day at a time.**
    a. Alcoholics Anonymous (AA)

b. Narcotics Anonymous (NA)

3. Psychotherapy: reality oriented; focused on coping without use of substances
4. Family therapy
   a. Improves communication
   b. Encourages members to define and maintain responsible self-functioning
5. Alcohol-deterrent therapy with disulfiram (Antabuse)
   a. Inhibits breakdown of alcohol in body
   b. Produces hypersensitivity reaction following alcohol ingestion
   c. Purpose: to discourage individual from taking alcohol
6. Methadone treatment: controlled use of opioid substitute methadone (Dolophine)
   a. Inhibits craving for heroin
   b. Some controversy about this treatment since methadone also causes dependence
7. Family support groups (eg, Al-Anon and Alateen): self-help organizations structured as a 12-step program to help family members focus on changing own behavior rather than trying to change behavior of substance-abusing member

II. Commonly abused substances and effects

A. Alcohol

1. **Central nervous system (CNS) depressant**
   a. **Immediate effects due to action on brain (acute intoxication)—causes slurred speech, incoordination and unsteady gait, impaired attention and memory. High doses may cause stupor and coma.**
   b. **Chronic use causes multisystem dysfunction**
2. **Withdrawal symptoms related to CNS excitation**
   a. Early phase (6 to 12 hours after last drink): anxiety and agitation, tremors, tachycardia and hypertension, diaphoresis, nausea and vomiting
   b. Delirium tremens: increased temperature, profuse diaphoresis, hypertension and tachycardia, seizures, perceptual disturbances such as illusions and hallucinations
3. Fetal alcohol syndrome
   a. Can occur in infants born to alcoholic mothers
   b. Causes intellectual deficits, physical abnormalities
   c. Requires infant withdrawal from alcohol
4. Treatment of withdrawal
   a. Anxiolytics such as chlordiazepoxide (Librium) and oxazepam (Serax) administered over 5 to 7 days in gradually decreasing doses
   b. Anticonvulsants such as phenytoin (Dilantin) or carba-

mazepine (Tegretol) for seizure prevention. Magnesium sulfate can also be used for seizure prevention caused by magnesium deficiency.

c. Use of measures to promote adequate nutrition and fluid and electrolyte balance

- Vitamin supplements including multivitamin preparations, vitamin B_1 (Thiamin) and folic acid
- Balanced diet with supplements as necessary
- Symptomatic treatment of nausea and vomiting
- Increased fluid intake

B. Amphetamines

1. CNS stimulant
   a. Immediate effects due to action on CNS: causes increased energy and euphoria; extreme vigilance, hostility, and impaired judgment; elevated blood pressure (sometimes to dangerous levels); tachycardia; dilated pupils; and nausea and vomiting
   b. **Chronic use can lead to psychosis with paranoid ideation; also can lead to infectious diseases related to intravenous drug use, such as human immunodeficiency virus (HIV) and acquired immune deficiency syndrome (AIDS) and hepatitis B, C, and D.**
2. Commonly abused drugs include dextroamphetamine (Dexedrine) and methamphetamine.
3. Withdrawal is characterized by severe depression, vivid dreams, insomnia or hypersomnia, and psychomotor agitation.
4. Treatment of withdrawal is symptomatic:
   a. Antidepressants to counteract severe depression
   b. Neuroleptics to treat any paranoia or psychosis
   c. Anxiolytics to treat psychomotor agitation

C. Cocaine

1. CNS stimulant and dopamine depletion
   a. Immediate effects due to action on CNS: causes euphoria, anxiety, or anger; impaired judgment and paranoid thinking; tachycardia; dilated pupils; elevated blood pressure; insomnia
   b. **Chronic use can lead to tolerance with need for increased amount of drug. Cocaine can also cause chronic fatigue, irritability, anxiety, mental confusion, paranoia, suicidal depression, and infectious disease related to intravenous use (see Section II.B.I.b), as well as symptoms of runny nose or damaged mucous membranes from chronic snorting of cocaine.**

2. Commonly abused drug forms include cocaine powder, which is snorted or injected, and crack crystal (cocaine derivative), which is usually smoked.
3. Withdrawal is characterized by severe depression, fatigue, vivid dreams and hypersomnia or insomnia, and psychomotor agitation.
4. Treatment of withdrawal
   a. Anxiolytics to treat psychomotor agitation
   b. Antidepressants to counteract depression
   c. Beta-adrenergic blockers to treat hypertension and tachycardia
   d. Dopamine receptor agonist, such as bromocriptine (Parlodel) to decrease cocaine craving from dopamine depletion
5. Cocaine crosses placental barrier and causes fetal addiction, possible brain damage, and seizure disorders in infant. Infant must go through cocaine withdrawal.

D. Cannabis

1. **Alters sensory perception due to active ingredient, tetrahydrocannibol (THC), which is a psychoactive substance.**
   a. Immediate effects: euphoria, sensation of slowed time, impaired motor coordination, social withdrawal, conjunctival irritation, increased appetite, dry mouth, tachycardia
   b. **Chronic use can cause decreased testosterone levels in males; may also cause chronic lung disease (emphysema and lung cancer)**
2. Commonly abused drug forms include marijuana and hashish.
3. Possible symptoms of withdrawal include irritable or anxious mood accompanied by physiologic changes such as tremor, perspiration, nausea, and sleep disturbance.
4. Cannabis crosses placental barrier and increases risk of low birth weight and smaller head circumference in infant.

E. Barbiturates, other sedatives and hypnotics, and anxiolytics

1. CNS depressants
   a. **Immediate effects due to action on CNS (similar to alcohol). Causes drowsiness, slurred speech, motor incoordination, mood lability, talkativeness, postural hypotension. At high doses causes respiratory depression, coma, death.**
   b. **Chronic use causes depression and paranoia.**
2. Commonly abused types
   a. Barbiturates: secobarbital (Seconal), pentobarbital (Nembutal)
   b. Sedative/hypnotics: methaqualone (Quaalude), chloral hydrate (Noctec)

c. Anxiolytics: lorazepam (Ativan), alprazolam (Xanax), diazepam (Valium), chlordiazepoxide (Librium)

3. Withdrawal

a. Occurs within 24 to 72 hours after last dose

b. Characterized by nausea, vomiting, high blood pressure, tachycardia, anxiety, depression, irritability, seizures (which may occur up to 2 weeks after withdrawal), possibly respiratory failure

4. Treatment of withdrawal

a. Anxiolytics in decreasing doses

b. Neuroleptics for psychotic-like symptoms

c. Anticonvulsants to prevent and/or treat seizures

F. Opioids

1. CNS depressants

a. **Immediate effects due to action on brain: causes euphoria, impaired attention and memory, apparent sedation (nodding out), psychomotor retardation, insensitivity to pain, apathy, pinpoint pupils, slurred speech, hypothermia. At high doses causes respiratory depression.**

b. **Chronic use can cause multiple infectious diseases related to intravenous drug use (HIV, hepatitis B, C, D).**

2. Commonly abused types include heroin, morphine, hydromorphone (Dilaudid), codeine, methadone.

3. Withdrawal

a. Occurs within a few hours after last dose of short-acting opioids; begins 2 to 3 days after last dose of longer-acting opioids

b. Characterized by dilated pupils, tearing, runny nose, sweating, nausea, vomiting, diarrhea, fever, insomnia, tachycardia, mild hypotension, restlessness

4. Treatment of withdrawal

a. Methadone for first 3 to 5 days

b. Clonidine hydrochloride (Catapres) to block withdrawal symptoms; may be given for 14 days

G. Hallucinogens

1. Mind-altering drugs affecting sensory perceptions

a. **Immediate effects include intensified perceptions; depersonalization; heightened response to color, textures, and sounds; illusions and hallucinations; anxiety and depression; dilated pupils, tachycardia, and sweating.**

b. **Chronic use may be characterized by paranoia. "Bad trips" may occur which can cause panic attacks. Flashbacks can occur at unpredictable times.**

c. Phencyclidine (PCP) dependence may be marked by extreme violent behavior followed by unresponsiveness.

2. Commonly abused drug types include PCP, lysergic acid (LSD), mescaline, and peyote.
3. No withdrawal symptoms described.

III. Nursing process in substance abuse

A. Assessment

1. Review client's history for characteristic stressors, which may include:
   a. Genetic-biologic vulnerability
   b. Difficult family relationships
   c. Environmental influences
   d. Peer and social influences

2. **Note physiologic responses to specific substance used:**
   a. Symptoms of acute intoxication (see specific substance)
   b. **Withdrawal symptoms which, in general, will be manifested as CNS excitation (see specific substance for characteristic symptoms)**
   c. Question client regarding patterns of substance use including frequency of use, length of time using, and whether needles have been shared. (Note: Clients with a history of substance abuse tend to underestimate usage.)
   d. Perform general physical assessment to determine state of client's health and signs of physical deterioration related to chronic substance abuse. Signs of possible infectious disease are also important to assess.
3. Assess client for typical behavioral responses to entering treatment for a substance abuse problem.
   a. Common feelings expressed include anxiety, anger, guilt, shame, despair, and depression.
   b. Common defense mechanisms include denial of substance abuse problem, rationalization about use, and projection of blame.
4. Assess client for impact of substance abuse on life functioning, including specific losses associated with abuse:
   a. Loss of jobs, financial security, homes
   b. Loss of personal relationships, including family and friends
   c. Loss of self-respect and self-esteem

B. Analysis and nursing diagnoses

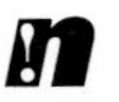

1. **Analyze extent to which substance abuse has affected all aspects of individual's life.**
2. Analyze potential for adverse consequences related to withdrawal symptoms.

3. Determine extent of individual's denial system related to substance abuse.
4. Analyze level of depression manifested, and determine potential for suicidal behavior.
5. Establish individualized nursing diagnoses for the client with a substance abuse disorder, including, but not limited to, the following:
   a. Ineffective Individual Coping
   b. Powerlessness
   c. Self Esteem Disturbance
   d. Altered Role Performance
   e. Sensory/Perceptual Alterations
   f. Anxiety
   g. Altered Nutrition: Less than body requirements
   h. Altered Thought Processes
   i. Altered Family Processes
   j. Sleep Pattern Disturbance
   k. Impaired Social Interaction
   l. Risk for Fluid Volume Deficit
   m. Knowledge Deficit
   n. Diversional Activity Deficit

C. Planning outcomes

1. Work with the client in setting realistic goals.
2. Establish desired outcome criteria for clients with a substance abuse disorder. The client will:
   a. Safely detoxify from substance abused.
   b. Demonstrate increased knowledge related to substance abuse.

   c. **Modify addictive lifestyle by changing people, places, and things associated with abuse.**
   d. Identify positive self-statements.
   e. Demonstrate effective coping mechanisms for handling anxiety.
   f. Follow balanced schedule of activities of daily living (ADLs).
   g. Increase appropriate social interaction.
   h. Identify with specific self-help group members and sponsor (AA and/or NA).
   i. Accept that family members participate in appropriate support group.

D. Nursing implementations

1. For the client going through *withdrawal*:

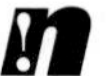

   a. **Monitor vital signs, daily weight, and intake and output.**

b. **Administer scheduled and prn medications according to specific detoxification schedule.**
c. **Encourage increased fluids and adequate nutrition.**
d. **Decrease environmental stimuli during initial acute withdrawal period.**
e. Maintain seizure precautions as indicated by individual client response.

2. **Maintain attitude of acceptance, avoiding judgmental behavior; be aware of personal biases that will affect treatment.**
3. Teach the client and significant others about substance abuse:
   a. Biopsychosocial symptoms and consequences of abuse
   b. Progressive course of dependence
   c. Phenomenon of relapse
   d. For the intravenous drug abuser, the risk of infections from contaminated needles, including HIV and hepatitis B
   e. For the alcohol abuser, effects of chronic abuse
   f. Review of the typical defense mechanisms used by client

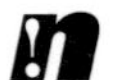

4. **Encourage the client to use self-help groups, such as AA and NA.**
5. Assist client to express anger in constructive manner.
6. Assist client to identify and express other feelings and emotions.
7. Assist client to examine maladaptive behavior.
8. **Assist client to identify strengths and utilize these in maintaining abstinence.**
9. **Review lifestyle changes needed to maintain life without abusing substances.**
10. Help client to focus on present reality.
11. Encourage development of adaptive social skills.
12. Teach assertive behavior.

E. Evaluation

1. Client admits substance abuse problem and identifies increased knowledge about symptoms and consequences of abuse.
2. Client demonstrates reduced or absent physiologic, behavioral, cognitive, and affective manifestations of substance dependence.
3. Client uses adaptive coping mechanisms rather than substance of abuse.
4. Client attends appropriate self-help group and follows 12-step program.
5. Family uses appropriate support group and reports increased coping ability.

Bibliography

American Psychiatric Association (1994). *Diagnostic and statistical manual of mental disorders (DSM IV)* (4th ed.). Washington, DC: American Psychiatric Association.

Gary, F., & Kavanagh, C. (1991). *Psychiatric mental health nursing.* Philadelphia: J. B. Lippincott.

Rawlins, R., & Heacock, P. (1993). *Clinical manual of psychiatric nursing* (2nd ed.). St. Louis: Mosby-Year Book.

Shives, L. (1994). *Basic concepts of psychiatric-mental health nursing* (3rd ed.). Philadelphia: J. B. Lippincott.

Townsend, M. C. (1993). *Psychiatric mental health nursing: Concepts of care.* Philadelphia: F. A. Davis.

Varcarolis, E. (1994). *Foundations of psychiatric-mental health nursing* (2nd ed.). Philadelphia: W. B. Saunders.

Wilson, H., & Kneisl, C. (1992) *Psychiatric nursing* (4th ed.). Menlo Park, CA: Addison-Wesley.

STUDY QUESTIONS

1. What is the difference between substance dependence and substance abuse?
   a. Substance dependence is less severe than substance abuse.
   b. Substance dependence is characterized by withdrawal, whereas substance abuse is not.
   c. Substance dependence involves continued use of the substance for at least 1 month; substance abuse does not.
   d. Substance dependence is not characterized by increased tolerance, whereas substance abuse is.
2. An RN entered treatment after being fired because of theft of morphine. The fired RN tells the unit RN, "I was framed." The other nurse responds, "That kind of thing happens often." This response would be
   a. helpful, because it provides support for the client
   b. not helpful because it increases stress
   c. helpful because it paves the way for a therapeutic relationship
   d. not helpful because it supports the client's defenses
3. Which of the following nursing diagnoses would be appropriate for the client described in question 2?
   a. Impaired Verbal Communication
   b. Sensory/Perceptual Alteration
   c. Knowledge Deficit
   d. Impaired Physical Mobility
4. The initial plan of care for the client described in question 2 should involve
   a. making appropriate outpatient referrals
   b. providing assertiveness training
   c. teaching about the risk of losing one's nursing license
   d. promoting a safe environment devoid of illicit substance use
5. Defense mechanisms commonly associated with substance dependence include
   a. repression and reaction formation
   b. denial and projection
   c. rationalization and sublimation
   d. regression and displacement
6. A client reports a need to drink 4 to 5 glasses of wine after work and to take a couple of sleeping pills before bedtime. The client also reports chain smoking and taking diazepam (Valium) frequently "to calm my nerves." On one hand, the client is concerned about a reduced ability to censor behavior and an inability to concentrate and attend to work. On the other hand, the client does not perceive the current status of substance use as being related to current concerns. The nurse recognizes that this client has
   a. polysubstance dependence because of equal dependence on three substances
   b. polysubstance dependence because of primary dependence on a tranquilizer
   c. alcohol dependence because of a primary problem with alcohol
   d. benzodiazepine dependence because of a primary problem with Valium use
7. The symptoms reported by the client in question 6 are typical of
   a. barbiturate dependence
   b. hypnotic dependence
   c. CNS depression
   d. antianxiety agent dependence
8. The nurse should inform a client who abuses alcohol, diazepam (Valium), and sleeping pills that using this combination of substances can lead to
   a. loss of employment
   b. loss of respect from significant others
   c. death
   d. reduced self-esteem
9. The nurse's *initial* plan for a client who abuses substances would be to assist the client to

a. recognize depression
b. develop health-promoting coping strategies
c. understand the dynamics of substance dependence
d. learn about the biopsychosocial consequences of substance dependence

10. A client recognizes the need to discontinue substance use and asks the nurse, "What should I do first?" The nurse recommends which of the following?
a. attending Alcoholics Anonymous
b. signing in for inpatient treatment
c. beginning family therapy
d. accepting crisis intervention

11. A slightly obese client was admitted to a psychiatric unit after exhibiting bizarre, suspicious behavior. The client was extremely agitated but told the nurse about taking pills to promote weight loss. The client was most likely taking
a. LSD
b. barbiturates
c. phencyclidine
d. amphetamines

12. The nurse would recognize that the type of substance abused by a client who exhibits extremely unpredictable behavior and who vacillates between extreme violence and unresponsiveness would be
a. marijuana
b. barbiturates
c. phencyclidine
d. amphetamines

13. The nurse plans to minimize a client's withdrawal symptoms after the client is admitted for treatment of dependence on amphetamines. This plan is necessary because withdrawal from amphetamines
a. results in delirium tremens
b. can be life threatening
c. is psychologically uncomfortable
d. mimics flu symptoms

14. The nurse would evaluate progress as positive for a client who abuses drugs if the client makes which of the following statements?
a. "I'm ready for discharge."
b. "I don't need to be here with these crazy people."
c. "I only used the pills to be able to sleep."
d. "Taking those pills got out of control."

ANSWER KEY

1. ***Correct response: b***
Substance dependence is characterized by withdrawal and increased tolerance and is more severe than substance abuse. Both substance dependence and abuse have durations of at least 1 month.
a, c, and d. These responses are all inaccurate descriptions.
Comprehension/Physiologic/ Analysis (Dx)

2. ***Correct response: d***
This statement would not be helpful because it would fail to assist the client in identifying defense mechanisms and how these defenses foster continued substance use.
a and c. These responses would support the client's defenses and therefore are not therapeutic.
b. This statement would remove any pressure for the client to begin the change process.
Analysis/Psychosocial/Implementation

3. ***Correct response: c***
From the information presented in this situation, it is apparent that the client demonstrates impaired judgment and impaired insight.
a, b, and d. Not enough information is provided to justify a diagnosis of impaired communication, altered sensory perception, or impaired physical mobility.
Application/Psychosocial/Analysis (Dx)

4. ***Correct response: d***
During the initial treatment period, when withdrawal is likely to occur, providing a safe environment is essential. Monitoring for client attempts to obtain their drug of choice would also be important during treatment.
a, b, and c. These options may be necessary for intermediate or long-term planning.
Application/Psychosocial/Planning

5. ***Correct response: b***
Defenses commonly employed in substance dependence include denial, projection, and rationalization.
a, c, and d. Repression, reaction formation, sublimation, regression, and displacement are not commonly used in substance dependence.
Knowledge/Psychosocial/Assessment

6. ***Correct response: a***
Polysubstance dependence is characterized by equal dependence on at least three substances, excluding nicotine.
b. Client is dependent on at least three substances.
c and d. Neither benzodiazepines nor alcohol alone comprise the primary problem.
Analysis/Psychosocial/Analysis (Dx)

7. ***Correct response: c***
The substances this client is using all belong to the CNS depressant category. The symptoms are typical for this category of substances.
a, c, and d. These substances are all subsumed under the CNS depressant category.
Application/Psychosocial/Analysis (Dx)

8. ***Correct response: c***
Alcohol, sleeping pills, and minor tranquilizers enhance each other's depressive qualities, thus making the combination much more potent than the single substance. This potentiating effect can be dangerous and can inadvertently lead to a lethal overdose.
a, b, and d. Even though these problems may result from the client's polysubstance dependence, they do not constitute the primary danger. The client needs to learn that these substances taken together can be lethal.
Application/Health promotion/ Implementation

9. ***Correct response: d***

During the initial treatment phase, the client needs to learn about the effect of substance use on every part of one's life.

a. As part of ongoing treatment, the client will be evaluated for the presence of depression.

b. Once the client becomes aware of substance use as a method of coping, treatment can focus on developing new coping strategies.

c. Depending on the type of treatment, this issue may or may not be addressed.

Application/Health promotion/Planning

10. ***Correct response: b***

Inpatient treatment would provide a complete medical workup, detoxification if needed, multiple treatment approaches (eg, group and individual therapy, self-help groups), and a safe, structured milieu.

a. AA would be recommended, if appropriate, after detoxification.

c. Family therapy may be included as part of the treatment program following detoxification.

d. Crisis intervention would not be applicable in this situation.

Application/Health promotion/Evaluation

11. ***Correct response: d***

Amphetamines, which are sometimes used to induce weight loss, produce the side effects described in the scenario.

a and c. Although the side effects of these substances can be similar to the ones described in this situation, neither is taken to promote weight loss.

b. This CNS depressant generally does not induce bizarre, suspicious behavior.

Application/Psychosocial/Analysis (Dx)

12. ***Correct response: c***

Persons taking phencyclidine (PCP) display unpredictable behavior, vacillating between unresponsiveness and violence. These persons are considered dangerous to themselves and to others.

a, c, and d. None of these substances involves the same degree of dangerousness (violence) as phencyclidine.

Application/Psychosocial/Analysis (Dx)

13. ***Correct response: c***

Amphetamine dependence results in a strong psychologic craving, and withdrawal is characterized by a depressive episode.

a, c, and d. These withdrawal symptoms are typically found in alcohol, barbiturate, and heroin dependence, respectively.

Application/Safe care/Planning

14. ***Correct response: d***

This response indicates that the client has some understanding of the dynamics of substance dependence.

a, b, and c. These responses demonstrate a lack of insight and would not indicate progress in treatment.

Application/Psychosocial/Evaluation

Family Violence

9

I. Overview

A. Definitions

1. Violence: physical force exerted for purpose of violating or damaging; unjust exercise of power often resulting in physical injury
2. Abuse: willful infliction of physical injury or mental anguish and deprivation by provider of essential services
3. Offender or perpetrator: person who inflicts violence or abuse on another
4. Victim: person who is scapegoat, target, recipient of abuse or violence

B. Types

1. Physical
   a. Beating, hitting, cutting, shooting, burning, raping
   b. Withholding personal care, neglecting basic needs for:
      - Food, water, warmth, cleanliness
      - Health care, including preventive care
      - Social contact
      - Education and supervision for children
2. Psychologic
   a. Verbal assault and threats of physical harm, usually to intimidate and manipulate
   b. Sarcasm, humiliation, devaluing, criticism
   c. Disturbed, inconsistent communication patterns, including withdrawal and silence

3. Material
   a. Theft of money or property
   b. Misuse of money or property
4. Social
   a. Violation of personal rights (family and friends, social activities)
   b. Isolation of victim
5. Sexual
   a. Pressured or forced sexual activity
      - Sexually stimulating talk or actions
      - Inappropriate touching or intercourse
      - Rape
   b. Incest: sexual behavior between blood relatives

C. Etiology

1. **No single cause accounts for family violence; multiple factors interact in any situation of family violence or abuse.**
2. Biologic theory
   a. Humans possess natural instinct for fighting.
   b. Limbic system and neurotransmitter irregularities precipitate violence.
3. Family theory
   a. Family systems theory: Violence is the outward manifestation of tension produced in an undifferentiated family system. Violence occurs through multigenerational transmission process.
   b. Structural family theory: Violence occurs in dysfunctional families with problems such as unclear boundaries and enmeshment of individuals and roles.
4. Behavioral theory: Violence is learned and becomes reinforced by the environment.
5. Psychodynamic theory: Family violence is linked to personal histories and conflicts influencing lack of ego strength, impulse controls, and nurturing capacities.
6. Social learning theory: Child learns behavior pattern in family setting by taking violent parent as role model.

D. Incidence

1. **Family violence is a primary public health issue in the United States.**
2. **It is estimated that half of all Americans have experienced violence in their families.**
   a. Occurs across many boundaries: affects all socioeconomic levels, both genders, all geographic areas, and all races, reli-

gions, and occupations. Occurs across life span: fetus, infant, child, adolescent, adult, and elderly populations.

b. Battering is single largest cause of injury to women in United States. Pregnancy is time of increased risk for abuse: 1 in 50 pregnant women is physically abused.

c. Infant abuse is a leading cause of infant mortality.

d. Annually more than 1 million older Americans are mistreated.

e. In three of five families, a child is physically abused by an adult.

f. One in seven married women reports marital rape. One in six couples will experience abuse each year.

g. Sibling abuse is considered by some experts to be the most common and unrecognized form of domestic violence.

3. Prevalence difficult to determine accurately because of underreporting

a. Estimated 10 to 20 unreported cases for each reported case

b. Family violence difficult for outsiders to recognize and validate

c. Since January 1993, the Joint Commission on Accreditation of Health Care Organizations (JCAHO) has required emergency services and staff education in domestic violence and elder abuse as well as policies and procedures for client treatment.

E. **Family characteristics**

1. Family is a closed system with members who are poorly differentiated and under increased stress from various sources.

a. One or more members become focal point for family anxiety and often are blamed for problems (family projection process).

b. Contagious anxiety increases conflict and reduces family's coping. Family system breaks down and outcome is violent behavior.

2. Family roles are stereotypic with rigid traditional sex roles and strong power differential between parent(s) and children.

a. Rules are inflexible with authoritarian behavior

b. Relationships emphasize control and power differentials

c. Dependence and enmeshment occur

d. Relationships characterized by mistrust

e. Family is secretive and isolated from outsiders

f. Communication patterns are dysfunctional (eg, denial and conflict avoidance, double-bind patterns, conditional loving, rationalization of abuse)

3. Characteristics of abuse-prone individual and of victim are discussed in Table 9-1.
4. Characteristic battered wife response to abuse:
   a. Believes that abuser will reform; rationalizes that abuser is not really responsible
   b. Fears leaving due to threats from abuser (the abuser is usually most dangerous when threatened with separation); women who do leave at high risk of murder by spouse
   c. Views relationship with spouse as male dominant (learned helplessness)
   d. Isolates self from other relationships due to spouse's extreme jealousy
   e. Feels inadequate, accepts self-blame for abuser's actions
5. Characteristic child responses to abuse
   a. Exhibits behavioral extremes, either very aggressive or very submissive; signs of regressive behavior include school phobia, panic, symbiotic behavior
   b. Fears parent or caretaker
   c. Becomes hyperactive, distractible, irritable
   d. Performs poorly in school, exhibits regression
   e. Thinks in disorganized manner; behaves in self-injurious way
   f. Manifests severe depression or suicidal behavior

TABLE 9-1.
General Characteristics of Abuser and Victim

CHARACTERISTIC	ABUSER	VICTIM
Behaviorial	Former victim of abuse Socially isolated History of drug/alcohol abuse Poor impulse control Involved in crisis situation	Lack of relationships with family/friends Financially dependent on abuser Socially isolated Fear of abuser—yet attempts to conceal this from others Efforts to please abuser/prevent from getting angry
Affective	Extremetly jealous and possessive Feels superior and in control when using violence	Depressed/anxious Feelings of guilt/self-blame Helplessness/fear
Cognitive	Perfectionistic standards for family members Rigid, obsessive regarding retaining control Inflexible with poor problem solving skills Narcissistic	Low self-esteem Sense of worthlessness Tendency to excuse abuser's behavior Hope that abuse will stop

g. Runs away from home, abuses drugs/alcohol, may engage in prostitution, may perform suicidal acts

h. Displays inability to form satisfactory peer relationships, sexually acts out if sexually abused

i. **Shows physiologic changes: enuresis, sleeping problems, encopresis**

6. Characteristics of elders who are abused

   a. Elders are usually parents of their abusers (the elder may have been an abuser when younger)

   b. Usually physically or mentally impaired

   c. May place stresses on family and primary caretakers (financial, emotional, physical, time)

   d. May be aggressive or submissive, creating emotional reaction in abuser

   e. Unwilling or unable to report abuse

F. **Cycle of violence:** Violent acts do not occur randomly, but constitute a predictable, three-phase cycle.

   1. Tension building phase: Abuser blames victim for problems in abuser's life.
   2. Serious abusive incident phase: Abuser's tension is relieved.
   3. Honeymoon phase: Abuser becomes kind and contrite.

II. Nursing process in family violence

A. Assessment

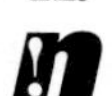

1. **Review family history for precipitating stressors, which may include:**

   a. Generational cycle of abuse

   b. Closed family system with poor differentiation of members

   c. Rigid, stereotypic roles and relationships

   d. Poor communication patterns

   e. Current experience of increased stress on system from internal or external sources (stressful life events)

   f. Evidence of reduced family coping including going from crisis to crisis

   g. Evidence of psychopathology in members including impaired reality base; sociopathy or other personality disorder; substance abuse

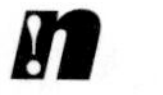

2. **Note characteristic signs and symptoms of family violence or abuse:**

   a. Evidence of physical injury: bruises and black eyes, broken bones and fractures in various stages of healing, burns, cuts, skin breakdown in sedentary individuals, complaints of pain or injury

   b. Evidence of abuse and neglect: untreated illness and absence of prophylactic care; person, clothing, environment, and dependents are unclean and unmaintained; inadequate or inconsistently met nutritional needs; lack of supervision for dependent members; reports of questionable events or practices from others; frequent unexplained absences from school or work; lack of social contacts, nonparticipation in activities

c. Evidence of child sexual abuse: chronic genitourinary infections; sexually transmitted disease symptoms; irritated or swollen genitalia and rectum (anal sex); sore throat, hyperactive gag reflex, vomiting (oral sex); weight gain or loss to affect attractiveness to abuser (by victim or observer); reports of incest or rape; sexual talk and behavior by young children

3. Inquire about situations often associated with family violence.
   a. Ask child, "What happens to you when you do something wrong?"
   b. Ask family member, "How do family disagreements affect you?"

4. Assess own feelings and responses to family violence and abuse.
   a. Personal memories may be reactivated by issues of violence and abuse.
   b. Negative feelings may emerge, such as anger, blame, denial, feeling overwhelmed, avoidance, frustration, hopelessness, fear, disgust.
   c. Positive feelings may emerge including hope, support, caring, helpfulness, commitment, understanding.
   d. Lack of confidence may be felt regarding professional ability to intervene.
   e. Seek support for self responses and feelings that interfere with ability to be therapeutic.

B. Analysis and nursing diagnoses

1. Analyze family's degree of dysfunction based on family dynamics, past history and current stressors, and evidence of violence and abuse.

2. Analyze family members' potential for violence and abuse.

3. Analyze family members' coping resources and abilities. (Include analysis of community resources available to assist family.)
   a. Nurses need to analyze strengths as well as weaknesses.
   b. Strengths of family can be used to promote change.

4. Establish nursing diagnoses for the family as well as the individual members, including but not limited to the following:

a. For the *victim*

- Impaired Tissue Integrity
- Risk for Infection
- Risk for Injury
- Altered Nutrition: Less [More] than body requirements
- Pain
- Sleep Pattern Disturbance
- Rape-Trauma Syndrome
- Fear

b. For the *family* system

- Altered Family Processes
- Altered Parenting
- Family Coping: Potential for Growth
- Ineffective Family Coping: Compromised
- Ineffective Family Coping: Disabling

c. For the *abuser*

- Risk for Violence: Directed at others
- Ineffective Individual Coping
- Impaired Adjustment
- Knowledge Deficit
- Noncompliance

d. For any *individual family member*

- Ineffective Individual Coping
- Social Isolation
- Impaired Social Interaction
- Diversional Activity Deficit
- Self Esteem Disturbance
- Anxiety
- Sexual Dysfunction
- Hopelessness
- Powerlessness

C. Planning outcomes

1. Work with individual members and family group in setting realistic goals.
2. Establish desired outcome criteria for the *family*. The family will:
   a. Identify intrafamily violence or abuse
   b. Remain safe and free from violence or abuse
   c. Accept assistance, follow through with referrals, and make use of community resources
   d. Implement coping strategies to prevent further violence or abuse
   e. Learn how to promote healthy growth and development of members

f. Parents will practice increased parenting skills.

3. Establish desired outcome criteria for the *victim* of abuse. The victim will:
   a. Demonstrate ventilation and catharsis
   b. Reestablish healthy self-concept
   c. Develop behaviors of a functioning survivor
   d. Demonstrate self-protective abilities and problem-solving strategies

4. Establish desired outcome criteria for the *abuser*. The abuser will:
   a. Demonstrate acceptance of responsibility for own behavior
   b. Establish and maintain impulse controls and coping strategies
   c. Cope with legal ramifications of abusive behavior, accepting court-determined punishment
   d. Cooperate with recommended treatment for mental illness, substance abuse
   e. Refrain from violence against others

D. Nursing implementations

1. Establish priorities for intervention for the victim of abuse.
   a. **Provide first aid or medical treatment to victim as needed.**
   b. **If violence or abuse is imminent, separate victim from aggressor.**
   c. **Provide reports to state protective services for child and elder abuse as required by law.**
   d. In instances of suspected sexual abuse, refer client to a community service which has developed a recognized chain-of-custody procedure to preserve evidence in case client goes into legal proceeding.
   e. Provide treatment before victim is returned to family environment.
   f. Promote ventilation and catharsis.
   g. Assist with integration of experience of abuse.
   h. Encourage reestablishment of healthy self-concept.
   i. **Assist client to move from victim role to that of functioning survivor.**
   j. Assist family to understand patterns and dynamics that permit or promote violence or abuse.
   k. **Provide support to victim for not tolerating abuse and taking steps toward growth.**
   l. **Provide support and assistance in coping with legal system to avoid revictimization.**

2. Establish priorities for interventions that focus on preventing violent behavior.

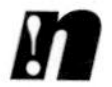

a. **Encourage acceptance of responsibility for abusive and violent behaviors.**
b. Provide support and assistance in accepting and coping with legal ramifications of behavior.
c. Assist abuser to establish and maintain impulse control.
d. Provide information about healthy functioning:

- Accepting responsibility for own needs
- Using problem-solving and coping strategies
- Accepting assistance from outside resources
- Learning effective parenting skills
- Demonstrating effective interpersonal relationships, communication, and role flexibility within family

e. Encourage acceptance of treatment for personal psychopathology.

3. Establish priorities for family interventions.
a. Assist family to identify intergenerational patterns.
b. Assist family to identify dysfunctional communication styles.
c. Explore relationships and roles.
d. Teach about healthy relationships.
e. **Provide support for attempts to change maladaptive behaviors.**
f. **Assist family to identify and use community and personal resources.**

- Community mental health centers
- Respite care services
- Protective services for children (foster home care)
- Emergency shelters for children, women
- Self-help groups such as Parents Anonymous
- Parent education classes

4. Act as responsible professional member of community by promoting social change.
a. Work to alleviate violence-promoting conditions:

- Poverty
- Inadequate housing, homelessness
- Underemployment
- Dysfunctional social attitudes
- Substance abuse

b. Work to develop and maintain resources for families so violence is prevented:

- Community mental health services, follow-up
- Respite care for elderly, mentally ill
- Child care services

- Foster care services
- Preventive education for children on appropriate interactions, avoiding abuse
- Volunteers, homemaker services
- Support groups

c. Support and promote legal and legislative efforts to eliminate family violence.

Bibliography

American Psychiatric Association (1994). *Diagnostic and statistical manual of mental disorders (DSM-IV)* (4th ed.). Washington, DC: American Psychiatric Association.

Farriery, S. J. (1994). Neutrality in a violent world. *Family Systems, I*(1), 44–55.

Fontaine, K., & Fletcher, J. (1995). *Essentials of mental health nursing* (3rd ed.). Redwood City, CA: Addison-Wesley.

Gary, F., & Kavanagh, C. (1991). *Psychiatric mental health nursing.* Philadelphia: J. B. Lippincott.

Keltner, N., Schwecke, L., & Bostrom, C. (1995). *Psychiatric nursing* (2nd ed.). St. Louis: Mosby-Year Book.

Rawlins, R., & Heacock, P. (1993). *Clinical manual of psychiatric nursing* (2nd ed.). St. Louis: Mosby-Year Book.

Shives, L. (1994). *Basic concepts of psychiatric-mental health nursing* (3rd ed.). Philadelphia: J. B. Lippincott.

Townsend, M. C. (1993). *Psychiatric mental health nursing: Concepts of care.* Philadelphia: F. A. Davis.

Varcarolis, E. (1994). *Foundations of psychiatric mental health nursing* (2nd ed.). Philadelphia: W. B. Saunders.

Wilson, H., & Kneisl, C. (1992). *Psychiatric nursing* (4th ed.). Menlo Park, CA: Addison-Wesley.

STUDY QUESTIONS

1. An 11-year-old walks into the school nurse's office at lunch complaining of nausea and dizziness. The child has a black eye that looks new. This is the fifth time in a month that the child has visited the nurse. Each time the child has vague complaints and explanations for various injuries. The school nurse first seeing this child would appropriately feel

a. concern about the child
b. anger because the nurse suspects child abuse
c. anxious about reporting suspicions of child abuse
d. all of the above

2. The school nurse's priority focus in assessing the child with the black eye, nausea, and dizziness would be

a. Decide how quickly child's mother can arrive to take child home.
b. Determine whether the black eye is self-inflicted or caused by accident or assault.
c. Question the child about ability to concentrate on schoolwork after resting.
d. Determine whether signs of concussion (due to trauma) requiring treatment are present.

3. The school nurse contacts the mother of a child that the nurse suspects has been abused. The mother tells the nurse that her husband hit the child when he had been drinking. The mother explains she has almost talked her husband into contacting AA. She asks the nurse not to interfere so her husband doesn't get angry and refuse alcohol treatment. Which of the following would be the nurse's best response?

a. Agree not to interfere if the husband attends AA that night.
b. Commend the mother's efforts and agree to let her handle things.
c. Commend the mother's efforts and plan to contact protective services through established channels.
d. Confront the mother's failure to protect the child and plan to contact protective services through established channels.

4. A mother comes to the school nurse's office after being contacted concerning her 11-year-old child's black eye. The mother reports that her husband "disciplined" the child for not getting him breakfast, stating that the child "should have known" to do so on Saturday despite being told on Thursday never to prepare him food. Which of the following would be an appropriate response from the nurse?

a. Acknowledge that children should meet their parents' needs.
b. Teach the mother that children need consistent limits and structure.
c. Admit that the child deserved to be hit but state that the husband went overboard by giving her a black eye.
d. Teach the mother that corporal punishment is appropriately administered to the buttocks, not the face.

5. In assessing a family in which child abuse has occurred, which of the following would be an unexpected finding?

a. flexible role functioning of parents depending on situation
b. increased stress levels within family
c. members who interact primarily with each other
d. relationships that emphasize control and power

6. A woman is admitted to the emergency department with a fractured right arm. The nurse doing her assessment asks the woman how she was injured. The woman explains that she provoked her husband when he was drunk and therefore got hurt when he pushed her. The nurse would analyze the client's statements as indicative of

a. a wife who appropriately accepts responsibility for dealing with an alcoholic spouse

b. an individual whose personality pattern is such that she can be an abuser as well as a victim
c. a battered wife who accepts blame for her abuser's actions
d. an atypical reaction of a wife who is abused

7. An adult daughter takes excellent care of her mother, who is bedridden. She voluntarily quit her part-time job to spend all of her time with her mother. Both women interact only with other family members. The daughter reports, "Mother can be difficult. She refuses to cooperate. In fact, during her bed bath yesterday, she slapped me." The daughter admits feeling guilty about her impulse to slap her mother back. She says, "You must think I'm awful. But then, I'm probably making a big deal out of nothing." The daughter's willingness to discuss this episode may stem from
a. her discomfort with her response to her mother
b. her need to ventilate frustration and helplessness
c. her trust in the nurse
d. all of the above

8. The nurse's best first response to the daughter described in question 7 would be
a. "Yes. After all, you didn't actually hit her."
b. "You have a difficult situation on your hands."
c. "You'd better not start slapping your mother."
d. "Have you thought about nursing home placement?"

9. The elderly mother in question 7 likely would benefit from
a. discussing her reasons for not cooperating
b. having more time alone to consider the effects of her behavior
c. being told that she could be charged with assault
d. being approached as if she were a recalcitrant child

10. Which of the following would impair an elderly person's ability to participate in problem-solving in a family situation?
a. organic mental disorder associated with aging
b. the desire to have suggestions written down
c. extreme old age
d. insisting the nurse visit after a favorite television program is over

11. A 16-year-old has been having trouble since she started 7th grade. She skips classes and acts sullen with adults, especially male teachers. She eats only one meal a day and sleeps poorly. When her mother entered the hospital recently for surgery, she went to stay at a friend's house but changed her mind after her friend's older brother came home. She then asked her neighbor, a nurse, if she could stay there, blurting, "I can't be home without Mom. Uncle Bill bothers me and won't stay in his own room." Based on this information, the nurse strongly suspects which of the following?
a. She is bothered by her uncle bothering her.
b. She prefers to have the house to herself.
c. She is psychotic.
d. She may be an incest victim.

12. Assuming that the girl in question 7 has been sexually abused, what would most likely be the significance of a change in eating habits, if she eats only one meal a day?
a. She is worried about her mother's illness.
b. It is not significant clinically.
c. She is attempting to make herself unattractive by losing weight.
d. It is of no significance unless she loses more than 5% of her body weight.

ANSWER KEY

1. ***Correct response: d***
The nurse should acknowledge all personal responses to this client and her situation, not just caring responses.
a, b, and c. All of these responses should be acknowledged.
Application/Health promotion/Assessment

2. ***Correct response: d***
The priority is to ensure physiologic health through referral for medical treatment if indicated. Psychosocial assessment is done when physical well-being is addressed.
a, b, and c. These responses are not of priority at this time. Of immediate concern is the severity of the injury.
Application/Physiologic/Assessment

3. ***Correct response: c***
Nurses belong to the group of professionals required by law to report child abuse.
a and b. The nurse is obligated by law to report all cases of child abuse.
d. Supporting family members' efforts at problem-solving yields better therapeutic effect than does a blaming or accusing response.
Comprehension/Safe care/Implementation

4. ***Correct response: b***
Providing information on effective parenting behaviors promotes psychologic security and safety for the child and improves parental coping skills.
a. This response would promote role blurring and perpetuate dysfunctional expectations.
c and d. These responses indicate approval of corporal punishment, which communicates that it is all right to hit someone to get what you want.
Application/Psychosocial/Implementation

5. ***Correct response: a***
Healthy families demonstrate flexibility in role function depending on the strengths of the individual members in a given situation.
b, c, and d. All of these factors are characteristic of dysfunctional families in which abuse may occur.
Knowledge/Psychosocial/Assessment

6. ***Correct response: c***
Characteristically, a battered wife blames herself for the abuse.
a. It is not appropriate to accept responsibility for another's behavior.
b. An abuser seldom acknowledges responsibility for his or her own behavior and usually will blame others.
d. It is typical of an abused wife to accept blame.
Knowledge/Psychosocial/Analysis (Dx)

7. ***Correct response: d***
All of these factors influence the nurse's ability to be available for intervention.
a, b, and c. All of these factors are significant.
Analysis/Psychosocial/Analysis (Dx)

8. ***Correct response: b***
This response offers empathic support, which encourages further discussion.
a. This response minimizes concerns and discourages problem-solving.
c. This response is critical and would interfere with developing an alliance. It also reflects doubt about continued coping abilities.
d. This response constitutes advice giving and would represent a premature intervention at this point.
Analysis/Psychosocial/Implementation

9. ***Correct response: a***
This approach provides assessment data and involves the mother in developing solutions to the problem.
b. This approach incorrectly recom-

mends further isolation for someone with already limited contacts.

c. This approach is threatening and could escalate a power struggle.

d. Interacting with elderly people as if they are children is a devaluing abuse in itself.

Analysis/Psychosocial/Planning

10. ***Correct response: a***

Many elderly victims or potential victims are psychologically impaired.

b and d. These offer ways to incorporate the mother's needs into the planning, and so are incorrect.

c. Old age in itself does not prevent problem solving.

Knowledge/Physiologic/Implementation

11. ***Correct response: d***

The evidence in this situation points to a possible incestuous situation.

a. The statement that Uncle Bill "doesn't stay in his room" points to a more serious problem than a "bother."

b. The teenager specifically states that Uncle Bill bothers her, suggesting that there is more involved than wanting to be alone.

c. Although data suggesting conduct disorder are provided, there is no reason to consider the adolescent psychotic.

Comprehension/Health promotion/Analysis (Dx)

12. ***Correct response: c***

Weight change (either loss or gain) is associated with body image and is a common response in incest victims.

a. This is a general statement regarding change in appetite. The question refers to sexual abuse and the relationship between this and changes in eating patterns.

b and d. Any unhealthy eating habit should be addressed as soon as it becomes apparent.

Application/Physiologic/Analysis (Dx)

10 Infant, Childhood, and Adolescent Disorders

I. Overview

A. Definitions

1. Infancy: usually defined as birth to about 12 months
2. Childhood: usually defined as beginning with toddlerhood (from 12 months to 36 months) and extending through the preschool years (3 to 5 years) and elementary and middle school period (up to age 12)
3. Adolescence: usually defined as beginning at age 12 or 13 years and extending through the teenage years, even to 20 or 21 years

B. Concepts

1. **Developmental theory is basic to understanding infant, childhood, and adolescent disorders. Deviation from developmental norms of behavior is considered significant in diagnosing these disorders (see Chap. 2 and Table 2-2 for developmental theories**
2. Whether or not infant, childhood, or adolescent behavior is indicative of emotional problems is usually difficult to determine. Some considerations include:
   a. Behavior is not age appropriate.
   b. Behavior deviates from cultural norms.

c. Behavior creates deficits or impairments in adaptive functioning.

3. **Emotional symptoms in infants, children, and adolescents may be related to family dynamics.**
4. General characteristics of infant, childhood, and adolescent disorders include:
   a. Impaired growth and development patterns (in infants: failure to thrive)
   b. Physical illness
   c. Lack of or unusual relationships with peers or significant others (in infants: symbiosis or anaclitic depression)
   d. Overachievement or underachievement
   e. Overinvolvement or underinvolvement with age-related activities
   f. Family system problems
   g. Expressions of self-disgust, sadness
   h. Impaired age-appropriate reality base
   i. Poor impulse control
   j. Sexual acting-out
   k. Aggressive and destructive behavior

C. Types

1. Developmental disorders
   a. Mental retardation
      - Subaverage intelligence (IQ of 70 or less)
      - Impaired social and communication skills, inability to be self-sufficient
      - Onset before age 18

   b. Pervasive developmental disorders: autistic disorders
      - Impaired interpersonal relationships; strong desire to be alone
      - Language used in an idiosyncratic manner; unconventional word meanings, continuous repetition of words (echolalia), and use of "I" for "you" and vice versa (pronoun reversal)
      - Likes things to stay the same, cannot tolerate change
      - Scope of interest: narrow and unimaginative, fascination with objects
      - Body movements: repetitive and restricted
      - Onset in the first 30 months of life

   c. Special developmental disorders
      - Developmental disorders in the areas of academics, language, and speech as well as in motor skills
      - Not attributable to mental retardation, pervasive developmental disorders, or educational deficiencies

2. Emotional disorders

a. Depression

- Prolonged sadness, apathy, crying
- Anhedonia (inability to experience pleasure)
- Low self-esteem, social isolation
- Poor concentration, reduced attention span, irritability
- Suicidal ideation
- Somatic complaints
- Acting-out behavior
- Reduced performance in school

b. Suicidal behavior

- Youth suicide increasing
- Second leading cause of death in ages 15 to 24
- Warning signs: depression and hopelessness, losses of significant others, stressful family environment

3. Anxiety disorders
   a. Separation anxiety disorders: characterized by excessive anxiety and worry related to separation; refusal to go to school and to be alone; duration of at least 2 weeks; onset before the 18th birthday
   b. Generalized anxiety disorder and social phobia, similar symptoms to those in adults

4. Schizophrenia
   a. In childhood, symptoms are similar to those in adults, except hallucinations and delusions are rare. Diagnosis usually not made before age 5 or 6, at which point child can communicate disruptions in thought processes.
   b. In adolescents, symptoms are similar to those in adults.

5. Substance abuse disorder
   a. Deterioration in social and academic functioning
   b. Changes in usual manner of behaving: bizarre behavior, aggressive behavior, extremely sedated behavior

6. Disruptive behavioral disorders
   a. Attention deficit-hyperactivity disorders

- Restlessness, short attention span, easy distractibility, impulsiveness, hyperactivity, poor concentration, failure to complete tasks, inability to wait
- Duration of at least 6 months
- Onset before age 7

b. Conduct disorders

- Disregard for the rights of others and for rules, physical aggressiveness, absence of guilt, irritability, low tolerance for frustration, low self-esteem, fire setting, stealing, running away, lying, sexual acting-out, trouble with the law

- ▸ Duration of at least 6 months
- ▸ Onset before age 18

c. Oppositional defiant disorders

- ▸ Argumentative, swearing, resentful and angry, low tolerance level, defiant, hostile
- ▸ Duration of at least 6 months
- ▸ Onset before age 18

D. Etiology

1. Biologic theory
   a. Genetic factors: Disorder can be related to mental impairment or mental retardation, as well as schizophrenia, autism, bipolar disorder, obsessive-compulsive disorder.
   b. Birth trauma: Decreased oxygen supply during birth affects infant's central nervous system (CNS) and is related to developmental deficits.
   c. Maternal factors (including drug and alcohol abuse) are related to developmental deficits (ie, fetal alcohol syndrome, cocaine-addicted neonates).
2. **Family systems theory: Severe emotional problems in children and teens are thought to involve family system elements.**
   a. Overanxious or rigid parenting
   b. Conflictual relationship
   c. Double-bind or inconsistent communication patterns
   d. Blurring of ego boundaries or enmeshed relationships; symbiosis in infancy; poor differentiation of individual identity
3. Behavioral theory: Maladaptive behavior is learned from reinforcement of maladaptive responses; appropriate behaviors are not reinforced.
4. **Sociocultural theory: Environmental factors adversely affect normal growth and development.**
   a. Poverty: associated with premature birth with low birth weights from inadequate prenatal care and prenatal nutrition
   b. Family violence and abuse (see Chap. 9)
   c. Inadequate guidelines for children, healthcare, and parental supervision
   d. Lack of school success (both academic and peer related), which can negatively affect ego development

E. Management

1. Individual psychotherapy: focuses on specific problems, such as poor self-concept, depression, extreme dependency, poor communication

2. Family therapy: provides assistance for family as a whole; focuses on assisting members of family improve adaptive functioning
3. Group therapy: useful in child and adolescent disorders involving substance abuse, oppositional disorders, depression
4. **Play therapy: specialized form of treatment in which child (between ages 3 and 12) has opportunity to express feelings with play objects and with peers**
5. Behavioral therapy: focuses on specific aspects of maladaptive behavior that may be modified by changing reinforcements
6. Psychobiologic therapy: medications used to control hyperactivity or attention deficit/hyperactivity disorder, depression, and anxiety; methylphenidate (Ritalin) is a CNS stimulant used in children with attention deficit-hyperactivity disorder.

II. Nursing process in infant, childhood, and adolescent disorders

A. Assessment

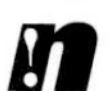

1. **Note growth and development patterns of client; compare to standard instruments such as Denver Developmental tool.**
2. **Identify abnormal physiologic responses associated with specific DSM-IV diagnostic criteria or those that deviate from age-appropriate responses.**
    a. Somatic complaints
    b. Substance-abuse symptoms
3. **Note behavioral responses indicative of infant, childhood, or adolescent disorders (include direct observations of play activity, interaction with family and peers).**
    a. Discipline or conduct problems
    b. Sexual acting-out
    c. Withdrawal or social isolation
    d. Aggressive or destructive behavior
    e. Problems with peer relationships
    f. Academic problems or truancy
    g. Poor impulse control, rebellion and deviance
    h. Restlessness, hyperactivity
    i. Substance use or abuse
4. Identify abnormal cognitive responses, such as:
    a. Lack of reality base, misperception of reality
    b. Poor attention span, learning problems
    c. Language and speech problems
    d. Unusual thought processes, suspicion
5. Observe for such affective responses as:
    a. Mood swings (elation to sadness, mania to depression)
    b. Intense emotions (rage, devastation)
    c. Feelings of hopelessness; suicidal thoughts and feelings
    d. Lack of affect

6. **Identify family system dynamics, such as:**
   a. Increased anxiety levels
   b. Conflictual relationships among family members
   c. Communication patterns that are inconsistent
   d. Lack of ego boundaries among family members
7. **Identify particular family strengths.**

B. Analysis and nursing diagnoses

1. **Compare client's biopsychosocial development with norms for particular age.**
2. **Differentiate priorities of physical, behavioral, cognitive, and affective symptoms.**
3. Analyze relationship of client's identified symptoms with regard to particular family system dynamics.
4. **Analyze child's self-concept and activity level.**
5. Determine client's level of insight into current problems.
6. Establish individualized nursing diagnoses for client and family with childhood or adolescent disorder, including but not limited to the following:
   a. Ineffective Individual Coping
   b. Social Isolation
   c. Risk for Violence: Self-directed or directed at others
   d. Impaired Social Interaction
   e. Self Esteem Disturbance
   f. Anxiety
   g. Ineffective Family Coping: Compromised
   h. Ineffective Family Coping: Disabling
   i. Altered Family Processes
   j. Altered Parenting
   k. Altered Thought Processes

C. Planning outcomes

1. Work with client and family in setting realistic goals.
2. Establish desired outcome criteria for client and family with an infant, childhood, or adolescent disorder:
   a. Client and family will demonstrate decreased anxiety levels and increased coping abilities.
   b. Client will control impulsive or acting out behavior.
   c. Client will state improvement in mood.
   d. Client will demonstrate improved attention span, improved ability to participate in learning activities.
   e. Client will demonstrate improved interaction with peers.
   f. Family members will participate in treatment program and follow through with specific referrals.

D. Nursing implementations

1. **Provide instruction about the disorder. Include information about normal development and about current treatments and home management.**
2. **Assist parents to decrease feelings of guilt and blame.**
3. Encourage expression of feelings of helplessness, confusion.
4. Listen empathically; show concern and support.
5. Establish position of neutrality: do not take sides of either parent or child.
6. As appropriate, educate siblings and assist them to express feelings and concerns.
7. Support strengths of family members.
8. Promote clear, honest, straightforward communication.

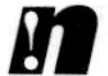

9. **Establish contracts with older children and adolescents to promote their sense of control and autonomy.**
10. Recognize own feelings (anger, sadness, frustration), and deal with them constructively.
11. Use the cognitive model to explain relationship between thoughts, feelings, and behavior (ie, thoughts lead to feelings and behavior, but person does not have to act on feelings or thoughts).
12. Participate in appropriate treatment plan on inpatient unit:
    a. Milieu therapy: Construct safe, structured environment with daily schedules and opportunity for client to increase functioning and self-esteem.
    b. Behavior modification program: Positively reinforce acceptable behavior with identified rewards.
13. Participate in play therapy for children:
    a. Provide safe environment for exploration and working through of conflicts and feelings.
    b. Use toys, paper, crayons, and other items as the medium of expression.
    c. Permit child to set the pace.
    d. Be facilitative and supportive.
14. **Make appropriate referrals:**
    a. Psychologic assessment
    b. Group psychotherapy
    c. Parental support group
    d. Family therapy
    e. Community resource agencies
    f. Big Brothers or Big Sisters organizations

E. Evaluation

1. The client and family exhibit improved coping skills.
2. Client controls impulsive behaviors.

3. Client participates in educational program, working at level of ability.
4. Client interacts socially with peer group.
5. Client and family participate in follow-up treatment program.

Bibliography

American Psychiatric Association (1994). *Diagnostic and statistical manual of mental disorders (DSM-IV)* (4th ed.). Washington, DC: American Psychiatric Association.

Gary, F., & Kavanagh, C. (1994). *Psychiatric mental health nursing.* Philadelphia: J. B. Lippincott.

Rawlins, R., & Heacock, P. (1993). *Clinical manual of psychiatric nursing* (2nd ed.). St. Louis: Mosby-Year Book.

Shives, L. (1994). *Basic concepts of psychiatric-mental health nursing* (3rd ed.). Philadelphia: J. B. Lippincott

Townsend, M. C. (1993). *Psychiatric mental health nursing: Concepts of care.* Philadelphia: F. A. Davis.

Varcarolis, E. (1994). *Foundations of psychiatric mental health nursing* (2nd ed.). Philadelphia: W. B. Saunders.

Wilson, H., & Kneisl, C. (1992). *Psychiatric nursing* (4th ed.). Menlo Park, CA: Addison-Wesley.

STUDY QUESTIONS

1. A 9-year-old girl was brought to the hospital after attempting to hang herself in her parents' basement. The nurse's first intervention should be to
- **a.** Talk to her parents alone to alleviate their fears.
- **b.** Talk to the child alone to provide immediate relief of her pain.
- **c.** Talk to the child and parents together for a brief period before spending time with the child alone.
- **d.** Talk to the child's teacher to obtain the child's academic record.

2. The next day, the nurse brings the child in question 1 several toys, including a doll house, a mother doll, a father doll, a child doll, and papers and pencils. The nurse's decision is based on the assumption that children
- **a.** communicate better verbally
- **b.** express their conflict nonverbally through their play
- **c.** need to be preoccupied with things
- **d.** have more fun when they are playing

3. The child in question 1 begins play therapy. She rearranges some of the furniture in the doll house and places the child doll in a room by itself. The nurse should say
- **a.** "No! Place the doll with her parents."
- **b.** Nothing; just observe the client's play.
- **c.** "Why is the child doll by herself?"
- **d.** "Let me read you a story."

4. A 13-year-old boy frequently fights with other children, lies, steals, and breaks rules. Which of the following nursing diagnoses is most appropriate for this boy?
- **a.** Risk for Violence: Directed at others
- **b.** Social Isolation
- **c.** Altered Thought Processes
- **d.** Body Image Disturbance

5. Even though the boy described in question 4 is chronologically in Erikson's identity vs. role confusion stage, his behavior is most typical of which of the following stages?
- **a.** trust vs. mistrust
- **b.** initiative vs. guilt
- **c.** autonomy vs. shame and doubt
- **d.** industry vs. inferiority

6. The nursing care plan includes this short-term goal for the client described in question 4: The client will eat all meals in his room. Which of the following statements best describes this goal?
- **a.** It doesn't address the client's defiant acting-out behavior.
- **b.** It addresses the client's problem by providing time out from an overstimulating environment.
- **c.** It addresses the client's problem by allowing for development of self-control.
- **d.** It doesn't address the client's problem of social isolation.

7. An appropriate initial nursing intervention for a child with a tendency to fight would be
- **a.** Talk to the child each time he or she hits another child.
- **b.** Anticipate and neutralize all potentially explosive situations.
- **c.** Take away the child's privileges.
- **d.** Ignore small infractions of the rules.

8. The nurse would evaluate intervention as successful if a client who has a tendency to fight
- **a.** eats meals
- **b.** talks to peers
- **c.** sits alone watching television
- **d.** plays cooperatively without fighting

9. A 7-year-old child has attention deficit-hyperactivity disorder. The child is most likely to exhibit which of the following symptoms?
- **a.** restlessness, decreased attention span, and distractibility
- **b.** hyperactivity, failure to complete tasks, and physical aggressiveness

c. impulsiveness, anhedonia, and shyness
d. poor concentration, decreased attention span, and somatic complaints

10. After obtaining information about a child's symptoms and observing the child's interactions with people and objects, the nurse says to the parents, "Often parents try many things to help their child before they come to the hospital. What things have you tried?" This intervention is
a. not therapeutic because it will not provide useful assessment data
b. not therapeutic because the parents are not in treatment
c. therapeutic because it reduces the overwhelming tension the nurse is experiencing
d. therapeutic because it provides information about the impact of the symptoms on the family

11. The parents of a newly admitted child with attention deficit-hyperactivity disorder say they have tried everything to calm their child, and nothing seems to work. They add that they are becoming irritable and are blaming each other for the child's behavior. Which of the following actions would be most appropriate for the nurse to take at this time?
a. Listen to the parents' concerns but quickly disengage.
b. Encourage the parents to talk to the physician.
c. Refer the parents for education about psychiatric disorders and management.
d. Tell the parents that they are overreacting.

12. The treatment team's recommendations for the parents of a child with attention deficit-hyperactivity disorder likely would include which of the following?
a. Give the child clear and simple directions.
b. Talk to the child for at least 1 hour each day.
c. Encourage more peer interaction for the child.
d. Encourage the parents to plan more family activities.

13. A safe, structured environment that provides daily schedules and promotes growth and development through constant and consistent feedback describes
a. supportive therapy
b. milieu therapy
c. psychoanalytic therapy
d. dynamic therapy

ANSWER KEY

1. ***Correct response: c***
   This allows the nurse to observe the family as a unit and to obtain some general information before spending time with the client alone.
   a and b. The nurse needs to be seen as a neutral intervener who is interested in the family as an adaptive functioning unit.
   d. Even though the client's academic records will be useful at a later point in assessment, they are not of primary concern initially.

Application/Psychosocial/Implementation

2. ***Correct response: b***
   Play therapy provides a medium for the child to nonverbally explore and develop strategies for dealing with conflict.
   a. Children often have problems verbalizing their pain.
   c and d. The purpose of play therapy is to enhance health development, not to keep the child busy or provide entertainment.

Application/Psychosocial/Implementation

3. ***Correct response: b***
   The nurse communicates acceptance and a desire to understand by allowing the child to set the pace during play therapy. In addition, the nurse needs to observe for patterns in the child's play.
   a, c, and d. These responses would not permit the child to establish the pace. Response *a* is placing a value judgment on the child's play, while choice *c* may be threatening to the child. Choice *d* interrupts the child's play and will change the focus of the child's attention.

Application/Psychosocial/Implementation

4. ***Correct response: a***
   The symptoms described are typically found in children with conduct disorder and the potential for violent behavior.
   b and d. Social isolation and disturbed body image are not typically characteristic of conduct disorder.
   c. There is no evidence of a thought disorder.

Comprehension/Psychosocial/
Analysis (Dx)

5. ***Correct response: c***
   Defiance is more characteristic of the autonomy vs. shame and doubt stage than of the stages mentioned in responses *a, b,* and *d.*
   a, c, and d. Defiance is not characteristic of these stages.

Comprehension/Psychosocial/
Analysis (Dx)

6. ***Correct response: a***
   Planning to have the boy eat in his room doesn't help him to develop more effective coping strategies.
   b and c. Neither of these actions would contribute to the client learning adaptive behaviors.
   d. This action would be inappropriate because the client is not socially withdrawn.

Analysis/Psychosocial/Planning

7. ***Correct response: b***
   The nurse's responsibility is to create a safe environment by anticipating and neutralizing extraneous stressors.
   a and d. These actions would only reinforce the client's fighting behavior.
   c. This action would not provide alternative behavior for the client to practice. However, if this is part of a behavior modification program, this response may be appropriate in terms of that program.

Application/Safe care/Implementation

8. ***Correct response: d***
   A client's cooperative, nonviolent behavior would be indicative of adaptive behavior.

a, b, and c. These criteria do not evaluate the client's fighting behavior.

Application/Safe care/Evaluation

9. ***Correct response: a***

Attention deficit-hyperactivity disorder is characterized by all of these symptoms.

b, c, and d. Physical aggressiveness, anhedonia, shyness, and somatic complaints are not associated with attention deficit-hyperactivity disorders.

Knowledge/Psychosocial/Assessment

10. ***Correct response: d***

It is important to obtain assessment data on the family's perceptions and reactions to the child's symptoms. These data will assist the nurse in developing and individualized the treatment plan for the child.

a, b, and c. These descriptions are not applicable to this approach.

Analysis/Psychosocial/Assessment

11. ***Correct response: c***

Instruction about psychiatric disorders and their management provides the family with useful information about the child's condition and what the family can do to manage the child at home. It also addresses typical parental responses to the child's disorder, thereby helping to alleviate guilt and blame.

a, c, and d. These actions would communicate disinterest and could exacerbate the parents' confusion and sense of helplessness.

Application/Psychosocial/Implementation

12. ***Correct response: a***

Children who are hyperactive need simple, concrete directions to help them focus their attention.

b. Brief interactions generally are more effective than prolonged ones.

c and d. Social isolation is not the child's problem.

Analysis/Psychosocial/Implementation

13. ***Correct response: b***

Milieu therapy creates a structured environment that promotes growth.

a, c, and d. The focus on these therapeutic approaches is not on a therapeutic community but rather on a one-to-one therapeutic relationship.

Comprehension/Safe care/Implementation

Cognitive Impairment Disorders

11

I. Overview

A. Definitions

1. **Cognitive impairment disorders (formerly organic mental disorder): temporary or permanent neuronal damage that results in psychologic or behavioral dysfunction and characterized by:**
   a. Major deficits in cognition or memory
   b. Significant change from previous level of functioning
2. Primary mental disorder (formerly, functional disorder): Term used to indicate those mental disorders that are not due to a general medical condition and that are not substance induced
3. Cognition: ability to think and reason
4. Orientation: ability to relate self to the sphere of time, place, and person
5. Aphasia: loss of language ability; may be receptive, expressive, or global
6. Apraxia: impaired ability to carry out motor activities despite intact motor function
7. Agnosia: failure to recognize or identify common objects despite intact sensory functioning

8. Confabulation: filling in memory gaps with detailed fantasy believed by the teller
9. Sundowning: increased confusion manifested at night
10. Catastrophic reactions: responses of fear or panic with strong potential to harm self or others

B. Concepts

1. **Cognitive impairment disorders can affect any age group but are most common in elderly.**
2. **Psychosocial factors can affect severity of symptoms associated with cognitive impairment disorders. Factors include:**
   a. Losses experienced by elderly persons, may be associated with depressive symptoms
   b. Withdrawal and social isolation, especially in elderly clients
   c. Poverty and poor nutrition
   d. Substance misuse, abuse, and dependence

3. **Delirium is an acute cognitive impairment with rapid onset; with prompt treatment it can be reversible.**
4. **Dementia is a chronic cognitive impairment that has slow, insidious onset.**
5. **Amnestic disorders are relatively uncommon and are characterized by severe memory impairment.**
6. An estimated 2% to 4% of the population over age 65 are affected by Alzheimer's disease (the most common type of dementia). After age 85, the incidence increases to 20%.
7. Depression in elderly individuals may mimic cognitive impairment disorder. It is important to differentiate these disorders because treating depression can alleviate cognitive problems in some individuals.
8. Medical diagnosis of cognitive impairment disorder is made through:
   a. Mental status examination and neuropsychologic testing, which can identify abnormalities in cognitive and memory functions
   b. Laboratory findings: computed tomography (CT) or magnetic resonance imaging (MRI) which may reveal cerebral atrophy, focal brain lesions, or ischemic brain injury
   c. Associated signs and symptoms

9. **General characteristics of cognitive impairment disorders include:**
   a. **Deficits in orientation**
   b. **Deficits in memory, both recent and remote**
   c. **Deficits in intellectual functioning (problem solving, reasoning, organizing and planning)**
   d. **Deficits in judgment**
   e. **Deficits in affect**

C. Types

1. Delirium
   a. Impaired consciousness and cognition; reduced ability to maintain attention; confusion and fleeting levels of consciousness
   b. Hallucinations, illusions
   c. Incoherence
   d. Agitation or somnolence, disorientation and confusion
2. Dementia
   a. Dementia of Alzheimer's type: most common type of dementia (see Table 11-1 for stages and related symptoms)
   b. Vascular dementia
      - Memory impairment and cognitive disturbances including one or more of following: aphasia, apraxia, agnosia
      - Focal neurologic signs and symptoms
      - Laboratory evidence of cerebrovascular disease
   c. Dementia due to other medical conditions (similar memory and cognitive symptoms as with vascular dementia)
3. Amnestic disorder
   a. Impairment in short- and long-term memory
   b. Inability to learn new material
   c. Remote memory better than recent
   d. Confabulation
   e. Apathy, lack of initiative
   f. Emotionally bland

TABLE 11-1.
Specific Stages and Related Symptoms in Alzheimer's Disease

	BEHAVIORAL SYMPTOMS	AFFECT	COGNITIVE CHANGES
Stage 1	Decline in work or goal-directed activities. Difficulty completing common activities of daily living Decline in personal appearance	Anxious, depressed Feelings of helplessness and frustration Apathy	Recent memory loss Time disorientation Decreased ability to concentrate, make judgments
Stage2	Socially unacceptable behavior Self-care deficits (bathing, dressing, grooming) Wandering behavior	Labile moods Persecutory delusions Catastrophic reactions	Recent and remote memory loss Use of confabulation Disorientation to time, place, and person
Stage 3	Severe self-care deficits, including incontinence, decreased ability to walk, decreased swallowing	Agitation Paranoia	Agnosia Apraxia Aphasia

D. Etiology

1. Factors associated with delirium may include:
   a. Hypoxias resulting from anemia; occult bleeding; deficiencies of iron, folic acid, or thiamine; dehydration; hyperthermia or hypothermia; lung disease; hypotension or hypertension; or increased intracranial pressure
   b. Metabolic disorders resulting from hormonal imbalance, endocrine dysfunction (thyroid, pancreas, adrenal), or nutritional factors
   c. Toxins and infections resulting from kidney pathology, hepatic pathology, drug interactions, alcoholism, or viral or bacteriologic stressors
   d. Structural changes resulting from tumors, trauma, surgery, or childbirth
   e. Environmental factors resulting from sensory overload or deprivation, sensory changes caused by poor eyesight and hearing, or isolation
2. Factors associated with dementia may include:
   a. All of the above stressors for delirium, if untreated or untreatable
   b. Vascular diseases such as arteriosclerosis, and cerebrovascular accidents (stroke)
   c. Neurologic diseases such as Huntington's chorea, Parkinson's disease, neurosyphilis, Pick's disease, multi-infarctional dementia, and cerebral atrophy
   d. Human immunodeficiency virus (HIV) infections of central nervous system (CNS), called HIV encephalopathy or AIDS dementia complex
3. Factors associated with dementia, Alzheimer's type:
   a. Pathophysiology: loss of neurotransmitters (especially acetylcholine), causing nerve cell degeneration of cerebral cortex
   b. Theoretical causes
      - Increased aluminum concentration in brain
      - Autoimmune disorder of brain
      - Gene related (familial Alzheimer's disease with early onset)
      - Beta-amyloid build-up in brain (certain protein associated with brain pathology common to Alzheimer's disease)
4. Factors associated with amnestic disorder:
   a. Head trauma, hypoxia, encephalitis
   b. Thiamine deficiency, chronic alcoholism

E. Management

1. Identify and treat underlying cause of delirium or amnestic disorder.
2. For *dementia:*

a. Adult day care services, personal care living arrangements, nursing home care
b. Use of behavioral therapy to decrease environmental stimuli and provide consistent, structured activities of daily living (ADLs)
c. Support groups for family members (Alzheimer's Association)
d. Medication with tacrine (Cognex), which is an acetylcholinesterase inhibitor that will prevent or retard breakdown of acetylcholine

II. Nursing process in cognitive impairment disorders

A. Assessment

1. Review individual's history and physical examination findings for characteristic signs and symptoms associated with physiologic changes related to specific disorder.

2. Assess for characteristic behavioral responses including:
a. Inattention to self-care and ADLs
b. Socially unacceptable behaviors
c. Tendency to wander
d. Sundowning
e. Specific history or potential for catastrophic reactions

3. Assess for characteristic affective responses including:
a. Specific level of anxiety
b. Emotional lability
c. Depression or apathy
d. Irritability, defensiveness
e. Suspicion
f. Feelings of helplessness and frustration

4. Assess for characteristic cognitive responses including:
a. Disorientation to time, place, and person
b. Recent and/or remote memory loss
c. Impaired intellectual functioning; difficulties in problem solving, planning, organizing, abstracting
d. Deficits in judgment (eg, inappropriate social behavior, inability to make decisions)

5. Assess own reaction and response in dealing with a client with a cognitive impairment.

6. Assess available family or social support group:
a. Evidence of family coping abilities
b. Evidence of specific problems faced by individual family members
c. Use of community resources by family members

B. Analysis and nursing diagnoses

1. **Differentiate priorities of physical, behavioral, cognitive, and affective symptoms.**
2. Evaluate client's use of coping abilities, level of anxiety, potential for acting-out behaviors.
3. **Analyze degree of impairment related to specific cognitive disorder.**
4. Analyze resources available for affected client as well as for family members.
5. Establish nursing diagnoses for the client with a cognitive impairment disorder, including but not limited to the following:
   a. Altered Thought Processes
   b. Sensory/Perceptual Alterations
   c. Self Care Deficit: Toileting, Bathing, Grooming, Dressing, Feeding
   d. Impaired Verbal Communication
   e. Altered Nutrition: Less than body requirements
   f. Bowel Incontinence
   g. Altered Urinary Elimination
   h. Social Isolation
   i. Sleep Pattern Disturbance
   j. Risk for Violence: Self-directed or directed at others
6. Establish nursing diagnoses when working with the family of a client with a cognitive impairment disorder:
   a. Altered Family Processes
   b. Caregiver Role Strain
   c. Ineffective Family Coping: Compromised

C. Planning outcomes

1. Work with the client and family in setting realistic goals.
2. Establish desired outcome criteria for client with a cognitive impairment disorder.
   a. Client will remain safe and free from injury.
   b. Client will demonstrate decreased anxiety levels.
   c. With assistance, the client will remain oriented at level of ability.
   d. Client will maintain existing ability to perform ADLs.
   e. Client will not harm self or others.
   f. Client will follow established ADL schedule.
   g. Family members will identify and use available support services.

D. Nursing implementations

1. **Provide emergency measures as necessary (eg, for aspiration, asphyxia, injury from confused behavior or seizures); anticipate hazards and prevent injury.**

2. Respond to underlying organic disease processes (eg, provide hydration, antibiotics, vitamins, oxygenation as indicated).
3. Maintain fluid and electrolyte balance.
4. Maintain nutritional balance.
5. Promote structured elimination patterns; use disposable pants as needed to preserve client's dignity.
6. **Promote rest by active daily schedule, avoiding hypnotics.**
7. Minimize risk of cardiovascular problems (utilize medication, diet, exercise, rest, stress management measures).
8. Monitor drugs and drug interactions; titrate medications carefully.
9. **Support the client in doing as much as possible without frustration, either independently or with assistance. Be creative in assisting with ADLs.**
10. Promote involvement or inclusion in ADLs; provide positive reinforcement.
11. **Decrease environmental stimuli and call the client by name to focus attention; use short, clear messages.**
12. Encourage the family to include the client in family functions; support the client and family as they adjust to altered roles and inappropriate social behavior; refer to appropriate community resources (eg, support groups, day care, respite care).
13. Provide orienting information concerning time, place, person; use environmental supports such as clocks, calendars, and consistent routine, and sensory aids such as glasses or hearing aids, as needed.
14. Do not reinforce or agree with hallucinations and delusions; instead, focus on feelings being indirectly expressed.
15. **Do not approach the client rapidly or use touch if the client is irritable, agitated, or suspicious; use restraints as a last resort in accordance with legal guidelines.**
16. Support the client's memory with reminders, structured environment, routines, orientation boards.
17. Support the client in intellectual functions by avoiding stressful demands, supporting or limiting decision making, providing stimulation.
18. Assist in avoiding or limiting socially embarrassing situations; support the family in adjusting and accepting socially inappropriate incidents.
19. **Reduce excessive stimuli, reduce pace, avoid procedures if client is agitated. Make directions and communications simple.**
20. Assist client and family to express feelings of loss, grief, or frustration.

21. Use nonjudgmental, empathic approach with client and family.
22. **Deal with client agitation and disorientation by using an approach known as validation therapy, in which the nurse enters the client's reality to provide comfort.**

E. Evaluation

1. Client demonstrates decreased anxiety and increased feelings of security in structured environment.
2. Client maintains maximum degree of orientation within level of ability.
3. Client maintains abilities to perform ADLs within structured environment.
4. Client refrains from acting-out behavior.
5. Family members use all available support services and community resources.

Bibliography

American Psychiatric Association (1994). *Diagnostic and statistical manual of mental disorders (DSM-IV)* (4th ed.). Washington, DC: American Psychiatric Association.

Gary, F., & Kavanagh, C. (1991). *Psychiatric mental health nursing.* Philadelphia: J. B. Lippincott.

Rawlins, R., & Heacock, P. (1993). *Clinical manual of psychiatric nursing* (2nd ed.). St. Louis: Mosby-Year Book.

Shives, L. (1994). *Basic concepts of psychiatric-mental health nursing* (3rd ed.). Philadelphia: J. B. Lippincott.

Stolley, J. M. (1994). When your patient has Alzheimer's disease. *American Journal of Nursing, 94*(8), 34–39.

Townsend, M. C. (1993). *Psychiatric mental health nursing: Concepts of care.* Philadelphia: F. A. Davis.

Varcarolis, E. (1994). *Foundations of psychiatric mental health nursing* (2nd ed.). Philadelphia: W. B. Saunders.

Wilson, H., & Kneisl, C. (1992). *Psychiatric nursing* (4th ed.). Menlo Park, CA: Addison-Wesley.

STUDY QUESTIONS

1. The nurse performing a basic level of consciousness assessment would establish which of the following?
   a. cranial nerve functioning
   b. cerebellar functioning
   c. anxiety and stress levels
   d. orientation to time, place, and person
2. Dementia is *best* defined as which of the following?
   a. memory loss occurring as natural consequence of aging
   b. difficulty coping with physical changes in aging
   c. onset of cognitive impairment that occurs rapidly
   d. loss of intellectual abilities, impairing ability to perform ADLs
3. Nursing interventions that are of primary importance in working with clients experiencing dementia include
   a. speaking to the client with short words and simple sentences
   b. challenging the client with stimulating activities
   c. promoting increased socialization with a variety of people
   d. reinforcing client's altered thought patterns
4. A 75-year-old client has dementia, Alzheimer's type. This client confabulates. The nurse understands that the client
   a. denies confusion by being jovial
   b. pretends to be someone else
   c. rationalizes various behaviors
   d. fills in memory gaps with fantasy
5. In caring for a client in the early phase of Alzheimer's disease, the nurse would anticipate the client retaining which of the following abilities?
   a. remembering the daily schedule
   b. recalling events of the past
   c. coping with anxiety
   d. solving problems of daily living
6. At age 82 a client is admitted to the medical-surgical unit for diagnostic confirmation and management of probable delirium. Which of the following statements by the client's daughter best supports the diagnosis?
   a. "Maybe it's just caused by aging. This usually happens by age 82."
   b. "The changes in behavior seemed to come on so quickly! I wasn't sure what was happening."
   c. "Dad just didn't seem to know what he was doing. He would forget what he had for breakfast."
   d. "Dad has always been so independent. He's lived alone since Mom died 12 years ago."
7. An elderly client with Alzheimer's disease becomes agitated and combative when the nurse approaches to help with morning care. The most appropriate nursing intervention would be
   a. Firmly tell the client that it's time to get dressed and ready for the day.
   b. Obtain assistance to restrain client for safety.
   c. Remain calm and talk quietly to client.
   d. Call the physician and request order for sedation.
8. The most appropriate goal of nursing interventions for a client with delirium would be
   a. Assist the client with activities of daily living.
   b. Support existing sensory reception until cognitive status returns to previous level.
   c. Maintain vigorous reality orientation since restoration of cognitive level is likely to be limited.
   d. Initiate activities that are simple to complete.
9. Which of the following should the nurse avoid in constructing a plan of care for a client with a cognitive impairment disorder?
   a. daily structured schedule

b. increased environmental stimuli
c. increased rest periods
d. use of positive reinforcement for performing ADLs

10. In clients with a cognitive impairment disorder, the phenomenon of increased confusion in the early evening hours is called
a. aphasia
b. agnosia
c. sundowning
d. confabulation

11. The son of an 80-year-old client accompanies the client to the clinic. The son tells the nurse that the client's constant confusion, incontinence, and tendency to wander are intolerable. The client has been diagnosed as having a chronic cognitive impairment disorder. The nursing diagnoses most appropriate for the client's son would be
a. Risk for Violence
b. Sleep Pattern Disturbance
c. Caregiver Role Strain
d. Social Isolation

12. Which of the following outcome criteria would be appropriate for the client with dementia?
a. Client will return to adequate level of self-functioning.
b. Client will learn new coping mechanisms to handle anxiety.
c. Client will seek out resources in the community for support.
d. Client will follow established schedule for ADLs.

ANSWER KEY

1. ***Correct response: d***
The initial and most basic assessment for altered level of consciousness is orientation to time, place, and person.
a, b, and c. All of these aspects may affect client's level of consciousness; however, the required data are those described in *d.*
Application/Physiologic/Assessment

2. ***Correct response: d***
Self-care ability is an important measure of the progression of dementia, as well as the loss of intellectual ability.
a. Loss of memory leading to dementia is not necessarily a natural consequence of age, but rather reflects underlying physical, metabolic, and pathologic processes.
b. This statement is incorrect.
c. Cognitive impairment in dementia occurs slowly, with insidious onset.
Comprehension/Psychosocial/Analysis (Dx)

3. ***Correct response: a***
Short sentences and simple words minimize client confusion and enhance communication.
b and c. These interventions would increase the confusion common to clients with dementia and would be inappropriate.
d. Reality orientation would be the first appropriate intervention when a client has altered thought patterns. If this increases client's level of agitation, then the technique of validation therapy may be used.
Application/Safe care/Implementation

4. ***Correct response: d***
Confabulation is the communication device used to compensate for memory gaps in dementia.
a, b, and c. These are not correct explanations of confabulation.
Knowledge/Psychosocial/Assessment

5. ***Correct response: b***
Recent memory loss is the characteristic sign of cognitive difficulty in early Alzheimer's disease. Recalling events of the past is usually retained until the later phases of this disorder.
a, c, and d. These would all be areas that would pose difficulty in the early phase of Alzheimer's disease.
Comprehension/Psychosocial/Analysis (Dx)

6. ***Correct response: b***
Delirium is an acute process characterized by abrupt, spontaneous cognitive dysfunction.
a. Cognitive impairment disorders (dementias or delirium) are not normal consequences of aging.
c. This would be characteristic behavior in dementia.
d. Although this detail provides background data about the client, it is unrelated to the current problem of delirium.
Application/Psychosocial/Assessment

7. ***Correct response: c***
It is important to maintain a calm approach when intervening with an agitated client.
a. This may increase client agitation, especially if the nurse touches the client.
b. Restraints are a last resort to ensure client safety and are not appropriate in this situation.
d. Sedation should be avoided if possible, because it will interfere with CNS functioning and may contribute to client confusion.
Application/Safe care/Implementation

8. ***Correct response: b***
Clients who have delirium are expected to return to a previous level of functioning after the underlying problem is identified and treated.

a and d. These would be appropriate interventions but not *the most appropriate* goal of intervention.

c. This is inappropriate. By definition, the client with delirium has reality impairment that is not corrected by vigorous reality orientation. Cognitive return is likely to be complete after successfully treating the underlying cause.

Application/Psychosocial/Planning

9. *Correct response: b*

This action would be inappropriate because a client with a cognitive impairment disorder requires a nonstimulating, predictable environment to maintain existing abilities.

a, c, and d. These are all appropriate interventions.

Application/Safe care/Planning

10. *Correct response: c*

Sundowning is a common phenomenon that occurs after daylight hours in a client with a cognitive impairment disorder.

a, c, and d. These are incorrect responses, although all may be seen in the client with these disorders.

Knowledge/Psychosocial/Assessment

11. *Correct response: c*

The son is describing a common problem for the primary caregiver of a client with a cognitive impairment disorder.

a, b, and d. Although these nursing diagnoses are possibilities, the scenario does not provide enough information to validate any of these.

Comprehension/Psychosocial/Analysis (Dx)

12. *Correct response: d*

Following established activity schedules is a realistic expectation for clients with dementia.

a, b, and c. All of these outcome statements require a higher level of cognitive ability than can be realistically expected for clients with dementia.

Comprehension/Psychosocial/Evaluation

12 Treatment Modalities: Crisis Intervention

I. Overview

A. Definitions

1. **Crisis: an overwhelming emotional reaction to a threatening situation in which usual problem-solving skills and coping mechanisms are not adequate to maintain equilibrium**
2. **Crisis situations are life transitions (life events) or stressful circumstances (internal or external stressors).**

B. Types of crises

1. Developmental-maturational crises include:
   a. Birth of a child
   b. Beginning school
   c. Puberty
   d. Old age
2. Developmental-transitional crises include:
   a. Birth of siblings
   b. Marriage

c. Death of significant other
d. Divorce
3. Situational crises include:
a. Loss of job; failure in school
b. Accidents
c. Illness
4. Adventitious (disaster) crises include:
a. Natural disasters (floods, earthquakes)
b. National disasters (wars, riots)
c. Crimes of violence (murder, rape)

C. Sequence of crisis development

1. Precrisis period
a. Emotional equilibrium
b. Effective coping mechanisms

2. Crisis period
a. Upset in steady state; experience of particular stressor
b. Increased anxiety; increased use of usual coping mechanisms
c. Usual coping mechanisms not successful

- **Relief behaviors such as withdrawal or flight**
- **Individual may become disorganized**

3. Postcrisis period
a. Return to (or increase or decrease in) usual level of functioning
b. Resolution of crisis

D. Loss and grief

1. Crisis intervention theory emerged from research on the grieving process.
2. Death is a universal experience anticipated with anxiety.
3. Grieving is an experience related to loss of a loved one or a valued object, ideal, position, or status.
4. Phases of grieving
a. First phase: shock and disbelief
b. Second phase: developing awareness of loss and emotional pain
c. Third phase: resolution, reorganization (takes up to 2 years)
5. Indicators of pathologic mourning include:
a. Inability to experience or express painful feelings about loss
b. Failure to acknowledge and accept loss
c. Anniversary reactions: becoming depressed on anniversary dates of loss
d. Prolonged and serious alterations in social adjustment

e. Development of agitated depression or suicidal thoughts or behavior

E. Factors affecting equilibrium

1. **Perception of the event involves:**
   a. **How crisis event is appraised**
   b. **Coping behaviors**
2. **Situational supports include:**
   a. **Persons on whom the person in crisis can depend**
   b. **Other resources (eg, money, housing, social services)**
3. **Coping skills depend on:**
   a. **Use of defense mechanisms (see Chap. 2 and Table 2-1)**
   b. **Handling of previous crises**
   c. **Problem-solving ability**
   d. **Current number of stressors in life**

F. Characteristics of crisis situations

1. **Crisis situations may produce such physiologic and psychologic effects as:**
   a. Physiologic symptoms of anxiety: diarrhea, dizziness, shortness of breath, palpitations
   b. Sleep disturbances
   c. Restlessness, lack of concentration
   d. Irritability, outbursts of anger
   e. Agitation, crying
   f. Inability to make decisions
   g. Paranoid thoughts, feelings of isolation
   h. Suicidal or homicidal ideation
2. Crisis situations have the following in common:
   a. Crisis occurs in all individuals at one time or another.
   b. Crisis is not necessarily pathologic.
   c. Individual's perception of problem determines crisis.
   d. Crisis is an acute situation which will be resolved one way or another within a brief period.
   e. Crisis situation contains possibility for growth or for deterioration.

3. **Because a client in crisis feels overwhelmed and unable to cope, effective crisis intervention must build on the client's existing strengths and resources.**

II. Principles of crisis intervention

A. Goal: to return to precrisis level of functioning

B. Specific guidelines

1. Assess strengths and weaknesses of family and/or support system as well as of client experiencing acute disorganization.

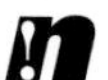

   a. **Define extent of crisis.**

b. **Determine cognitive, affective, behavioral manifestations.**

2. Utilize Maslow's hierarchy of needs to determine priorities for intervention, for example:
   a. Physical resources necessary for survival, such as food and shelter
   b. Psychologic resources necessary for self-esteem, such as love and security
   c. Social resources that encourage self-actualization necessary for fulfillment
3. **Collaborate with client and/or crisis worker in developing plan of action.**
   a. Crisis worker may take active, directive role, if necessary.
   b. Suggestions may be made, but avoid coercive direction.
   c. Solutions must be acceptable to client as well as to client's family.
4. Offer hope. Because every crisis eventually comes to a conclusion, this assurance is realistic.
5. Make use of community resources during and after crisis resolution for support.

III. Nursing process in crisis intervention

A. Assessment

1. **Identify precipitating event and explore the following:**
   a. Circumstances that brought on crisis
   b. Event's chronology
   c. Factors affecting client's ability to solve crisis
2. **Explore client's perception of crisis, including the following:**
   a. Themes and memories that reveal meaning of crisis to client
   b. Underlying needs threatened by crisis
   c. Degree of life disruption caused by crisis
3. **Assess support systems, including the following:**
   a. Living situation (ie, client lives alone or with family or friends)
   b. Persons available to help the client
   c. Effect of crisis on family and support persons
   d. Other resources available (eg, financial, religious, social, community)
4. **Assess client's coping skills, including the following:**
   a. How client has handled previous crises
   b. Personal strengths and weakness
   c. Adaptive coping skills used
   d. Defense mechanisms used

B. Analysis and nursing diagnoses

1. Nurse should recognize potential crises in various nursing practice areas, including:
    a. Maternal-child: birth of premature infant, stillborn infant, birth anomalies, miscarriage or abortion
    b. Pediatrics: onset of a serious illness, chronic or debilitating illnesses, severe accidents, a dying child
    c. Medical-surgical: learning about a serious diagnosis, debilitating illness, hospitalization for acute problem, loss of body part or functions, death and dying
    d. Gerontology: cumulative losses, debilitating illness, dependency, nursing home placement
    e. Emergency: physical trauma, acute illness, rape, death
    f. Psychiatry: being hospitalized with a psychiatric disorder, life stressors for the chronically mentally ill, suicide
2. Analyze impact of crisis situation on client and family.
3. **Analyze adequacy of client's coping skills and potential personal, social, and environmental supports.**
4. Determine individualized nursing diagnoses for client and family, including but not limited to:
    a. Ineffective Individual Coping
    b. Altered Thought Processes
    c. Fear
    d. Anxiety
    e. Dysfunctional Grieving
    f. Altered Role Performance
    g. Altered Family Processes
    h. Rape-Trauma Syndrome
    i. Post-Trauma Response
    j. Powerlessness

C. Planning outcomes

1. Assist the client in setting realistic, short-term goals.
2. Establish desired outcome criteria.
    a. Client will verbalize meaning of crisis situation.
    b. Client will discuss possible options for resolving crisis.
    c. Client will choose strategy for coping with current crisis.
    d. Client will implement measures to bring about crisis resolution.

D. Nursing implementations

1. Use effective problem-solving processes with the client, including:
    a. Assisting him or her to gain understanding of the crisis; dividing crisis down into component problems
    b. Helping correct misperceptions about the crisis

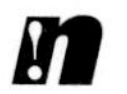

    c. **Promoting expressions of feelings**

d. **Supporting adaptive coping mechanisms through reinforcement**
e. **Employing active listening and reflection as tools to support client in identifying options for resolution.**

2. Intervene to deter any plans for suicide or homicide by:
   a. **Taking warning signs seriously**
   b. Determining the concreteness of the plan (a concrete plan increases the likelihood of an attempt)
   c. Removing dangerous and potentially lethal materials or objects as possible
   d. **Placing client in safe, protective environment and monitoring closely and consistently or mobilizing support**
   e. Communicating your presence and desire to protect client from harming self or others
   f. Encouraging client to talk about stressors: feelings of pain, anger, and anguish; and suicide or homicide plans
   g. Listening empathically
   h. Reinforcing client's desire to resolve problems and to live
   i. Referring client for follow-up treatment
3. Raise the client's self-esteem by:
   a. Acknowledging his or her strengths
   b. Empathizing with client and his or her situation
   c. Mobilizing client to constructive actions
   d. Offering support in an active way; staying with client, expressing caring and concern
4. **Mobilize the client's support systems by:**
   a. **Helping him or her contact family or friends who will be supportive**
   b. Referring him or her to appropriate social or community services
5. Provide anticipatory guidance and follow-up, including:
   a. Reviewing various consequences for each possible solution
   b. Providing opportunity to rehearse what might be done now and in future crises
   c. Providing support for client anticipating potentially stressful situation (eg, surgery, childbirth)
   d. Providing support for client who has experienced stressful event (eg, rape, child abuse, natural disaster)
   e. Teaching client relaxation techniques, prescribed treatment modalities, stress management strategies

D. Evaluation

1. Client identifies relationship between stressors and psychologic/physiologic symptoms experienced in crisis.
2. Client evaluates possible solutions to crisis.

3. Client selects option for solution to crisis.
4. Client exhibits return to precrisis state or improved situation or behavior.

Bibliography

American Psychiatric Association (1994). *Diagnostic and statistical manual of mental disorders (DSM-IV)* (4th ed.). Washington, DC: American Psychiatric Association.

Gary, F., & Kavanagh, C. (1991). *Psychiatric mental health nursing.* Philadelphia: J. B. Lippincott.

Rawlins, R., & Heacock, P. (1993). *Clinical manual of psychiatric nursing* (2nd ed.). St. Louis: Mosby-Year Book.

Shives, L. (1994). *Basic concepts of psychiatric-mental health nursing* (3rd ed.). Philadelphia: J. B. Lippincott.

Stolley, J. M. (1994). When your patient has Alzheimer's disease. *American Journal of Nursing, 94*(8), 34–39.

Townsend, M. C. (1993). *Psychiatric mental health nursing: Concepts of care.* Philadelphia: F. A. Davis.

Varcarolis, E. (1994). *Foundations of psychiatric mental health nursing* (2nd ed.). Philadelphia: W. B. Saunders.

Wilson, H., & Kneisl, C. (1992). *Psychiatric nursing* (4th ed.). Menlo Park, CA: Addison-Wesley.

STUDY QUESTIONS

1. After a happy childhood, a 13-year-old girl is having a difficult adolescence. She grew 5 inches taller in the last year and developed large breasts. One day after some boys in her class teased and intimidated her, she went to the school nurse in tears. She is so affected by the teasing and intimidation that she starts to withdraw and perform less effectively in her school work. Based on this information, the school nurse would conclude that this client is experiencing what type of crisis?
   - **a.** developmental-maturational
   - **b.** developmental-transitional
   - **c.** situation-victim
   - **d.** combination of situational and developmental
2. What is the first step the school nurse should take in the situation described in question 1?
   - **a.** Call the client's family and report the problem.
   - **b.** Encourage the client to tell in detail what happened.
   - **c.** Ask the client who her best friends are.
   - **d.** Take the client's temperature, pulse, and blood pressure.
3. As the client described in question 1 talks about the events that precipitated her crisis, the nurse learns that she is a lonely girl with few friends. Which of the following actions would be most appropriate for the nurse to take at this time?
   - **a.** Suggest that the client transfer to another nearby school.
   - **b.** Suggest that the client ask the boys in her class to stop teasing her.
   - **c.** Suggest that the client volunteer to help others.
   - **d.** Suggest that the client visit the nurse on a regular basis.
4. Which of the following questions would best help the nurse to clarify the client's perception of the crisis event described in question 1?
   - **a.** "Do you know the boys who teased you?"
   - **b.** "Have you noticed that other girls get teased also?"
   - **c.** "Can you tell me what happened first?"
   - **d.** "Do you think the boys meant to hurt your feelings?"
5. As the client in crisis comes to trust the nurse, which of the following nursing actions most likely would enhance the client's ability to deal with the situation described in question 1?
   - **a.** Explore ways to deal with teasing of classmates.
   - **b.** Talk to the school principal about the teasing.
   - **c.** Discuss aspects of adolescent development.
   - **d.** Express empathy for the trauma the client has experienced.
6. A 17-year-old girl was raped by a man in her neighborhood. She is in the emergency department for treatment and requires laboratory tests. After the procedures are completed, a psychiatric clinical nurse specialist takes the client into the conference room for rape counseling. Implementing a system of routine counseling for a rape victim represents
   - **a.** assessment
   - **b.** anticipatory crisis intervention
   - **c.** empathic concern
   - **d.** unwarranted intrusion
7. During the assessment process, which of the following actions would be appropriate for the situation described in question 6?
   - **a.** Have the client recount the events of the rape.
   - **b.** Encourage the client to talk about her early childhood.
   - **c.** Allow the client to call her boyfriend.
   - **d.** Ask the client to describe the rapist.
8. The client expresses her belief that the

rape was her fault because she walked down the alley on her way to school. Which of the following actions should the nurse take to address this perception?

a. Ask the client what other behaviors may have contributed to the rape.
b. Suggest that the client walk to school with a group of classmates.
c. Agree that taking the alley to school is risky behavior.
d. Emphasize that the rapist, not the client, is responsible for the rape.

9. The client who has been raped wants to go home from the emergency department by herself. What would be the best way for the nurse to respond to the client's wish?

a. Ask the client how she will get home.
b. Offer to call a family member for the client before she leaves.
c. Drive the client home using the nurse's car.
d. Let the client do as she wishes.

10. A man with a chronic mental illness lives in a halfway house where meals and medications are provided. Each day he takes the bus 5 miles to his job as an assistant janitor for a large apartment building. One day, he loses his wallet on the bus. He becomes extremely upset, gets off the bus, and starts to walk back to the halfway house. It starts to snow heavily, and he becomes confused about directions and gets lost. He finally wanders into a store and asks the owner to call the police. Based on this information, the nurse could make which of the following analyses about this client?

a. He has a deficit in coping skills that predisposes him to crises.
b. He should not be allowed to travel on his own via public transportation.
c. He is not in crisis because he is chronically mentally ill.
d. He is a victim of circumstances.

11. In the scenario in question 10, which of the client's actions indicates a coping strength?

a. deciding to walk home
b. not telling anyone about the lost wallet
c. becoming extremely upset about the lost wallet
d. calling the police

ANSWER KEY

1. *Correct response: d*
   Adolescence presents a time of crisis for this client; having the boys in her class tease her poses a situational-victim type of crisis.
   a and c. Although these are also correct, they are incomplete answers since the external teasing adds the dimension of a situational crisis for this girl.
   b. Transitional crises refer to major transitions such as marriage and the birth of a child.

Comprehension/Psychosocial/Assessment

2. *Correct response: b*
   The first step in crisis intervention is to obtain the client's perception of the crisis event.
   a and c. These refer to situational supports, which are mobilized later in the intervention process, after consultation with the client.
   d. There are no physiologic indicators pointing to the need for this action.

Application/Psychosocial/Assessment

3. *Correct response: d*
   By becoming directly available to the client, the nurse raises the client's self-esteem. The nurse becomes involved in an active way, which is appropriate in crisis intervention.
   a, b, and c. These responses avoid direct involvement with the client in crisis and also they are premature solutions selected by the nurse without discussing with client the acceptability of these options.

Analysis/Psychosocial/Implementation

4. *Correct response: c*
   Placing the events in chronological sequence helps to clarify what happened.
   a, c, and d. These are less useful questions and also are closed-ended. It would be better to help the client get started by using open-ended questions.

Application/Psychosocial/Assessment

5. *Correct response: a*
   Once trust has developed, the nurse can help the client think of alternative coping skills to deal with the problems she encounters.
   b. Through this action, the nurse would be attempting to solve the problem for the client rather than helping her learn new coping skills.
   c. This action addresses understanding rather than problem solving.
   d. Although empathy is very important, it is used for building trust and rapport and does not address problem solving.

Analysis/Psychosocial/Implementation

6. *Correct response: b*
   Anticipatory guidance is part of the crisis intervention model. Certain stressful events, such as rape, make a person more vulnerable to crisis. Counseling at the time of the stressful event can strengthen the client's coping skills and prevent a full-blown crisis from occurring.
   a, c, and d. These responses do not describe the intervention.

Comprehension/Health promotion/ Implementation

7. *Correct response: a*
   Crisis intervention begins with having the client talk about the precipitating event in detail. In this way, the nurse can assess how the client perceives the event.
   b. Early childhood exploration is not a usual component of crisis intervention.
   c and d. These aspects might be addressed later on in the counseling session.

Application/Psychosocial/Assessment

8. ***Correct response: d***

Through exploring the precipitating events, the nurse observes for and corrects apparent misperceptions about the event. In this case, the client sees the rape as her fault. The nurse helps the client arrive at a more realistic perception.

a, b, and c. These actions lay the responsibility for the rape on the client.

Application/Psychosocial/Implementation

9. ***Correct response: b***

Crisis intervention should mobilize the client's support system. By offering to call the family, the nurse remains involved in an active way.

a and d. The client needs the support of family or friends after experiencing such a traumatic event.

c. This service would be better provided by a family member, a volunteer, or even the police.

Application/Safe care/Implementation

10. ***Correct response: a***

Chronically mentally ill clients such as this client are vulnerable to crises because their coping skills are less adaptive. When the client lost his wallet, he panicked and got off the bus.

b. The client has been able to handle the bus trip on a regular basis; continued independence should be encouraged.

c. Just the opposite is true; chronically mentally ill clients are very vulnerable to crises.

d. The client could have handled things differently.

Analysis/Psychosocial/Analysis (Dx)

11. ***Correct response: d***

By calling the police, the client demonstrated sufficient understanding of his situation to know that he needed help. He contacted an appropriate social institution to mobilize support on his behalf.

a, b, and c. These are all indicators of poor problem-solving skills.

Application/Psychosocial/Assessment

13 Treatment Modalities: Group Therapy

I. Overview

A. Definitions

1. **Group: collection of individuals whose association is based on shared common interests, values, norms, or purpose**
   a. Average group size is 6 to 12 members (small groups).
   b. Members have something in common.

2. **Group dynamics: interactions and relationships existing within the group**
3. Group therapy: a therapy group, founded in a specific theoretical framework, and led by a person with an advanced degree in psychology, social work, nursing, or medicine

B. Stages of group development

1. Most groups proceed through fairly well-anticipated phases:
   a. Orientation phase (beginning stage)
   b. Working phase (middle stage)
   c. Termination phase (ending stage)
2. Expected client behaviors in the orientation phase include:
   a. High anxiety

b. Hesitancy, uncertainty
c. Unclear contract expectations
d. Superficial sharing; focus on self
e. Testing of therapist and other group members

3. Expected client behaviors in the working phase include:
a. Increased self-disclosure
b. Developing sense of group feeling, evolving concern for other members
c. Working on problem or concerns
d. Possible in-depth exploration of a topic or problem

4. Expected client behaviors during the termination phase include:
a. Expression of varying feelings about termination (eg, anger, sadness, joy, rejection)
b. Possible increased testing of therapist
c. Possible sense of loneliness or fear

C. Group dynamics

1. Group *content* refers to verbal communication among members.

2. Group *process* refers to what occurs within the group, including:
a. **Nonverbal communication among members**
b. **Relationships or interchanges among members**
c. **Body language, gestures**
d. **Seating arrangements**
e. **Speaking patterns or tones**
f. **Group themes: may be expressed overtly or covertly**

3. Group *cohesiveness* refers to the sense of belonging, of unity, of "groupness"; it involves:
a. Loyalty and allegiance to the group
b. High degree of participation and sharing among members
c. Nonjudgmental attitudes among members
d. Maintenance of group norms
e. High member attendance and low dropout rate
f. High tolerance for conflict or disagreement
g. Effective problem-solving mechanisms
h. Sense of group togetherness

4. Group *norms* refer to implicit or explicit rules defining members' behavior; types include:
a. Productive norms, which enhance cohesiveness (eg, all members' opinions respected, only one person speaks at a time)
b. Nonproductive norms, which inhibit cohesiveness (eg, no disagreements allowed, absenteeism or tardiness accepted)

5. Group *roles* refer to the parts various members play within one group. Each member may adopt more than one role, and may change roles according to the situation.
a. Initiator: suggests innovative ideas, starts the interactions

b. Coordinator: organizes and integrates
c. Evaluator: appraises group performance
d. Information-seeker: elicits facts
e. Gatekeeper: screens input and maintains open communication
f. Encourager: praises and accepts
g. Harmonizer: maintains peace through compromise, alternatives
h. Commentator: processes the group interaction
i. Blocker: inhibits the group's advancement
j. Recognition-seeker: self-aggrandizes
k. Monopolizer: controls by endless talking
l. Self-confessor: discloses personal information inappropriately

6. Leadership refers to the therapist's and members' responsibilities for guiding the group (Table 13-1). Types of small group leadership include:
   a. Authoritarian
   b. Democratic
   c. Laissez-faire
7. **Generally, a group functions best when leadership is shared among members, particularly during the middle stage (working phase).**
8. **Power refers to the ability to influence others. A successful group power structure helps all members meet their needs. Some groups may experience ongoing realignment or struggles for power.**

D. Advantages and disadvantages of group therapy

1. Advantages include:
   a. Helps group members learn that their problems are not unique
   b. Promotes interpersonal relationships through actual participation
   c. Facilitates group members' participation in problem solving of personal and others' problems
   d. Provides multiple sources of feedback and reality testing
   e. Instills hope that participant's own problems can also be resolved
   f. Imparts knowledge through formal instruction as well as sharing of advice and suggestions among group members
2. Disadvantages include:
   a. Reduces individual attention from the leader
   b. Necessitates reduced intensity of focus on, or support for, an individual's problems or pain
   c. May create a lack of confidence in confidentiality

TABLE 13-1.
Common Group Styles

STYLE	CHARACTERISTICS
Authoritarian	The leader —Exerts total control —Makes the decisions, establishes policies, and decides goals and purposes —Discourages communication and sharing among members; all communication is directed to the leader —Is task-oriented Group members —May be frustrated and angry —Act out by scapegoating or exhibiting passive–aggressive behavior The group atmosphere generally is tense. This style may be effective for large groups and when quick decisions are needed.
Democratic	The leader —Encourages member involvement and collaboration —Promotes group cohesiveness and the development of productive norms —Facilitates individual input and growth —Promotes open communication Group members generally like the group. The atmosphere tends to be more comfortable
Laissez-faire	The leader —Functions as a consultant/resource person —Provides minimal direction —Promotes minimal interpersonal interactions among members Group members —May feel lost without directions —May be disorganized —May be apathetic —Tend to be self-focused Productivity is reduced. The atmosphere is haphazard. This style may be effective for groups of highly self-directed persons.

E. Characteristics of groups

1. In cohesive groups:
   a. Group norms are maintained (eg, attendance is high, and members arrive on time).
   b. Trust has been established.
   c. Participation is high and on a deep-feeling level.
   d. Commitment or loyalty to the group increases over time; members stay in group.
   e. Mutual support is offered.
   f. Member-to-member influence is present.
   g. Productivity ("work") is evident.
   h. Group concerns ("we") become more pronounced than individual concerns.

   i. Leadership usually is democratic and shared to some extent among members.
2. In noncohesive groups:
   a. Group norms are lacking or violated (eg, absenteeism, tardiness).
   b. There is lack of trust, uncertainty, or suspicion among members.
   c. Participation is minimal and sporadic.
   d. There is poor loyalty to the group, individual competition among members, and a high dropout rate.
   e. There is a lack of interpersonal concern among members.
   f. There is member-to-member criticism, competition.
   g. Productivity and work achievement are lacking.
   h. There are pronounced individual concerns ("I") as compared to those of the group.
   i. There is usually an autocratic or laissez-faire leadership style; therapist-dominated.

F. Role of the nurse in group therapy

1. **Specific role of nurse in group therapy is a function of educational level and experience.**
2. American Nurses Association (ANA) sets standard for specific nursing role related to group work.
   a. Basic level: Psychiatric-Mental Health Registered Nurse—may be involved in working with therapeutic groups "on a problem representing an immediate difficulty related to health or well being" (ANA, 1994, p. 15).
   b. Advanced level: Psychiatric-Mental Health Clinical Specialist—"in the role of group therapist, the certified psychiatric-mental health nursing specialist utilizes knowledge of behavior at the intrapersonal, interpersonal, and group levels" (ANA, 1994, p. 18).

II. Types of groups

A. Therapy and support groups

1. Group psychotherapy may focus on:
   a. Personality reconstruction
   b. Insight, self-awareness
   c. Remotivation
   d. Problem solving
   e. Reeducation
   f. Support
2. Therapeutic (primary prevention, crisis intervention) groups may provide:
   a. Prevention
   b. Education
   c. Support

3. Self-help groups (led by group members) may be aimed at providing:
    a. Behavioral improvement
    b. Stress reduction
    c. Self-esteem, maintained social integration

B. Other types of groups

1. Task-oriented groups (eg, committees) focus on:
    a. Performance of specific job or assignment
    b. Achievement of mission or goals for a larger group
2. Teaching-learning groups focus on:
    a. Skill acquisition
    b. Information sharing
3. Social groups convene for:
    a. Recreation, relaxation
    b. Fun, pleasure
    c. Companionship
    d. Satisfaction, acquisition of social skills

III. Nursing process in group therapy

A. Assessment

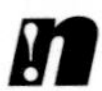

1. **Evaluate individual client's behavior in the group context.**
2. Assess verbal content in the group setting.
3. Assess group processes, noting:
    a. Where members sit
    b. Who talks with whom and about what
    c. Tones of voice used by members
    d. Response to group norms
    e. Congruence of verbal content and process
    f. Roles assumed by members
    g. Evolution of group cohesiveness

B. Analysis and nursing diagnoses

1. Recognize effects of behavior of group and self on group members.
2. Analyze group dynamics.
3. Determine individualized nursing diagnoses for client within group, including but not limited to:
    a. Ineffective Individual Coping
    b. Impaired Social Interaction
    c. Anxiety
    d. Impaired Adjustment
    e. Dysfunctional Grieving

C. Planning outcomes

1. Work with group members in setting realistic goals.
2. Establish desired outcome criteria for group.
    a. Individual members will participate in group activities.

b. Group members will demonstrate group feeling and concern for individual members.
c. Group members will focus on identified purpose related to specific type and task of group.
d. Individual members will demonstrate improved problem-solving skills in coping with life issues.

D. Nursing implementations

1. During the orientation phase:
   a. Be directive and active.
   b. Establish contract for meetings and relationships.
   c. Promote productive norms and group cohesiveness.
   d. Encourage open communication and exploration of feelings and ideas.

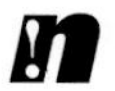

   e. **Listen, observe, and give therapeutic feedback.**
   f. Comment on behavior that enhances or hinders constructive group process.
   g. Assist individual members and the group to evaluate behaviors.
2. During the working phase:
   a. Assume the roles of consultant and facilitator.
   b. Recognize conflicts; label them and explore meanings.

   c. **Assist the group to deal constructively with conflicts and problems.**
   d. Assist the group to examine the impact of subgroups, scapegoating, absenteeism, and passive-aggressive behavior, as applicable.
3. During the termination phase:
   a. Assume a more direct, supportive role.
   b. **Assist members to verbalize and explore feelings and thoughts about termination.**
   c. Encourage evaluation of group and individual members' progress.
   d. Provide adequate time for members to deal with termination.
   e. Refer those whose needs were unmet by the group for further evaluation and care, as appropriate.

E. Evaluation

1. Group
   a. The group exhibits cohesiveness; members demonstrate shared allegiance and responsibility to the group.
   b. Norms are productive and enhance members' emotional development.
   c. Group maintenance and group task roles are predominant.

   d. Communication occurs among members and not just between the leader and members.
   e. Leadership is shared among members.
   f. Members work together as a team to reach goals and to resolve problems and conflicts.
2. Individual
   a. The client demonstrates improved communication ability.
   b. The client exhibits improved problem-solving skills.
   c. The client reports improved coping with life issues.

Bibliography

American Nurses Association (1994). *Statement on psychiatric-mental health clinical nursing practice and standards of psychiatric-mental health clinical nursing practice.* Washington, DC: American Nurses Publishing.

American Psychiatric Association (1994). *Diagnostic and statistical manual of mental disorders (DSM-IV)* (4th ed.). Washington, DC: American Psychiatric Association.

Gary, F., & Kavanagh, C. (1991). *Psychiatric mental health nursing.* Philadelphia: J. B. Lippincott.

Rawlins, R., & Heacock, P. (1993). *Clinical manual of psychiatric nursing* (2nd ed.). St. Louis: Mosby-Year Book.

Shives, L. (1994). *Basic concepts of psychiatric-mental health nursing* (3rd ed.). Philadelphia: J. B. Lippincott.

Stolley, J. M. (1994). When your client has Alzheimer's disease. *American Journal of Nursing, 94*(8), 34–39.

Townsend, M. C. (1993). *Psychiatric mental health nursing: Concepts of care.* Philadelphia: F. A. Davis.

Varcarolis, E. (1994). *Foundations of psychiatric mental health nursing* (2nd ed.). Philadelphia: W. B. Saunders.

Wilson, H., & Kneisl, C. (1992). *Psychiatric nursing* (4th ed.). Menlo Park, CA: Addison-Wesley.

STUDY QUESTIONS

1. During a community meeting in a psychiatric unit, the nurse is having difficulty getting the members to take their seats and settle down. The nurse asks Client A, the community president (an officer elected by the group), to start the meeting. Not 5 minutes into the meeting, Client B shouts to Client C on the other side of the room, "Can I have a cigarette?" The nurse should best deal with this situation by
   a. telling Client A to proceed
   b. asking the group to examine what has just happened
   c. apologizing to Client A
   d. ignoring the interaction
2. The appropriate intervention in the above situation is based on the nurse's plan to improve
   a. individual members' coping skills
   b. member interest in group
   c. group members' commitment to group norms
   d. group members' decision-making abilities
3. Based on a nursing needs assessment revealing that parents in a clinic have misconceptions about child development that affect their ability to discipline, the nurse decides to form a teaching-learning group. The nurse chose a teaching-learning group over a support group because the focus should be on
   a. information, not feelings
   b. socialization, not insight
   c. insight, not information
   d. feelings, not socialization
4. A neighborhood group that meets monthly to promote safety in the neighborhood is what type of group?
   a. task-directed group
   b. socialization group
   c. insight-oriented group
   d. teaching-learning group
5. A group that meets every 2 weeks has a high rate of absenteeism and minimal participation by members. This group is not cohesive because it
   a. doesn't have a designated leader
   b. has no group content
   c. has no group loyalty
   d. has no gatekeeper
6. Select the group behavior indicating that a group is in the orientation phase.
   a. expression of feelings about termination
   b. increased disclosure of self
   c. working on problems and concerns
   d. unclear contract expectations
7. A therapist leads a group of adolescents in a biweekly meeting. The therapist provides strong direction and discourages communication among group members. This leadership style is characterized as
   a. democratic leadership
   b. laissez-faire leadership
   c. authoritarian leadership
   d. distributed leadership
8. In the group described in question 7, members would most likely
   a. be confused
   b. form a cohesive bond
   c. scapegoat another member
   d. demonstrate good productivity
9. To determine a group's effectiveness, the nurse would do all of the following except
   a. measure group members' participation in problem solving
   b. obtain only the leader's opinion
   c. observe group members' flow of communication
   d. look at the group's strategies for resolving conflict
10. Which of the following would be an appropriate reason to establish unit meetings on an inpatient psychiatric unit?
   a. to provide an arena for the clients' complaints
   b. to promote involvement in unit management

c. to address staff members' concerns
d. to focus on survival on the outside

11. The purpose of screening candidates for group therapy is to determine
a. friendliness
b. sociability
c. motivation
d. intelligence

ANSWER KEY

1. ***Correct response: b***
Assisting the group to look at its behavior focuses members on the exploration, the analysis, and the resolution of disruptive interpersonal relationships.
a and c. These actions would hinder group development because the nurse is taking control.
d. Ignoring the situation would miss an opportunity for the group to examine and analyze behavior.
Application/Psychosocial/Implementation

2. ***Correct response: c***
The problem exemplified in this situation is a disruptive situation in which group norms of one member speaking at a time and respect for individual members is violated. Therefore, the nurse's plan is to use the group to help reinforce these norms.
a, c, and d. None of these goals are relevant to the problem.
Analysis/Psychosocial/Planning

3. ***Correct response: a***
These parents need didactic information to correct their misperceptions about child development.
b, c, and d. There is no indication from this example that a support group or an insight-oriented group would be needed.
Comprehension/Health promotion/Planning

4. ***Correct response: a***
This group's purpose is promotion of a safer neighborhood.
b, c, and d. The purpose is not promotion of effective social skills, development of personal insight, or dissemination of factual information, respectively.
Comprehension/Psychosocial/Assessment

5. ***Correct response: c***
Group loyalty, a measure of group cohesiveness, is not evident in this group, in which absenteeism is high and group participation is minimal.
a, c, and d. These factors are not used to measure group cohesiveness.
Analysis/Psychosocial/Assessment

6. ***Correct response: d***
In the orientation phase of group development, the group members can have unclear contract expectations.
a. This behavior would occur in the termination phase.
b and c. These behaviors characterize the working phase of a group.
Comprehension/Psychosocial/Assessment

7. ***Correct response: c***
An authoritarian leadership style involves exerting complete and total control over group members.
a, c, and d. None of these leadership styles involves the type of control described in the scenario.
Comprehension/Psychosocial/Assessment

8. ***Correct response: c***
In this scenario, group members likely would become frustrated and angry. Scapegoating is one way of acting-out frustration and anger.
a, c, and d. These would not be expected responses in the scenario described.
Comprehension/Psychosocial/Evaluation

9. ***Correct response: b***
Talking only to the authorized leader would give the nurse a skewed picture of the group.
a, c, and d. All of these actions would help provide a more comprehensive and accurate picture of the group's effectiveness.
Application/Psychosocial/Evaluation

10. ***Correct response: b***
Community meetings are designed to increase clients' involvement in the everyday management of their living environment.

a, c, and d. Although these aims can be components of the community meetings, none is the primary purpose of holding the meetings.

Knowledge/Psychosocial/Implementation

11. ***Correct response: c***

The candidate's motivation for group therapy is of utmost importance to the success he or she will experience in the group.

a, c, and d. None of these are typical screening criteria.

Knowledge/Psychosocial/Assessment

14 Treatment Modalities: Family Therapy

I. Overview

A. Definitions

1. **Family: a group of people living in one household who have emotional attachment, regular interaction, and shared concerns and responsibilities**
2. Types of families:
   a. Traditional, nuclear family: married couple and their child or children by birth or adoption
   b. Single-parent family: lone parent and child or children by birth or adoption
   c. Blended family: married or not married couple, one or both of whom were married previously, and his, her, or their child or children
   d. Alternative family: persons with or without blood or marital ties who live together to achieve common goals

3. **System: a set of elements that have reciprocal interactions or relationships among themselves; types and associated concepts include:**

a. Supra system: a bigger system in which the family system functions (eg, church, school, neighborhood, cultural group)
b. Subsystem: smaller subsets of the family system (eg, siblings, parents, parent-child, intergenerational)

c. **Boundaries: parameters defining who is inside and outside the system and the rules governing the system; may be open, closed, or diffused or unclear**
d. Homeostasis: maintenance of system continuity, constancy, equilibrium
e. Synergy: cooperative action among members of a system such that the whole is greater than the sum of the parts (eg, greater results are possible through unified family effort than through individual member's effort)

B. Family systems

1. **In a family, all members operate to maintain characteristic behavior, roles, and relationship patterns.**
2. **Relationships are characterized by a continuous cycle of interaction (circular cause-and-effect, not linear cause-and-effect).**
3. **Change in any part of the family system creates change in all other parts and in the whole system.**
4. A person's family system is likely the most emotionally intense of all the systems in which he or she is involved.
5. Coalitions (eg, dyad between two people) formed among members of the system may become problematic. For example, an intergenerational dyad may hinder intragenerational communication.
6. Triangles also may become problematic; examples include:
   a. Three people
   b. Two people and an issue
   c. Two people and a group
7. Inappropriate distribution of power within the family also can create problems.

C. Developmental issues of families

1. Phases of family development (particularly pertinent to traditional nuclear and blended families) include:
   a. Coupling or marriage
   b. Childbearing
   c. Preschool-age children
   d. School-age children
   e. Teenage children
   f. Launching children
   g. Middle age
   h. Aging family members

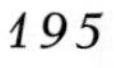

2. Developmental tasks of family systems include:
    a. Physical maintenance: food, shelter, clothing
    b. Physical and emotional resource allocation: expenses, goods, space, emotional support
    c. Division of labor: financial, household management, child rearing
    d. Socialization of members: physical, emotional, social, spiritual guidelines or rules
    e. Entry and release of members: birth, adoption, moving out, visitation, living-in
    f. Order: conformity to family or societal rules, standards, and norms
    g. Interaction with larger systems: relationship with church, school, neighborhood, society
    h. Motivation and morale: guiding philosophy, family loyalty, reinforcement and rewards, traditions

D. Communication in families

1. **In family systems, important communication occurs on both verbal and nonverbal levels.**
2. Verbal communication (eg, who talks to whom, what is said, how something is said) helps define relationships within the system.
3. Nonverbal communication (eg, body language, gestures, tone of voice, seating arrangements, timing of verbal feedback) helps define relationships within the system.
4. **In good family communication, family members openly encourage, on a verbal and nonverbal level, clear, direct discussion of issues and feelings.**
5. **In maladaptive family communication, family members on a verbal and nonverbal level discourage open discussion of issues and feelings; both the message and the target of the message are unclear and confusing.**
6. Pathologic communication patterns include:
    a. Incongruence: relaying two conflicting messages at the same time (eg, verbal and nonverbal messages do not match)
    b. Double-bind: an incongruent message wherein the recipient is a victim and cannot "win" (eg, "Do what I tell you; be more independent.")

E. Basic concepts: the individual in families

1. **Individuation (the process of differentiating oneself, developing autonomy) occurs within the family group.**
2. Problems associated with individuation include:
    a. Enmeshment: overinvolvement of family members, interference with individuation

b. Disengagement: underinvolvement of family members, leads to estrangement of individuated members

3. Projection of family problems or expectations onto individual members includes:
   a. Scapegoating: One member is blamed or made to suffer for problems in the family.
   b. Identified client: One family member develops more outward symptoms of dysfunction as a result of family problems.
   c. Labeling: Members are identified by one or more characteristics (eg, "good" one, "bad" one, "cheerful" one).
   d. Schismatic situation: Schism exists in the couple's relationship, creating a situation wherein the child or children must "take sides."
   e. Skewed situation: Skew exists in the marriage relationship because one member is dysfunctional, leading to an imbalance of roles or wellness in family relations.

II. Functional and dysfunctional families

A. Functional families

1. A functional family is one that possesses most characteristics of functional families over an extended period.

2. **In a functional family, members effectively shift roles, responsibilities, and interaction during periods of stress.**
3. **A functional family may exhibit problematic symptoms during prolonged stress but will rebalance with support of each member.**
4. Specific characteristics of a functional family include:
   a. Communicates in a clear, direct manner; encourages discussion of issues, even issues that evoke conflict
   b. Has clearly defined boundaries among the family subsystems and clearly but not rigidly defined boundaries delineating the family from the suprasystem
   c. Is flexible
   d. Maintains a balance between change and stability
   e. Develops basic belief patterns that are supported by facts; members are cognizant of their belief patterns and willing to discuss them
   f. Promotes and encourages individual autonomy and growth of members
   g. Resolves problems: clearly defines and names the problem, explores alternative solutions, implements and evaluates the selected solution, and is willing to try another solution if the selected solution does not work
   h. Defines family members' roles and responsibilities (who does what, when, where, and how)

B. Dysfunctional families

1. **A dysfunctional family lacks one or more characteristics of the functional family.**
2. **Symptoms arise over time or with stress, during family development, and at life transitions; predisposing factors include:**
   a. **Marital conflict**
   b. **Parent-child conflict**
   c. **Sibling conflict**
   d. **Acting-out of child (children)**
   e. **Symptoms in individual (identified client)**
3. **Dysfunction may be transmitted across generations.**
4. In contrast to a functional family, a dysfunctional family:
   a. Communicates in a confusing and indirect manner (neither the message nor the target of the communication is clear)
   b. Has unclear and diffuse boundaries delineating family subsystems and either diffuse or rigidly delineated suprasystem boundaries
   c. Is inflexible
   d. Resists change
   e. Develops belief patterns based on stereotypes, myths, and biases; members may or may not be cognizant of belief patterns and cannot accept challenges to belief patterns
   f. Does not encourage or support individual autonomy among members; experiences enmeshment, disengagement, or triangulation
   g. Experiences difficulty in resolving problems; may have trouble defining and naming a problem, exploring alternative solutions, and implementing a solution
   h. Has unclear definitions of family members' roles and responsibilities

III. Family therapy

A. Purposes

1. **Uses the family strengths to assist family in identifying problems and setting goals for change**
2. **Helps family members gain insight into their problems and change behavior from dysfunctional to functional**
3. Fosters open communication of thoughts and feelings among members
4. Assists one or more individuals within the family to individuate (differentiate)

B. Types

1. Psychoanalytic: intensive over long periods and focuses on cog-

nitive, affective, and behavioral components of family interaction

2. Family systems (Bowen approach): aims to help each member to avoid being dominated by emotional reactivity and to achieve better differentiation of self
3. Structural (Minuchin approach): endeavors to change family organization and develop clear boundaries for individual members
4. Interactional (Satir approach): strives to identify invisible, unspoken laws governing family relationships and use communication theory to promote improved relationships among members
5. Behaviorist: promotes change by implementing principles of learning theory and reinforcing positive, healthy behavior.

C. Role of the nurse

1. Specialist: Psychiatric-mental health nursing at the advanced level demands expertise in psychotherapeutic methods. According to the American Nurses Association (ANA) statement on mental health practice, "The certified specialist acting as family therapist can use a variety of approaches to enhance the function of family."
   a. Family diagnosis
   b. Psychotherapeutic interventions
   c. Outcome evaluations

2. **Generalist: applies nursing process with families:**
   a. **Assesses family functioning, establishing standard North American Nursing Diagnosis Association (NANDA) nursing diagnoses**
   b. **Promotes and fosters healthy behaviors**
   c. **Assists families to regain or improve coping skills**
   d. **Participates in programs that teach healthy parenting and focus on preventing family violence**

IV. Nursing process in families

A. Assessment

1. Identify phase and tasks of individual family development.
2. Determine ethnic and cultural background, beliefs, and practices.
3. **Assess family strengths and support systems.**
4. **Identify family perception of problem.**
5. Recognize communication patterns among members.

B. Analysis and nursing diagnoses

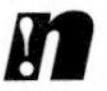

1. **Analyze family behaviors considered functional.**
2. **Analyze family behaviors considered dysfunctional.**
3. Determine nursing diagnoses applicable to families, for example:

a. Ineffective Family Coping: Compromised
b. Ineffective Family Coping: Disabling
c. Family Coping: Potential for Growth
d. Altered Family Processes

C. Planning outcomes

1. Work with family members to establish realistic goals.
2. Establish desired outcome criteria for intervention.
   a. Family group will identify resources within itself to deal with situation.
   b. Family members will practice open communication of thoughts and feelings.
   c. Family members will determine appropriate roles and responsibilities based on situation.
   d. Family members will encourage individual autonomy and growth of members.

D. Nursing implementations

1. **View family as a system. Keep in mind that no one member of the family is the problem (no identified client); rather, the problem exists within the family and is a family problem.**
2. **Remain neutral and objective; avoid taking sides.**
3. Focus on "here and now" problems and relationships.
4. Model clear, congruent verbal and nonverbal communication.
5. Assist family to understand "who owns the problem" and who is responsible for resolution.
6. Assist family to develop effective communication skills including active listening, "I" messages, and problem-solving techniques.
7. Identify possible support groups available in community for family members.
8. Assist family to identify coping skills being used and how these skills are or are not helping them deal with situations.
9. Refer family to qualified family therapist when problems are beyond scope of nursing intervention at the generalist level.

E. Evaluation

1. Family members verbalize coping strategies to be used.
2. Family members openly communicate thoughts and feelings, respecting members' differences.
3. The family exhibits functional family behaviors (see Section II.A).

Bibliography

American Nurses Association (1994). *A statement on psychiatric-mental health clinical nursing practice and standards of psychiatric-mental health clinical nursing practice.* Washington, DC: American Nurses Association Publishing.

Doenges, M. E., & Moorhouse, M. F. (1993). *Nurse's pocket guide: Nursing diagnoses with interventions* (4th ed.). Philadelphia: F. A. Davis.

Shives, L. R. (1994). *Basic concepts of psychiatric-mental health nursing* (3rd ed.). Philadelphia: J. B. Lippincott.

Townsend, M. C. (1993). *Psychiatric-mental health nursing: Concepts of care.* Philadelphia: F. A. Davis.

Varcarolis, E. (1994). *Foundations of psychiatric-mental health nursing* (2nd ed.). Philadelphia: W. B. Saunders.

STUDY QUESTIONS

1. A family reports being referred to the clinic by a teacher who is concerned because the 8-year-old family member's grades recently dropped significantly and the child is having fights with classmates. When assessing this family, the nurse would want to elicit which of the following information?
   a. detailed explanation of the difficulties with classmates
   b. the parents' perception and explanation of the problem
   c. explanation of the teacher's attempts to help solve the problem
   d. the child's thoughts and feelings about school
2. The parents tell the nurse that they are planning to divorce but haven't yet communicated this decision to their child. In applying principles of family theory, the nurse understands that the child's current behavior is
   a. characteristic of a schismatic situation in the family
   b. related to double-bind communication from parents
   c. reflective of tension and conflict in parental relationship
   d. typical of a child's developing autonomy and independence from parents
3. The nurse establishes the diagnosis, Ineffective Family Coping: Compromised, related to situational crisis of planned divorce. An appropriate outcome-based goal statement for this diagnosis would be: The parents will
   a. openly discuss thoughts and feelings about current crisis
   b. continue to protect child from unpleasant reality
   c. agree to remain together for sake of child
   d. allow child to determine future plans independently
4. The example of the child's problem behavior described in question 1, when viewed from a family perspective, can be analyzed as follows:
   a. The child has been labeled as a scapegoat.
   b. The parents and child are in a situation of disengagement.
   c. The child has the role of the identified client for a family problem.
   d. The parents are creating a schismatic situation with their child.
5. The nurse observing a father-daughter interaction hears the father say to his daughter (hospitalized with a diagnosis of schizophrenia, undifferentiated type), "I want you to make your own decisions about where to live after discharge, but come home with me so you'll have time to think about your future." The nurse analyzes this interchange as an example of
   a. double-bind communication
   b. parent-child conflict
   c. scapegoating of daughter
   d. skewed family interaction
6. The school nurse has been asked to conduct a program with the Parent-Teacher Association. The topic is parent-child relationships. In planning to focus on conflict resolution, the nurse would incorporate which of the following principles in promoting healthy family functioning?
   a. Parents need to communicate their ideas about solving problems to their children.
   b. Children can be encouraged to follow parental advice when having problems.
   c. Conflict is a reflection of poorly functioning family systems.
   d. Conflictual issues can be discussed in a direct, clear way among all family members.
7. According to family theory, the process of differentiation can best be described as

a. incongruent messages wherein the recipient is a victim
b. developing autonomy within the family group
c. cooperative action among members of a family
d. maintenance of system continuity or equilibrium

8. The nurse is interacting with a family group consisting of parents and a hospitalized adolescent who has an alcohol addiction. The nurse agrees with the adolescent's view about family rules. Which of the following implementations would be *best* in this situation?
   a. Remain neutral and objective; avoid taking sides.
   b. Align self with adolescent who is family scapegoat.
   c. Encourage parents to view situation from adolescent's side.
   d. Encourage adolescent to view situation from parental side.

9. In the above situation, the nurse establishes which of the following nursing diagnoses?
   a. Altered Family Processes, related to intergenerational conflict
   b. Ineffective Individual Coping: Compromised, related to lack of parental support
   c. Impaired Social Interaction, related to family conflict
   d. Ineffective Family Coping: Disabling, related to substance abuse in adolescent

10. A 16-year-old is hospitalized for treatment of anorexia nervosa. The parents are very upset and tell the nurse they have tried "everything" to get the teenager to eat. They explain that their child has always done everything to please them. They cannot understand this current stubbornness about eating. The nurse understands that this family situation is characteristic of
   a. enmeshment
   b. disengagement
   c. differentiation
   d. scapegoating

11. An appropriate outcome for the family described in the above situation would be
   a. Parents will use the love of their child to encourage appropriate eating.
   b. Parents will accept more independent functioning of their teenager.
   c. Parents will recognize that their teenager has a medical problem.
   d. Parents will maintain high standards and expectations of their teenager.

ANSWER KEY

1. ***Correct response: b***
It is imperative to understand the presenting problem from the family's perspective. This will aid in developing intervention strategies.
a, c, and d. Detailed investigation into these areas would not enhance the nurse's understanding of the presenting problem.
Application/Psychosocial/Planning

2. ***Correct response: c***
The family is a unified system whereby change in any part of the system creates change in all other parts. The child's school problems are a response to parental tension.
a and b. These problems are not evident in the description of the family.
d. An 8-year-old would not normally develop autonomy in this manner.
Analysis/Psychosocial/Analysis (Dx)

3. ***Correct response: a***
The parents are not currently communicating in an open manner. The crisis of divorce is not being dealt with by this family; the attempt to protect the child is not realistic.
b, c, and d. These would all be inappropriate responses to a family crisis of divorce. The parents may need intervention to assist them in taking appropriate responsibility for their own behavior as well as help in communicating realistically with their child.
Application/Psychosocial/Planning

4. ***Correct response: c***
Often, when parents cannot resolve issues between themselves, the child becomes the focus for the tension and anxiety. A child thus focused upon may develop problem behaviors.
a. The parents are not currently blaming their child for their difficulties.
b and d. These are not accurate explanations for the current family dynamics.
Comprehension/Psychosocial/Analysis

5. ***Correct response: a***
This is a classic example of a double-bind communication in which conflicting messages are delivered by a person in a position of authority.
b. Although conflict may exist between the father and daughter, the situation does not describe this.
c and d. There is insufficient information to make these determinations.
Application/Psychosocial/Analysis

6. ***Correct response: d***
In families, the ability to discuss difficult issues openly among members reflects healthy behavior.
a and b. Communication needs to be reciprocal between parents and children. Whoever "owns" the problem should be the one to decide solutions.
c. Conflict is normal among members of a family. The way in which conflict is resolved is a good indication of whether the family is functional or dysfunctional.
Knowledge/Psychosocial/Implementation

7. ***Correct response: b***
Differentiation is the process of developing autonomy.
a, c, and d. These are not related to the concept of differentiation.
Knowledge/Psychosocial/Assessment

8. ***Correct response: a***
Maintaining objectivity is vital for the nurse to communicate respect for each family member. The nurse maintains a nonjudgmental attitude.
b, c, and d. All of these implementations involve taking sides and would negate the nurse's position as a neutral party who actively listens to each person's viewpoint.
Application/Psychosocial/Implementation

9. ***Correct response: d***
This family is currently experiencing a

crisis situation whereby the teenager is hospitalized for substance abuse.

a. The data show no evidence of this conflict.

b and c. Although these diagnoses may apply to the adolescent with a substance abuse problem, there is no evidence given in this situation.

Analysis/Psychosocial/Analysis (Dx)

10. ***Correct response: a***

The parents are overinvolved in the teenager's life and provide little freedom for the adolescent to begin making autonomous decisions. Often, the adolescent with anorexia nervosa exerts control only over his or her own eating.

b, c, and d. There is no evidence of these problems in this situation.

Knowledge/Psychosocial/Assessment

11. ***Correct response: b***

If the parents can decrease their overinvolvement, the adolescent can begin to function in a more autonomous manner.

a and d. These behaviors can contribute to anorexia nervosa in the adolescent.

c. The parents are aware that not eating is a medical problem and have expressed concern about this behavior.

Application/Psychosocial/Planning

15 Treatment Modalities: Somatic Therapies

I. Overview

A. Definitions

1. Psychotropic (psychoactive) drugs: chemicals that affect the brain and nervous system; alter feelings, emotions, and consciousness in various ways

2. **Neurotransmitters: highly specialized chemicals that allow transmission of electrical impulses from one neuron to another across the synapse. Alterations in neurotransmitters have been implicated in various mental disorders.**
3. Extrapyramidal system: tracts of motor neurons from the brain to parts of the spinal cord; this system has complex relays and connections to areas of the cortex, cerebellum, brain stem and thalamus. The extrapyramidal system helps maintain equilibrium and muscle tone. Side effects of some psychotropic drugs can involve the extrapyramidal system.
4. Neuroleptic malignant syndrome: a rare, but potentially fatal complication of treatment with antipsychotic drugs. Symptoms include severe muscle rigidity, elevated temperature, hypertension, tachycardia, diaphoresis, and elevated creatinine phosphokinase (the enzyme associated with muscle activity) levels.

5. **Electroconvulsant therapy (ECT): the induction of a tonic-clonic (generalized) seizure through the application of electrical current to the brain**

B. Major concepts

1. Psychotropic medications are not intended to "cure" the mental illness. Although their contribution to psychiatric care cannot be minimized, these medications only relieve physical and behavioral symptoms.

2. **Biologic therapies (ie, psychotropic medications and ECT) may promote healing because they produce changes in cell function in the central nervous system (CNS). These changes permit new behaviors to emerge.**
3. Selected neurotransmitters and relationships to mental disorders
   a. Dopamine: Excessive dopamine activity has been implicated in schizophrenia. Increased dopamine causes nerve impulses in the brain stem to be transmitted faster than normal. Some experts believe that strange thoughts, hallucinations, and bizarre behaviors are the result.
   b. Serotonin and norepinephrine: These neurotransmitters have been studied since the 1960s as causal factors in mania and depression. Current researchers think mood disorders are the result of complex interactions between various chemicals, including neurotransmitters and hormones.
   c. Gamma-aminobutyric acid (GABA): This neurotransmitter is believed to exert an inhibitory effect on anxiety.
   d. Acetylcholine: Some theorists propose that the cognitive deficits that are common in Alzheimer's disease result from a reduction in acetylcholine available to the brain.

   e. Monoamine oxidase: an enzyme responsible for certain neurotransmitter destruction
4. Periodic recognition of the contribution of ECT in treating mental illness has been evident in the United States. Some depressed individuals show improvement with ECT after failing to respond to other forms of therapy.
5. Major classifications of psychotropic drugs
   a. Antipsychotics
   b. Antidepressants
   c. Antimanic agents
   d. Anxiolytics (antianxiety) agents
   e. Sedative-hypnotics

II. Antipsychotic agents

A. Types: Standard and atypical antipsychotic agents (also called neuroleptic agents) are discussed in Table 15-1.

B. Indications

1. Antipsychotic agents are used to treat the positive symptoms of schizophrenia (hallucinations, delusions, disor-

TABLE 15-1.
Antipsychotic Drugs

CLASS	GENERIC NAME	TRADE NAME	USUAL DAILY MAINTENANCE DOSAGE RANGE
Standard Antipsychotics			
Phenothiazines	Chlorpromazine	Throrazine	50–400 mg
	Thioridazine	Mellaril	50–400 mg
	Trifuoperazine	Stelazine	2–30 mg
	Perphenazine	Trilafon	8–24 mg
	Triflupromazine	Vesprin	60–150 mg
	Fluphenazine	Prolixin	2.5–20 mg
	Mesoxidazine	Serentil	30–150 mg
Butyrophenones	Haloperidol	Haldol	1–15 mg
Thioxanthenes	Thiothixene	Navane	6–30 mg
	Chlorprothixene	Taractan	50–400 mg
Dihydroindolones	Molindone	Moban	40–225 mg
Dibenzoxazepines	Loxipine	Loxitane	25–250 mg
Atypical Antipsychotics			
Other	Clozapine	Clozaril	300–450 mg
	Pimozide	Orap	300–450 mg
	Risperidone	Risperdal	4–6 mg

dered thinking, paranoia). The newer, atypical antipsychotic agents clozapine (Clozaril) and cisperiodone (Risperdal) help reduce the negative symptoms of schizophrenia (lack of motivation, anergia, impaired social interaction).

2. Antipsychotics can also be used to treat psychotic symptoms occurring in clients with bipolar disorder and cognitive impairment disorders.
3. Such symptoms as agitation, rage, overreactivity to sensory stimuli, hallucinations, delusions, paranoia, and combativeness may also be treated with antipsychotics.
4. Other indications include treatment of intractable vomiting, hiccoughs, and vertigo.

C. Mechanism of action

1. Antipsychotics create a postsynaptic dopamine-receptor blockade in the limbic system, hypothalamus, and cerebral cortex.
2. The same dopamine blockade occurs in the basal ganglia, causing extrapyramidal and other undesirable side effects.
3. The atypical antipsychotics act through a combination of dopamine and serotonin antagonism, although exact the exact mechanism of action is unknown. Many of the side effects of the standard antipsychotics are missing from these newer drugs.

D. General considerations

1. Principles of antipsychotic administration
   a. Initial treatment may require parenteral doses. These are changed to oral pill or concentrate forms as the behavior disturbance subsides. These drugs are rapidly absorbed through oral concentrates, suspensions, or intramuscular injections.
   b. Total doses are tailored to individual needs, and wide variation may exist among clients. Careful dosage titration is essential to target changes in symptoms.
   c. Divided doses are changed to a single dose, primarily at bedtime, as soon as practical to maximize effect of drug's sedative properties.
   d. Most clients require maintenance doses for sustained improvement.
   e. **Low-dose therapy is recommended for elderly clients. Adverse and side effects are more common in elderly clients because of their decreased kidney and liver function as well as decreased muscle mass compared to adipose tissue.**
   f. Serum half-life is about 24 hours. The drug accumulates in fatty tissue. When drug is discontinued, release from fatty tissue continues, and side effects may persist.
   g. Antipsychotics have a high therapeutic index and can be

given at high dose with minimal risk. Ordinarily, overdose is not life threatening.

h. These drugs are not addicting and do not produce euphoria, and the client does not develop tolerance to their antipsychotic effects.

i. Effects of antipsychotics on the fetus are not clear; use of antipsychotic drugs during pregnancy is not recommended.

2. Contraindications

a. Antipsychotics are contraindicated in clients with severe CNS depression resulting from excessive alcohol, barbiturate, or narcotic use; brain damage; or trauma.

b. These drugs should not be administered to clients with known sensitivity or severe allergic response to one of the antipsychotic drugs.

c. Clients with Parkinson's disease may experience an increase in symptoms.

d. Clients with a history of blood dyscrasias are more likely to develop dyscrasias as a side effect of drug therapy than are those with no such history.

e. These drugs should be used cautiously in clients with a history of liver damage or jaundice.

f. Clients with acute narrow-angle glaucoma and prostatic hypertrophy may experience increased intraocular pressure and urinary retention, respectively, because of the strong anticholinergic properties of these drugs.

E. Side effects and nursing interventions (standard antipsychotics)

1. Cardiovascular side effects (Table 15-2)

a. Hypotension and postural hypotension

- **Check client's blood pressure in lying, sitting, and standing positions. Hold dose in client with standing systolic pressure of 80 in accordance with healthcare facility policy.**
- Advise client to change position slowly from lying to sitting or standing position.

b. Tachycardia

- Be sure cardiac workup has been performed before client with preexisting cardiac problem starts taking antipsychotic medication.

2. Anticholinergic side effects

a. Urinary retention and hesitancy

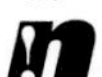

- **Monitor client's ability to void. Check bladder for distention if client complains of inability to void. Catheterization may be necessary.**

TABLE 15-2.
Managing Common Side Effects of Psychotropic Medications

SIDE EFFECT	NURSING IMPLEMENTATION
Anticholinergic	
Dry mouth	Suggest using sugarless gum/candy to relieve oral dryness.
Blurred vision	Caution client to avoid driving or operating heavy machinery until vision problem subsides.
Urine retention and constipation	Monitor client's elimination patterns. Assess for bladder distention. Encourage client to increase fluid intake, add fiber to diet, and exercise regularly.
Cardiovascular	
Postural hypotension	Monitor client's pulse rate and blood pressure. Take blood pressure with client in lying, sitting, and standing positions. Show client how to change positions safely and slowly.
Arrhythmias	Instruct client to report sensations of heart racing, dizziness, or feeling light-headed.
Photosensitivity	
Sunburn, rash	Instruct client to wear sunglasses and sunscreen when exposed to sunlight.
Sedation	
Drowsiness, lack of alertness	Advise client to take prescribed dose at bedtime and to avoid driving, operating machinery, or performing activities that require mental alertness while sedated.
Extrapyramidal symptoms (EPS)	
Pseudoparkinsonism, acute dystonic reaction, akathisia, tardive dyskinesia	Monitor for EPS effects using a standardized measuring device. Teach client to recognize possible EPS effects and to alert the nurse or physician. Administer anticholinergic or antihistamine agents as prescribed to counter EPS effects
Neuroleptic malignant syndrome	
Elevated temperature, muscle rigidity, hypertension, elevated CPK levels	Monitor for signs of neuroleptic malignant syndrome, withhold medications if client has signs and symptoms, and alert physician.

b. Constipation

- Encourage fiber-rich diet and increased fluids. Evaluate need for mild laxative or stool softener.

c. Blurred vision

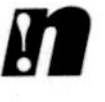

- **Advise client to avoid driving or operating machinery if vision is blurred. Blurred vision usually abates in 1 or 2 weeks.**

d. Nasal congestion, dry mouth

- Inform client that nasal decongestants may offer relief; body will adjust to drug in a few weeks. Use sugarless candy or gum to relieve dry mouth.

3. Extrapyramidal side effects

a. Pseudoparkinsonism (includes masklike facies, stiff and stooped posture, shuffling gait, drooling, tremors, "pill-rolling")

- Alert physician, who may lower dosage or prescribe an anticholinergic agent, such as trihexphenidyl (Artane), benztropine (Cogentin), or amantadine (Symmetrel). These anticholinergic agents may be prescribed prn (as needed) for clients taking antipsychotic drugs.

b. Acute dystonic reaction (includes acute contractions of tongue, face, neck, and back; also opisthotonos, in which tetanic arching of entire body occurs, and oculogyric crisis, in which eyes lock upward)

- **Alert physician. Administer antidote, either diphenhydramine (Benadryl) 25–50 mg IM or IV or benztropine (Cogentin) 1–2 mg IM or IV, as prescribed.**
- Remain with client; provide reassurance until medication counteracts the dystonia.

c. Akathisia (includes motor restlessness and excessive walking)

- Alert physician, who may lower dosage or prescribe antiparkinsonian agent. (*Note*: These symptoms may be misinterpreted as an increase in psychotic behavior. If symptoms result from agitation, they will worsen if antipsychotic dosage is decreased.)

d. Tardive dyskinesia (includes protruding and rolling tongue, blowing, smacking, licking. Spastic facial distortion and choreic or athetoid limb movements also can occur). This symptom is generally considered irreversible.

- **Monitor clients for signs of tardive dyskinesia and alert physician immediately. Many drugs have been tried to reverse tardive dyskinesia; none has been effective, but clozapine may prove beneficial according to reports in the *Medical Letter on Drugs and Therapeutics* (Abramowicz, 1994). An antipsychotic medication may be discontinued because of tardive dyskinesia.**
- **Monitor all clients receiving antipsychotic drugs for any adverse extrapyramidal side (EPS) effects. Assessment tools that help ensure consistent monitoring and evalua-**

tion of interventions for EPS effects include the Simpson Neurological Scale and the Abnormal Involuntary Movement Scale (AIMS). AIMS quantifies EPS effects on a scale of 0 (no effects) to 4 (severe effects) and measures involuntary movements of the face, mouth, extremities, and trunk.

4. Other side effects

a. Sedation

- If sedative effect of drug bothers client, contact physician, who may authorize administering a full dose of the medication at bedtime.

b. Skin changes (may include hives, contact dermatitis)

- Alert physician, who may discontinue drug or prescribe antihistamines.

c. Photosensitivity

- **Advise client to stay out of sunlight if possible. When in the sun, the client should be instructed to wear sunglasses, sunblock, long-sleeved clothing, and a protective wide-brimmed hat.**

d. Endocrine changes (including moderate breast enlargement and galactorrhea in women, gynecomastia in men; changes in sexual drive, usually loss of libido in both sexes; possibly, amenorrhea in women)

- Alert physician, who may change medication.

e. Increased weight

- Work with client to monitor weight gain and to maintain nutritionally sound diet.

5. Serious but rare side effects

a. Agranulocytosis (symptoms include sore throat, fever, malaise, mouth sores)

- Draw blood regularly for routine analysis to detect this adverse effect.
- **Notify physician immediately and withhold medication. Physician should order blood work to determine whether blood abnormalities constitute leukopenia or agranulocytosis. If test results indicate agranulocytosis, medication will be discontinued, and reverse isolation may be indicated to protect client.**

b. Cholestatic jaundice (symptoms include fever, nausea, abdominal pain, jaundice)

- ▸ Notify physician, and withhold drug. Liver function studies will be ordered and symptoms will be treated by conservative measures, such as bedrest, high-protein and high-carbohydrate diet, increased fluids.

c. Neuroleptic malignant syndrome

- ▸ **Immediately notify physician, stop medication, and transfer client to medical unit. Treatment is symptomatic and includes bromocriptine (Parlodel) for muscle rigidity; IV therapy with electrolyte replacements for hyperthermia; antiarrhythmic medications as necessary.**
- ▸ **Important: Detecting neuroleptic malignant syndrome in early stage increases client's chances for survival.**

F. Side effects and nursing interventions (atypical antipsychotics)

1. Agranulocytosis: 1% to 2% incidence in clients taking clozapine (Clozaril); see Section II.E.5.a for symptoms.
   - ▸ **Monitor client's white blood cell count weekly while client takes Clozaril. Explain importance of client complying with monitoring system.**
2. Seizures
   - ▸ **Notify physician, who may decide to reduce medication, stop drug, or administer anticonvulsants. Institute seizure precautions for client who is seizure prone.**
3. Other side effects (sedation, postural hypotension, constipation, EPS effects, neuroleptic malignant syndrome) and nursing interventions are similar to those associated with standard antipsychotic drugs (Table 15-2).

III. Antidepressant drugs

A. Types: for information on types of antidepressants, see Table 15-3.

B. Indications

1. **Used primarily to treat depressive disorders, these medications can positively alter degree of withdrawal, activity level, and the vegetative signs of depression.**
2. Antidepressants may also be used in treating anxiety disorders, enuresis and hyperactivity in children, and chronic pain.

C. Mechanism of action

1. The mechanism of action depends on the type of antidepressant (see Table 15-3).
2. Tricyclic antidepressants (TCAs): increase level of neurotrans-

TABLE 15-3.
Antidepressant Drugs

CLASS	GENERIC NAME	TRADE NAME	USUAL DAILY DOSAGE
Tricyclic antidepressants (TCAs)	Imipramine	Toframil	50–150 mg
	Amitriptyline	Elavil	50–100 mg
	Desipramine	Norpramin	75–200 mg
	Nortipamine	Pamelor	75–100 mg
	Protriptyline	Vivactyl	15–45 mg
	Doxepin	Sinequan	75–150 mg
	Maprotiline	Ludiomil	150–225 mg
	Clomimpramine	Anafranil	75–300 mg
Monoamine oxidase inhibitors (MAOIs)	Toranylcypromine	Parnate	10–30 mg
	Isocarboxazid	Marplan	10–30 mg
	Phenelzine	Nardil	15–90 mg
Nontricyclic	Venlafaxine	Effexor	150–375 mg
	Trazedone	Desyrel	150–400 mg
	Bupropion	Wellbutrin	200–450 mg
Serotonin reuptake inhibitor (SSRI), second generation antidepressants	Floxetine	Prozac	20–40 mg
	Sertraline	Zoloft	50–200 mg
	Paroxetine	Paxil	20–50 mg

mitters by blocking reuptake of norepinephrine and serotonin at presynaptic neuron

3. Monoamine oxidase inhibitors (MAOIs): inhibit monoamine oxidase, which is an enzyme responsible for neurotransmitter metabolism. This action then allows increased levels of neurotransmitters to remain in effect at synapse.
4. Atypical antidepressants or serotonin-specific receptor inhibitors (SSRIs): act specifically on the neurotransmitter serotonin by blocking its reuptake into the presynaptic cell

D. General considerations

1. TCAs are potentially lethal if taken in amounts of 10 to 30 times daily recommended dose.

2. **Client response to antidepressants may not occur until up to 3 weeks after first dose.**
3. Severely depressed clients with delusions or other psychotic symptoms may require an antipsychotic drug concurrently with an antidepressant.
4. Previously, a TCA was generally considered the drug of choice for treating nonpsychotic, nonbipolar depression. Currently, an SSRI may be the drug of choice.
5. MAOIs are effective antidepressants that can help some clients who cannot tolerate or fail to respond to a TCA or SSRI.

6. Clients receiving antidepressants should be monitored for suicidal ideation because the medications may increase client energy levels and ability to carry out plan.

E. Contraindications and precautions

1. TCAs
    a. Previously existing cardiovascular disease
    b. History of seizures
    c. Narrow-angle glaucoma
    d. Prostatic hypertrophy
    e. Pregnancy and lactation
2. Monoamine oxidase inhibitors (MAOIs)
    a. Lack of conformance to restricting foods containing tyramine (Display 15-1).
    b. History of cerebrovascular defects or cardiovascular disease
    c. Age (over 60)
    d. Liver disease
    e. Use of drugs (either over-the-counter or prescription) that will precipitate hypertensive crisis (see Display 15-1)
3. Serotonin-specific reuptake inhibitors (SSRIs)
    a. Hepatic or renal impairment
    b. Pregnancy or lactation

DISPLAY 15-1.
Avoiding Substances that Interact with MAOIs

The nurse needs to caution a client taking an antidepressant known as a monoamine oxidase inhibitor (MAOI) not only to avoid medications that may cause a harmful interaction but also to avoid food and beverages containing tyramine. Tyramine in combination with an MAOI can lead to hypertensive crisis.

Foods to avoid

- Products containing brewer's yeast*
- Broad beans, pickles, sauerkraut
- Bananas,* figs,* raisins*
- Cheddar or other aged cheeses, yogurt*
- Chicken liver, pickled herring, smoked salmon (lox), snails
- Chocolate,* licorice, soy sauce*

Beverages to avoid

- Beer, coffee,* tea,* wine (particularly Chianti)

Drugs to avoid

- Over-the-counter medications for colds, allergies, or congestion (particularly products containing ephedrine, phenylephrine, or phenylpropanolamine)
- Prescribed drugs, such as tricyclic antidepressants, narcotics, antihypertensives, sedatives, general anesthetics, stimulants (eg, amphetamines or cocaine)

*Currently, some experts think that these items can be allowed in moderation (Varcarolis, 1994).

c. History of seizures
d. Concurrent MAOI therapy
e. Clients at risk for suicide

F. Side effects and nursing implementations: TCAs (For specific symptoms and nursing implementations, see Table 15-2)

1. Anticholinergic effects
2. Cardiovascular effects
3. Sedation
4. Photosensitivity
5. Other uncommon side effects
a. Lower seizure threshold

▸ Alert physician; institute seizure precautions.

b. Decreased or increased libido: ejaculatory and erectile disturbances

▸ Alert physician, who may decide to change medication.

G. Side effects and nursing interventions: MAOIs

1. In addition to the side effects associated with TCAs, side effects of MAOIs may include diarrhea, abdominal pain, restlessness, insomnia, and dizziness.

2. The most serious potential side effect is hypertensive crisis; this occurs when tyramine-containing foods are consumed or when certain drugs are taken which will increase norepinephrine-like activity (Display 15-1).

3. Symptoms of hypertensive crisis include generalized headache,

TABLE 15-4.
Potential Drug Interactions with Lithium

DRUG	EFFECT WITH LITHIUM
Antipsychotics	Neurotoxicity
Antidepressants	Manic relapse
Aminophylline or theophylline Sodium bicarbonate or sodium chloride	Lower serum lithium level
Diuretics	Increased lithium reabsorption by renal mechanisms, which can precipitate toxicity
Tetracycline, streptomycin, or nonsteroidal antiinflammatory drugs (NSAIDs)	Increased serum lithium level
Muscle relaxants and anesthetics	Prolonged neuromuscular blockade related to succinylcholine and pancuronium. Lithium should be discontinued 48 to 72 hours before administering these agents and resumed when oral intake resumes after surgery.

nausea, vomiting, pallor, chills, stiff neck, muscle twitching, palpitations, and chest pain.

4. Treatment includes administering phentolamine mesylate (Regitine) slowly and promoting hydration and electrolyte balance.
5. Nursing interventions

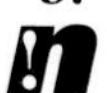

   a. **Instruct clients taking MAOIs about the need to restrict tyramine-containing foods—especially fermented or aged foods, such as cheese, red wine, dried sausages, pickled herring and other pickled or smoked meats, or fish, liver, and brewer's yeast. Inform clients that restricting tyramine-containing foods is essential for about 2 weeks after discontinuing an MAOI.**
   b. **Caution clients not to take over-the-counter medications (e.g. cough medicine) without consulting physician. Urge clients to inform all physicians, including dentists, that they are taking an MAOI.**
   c. **Teach clients to recognize signs and symptoms of undesired side effects, particularly hypertensive crisis.**

H. Side effects and nursing interventions: SSRIs

1. Similar to those of TCAs
2. Clients taking SSRIs have a lower incidence of anticholinergic side effects and less cardiotoxicity; however, SSRIs show less ability to lower the seizure threshold.

IV. Antimanic drugs

A. Indications

1. **Lithium carbonate and lithium citrate are antimanic agents used primarily for acute manic and hypomanic episodes and also for long-term prophylaxis of bipolar disorders. Antimanic drugs are particularly effective in preventing recurrent manic episodes.**
2. Used experimentally to treat other psychiatric disorders that involve mood disturbance, such as:
   a. Alcoholism
   b. Drug abuse
   c. Premenstrual syndrome
   d. Pathologic sexual behaviors and phobias

B. Mechanisms of action

1. The exact mechanism of action of antimanic drugs is unclear.
2. Studies indicate that antimanic drugs interfere with norepinephrine, dopamine, and serotonin metabolism.
3. These agents affect electrolyte balance in the brain and alter sodium transport in nerves and muscle cells.
4. Experts speculate that lithium corrects an ion exchange abnormality.

C. General considerations

1. Lithium is a naturally occurring salt found in minerals, seawater, plants, and animals.
2. It is readily absorbed after oral administration.
3. It competes with sodium for reabsorption in the proximal tubules of the kidney.

4. **Before receiving lithium therapy, a client must undergo a complete health history and physical examination, focusing on:**
   a. **Renal function: 24-hour creatinine clearance, blood urea nitrogen (BUN), and electrolyte levels; personal or family history of renal disease and diabetes mellitus; diuretic or analgesic use**
   b. **Thyroid function: blood test to evaluate thyroid function; personal or family history of thyroid disease**
5. Lithium has a success rate of 70% to 80% in treating bipolar disorder.
6. Lithium augments the effects of antidepressants and is effective in resolving and preventing recurrent major depression.

7. **Other drugs used as antimanic agents include the following anticonvulsants: carbamazepine (Tegretol), valproic acid (Depakene), clonazepam (Klonopin).**
   a. **Used if lithium is ineffective or cannot be tolerated**
   b. **Can also be used in combination with lithium**
   c. **Because these drugs are anticonvulsants, they cannot be abruptly discontinued because this may precipitate status epilepticus**
8. Antipsychotic drugs may be used concurrently with lithium in acute manic episodes to manage behavioral and psychotic manifestations.
9. Lithium therapy typically begins with 300 mg tid for several days, followed by increasing titrated doses until steady level is achieved.
10. During lithium stabilization, blood is drawn regularly to measure serum lithium levels until a therapeutic level is identified.
11. After symptom resolution, lithium is decreased for maintenance treatment to approximately one half to two thirds the acute dose. Blood levels are checked every 2 to 3 months or when there is reason to suspect a change.

D. Contraindications and precautions

1. **Lithium has a narrow therapeutic index; the therapeutic dose is only slightly less than the amount that produces toxicity.**
2. Administer cautiously in elderly or debilitated clients, those

with thyroid or renal disease or seizure disorders; or those taking incompatible medications (see Table 15-4).

3. Dehydration or sodium depletion can precipitate lithium toxicity.

E. Side effects and nursing interventions

1. Side effects include the following:

a. Nausea, abdominal discomfort, diarrhea, or soft stools (usually benign and temporary)

b. Tremors (ranging from fine to coarse)

c. Thirst

d. Weight gain

e. Muscle weakness and fatigue (usually benign and temporary)

f. Hair loss (usually temporary)

g. Polyuria (usually benign but possibly progressing to diabetes insipidus)

h. Lithium toxicity (serum lithium levels exceeding 2.0 mEq/L)

- Mild toxicity (serum lithium level about 1.5 mEq/L): slight apathy, lethargy, diminished concentration, mild ataxia and muscle weakness, coarse hand tremors, slight muscle twitching
- Moderate toxicity (serum lithium level between 1.5 and 2.5 mEq/L): severe diarrhea, nausea and vomiting, mild to moderate ataxia and incoordination, slurred speech, tinnitus, blurred vision, frank muscle twitching, ataxia, irregular tremors
- Severe toxicity (serum lithium level exceeding 2.5 mEq/L): nystagmus, muscle fasciculations, deep tendon hyperreflexia, visual or tactile hallucinations, oliguria or anuria, severely impaired level of consciousness, grand mal seizure, coma, death

2. Nursing interventions include the following:

a. For *GI symptoms*: Administer lithium with meals, snacks, or milk or instruct the client to do so. If symptoms persist, consult with physician, who may decide to decrease the dose or prescribe another lithium preparation.

b. For *tremors:* Advise the client to restrict caffeine intake. Also consult with physician, who may reduce dosage or prescribe propranolol (Inderal) for severe or incapacitating tremors.

c. For *thirst:* encourage the client to maintain stable fluid intake of six to eight glasses of water daily.

d. For *weight gain:* obtain a diet history, advise against fluid and sodium restriction, and encourage a moderate restriction of calories combined with an exercise regimen.

e. For *muscle weakness and fatigue:* assess rest and activity pattern; protect the client from exhaustion by limiting stimuli; promote safety by discouraging smoking alone; and discourage the client from operating a motor vehicle or machinery requiring alertness.
f. For *hair loss:* review laboratory data assessing thyroid function for hypothyroidism; notify physician of abnormal results. Advise client that if hair loss persists, lithium may need to be discontinued.
g. For *polyuria:* monitor intake and output; conduct 24-hour urine collection for analysis.
h. For *lithium toxicity*
   - **Teach client to take preventive steps, such as maintaining normal sodium intake and adequate fluid intake (48 to 64 oz water daily) and replacing fluids and electrolytes lost during exercise, prolonged heat exposure, or GI illness. Explain that common causes of elevated lithium levels include decreased sodium intake; fluid and electrolyte loss associated with severe sweating, dehydration, or diarrhea; diuretic therapy; medical illness; and overdose.**
   - Rapidly assess clinical symptoms; trust clinical judgment even if serum lithium level is within or slightly above therapeutic range. Hold lithium and alert physician of assessment findings.
   - Monitor vital signs and level of consciousness.
   - As prescribed, draw blood to measure serum lithium, electrolyte, BUN, and creatinine levels; to perform complete blood count (CBC) profile; and to monitor cardiac status.
   - Assist in further support measures as indicated by client's status or as prescribed by physician.
   - Caution client that combining lithium with certain other medications may cause problems (Table 15-4).

V. Antianxiety (anxiolytic) and sedative-hypnotic drugs

A. Indications

1. **These agents are used primarily to treat anxiety and sleep disorders (Table 15-5 and Table 15-6).**
2. Anxiety that requires drug treatment and that is unrelated to a more specific syndrome is usually treated with a benzodiazepine, according to reports in the *Medical Letter on Drugs and Therapeutics* (Abramowicz, 1994).
3. Drugs that are classified as sedative-hypnotics can be used to relieve anxiety or induce sleep, depending on drug dosage.
4. They also may be used as tools for alcohol and drug withdrawal management, as preoperative medications, and as muscle relaxants or anticonvulsant agents.

TABLE 15-5.
Antianxiety (Anxiolytic) Drugs

CLASS	GENERIC NAME	TRADE NAME	USUAL DAILY DOSE
Benzodiazepines	Flurazepam	Dalmane	used as hypnotic
	Chlordiazepoxide	Librium	5–25 mg
	Diazepam	Valium	2–10 mg
	Oxazepam	Serax	10–30 mg
	Chorazepate	Tranxene	15–60 mg
	Lorazepam	Ativan	2–6 mg
	Alprazolam	Xanax	0.5–1.5 mg
	Clonazepam	Klonopin	1.5–10 mg
	Prazepam	Centrax	30–60 mg
Diphenylmethane	Hydroxyzine HC	Atarax	200–400 mg
Antihistamines	Hydroxyzine pamonte	Vistaril	200–400 mg
Other	Busiprone	BuSpar	15–30 mg
Beta-adrenergic blocker	Propranolol	Inderal	30–80 mg

TABLE 15-6.
Sedative-Hypnotic Drugs

CLASS	GENERIC NAME	TRADE NAME	USUAL SEDATIVE DOSE (3–4 times/day)	HYPNOTIC DOSE
Barbiturates	Secobarbital	Seconal	30–50 mg	100–200 mg
	Pentobarbital	Nembutal	30 mg	100–200 mg
	Amobarbital	Amytal	30–50 mg	100–200 mg
	Butabarbital	Butisol	15–30 mg	100–200 mg
	Phenobarbital	Luminal	16–32 mg	100–200 mg
	Thiopental	Pentothal	30–90 mg	100–200 mg
	Methohexital	Brevital	used for anesthesia, ultra-short acting	100–200 mg
Non-barbiturates	Glutethimide	Doriden	500 mg	250–500 mg
	Methyprylon	Noludar	—	200–400 mg
	Chloral hydrate	Noctec	250 mg	0.5–2 gm
	Ethchlorvynol	Placidyl	—	500–750 mg
Benzodiazepines (used as hypnotics)	Temazepam	Restoril	—	15–30 mg
	Triazolam	Halcion	—	0.25–0.5 mg
	Zolpidem	Ambien	—	5–10 mg
	Flurozepam	Dalmane	—	15–30 mg

5. Barbiturates may be used to treat seizure disorders or as preoperative sedatives.
6. Beta blockers may treat stress or specific anxiety resulting in such autonomic symptoms as trembling, palpitations, diaphoresis, and tachycardia.

B. Mechanism of action

1. **Benzodiazepines are thought to potentiate neurotransmitter gamma aminobutyric acid (GABA), producing muscle relaxation and anxiety relief.**
2. Barbiturates and nonbarbiturate sedative-hypnotic drugs produce CNS depression.
3. Beta blockers induce a peripheral beta-adrenergic blockade and possibly exert some CNS effects.
4. Antihistamines used for anxiety act as CNS depressants at the subcortical level.

C. General considerations

1. Benzodiazepines, the most widely prescribed drugs in the world, generally are regarded as the drug of choice for anxiety and sleep disorders.

2. **Benzodiazepines and sedative-hypnotics produce tolerance to their effects within days; cross-tolerance among drugs also may develop.**
3. **Continued use may lead to emotional and physical dependency; withdrawal symptoms may occur with abrupt discontinuation of therapy.**
4. **Barbiturates, although inexpensive, have a narrow margin of safety; doses as low as 10 to 15 times the therapeutic dose have proven lethal.**
5. Experts generally recommend that an antianxiety agent and sedative-hypnotic therapy be brief, prescribed for a specific stressor, and used as an adjunct to psychotherapy and other therapeutic modalities in treating anxiety disorders.
6. Benzodiazepines are generally given orally; an IM form is also available.
7. All benzodiazepines, regardless of half-life, should be tapered for safe discontinuation.
8. Sedative-hypnotic agents typically are used at bedtime. A repeated dose is possible if client doesn't fall asleep within designated period.

D. Contraindications and precautions

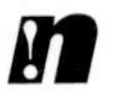

1. **In general, avoid administering benzodiazepines to clients with a history of alcohol or drug abuse because of the possibility of cross-tolerance and the increased risk for abuse.**

2. Clients with uremia or hepatic insufficiency should not take benzodiazepines or barbiturates.
3. Anxiolytics or sedatives are not recommended for pregnant or lactating women.
4. Propranolol (Inderal) is contraindicated in clients with certain cardiac and pulmonary diseases.

E. **Side effects and nursing interventions**

1. **Clients who combine benzodiazepines with other CNS depressants, particularly alcohol, may experience hazardous CNS depression.**

   ▸ **Alert physician to CNS depression. The physician may reduce dosage or discontinue drug.**

2. Symptoms of benzodiazepine withdrawal include tremulousness, insomnia, headache, tinnitus, anorexia, and vertigo.

   ▸ **Inform client that discontinuing anxiolytic or sedative-hypnotic agents requires gradually reducing the dosage (tapering) rather than abruptly stopping the drug. If withdrawal symptoms occur, the physician should be notified. In such cases, the physician can reinitiate drug administration and then taper the dosage.**

3. Side effects associated with barbiturates: suppression of rapid eye movement (REM) phase of sleep, daytime drowsiness, and a hangover effect in the morning

   ▸ Monitor client's sleep patterns. Instruct client to notify physician if side effects occur.

4. Propranolol may cause insomnia, hallucinations, impaired metabolism of other drugs, lethargy, or depression.

   ▸ Teach client to recognize side effects and alert physician if effects occur.

5. Antihistamines may produce sedation, anticholinergic side effects, and decreased seizure threshold.

   ▸ **Inform client about sedative effect. Caution client to avoid activity requiring alertness and concentration (see nursing interventions for anticholinergic side effects and decreased seizure threshold in the antipsychotic drug section).**

VI. Electroconvulsant therapy (ECT)

A. **Indications**

1. **Treatment of clients who have severe depression; who are**

acutely suicidal; or who are unwilling to eat, do not respond to antidepressants, and cannot tolerate medication

2. May also be indicated in manic clients whose conditions are resistant to lithium and antipsychotic drugs and in clients whose systems cycle drugs rapidly ("rapid cyclers")

B. Mechanism of action

1. Exact mechanism by which ECT effects a therapeutic response is unknown.

2. **Several experts have demonstrated that electric stimulation results in significant increases in circulating levels of several neurotransmitters.**

C. Contraindications and precautions

1. The only absolute contraindication for ECT is increased intracranial pressure.
2. Other conditions that place clients at high risk include cardiovascular disorders, aortic or cerebral aneurysms, severe hypertension, severe osteoporosis, acute and chronic pulmonary disorders, and pregnancy.

D. Nursing process in ECT

1. Assessment

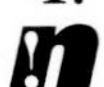

   a. **Review completed physical exam of client, including thorough assessment of cardiovascular and pulmonary status.**
   b. **Ensure that client's signed informed consent form is on file.**
   c. **Determine client's baseline status including mood, evidence of suicidal ideation, level of anxiety, current short and long-term memory condition.**
   d. Determine what client knows about ECT.

2. Analysis and nursing diagnoses
   a. Analyze client's degree of depression and anxiety.
   b. Analyze client and family concerns regarding ECT.
   c. Determine appropriate nursing diagnoses, for example:

   - Anxiety
   - Knowledge Deficit
   - Risk for Injury
   - Self Care Deficit

3. Planning outcomes
   a. Work with client in establishing realistic goals.
   b. Establish desired outcome criteria for clients having ECT therapy.

- Client will verbalize understanding of rationale, side effects, and risks of ECT.
- Client will experience no adverse effects (eg, injury, aspiration) during ECT.
- Client will be monitored after ECT for status of vital signs, level of orientation, swallowing and gag reflexes.
- Client will be positioned after ECT to facilitate breathing and prevent aspiration.
- Client will maintain orientation to reality after ECT.

4. Nursing implementations

a. Before ECT

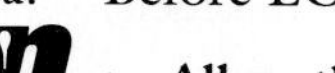

- **Allow the client no food or fluids at least 4 hours before ECT.**
- **Ensure that informed consent form, laboratory data, health history, and physical examination findings are recorded on client's chart.**
- **Establish and record baseline vital signs.**
- **Have client void before procedure.**
- **Remove client eyeglasses or contact lenses, dentures, jewelry, hairpins and the like.**
- **Administer prescribed medications to decrease secretions and to promote relaxation.**

b. During ECT

- **Ensure client has patent airway; provide suctioning as needed.**
- Assist anesthesiologist with oxygenation as required.
- Observe data displayed on vital signs and cardiac monitors.
- Support client's arms and legs during seizure.

- **Observe and document type and amount of movement induced by seizure.**

c. After ECT

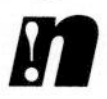

- **Monitor vital signs every 15 minutes for the first hour after ECT.**
- Position client on side to prevent aspiration.
- Orient client to time and place, informing client that procedure has been completed.
- Reassure client that memory loss is transient.
- Offer fluids and food when gag and swallow reflexes resume.

5. Evaluation

a. Client maintains anxiety at manageable level.

b. Client and family verbalize understanding of procedure, side effects, and risks.

c. Client completes treatment without experiencing injury or aspiration.
d. Client maintains adequate tissue perfusion during and after ECT.
e. Client regains orientation to time and place after treatment.

Bibliography

Abramowicz, M. (Ed.). (1994). Drugs for psychiatric disorders. *Medical letter on drugs and therapeutics, 36*(933), 89–96.

Deglin, J. H., & Vallerand, A. H. (1995). *Davis's drug guide for nurses* (4th ed.). Philadelphia: F.A. Davis.

Townsend, M. C. (1993). *Psychiatric mental health nursing: Concepts of care.* Philadelphia: F. A. Davis.

Varcarolis, E. (1994). *Foundations of psychiatric-mental health nursing* (2nd ed.). Philadelphia: W. B. Saunders.

Wilson, H., & Kneisl, C. (1992). *Psychiatric nursing* (4th ed.). Menlo Park, CA: Addison-Wesley.

STUDY QUESTIONS

1. A client has been diagnosed with bipolar disorder and has been taking lithium carbonate for the past month. While on pass, the client went to the beach to enjoy the warm July weather. On returning to the unit, the client complains of apathy, vague GI symptoms, and decreased attention span. What further data would the nurse collect to assess the client's present symptoms?
   a. the last time she ate
   b. the presence of hypomanic symptoms
   c. the level of anxiety experienced
   d. her fluid intake while on pass
2. The nurse is working with a paranoid schizophrenic client to improve compliance with the antipsychotic medication regimen. Which of the following issues should the nurse explore with the client?
   a. the nurse's frustrations concerning the client's unwillingness to cooperate
   b. the meaning the client attaches to taking medication
   c. whether or not the client really needs to take medication
   d. the possibility that the client may need hospitalization
3. Which of the following vital signs readings would cause the nurse to consult with the physician about changing a client's scheduled morning dose of haloperidol (Haldol)?
   a. BP 124/84, P 92 (supine); BP 126/90, P 84 (standing)
   b. BP 112/62, P 84 (supine); BP 114/80, P 78 (standing)
   c. BP 122/70, P 80 (supine); BP 90/60, P 112 (standing)
   d. BP 130/80, P 100 (supine); BP 120/68, P 110 (standing)
4. A client is taking thiothixene (Navane) 6 mg PO tid. The nurse would teach which of the following if the client is planning to spend several hours at the zoo with his family?
   a. Drink extra fluids.
   b. Use plenty of sunscreen.
   c. Use extra sodium.
   d. Avoid any caffeine.
5. Which of the following statements accurately explain the rationale for blood pressure monitoring in clients taking antipsychotic drugs?
   a. Orthostatic hypotension is a common side effect
   b. Elevated blood pressure can occur as a side effect.
   c. Intake of foods containing amines can affect blood pressure when taking antipsychotics.
   d. Altered blood pressure readings can indicate need for antiparkinsonian drugs.
6. Isocarboxazid (Marplan), one of the MAOI antidepressants, has been prescribed for a client who was diagnosed with major depression. The client, who has been taking the drug for 1 week, complains that she feels the same, with no improvement. Which of the following principles would be the basis for the nurse's response to this client?
   a. Supplemental drug therapy may increase effectiveness of this antidepressant.
   b. Clients with major depression may need longer to experience relief with antidepressants.
   c. The client may need to take an MAOI for several weeks before a response occurs.
   d. MAOIs are usually not as effective as other antidepressants.
7. When monitoring a client taking the MAOI phenelzine (Nardil), the nurse would assess for compliance with
   a. regular laboratory testing
   b. adequate fluid intake
   c. correct frequency of doses
   d. maintenance of tyramine restriction

8. The nurse understands that clients taking which of the following drugs should be taught about anticholinergic side effects?

- **a.** antipsychotics and anxiolytics
- **b.** antidepressants and antipsychotics
- **c.** lithium and anxiolytics
- **d.** sedative-hypnotics and lithium

9. A client has been taking fluphenazine (Prolixin) and experiences an acute dystonic reaction. Which of the following prescribed medications would the nurse administer prn to this client?

- **a.** diphenhydramine (Benadryl) 25 mg IM
- **b.** thiothixene (Navane) 6 mg PO or IM
- **c.** acetaminophen (Tylenol) 325 mg PO
- **d.** milk of magnesia (MOM) 30 mL PO

10. The nurse assessing a client taking an antipsychotic drug notes an elevated temperature, elevated blood pressure, and diaphoresis. Which of the following nursing interventions would be a priority?

- **a.** Collect further assessment data before intervening.
- **b.** Encourage bedrest and increased fluids.
- **c.** Hold medication and notify physician.
- **d.** Monitor vital signs every 30 minutes.

11. A client has been diagnosed with chronic undifferentiated schizophrenia. The physician prescribes clozapine (Clozaril) for this client. It is most important to teach the client and the client's family about

- **a.** food restrictions with this medication
- **b.** frequent blood pressure monitoring
- **c.** the possibility that the client may not notice a response to this medication for at least 3 weeks
- **d.** the importance of monitoring the client's white blood cell count

12. In teaching a client about side effects of the benzodiazepine alprazolam (Xanax) prescribed to treat social phobia, the nurse emphasizes which of the following?

- **a.** daytime drowsiness, ataxia
- **b.** restlessness, increased racing thoughts
- **c.** dry mouth, constipation
- **d.** hypertension, tachycardia

13. The nurse should teach a client who is taking the benzodiazepine oxazepam (Serax) to avoid excessive intake of

- **a.** ibuprofen
- **b.** cheese
- **c.** shellfish
- **d.** coffee

14. For which of the following clients would benzodiazepines be contraindicated?

- **a.** A client with active alcoholism
- **b.** A client with a history of cholecystitis
- **c.** A client who just had a myocardial infarction
- **d.** A client who has anorexia nervosa

15. Which of the following nursing interventions would be appropriate immediately after ECT?

- **a.** monitoring for further seizures
- **b.** assessing vital signs and reorienting the client
- **c.** applying restraints to prevent injury
- **d.** administering previously held medications

16. Which of the following principles should the nurse keep in mind when planning care for clients receiving anxiolytic drugs?

- **a.** Orthostatic hypertension may occur.
- **b.** Increased mental alertness will be expected.
- **c.** Other CNS depressants will potentiate the drug's sedative action.
- **d.** Enhanced psychomotor coordination is expected.

17. A client has been receiving lithium for the past 2 weeks for treatment of bipolar disorder. When planning client teaching, the nurse understands that the client needs to know that

a. a low-sodium diet must be maintained
b. a diuretic should be taken with lithium
c. serum lithium levels will be monitored on a regular basis
d. a missed dose should be taken regardless of the time elapsed since the scheduled dose

18. Early signs of lithium toxicity include

a. torticollis
b. tinnitus
c. akathisia
d. diarrhea

19. Clients taking lithium must be particularly sure to maintain adequate intake of

a. protein
b. sodium
c. vitamin K
d. multivitamins

ANSWER KEY

1. ***Correct response: d***
The nurse would suspect that the client is dehydrated; decreased fluid intake or increased diaphoresis would result in a rise in lithium level.
a. There is no relationship between frequency of food intake and fluctuating lithium levels.
b. There are no data presented to suggest hypomania.
c. This is not relevant to the nurse's immediate assessment.

Analysis/Physiologic/Assessment

2. ***Correct response: b***
It is important to explore this issue because a client's misconceptions about the need for drug therapy may lead to noncompliance.
a. The nurse does not need to explore this issue with the client.
c. The assumption is made that antipsychotic medication is the drug of choice for treating schizophrenia.
d. This would be a last resort; efforts should be directed toward promoting compliance in the community setting.

Application/Psychosocial/Evaluation

3. ***Correct response: c***
A rise in pulse rate of 30 beats/minute or a drop in blood pressure of 30 mm Hg when changing position from lying to sitting or sitting to standing is considered indicative of orthostatic hypotension.
a, c, and d. These values do not indicate orthostatic hypotension.

Application/Physiologic/Implementation

4. ***Correct response: b***
Photosensitivity in clients taking antipsychotic drugs may result in severe sunburn if the client spends time in the sun without protection.
a. Extra fluid intake will not protect against side effect of photosensitivity.
c and d. Neither sodium intake nor coffee intake has relevance to the nurse's instructions concerning the side effects of Navane.

Application/Safe care/Implementation

5. ***Correct response: a***
Orthostatic hypotension is relatively common, particularly during the first few weeks of treatment.
b. The opposite is true generally.
c. This has no relevance to the rationale for taking clients' blood pressure.
d. The need for an antiparkinson drugs is indicated by other adverse effects, such as akathisia or other extrapyramidal symptoms.

Comprehension/Physiologic/ Analysis (Dx)

6. ***Correct response: c***
Response to antidepressant medications usually does not occur for about 3 weeks after therapy begins.
a. The antidepressants do not require supplemental drugs to ensure effectiveness of therapy.
b. Response to antidepressants usually takes up to 3 weeks, regardless of the severity of depression.
d. This has no bearing on the effectiveness of and response time to the antidepressants.

Comprehension/Health promotion/ Implementation

7. ***Correct response: d***
Consumption of foods containing tyramine can cause a hypertensive crisis.
a. This is not necessary when taking MAOIs.
b. Although this is a healthy practice, it is not crucial to effectiveness of MAOIs.
c. Although this is an important issue, it is of critical importance that client's diet be monitored during this time so as not to compromise

treatment or precipitate hypertensive crisis.

Analysis/Safe care/Evaluation

8. ***Correct response: b***

This is largely due to these drugs' anticholinergic actions including dry mouth, blurred vision, urine retention, and constipation.

a, c, and d. Few common side effects are shared by agents in these major drug classifications.

Analysis/Physiologic/NA

9. ***Correct response: a***

Diphenhydramine (Benadryl) is commonly used to counteract an acute dystonic reaction.

b. Another antipsychotic drug would only increase the severity of the dystonic response and would be contraindicated.

c and d. Neither of these drugs would have an effect on a dystonic response. Oral medications would be contraindicated until the dystonic response is reversed because swallowing may be impaired.

Knowledge/Safe care/Implementation

10. ***Correct response: c***

These symptoms can indicate neuroleptic malignant syndrome. The next dose should be held and the physician should be notified immediately so that treatment measures may be implemented.

a. Although other assessment data can be collected, the priority is to notify the physician.

b. These measures are inadequate for treating neuroleptic malignant syndrome.

d. Vital signs will be monitored frequently, however, the physician must be notified.

Analysis/Safe care/Implementation

11. ***Correct response: d***

Agranulocytosis is a major concern when clients take clozapine (Clozaril). Weekly monitoring of the white blood cell count is essential.

a, b, and c. These items are not related to treatment with Clozaril.

Knowledge/Health promotion/Implementation

12. ***Correct response: a***

Alprazolam (Xanax) is a CNS depressant and may cause side effects such as drowsiness and, possibly, ataxia.

b. This would be an unexpected reaction to a benzodiazepine.

c and d. These are not side effects of benzodiazepines.

Knowledge/Safe care/Implementation

13. ***Correct response: d***

The effectiveness of benzodiazepines is diminished when they are combined with excessive intake of caffeine or tobacco.

a, b, and c. No known adverse interactions with these substances have been reported.

Knowledge/Health promotion/Implementation

14. ***Correct response: a***

Alcohol potentiates the action of benzodiazepines; abuse may occur as a result of cross-tolerance between these drugs.

b, c, and d. No evidence suggests that benzodiazepines are contraindicated in clients with cholecystitis, myocardial infarction, or anorexia nervosa.

Analysis/Physiologic/Analysis (Dx)

15. ***Correct response: b***

The client should be monitored for changes in vital signs just as any client who has had an anesthetic for a short procedure. Reorientation is necessary because a period of confusion occurs after ECT-induced seizure.

a. Grand mal seizures do not occur after the procedure, just during procedure.

c. Restraints are not indicated unless the client becomes agitated.

d. Medications are not given until the client regains consciousness and swallowing and gag reflexes.

Comprehension/Safe care/Implementation

16. ***Correct response: c***

CNS depressants, such as alcohol, potentiate the action of sedative-hypnotics and antianxiety drugs.

a. This simply does not occur with this classification of drugs.

b and d. The converse would be true.

Application/Physiologic/Planning

17. ***Correct response: c***

Because lithium is a potentially dangerous and toxic medication, serum drug levels must be evaluated regularly to ensure that lithium levels are maintained within a therapeutic range.

a. A low-sodium diet would raise the lithium level.

b. Diuretic use may cause dehydration, which may promote lithium toxicity.

d. Because of the potential toxicity of lithium, missed doses should not be made up later than 2 hours after the scheduled dosage time.

Comprehension/Health promotion/Planning

18. ***Correct response: d***

GI discomfort is usually the first symptom of lithium toxicity.

a. Torticollis is a dystonic reaction that occurs only with the antipsychotic drugs.

b. Tinnitus is a symptom of moderate toxicity.

c. Akathisia is also an extrapyramidal side effect that occurs with antipsychotic medications.

Comprehension/Safe care/Assessment

19. ***Correct response: b***

Because lithium competes with sodium in the distal tubules of the kidney, a fluctuating sodium level results in a fluctuating lithium level. Therefore, "normal" intake of sodium is necessary to keep lithium from accumulating at toxic levels in the body.

a. Variances in protein intake have no bearing on lithium level.

c. This has no relevance to maintaining a stable lithium level.

d. The client taking lithium has the same need for multivitamins as does a person not taking lithium.

Application/Health promotion/Implementation

COMPREHENSIVE TEST—QUESTIONS

1. When a client is in a psychiatric facility under a voluntary admission, which of the following statements is true?
   a. The client has been judged dangerous to self or others.
   b. A written request must be submitted for the client to leave before discharge.
   c. The client will lose his or her civil rights during psychiatric inpatient treatment.
   d. The client must remain in the hospital for at least 5 days.
2. The nurse who wishes to provide culturally sensitive care would understand that membership in a particular cultural group can affect the client in which of the following ways?
   a. It will affect the client's view of authority and compliance with treatment.
   b. It will affect client's thinking, feeling, and behavior.
   c. It will influence client's specific dietary practices.
   d. It will influence client's specific diagnosed mental illness.
3. When a nurse is assigned to care for a client who speaks another language, an important intervention to facilitate communication with the client would be
   a. relying on gestures and other forms of nonverbal communication
   b. using validation as a therapeutic tool
   c. using an interpreter
   d. using simple pictures
4. A Native American has been hospitalized on the psychiatric unit and requests that the tribal shaman be involved in treatment. The nursing implementation that would be most appropriate in this situation would be
   a. Explain to the client that this is not appropriate in psychiatric treatment.
   b. Facilitate the client's request by reporting to the treatment team.
   c. Ignore the client's request as it is not possible to do this.
   d. Reflect that the client is seeking magical healing rather than relying on self.
5. A nurse and client are talking comfortably about the client's progress and feelings about the therapeutic relationship. This is typical of which phase in the therapeutic relationship?
   a. assessment
   b. orientation
   c. working
   d. termination
6. The nurse working as a team member in a facility that provides partial hospitalization for a client recently discharged from an inpatient psychiatric unit provides which of the following levels of preventive care?
   a. primary
   b. secondary
   c. tertiary
   d. premorbid
7. The nurse says to the client, "I'm here to help you." The client states, "I don't want to talk," and turns away from the nurse. Basing your answer on knowledge about the structural model of communication, which of the following statements about the situation is correct?
   a. No feedback loop exists because the client did not respond.
   b. The client's verbal and nonverbal behavior constitutes a feedback loop.
   c. The nurse's message is the feedback loop.
   d. A feedback loop is not illustrated in this situation.
8. A client states, "People think I'm no good, if you know what I mean." Which of the following responses by the nurse would be most therapeutic for this client?

a. "Well, people don't always mean what they say about you."
b. "I think you're good. So you see, there's one person who likes you."
c. "I'm not sure what you mean. Tell me more about that."
d. "What have you done to create this impression on people?"

9. A client with depression is scheduled for voluntary admission to an open psychiatric unit. However, at arrival time, no bed is available. The alternative is to place the client temporarily on the high-security locked unit. However, this action violates the client's right to
a. privacy
b. receive treatment in the least restrictive setting
c. retain his or her civil rights
d. communicate with people outside the hospital

10. A nurse on the unit is observed as routinely responding to clients in an autocratic, controlling manner with little consideration for their dignity and rights. After attempts to directly acknowledge the situation with the nurse in question, the nurse's colleagues plan to meet with the supervisor to express their concern about the nurse's unprofessional manner. The plan to go to the supervisor is
a. appropriate, because peer review is a professional activity to maintain quality care
b. appropriate, because the nurse is probably looking for limits to be set on his or her behavior
c. inappropriate, because it is up to the supervisor to evaluate the nurse
d. inappropriate, because each nurse is responsible only for her or his own practice

11. A client comes to the mental health clinic in crisis. The client was recently evicted and spent 2 weeks living with a friend who no longer wants a roommate. The nurse who plans interventions according to a hierarchy of the client's needs is following which of the following developmental theorists?
a. Freud
b. Sullivan
c. Maslow
d. Erikson

12. The nurse would understand that the theoretical framework that describes maladaptive behavior as learned would be which of the following?
a. behavioral
b. educational
c. psychodynamic
d. cognitive

13. A client with psychotic symptoms is given prescribed medications and agrees to a contract specifying behavior that is acceptable and behavior that will result in a loss of privileges. The nurse understands that this treatment plan is based on which frameworks for psychiatric care?
a. cognitive and behavioral
b. behavioral and psychobiologic
c. psychodynamic and psychobiologic
d. interpersonal and humanistic

14. A nurse who explains a client's psychotic behavior as being unconsciously motivated understands that the client's disordered behavior arises from which of the following?
a. abnormal thinking
b. altered neurotransmitters
c. internal needs
d. response to stimuli

15. A nurse observes that a mother seems highly anxious when caring for her infant. Which theorist would say that the mother's anxiety is internalized by the infant?
a. Freud
b. Sullivan
c. Maslow
d. Erikson

16. A client with depression has been hospitalized for treatment after taking a leave from a company that expects the client to return to work following inpatient treatment. The client constantly tells the nurse, "I'm no good. I can't even work. I'm a failure." The nurse who understands cognitive theory recognizes that the client's self comments are an example of

a. thought processes that maintain the depression
b. punitive superego and weak id
c. learned behavior requiring modification
d. use of projection and reaction formation

17. A couple just had their first child and moved into a new home, shortly after which the wife's mother dies. Which of the above events would be considered stressors on the family?

a. the move into a new home, the mother's death
b. having their first child, the mother's death
c. having their first child, move into new home
d. moving into new home, birth of child, mother's death

18. The nurse would use Selye's general adaptation theory in which of the following ways?

a. to teach clients stress-reduction techniques
b. to help clients develop awareness of stressors
c. to look at life events that require adaptation
d. to explain how the body adapts to stress

19. The nurse observes a client pacing in the hall. To help the client recognize anxiety, the nurse may say which of the following?

a. "I guess you're worried about something, aren't you?"
b. "Can I get you some medication to help calm you?"
c. "Have you been pacing for a long time?"
d. "I notice that you're pacing. How are you feeling?"

20. A client who is a Vietnam war veteran suffers from nightmares and flashbacks about his war experience. He has been diagnosed with post-traumatic stress disorder. Which of the following nursing diagnoses would be most appropriate?

a. Fear, related to intrusive images from past experiences
b. Ineffective Individual Coping: Compromised, related to failure to establish role responsibilities
c. Anxiety, related to fear of the unknown
d. Self Esteem Disturbance, related to past experiences of inadequacy in combat

21. A client is diagnosed with hypochondriasis. During the nursing assessment, the client makes all of the following statements. Which statement is most typical of a client with this diagnosis?

a. "I feel tired almost all the time."
b. "I think I have stomach cancer."
c. "Nobody understands my problems."
d. "I haven't been able to concentrate."

22. The nurse describes a client as anxious. Which of the following statements about anxiety is true?

a. Anxiety is usually pathologic.
b. Anxiety is directly observable.
c. Anxiety is usually harmful.
d. Anxiety is a response to threat.

23. A client with a phobic disorder is treated by systematic desensitization. The nurse understands that this approach will do which of the following?

a. Help the client execute actions that he or she fears and avoids.
b. Help the client develop insight into irrational fears.
c. Help the client substitute fears.
d. Help the client decrease anxiety.

24. A client with obsessive-compulsive disorder is hospitalized. Which of the following nursing responses is most thera-

peutic in regard to the client's compulsive checking behavior?
   a. challenging this behavior
   b. preventing this behavior
   c. accepting this behavior
   d. rejecting this behavior

25. A client with generalized anxiety disorder would be assessed by the nurse for which of the following symptoms?
   a. suspicion, withdrawal from others, anger
   b. blank affect, echolalia, feelings of unreality
   c. sadness, lack of hope, poor self-esteem
   d. restlessness, sleep disturbance, difficulty concentrating

26. A child who is hospitalized following a history of abuse develops another personality that emerges in times of stress. The nurse understands that which of the following explanations best fits this phenomenon?
   a. The child dissociates from the self as a way of coping.
   b. The child develops another personality for companionship.
   c. The child has poor ability to concentrate and focus on reality.
   d. The child assumes a complete, new, and permanent identity.

27. A 45-year-old woman with a history of depressive episodes now complains of marital and sexual concerns. She has difficulty with sexual arousal and situational preorgasmia. She is slightly overweight and diets frequently. She reports her marital relationship is somewhat supportive. The nurse knows that all the following information may be compiled in a sexual assessment of this client. However, the least important would be
   a. physical examination
   b. medication evaluation
   c. sex history
   d. work history

28. A client reveals a history of sexual molestation by a female friend of the family when she was 9 years old. The family has no knowledge of this. The client has dated boys since she was 15 and states she wants to continue. She also discusses fantasies focused on a close female friend with whom she has had sexual activity. With this information in mind, the nurse would select which of the following as the most significant evaluation criteria?
   a. Client will explore feelings, fantasies, and sexual behaviors regarding both heterosexual and homosexual experiences.
   b. Client will tell parents about sexual experience at age 9.
   c. Client will continue to date boys, identify attraction to them, and receive reinforcement from staff and family for this.
   d. Client will explore lesbian subculture to gain support.

29. Because the client with a borderline personality disorder often expresses intense emotions, the nurse should plan which of the following?
   a. awareness of and support for the nurse's own feelings and reactions
   b. group interactions where client can ventilate intense feelings to several persons
   c. isolation room experience where client can express intense feelings without harm to others
   d. dealing only with content expressed rather than intense emotions

30. The nurse would evaluate which of the following as successful outcome criteria for the client with an antisocial personality?
   a. statements of self-satisfaction and good self-esteem
   b. charming behavior directed toward others
   c. statements that guilt and anxiety are not useful
   d. increased impulse control and ability to delay gratification

31. In performing a physical assessment of a client with anorexia nervosa, the nurse would expect to find which of the following?

a. hypertension, fluid retention, intolerance to cold
b. hypotension, tachycardia, intolerance to heat
c. tachycardia, diarrhea, irregular menses
d. bradycardia, constipation, amenorrhea

32. Which of the following nursing diagnoses is most appropriate for a client with anorexia nervosa who expresses feelings of guilt about not meeting family expectations?

a. Anxiety
b. Body Image Disturbance
c. Defensive Coping
d. Powerlessness

33. Which of the following nursing implementations would be most appropriate for a client with anorexia nervosa during initial hospitalization on a behavioral therapy unit?

a. Emphasize the importance of good nutrition to establish normal weight.
b. Ignore client's mealtime behavior and focus instead on issues of dependence and independence.
c. Help establish plan using privileges and restrictions based on compliance with re-feeding.
d. Teach client information about anorexia and its long-term physical complications.

34. A client with rheumatoid arthritis is treated with both medical and nonmedical interventions. The nurse may teach this client about which of the following to increase the client's sense of control over the symptoms?

a. biofeedback measures
b. medication side effects
c. pathophysiology of disease process
d. management of stress

35. In planning care for the client with a somatoform disorder, the nurse would avoid which of the following?

a. evaluating physical complaints
b. reinforcing secondary gains
c. limiting manipulative behavior
d. teaching relaxation techniques

36. The nurse would evaluate therapy with the family of a client with anorexia nervosa as successful if which of the following occurred?

a. Parents reinforce increased decision making by client.
b. Parents clearly verbalize expectations of client.
c. Client verbalizes that family meals are now enjoyable.
d. Client tells parents about feelings of low self-esteem.

37. The nurse typically establishes which of the following outcome goals when working with a client with a somatoform disorder?

a. Client will recognize signs and symptoms of physical illness.
b. Client will cope with physical illness.
c. Client will take prescribed medications.
d. Client will express anxiety verbally rather than by physical symptoms.

38. The nurse understands that the most distinguishing feature of a client with an antisocial personality disorder is

a. attention to detail and order
b. bizarre mannerisms and thoughts
c. submissive, dependent behavior
d. disregard for social and legal norms

39. A male client in the unit is charming and manipulative. He is especially flattering and flirty today. He pays special attention to one female nurse, getting her coffee and holding her chair. Which of the following would be this nurse's best approach to this situation?

a. Accept the client's efforts to practice socially acceptable behavior.
b. Reinforce the client's attentions to others rather than himself.

c. Ask the client directly what he wants from her.
d. Tell the client matter-of-factly that he does not need to flatter to get her attention, and explore other ways of relating.

40. Evaluation is especially difficult in clients with personality disorders for which of the following reasons?
a. Clients are often withdrawn even after therapy and may not share results openly.
b. Typically, few changes in behavior may be identified over time.
c. Nurses have personality disorders of their own and may overidentify with these clients.
d. Clients improve rapidly and wish to move on with their lives rather than focus on improvements made.

41. A client is admitted to the psychiatric unit with a diagnosis of major depressive disorder. The nurse should assess for which of the following physiologic signs of depression?
a. complaints of restlessness and anxiety
b. complaints of rapid heart rate and dizziness
c. significant appetite and sleep pattern changes
d. significant increase in thirst and urinary frequency

42. The nurse will use which of the following methods to determine a client's potential risk for suicide?
a. Allow client to bring up the subject of suicide.
b. Observe client behavior for cues of suicidal ideation.
c. Question client directly about suicidal thoughts.
d. Question client about plans for the future.

43. A client with a diagnosis of dysthymic disorder reports feeling hopeless and expects that life will never get better. The nurse's most therapeutic response would be
a. Accept client's painful feelings.
b. Challenge accuracy of the client's feelings.
c. Deny that the situation is hopeless.
d. Cheer client by focusing on positives.

44. A client with a diagnosis of major depression attempts to stay in the room most of the day and remains socially isolated. The nurse initially intervenes in which of the following ways?
a. Explain that hospital policy does not allow clients to stay in their room.
b. Spend brief periods of time with the client throughout the day.
c. Approach the client in an upbeat mood to enhance conversation.
d. Reassure the client that everything will be okay.

45. The client tells the nurse, "Everyone would be better off if I weren't alive." Keeping this statement in mind, the nurse would make which of the following nursing diagnoses?
a. Altered Thought Processes
b. Ineffective Individual Coping
c. Risk for Violence: Self-directed
d. Impaired Social Interaction

46. A client with a bipolar disorder exhibits manic behavior. The nursing diagnosis is Altered Thought Processes, related to difficulty concentrating secondary to flight of ideas. Which of the following outcome criteria would indicate improvement in the client?
a. Client will verbalize feelings directly during treatment.
b. Client will verbalize positive self statements.
c. Client will speak in coherent sentences.
d. Client will report increased feelings of calm.

47. The nurse's discharge plans for a client diagnosed with depression should include
a. discussion of outpatient treatment
b. discussion of inpatient treatment

c. discussion of work setting
d. discussion of staff's effectiveness

48. A recently admitted female client exhibits manic behavior. She flirts with men on the unit and wears excessive make-up as well as provocative clothes. The most appropriate nursing response would be
 a. "You are not acting like a lady. Get control of yourself."
 b. "Your family would not approve of this behavior."
 c. "Let's look through your things to find some clothing that goes better with this setting."
 d. "You look really great today, are you planning on going anywhere special?"

49. A family member of a client with a schizophrenic disorder questions the nurse about the cause of schizophrenia. The nurse bases the response on which of the following statements regarding what is known about schizophrenia?
 a. The disorder is thought to result from disturbed family relations and communication problems.
 b. The disorder is thought to be caused by brain alterations in the frontal lobe.
 c. The disorder is thought to be caused by a combination of biologic and psychosocial factors.
 d. The disorder is thought to be caused by altered dopamine transmission within the brain.

50. When formulating a nursing diagnosis of Sensory/Perceptual Alterations for a client diagnosed with schizophrenia, the nurse must differentiate psychotic responses. This means the nurse must assess
 a. how the client experiences and interprets the environment
 b. the number of psychotic symptoms the client exhibits
 c. the client's ability to establish trust
 d. the inappropriate use of defense mechanisms

51. For a paranoid client who distorts the events in his or her daily environment on the unit, which of the following outcome goals would be most important to consider?
 a. The client will demonstrate realistic interpretation of daily events in the unit.
 b. The client will perform daily hygiene and grooming without assistance.
 c. The client will take prescribed medications without supervision.
 d. The client will leave the milieu if events become too stimulating.

52. A client with paranoid schizophrenia often directs brief, hostile verbal outbursts toward the nursing staff. Of the nursing actions below, which one is most likely the best way to deal with this problem?
 a. Place the client in seclusion when these episodes occur.
 b. Administer antipsychotic medications, as needed, when verbal outbursts occur.
 c. Set limits and provide a structured, predictable environment.
 d. Minimize the outbursts by walking away when they occur.

53. Which of the following activities would be appropriate for the nurse to implement with a severely withdrawn client?
 a. art activity with a staff member
 b. board game with a small group of clients
 c. team sport in the gym
 d. no activity

54. The client looks frightened and says, "The unit is wired up to the FBI, and they're taking my thoughts away." Which of the following responses by the nurse would be most therapeutic?
 a. "These thoughts aren't real; they're part of your illness."
 b. "I don't believe this is so, but you seem scared."
 c. "How long have you been thinking this?"

d. "Let me show you that the unit is not wired up."

55. A client who has undifferentiated schizophrenia reports that her body is made of wood and her arms do not work. The nurse understands that the client is manifesting the symptom of

a. autism
b. ambivalence
c. depersonalization
d. regression

56. A client who has cirrhosis of the liver initially denies having a drinking problem but later admits drinking more and experiencing blackouts. The client reports the ability to stop drinking at any time but plans to continue at present because of spousal nagging. From this information, the nurse could logically conclude that this client

a. is dependent on alcohol
b. lacks control over drinking
c. abuses alcohol
d. has developed tolerance

57. The client who blames drinking on a nagging spouse is demonstrating

a. displacement
b. projection
c. rationalization
d. sublimation

58. A client with a substance use disorder denies that the substance use creates problems in daily life. The nursing diagnosis of Ineffective Denial has been established. Which of the following outcome statements would indicate successful intervention?

a. Client describes the types and amounts of substances used.
b. Client verbalizes association of substance use and personal problems.
c. Client acknowledges experiencing withdrawal symptoms.
d. Client participates in group therapy with other substance abusers.

59. A client has developed tolerance to CNS depressants. To the nurse this means

a. concurrent abuse of two different substances
b. continued use of substance despite life problems
c. need to increase dose to obtain desired effect
d. physiologic symptoms occur when drug is discontinued

60. The nurse assessing a client for alcohol withdrawal symptoms watches for which of the following?

a. agitation, increased pulse rate and blood pressure
b. drowsiness, decreased pulse rate and blood pressure
c. euphoria, increased energy, hostility
d. slurred speech, incoordination, memory loss

61. A pregnant woman has abused heroin for the past 3 years. She is unemployed and obtains money by prostitution and stealing. What would be the most important initial nursing intervention for this client?

a. Counsel the client about her lifestyle and needed changes.
b. Assess nurse's own personal attitudes about heroin addiction and prostitution.
c. Identify the legal implications of stealing, the health risks associated with prostitution, and the effects of drugs on the fetus.
d. Review literature on substance dependence and its impact on women.

62. The nurse would understand that if a client continues to be dependent on heroin throughout her pregnancy, her baby will be at high risk for

a. mental retardation
b. heroin dependence
c. addiction in adulthood
d. psychologic disturbances

63. The nurse is planning care for a family in which violence commonly occurs. Which of the following statements about nonvictim members of violent families is correct?

a. They do not require intervention because they are not involved.
b. They often experience more trauma than do actual victims.
c. The should be encouraged to seek alternative living arrangements.
d. They commonly experience fear and guilt from their exposure to family violence.

64. The violent family with severe communication problems could best be helped with
a. individual art therapy for the child victims
b. one-to-one behavior modification sessions for the abuser
c. group sessions guided by a family systems model
d. long-term marital counseling for the parents

65. The nurse applying psychodynamic theory to understand sexual abuse knows which of the following factors are associated with this problem?
a. personal history of abuse for the abuser, diminished ego strength
b. observation of incest in childhood, poor adult role models
c. overcoming internal controls to abuse
d. a belief that women and children are property

66. The assessment of whether an abuse victim of family violence can remain safely in the home would not depend on which one of the following factors?
a. the availability of appropriate community shelters
b. the ability of the nonabusing caretaker to intervene on the client's behalf
c. the client's possible response to relocation of the abuser only
d. the family's socioeconomic status

67. An 11-year-old child is admitted to a psychiatric unit for treatment. The client is diagnosed with conduct disorder. The nurse will assess the client for which of the following behaviors?
a. restlessness, short attention span, hyperactivity
b. physical aggressiveness, low stress tolerance, disregard for rights of others
c. deterioration in social functioning, excessive anxiety and worry, bizarre behavior
d. sadness, poor appetite and sleeplessness, loss of interest in activities

68. Which of the following theories are essential for the nurse to understand in working with childhood and adolescent psychiatric disorders?
a. developmental theory
b. learning theory
c. educational theory
d. psychodynamic theory

69. The nurse plans to work with the parents of a child diagnosed with a depressive disorder. The parents and child validate that they rarely agree on rules appropriate for the child. Which of the following would be an inappropriate nursing response?
a. Encourage expression of feelings of all family members.
b. Support family strengths.
c. Provide education about age-appropriate development.
d. Take the side of the child.

70. The nurse would expect a client with early Alzheimer's disease to have problems in which of the following areas?
a. balancing a checkbook
b. operating a washing machine
c. relating to family members
d. remembering own name

71. The nurse would differentiate the cognitive impairment disorders of delirium and dementia in which of the following ways?
a. Delirium occurs slowly and responds to treatment.
b. Delirium has a rapid onset and may be reversed.
c. Dementia has a rapid onset and can be reversed.

d. Dementia occurs slowly and responds to treatment.

72. A client with Alzheimer's disease has frequent episodes of emotional lability. The nurse implements which of the following?

a. logic to point out reality factors
b. humor to alter mood
c. exploration of reasons for altered mood
d. reduction in environmental stimuli to redirect client's attention

73. The nurse understands that the pathophysiologic factor thought to be related to Alzheimer's disease is

a. deficiency of epinephrine
b. deficiency of acetylcholine
c. excess amount of serotonin
d. excess amount of dopamine

74. The daughter of a client with Alzheimer's disease reports feeling chronic fatigue and mild depression. Further assessment reveals that this daughter has been feeding, cleaning, and doing laundry for the parent while maintaining a full-time job and caring for two teenagers. The nurse establishes which nursing diagnosis for the client's daughter?

a. Altered Family Process
b. Ineffective Family Coping
c. Caregiver Role Strain
d. Social Isolation

75. The nurse guided by a crisis intervention model would assess which of the following?

a. communication patterns, coping skills, problem solving
b. situational support, expression of feelings, anxiety
c. perception of event, situational support, coping skills
d. coping skills, reality testing, cognitive distortions

76. A seriously ill client dies much sooner than expected. Family members are called in and, when they arrive, are told about the death. At this time, the nurse can expect family members to initially

a. demonstrate shock and disbelief
b. exhibit helplessness and withdrawal
c. share fond memories about the deceased
d. state how much they miss their family member

77. If a crisis remains unresolved for more than 3 months, what might be a more appropriate analysis of the client's situation?

a. The client has not received adequate support.
b. The client may be experiencing an adjustment disorder.
c. The client is not amenable to crisis intervention.
d. The client is not cooperating well with therapy.

78. The nurse evaluates a client's response to crisis intervention as favorable if the client

a. changes coping skills and behavioral patterns
b. develops insight into reasons why crisis occurred
c. learns to relate better to others
d. returns to previous level of functioning

79. Two nurses are co-leading group therapy for seven clients in the psychiatric unit. The leaders observe that the group members are anxious and look to them for answers. The group is in which phase of development?

a. conflict resolution phase
b. initiation phase
c. working phase
d. termination phase

80. The nurse who is leading a therapeutic group tells the members, "This is our group and we meet to learn different ways of talking to people. It is important that we practice listening. Our group is designed to help with talking and listening." This response is

a. nontherapeutic because it restricts group spontaneity
b. therapeutic because it enhances cohesiveness

c. nontherapeutic because it does not address norms
d. therapeutic because it prevents the development of conflict

81. The nurse responsible for leading a therapy group evaluates the group as being in the working phase if the group members

a. begin to comment on their behavior in group
b. ask the nurse for advice regarding problems
c. talk about someone outside the group
d. focus on their past relationships

82. Group members have worked very hard, and the nurse reminds them that termination is approaching. Termination is considered successful if group members

a. decide to continue
b. evaluate group progress
c. focus on positive experiences
d. stop attending before termination

83. A homosexual couple has lived together for the past 5 years. They tell the nurse that their relationship is deteriorating. The nurse should first

a. tell them to separate if their feelings are mutual
b. recognize his or her own feelings about homosexuality
c. teach them adaptive ways of dealing with heterosexuals
d. discuss benefits of discontinuing their relationship

84. The nurse assesses a family's communication skills. Which of the following data validate good communication skills?

a. evidence that children accept and adopt parental value system
b. family members who express agreement on issues and problems
c. open and clear discussion of issues and feelings among members
d. parents who state that they have no problem communicating with their children

85. A nurse working with families understands that only one of the following events does not increase stress on the family system. It is

a. adolescent leaving home
b. birth of a child
c. death of a grandparent
d. parental disagreement

86. The nurse providing care for an adolescent hospitalized for depression is asked by the parents to encourage the adolescent to attend college. The nurse can intervene most therapeutically by

a. encouraging each family member to discuss his or her feelings on this issue
b. explaining to the parents that the adolescent can make the decision about college
c. talking to the adolescent about the advantages of education
d. refusing to get involved in this issue

87. A client hospitalized with a diagnosis of schizophrenia recently started taking oral trifluoperazine (Stelazine) 2 mg tid. The client complains of progressively stiff, painful, and tense neck muscles. Given these data, the nurse suspects that the client is experiencing

a. increased tension related to the illness
b. an acute dystonic reaction
c. symptoms of pseudoparkinsonism
d. toxic effects of an antipsychotic medication

88. A client starts taking lithium carbonate (Eskalith) 300 mg tid. The nurse needs to caution the client about concurrent use of medications that may increase the risk of lithium toxicity. Which of the following drugs would increase this risk?

a. antacids
b. diuretics
c. stool softeners
d. antibiotics

89. A client has been taking haloperidol (Haldol) 5 mg tid to treat schizophrenia. The nurse routinely assesses for extrapyramidal side effects. Which of the following does not an indicate extrapyramidal effects?

- **a.** dry mouth, urine retention
- **b.** eyes rolling upwards uncontrollably
- **c.** excessive motor restlessness
- **d.** tremors, shuffling gait

90. A client with generalized anxiety disorder has been taking diazepam (Valium) 5 mg tid for the past 2 weeks. At the outpatient clinic, the nurse assesses the client's knowledge about drug therapy. Which of the following statements made by the client indicates the need for further instruction?

- **a.** "I know this drug can be addicting."
- **b.** "I understand that when I no longer need this drug, I'll have to gradually stop taking it."
- **c.** "I won't drink alcohol while I'm taking this drug."
- **d.** "I understand that this drug will help decrease my depression."

91. The nurse is to administer chlorpromazine (Thyroxin) 50 mg IM to a client with agitation. Which of the following implementations would be essential before giving this drug?

- **a.** assess skin color and sclera
- **b.** obtain radial pulse
- **c.** take blood pressure
- **d.** ask client to void

92. The nurse is to administer clozapine (Clozaril) to a client with schizophrenia. Evaluation of the effectiveness of this medication would be based on data indicating which of the following?

- **a.** increased motivation and improved social interaction
- **b.** decrease in hallucinations and paranoid thinking
- **c.** decreased agitation and excitement levels
- **d.** decreased depression and improved appetite and sleep patterns

93. A client taking the monoamine oxidase inhibitor (MAOI) antidepressant isocarboxazid (Marplan) is instructed by the nurse to avoid which of the following foods containing tyramine?

- **a.** aged cheese, caffeinated beverages
- **b.** milk products, green leafy vegetables
- **c.** citrus fruits, nuts
- **d.** lean red meats, dried fruits

94. A client who has been taking amitriptyline (Elavil) for depression for the past 7 days reports no improvement from this drug and wonders if it should be should be continued. The nurse's response would be based on which of the following data?

- **a.** The drug's onset of action is 24 to 48 hours.
- **b.** The drug's onset of action is 2 to 3 weeks.
- **c.** The drug's effect may be diminished in major depression.
- **d.** The drug's effect may not always be reliably observed by the client.

95. The nurse would consider which of the following as a potential nursing diagnosis for an elderly man taking imipramine (Tofranil) for depression?

- **a.** Ineffective Airway Clearance
- **b.** Risk for Infection
- **c.** Altered Urinary Elimination
- **d.** Fluid Volume Deficit

Answer Sheet for Comprehensive Exam

With a pencil, blacken the circle under the option you have chosen for your correct answer.

No.				
1.	A ○	B ○	C ○	D ○
2.	A ○	B ○	C ○	D ○
3.	A ○	B ○	C ○	D ○
4.	A ○	B ○	C ○	D ○
5.	A ○	B ○	C ○	D ○
6.	A ○	B ○	C ○	D ○
7.	A ○	B ○	C ○	D ○
8.	A ○	B ○	C ○	D ○
9.	A ○	B ○	C ○	D ○
10.	A ○	B ○	C ○	D ○
11.	A ○	B ○	C ○	D ○
12.	A ○	B ○	C ○	D ○
13.	A ○	B ○	C ○	D ○
14.	A ○	B ○	C ○	D ○
15.	A ○	B ○	C ○	D ○
16.	A ○	B ○	C ○	D ○
17.	A ○	B ○	C ○	D ○
18.	A ○	B ○	C ○	D ○
19.	A ○	B ○	C ○	D ○
20.	A ○	B ○	C ○	D ○
21.	A ○	B ○	C ○	D ○
22.	A ○	B ○	C ○	D ○
23.	A ○	B ○	C ○	D ○
24.	A ○	B ○	C ○	D ○
25.	A ○	B ○	C ○	D ○
26.	A ○	B ○	C ○	D ○
27.	A ○	B ○	C ○	D ○
28.	A ○	B ○	C ○	D ○
29.	A ○	B ○	C ○	D ○
30.	A ○	B ○	C ○	D ○
31.	A ○	B ○	C ○	D ○
32.	A ○	B ○	C ○	D ○
33.	A ○	B ○	C ○	D ○
34.	A ○	B ○	C ○	D ○
35.	A ○	B ○	C ○	D ○
36.	A ○	B ○	C ○	D ○
37.	A ○	B ○	C ○	D ○
38.	A ○	B ○	C ○	D ○
39.	A ○	B ○	C ○	D ○
40.	A ○	B ○	C ○	D ○
41.	A ○	B ○	C ○	D ○
42.	A ○	B ○	C ○	D ○
43.	A ○	B ○	C ○	D ○
44.	A ○	B ○	C ○	D ○
45.	A ○	B ○	C ○	D ○
46.	A ○	B ○	C ○	D ○
47.	A ○	B ○	C ○	D ○
48.	A ○	B ○	C ○	D ○
49.	A ○	B ○	C ○	D ○
50.	A ○	B ○	C ○	D ○
51.	A ○	B ○	C ○	D ○
52.	A ○	B ○	C ○	D ○
53.	A ○	B ○	C ○	D ○
54.	A ○	B ○	C ○	D ○
55.	A ○	B ○	C ○	D ○
56.	A ○	B ○	C ○	D ○
57.	A ○	B ○	C ○	D ○
58.	A ○	B ○	C ○	D ○
59.	A ○	B ○	C ○	D ○
60.	A ○	B ○	C ○	D ○

61.	A ○	B ○	C ○	D ○	**73.**	A ○	B ○	C ○	D ○	**85.**	A ○	B ○	C ○	D ○
62.	A ○	B ○	C ○	D ○	**74.**	A ○	B ○	C ○	D ○	**86.**	A ○	B ○	C ○	D ○
63.	A ○	B ○	C ○	D ○	**75.**	A ○	B ○	C ○	D ○	**87.**	A ○	B ○	C ○	D ○
64.	A ○	B ○	C ○	D ○	**76.**	A ○	B ○	C ○	D ○	**88.**	A ○	B ○	C ○	D ○
65.	A ○	B ○	C ○	D ○	**77.**	A ○	B ○	C ○	D ○	**89.**	A ○	B ○	C ○	D ○
66.	A ○	B ○	C ○	D ○	**78.**	A ○	B ○	C ○	D ○	**90.**	A ○	B ○	C ○	D ○
67.	A ○	B ○	C ○	D ○	**79.**	A ○	B ○	C ○	D ○	**91.**	A ○	B ○	C ○	D ○
68.	A ○	B ○	C ○	D ○	**80.**	A ○	B ○	C ○	D ○	**92.**	A ○	B ○	C ○	D ○
69.	A ○	B ○	C ○	D ○	**81.**	A ○	B ○	C ○	D ○	**93.**	A ○	B ○	C ○	D ○
70.	A ○	B ○	C ○	D ○	**82.**	A ○	B ○	C ○	D ○	**94.**	A ○	B ○	C ○	D ○
71.	A ○	B ○	C ○	D ○	**83.**	A ○	B ○	C ○	D ○	**95.**	A ○	B ○	C ○	D ○
72.	A ○	B ○	C ○	D ○	**84.**	A ○	B ○	C ○	D ○					

COMPREHENSIVE TEST—ANSWER KEY

1. ***Correct response: b***
Under voluntary admission it is still necessary for a person to submit a written notice of intent to leave before formal discharge. This safeguard allows the treatment facility time to file for involuntary admission if the person is judged dangerous to self or others.
- **a.** This is the usual criteria for involuntary admissions.
- **c.** An individual retains his or her civil rights during any type of psychiatric admission.
- **d.** This is the usual period for emergency involuntary admission.

Application/Psychosocial/Analysis

2. ***Correct response: b***
Members of a particular cultural group share similar patterns of behavior, values, and beliefs. This in turn affects a client's thinking process, feeling responses, and manner of behavior.
- **a and c.** Although these may be true, they are not a complete answer. Choice *b* encompasses both of these choices.
- **d.** Although some diagnosed mental illnesses are more common in members of a particular cultural *group*, this fact will not help the nurse provide culturally sensitive care.

Comprehension/Psychosocial/Analysis

3. ***Correct response: c***
When a client speaks another language, an interpreter will help facilitate communication.
- **a.** Nonverbal communication is important; however, the client also needs to be able to verbalize thoughts and feelings to the nurse.
- **b.** Validating is an important therapeutic technique when relating to persons of a different culture. However, the technique requires verbal communication.
- **d.** Pictures can aid in communication of basic needs; however, they do not facilitate communication in other areas.

Application/Safe care/Assessment

4. ***Correct response: b***
Native Americans often believe in the special healing abilities of a religious shaman. The client's request is congruent with cultural beliefs and should be honored. The nurse can help facilitate this request by acting as the client's advocate.
- **a.** This is a value judgment on the nurse's part. It is not appropriate to tell the client this.
- **c.** Ignoring this request would be disrespectful and nonaccepting of the client's beliefs. This would damage the nurse-client relationship.
- **d.** This would be an interpretive response based on the nurse's belief system. It does not accurately reflect the client's culture.

Application/Psychosocial/Implementation

5. ***Correct response: d***
Termination is an important phase in the therapeutic relationship, during which the nurse and client reassess the client's progress, evaluate goal attainment, and explore how the therapeutic relationship was experienced. It is also important to deal with feelings about termination during this phase.
- **a.** Assessment would be an ongoing part of the therapeutic relationship and would occur in all phases.
- **b and c.** These phases of the relationship are characterized by establishing trust (orientation) and planning outcomes and interventions to assist the client to meet goals (working).

Comprehension/Psychosocial/Implementation

6. ***Correct response: c***
Tertiary prevention involves minimizing long-term residual effects of illness. Such things as rehabilitation programs,

vocational training, aftercare support, and partial hospitalization programs all provide this level of care.

a. Primary prevention involves altering causative or risk factors to prevent the development of illness.

b. Secondary prevention focuses on reducing or minimizing effects of illness in acute stages.

d. Premorbid refers to a state before the onset of an illness. This is not a classified level of care.

Application/Health promotion/Evaluation

7. ***Correct response: b***

The structural model of communication consists of sender, receiver, message, context, and feedback loop. Feedback refers to the receiver's verbal and/or behavioral response.

a and d. The client's verbal and nonverbal behavior does constitute a response.

c. The nurse is the sender of the message.

Comprehension/Psychosocial/Assessment

8. ***Correct response: c***

When a client makes vague, global statements, the therapeutic approach is to seek clarification. Seeking clarification helps the client become more aware of thoughts, feelings, and ideas.

a, b, and d. None of these responses would be therapeutic.

Application/Psychosocial/Implementation

9. ***Correct response: b***

Placing a client in a treatment setting with more restrictions than necessary violates the client's rights.

a, c, and d. These also are client rights but are not applicable in this situation.

Comprehension/Safe care/Evaluation

10. ***Correct response: a***

The ANA's Standards of Psychiatric and Mental Health Practice call for peer review as a mechanism for maintaining quality care. In the situation described, it would be better if a formal peer review system were in place to evaluate the nurse's performance. However, the colleagues are correct in expressing their concerns to the supervisor.

b, c, and d. These responses do not address the nurses' responsibilities for upholding professional standards of practice.

Application/Safe care/Evaluation

11. ***Correct response: c***

Maslow views human development as a process of needs fulfillment. Basic physiologic and safety needs must be met before a person can grow toward psychologic and spiritual fulfillment. The nurse's first priority would be to help this client meet basic needs.

a, b, and d. These theorists view human development in terms of chronologic stages.

Application/Physiologic/Intervention

12. ***Correct response: a***

Behavioral theory views maladaptive behavior as a learned response that is reinforced in the environment.

b. Education is not a theoretical framework.

c. The psychodynamic framework views maladaptive behavior as an interpsychic or interpersonal process.

d. The cognitive framework views maladaptive behavior as the result of faulty thought patterns.

Comprehension/Psychosocial/Assessment

13. ***Correct response: b***

Using contracts specifying acceptable and unacceptable behavior involves behavioral framework. Using medications to alter neurotransmitter activity is a psychobiologic approach to treatment.

a, c, and d. These are other frameworks for care; they are not applicable to this situation.

Comprehension/Psychosocial/Analysis

14. ***Correct response: c***

The concept that behavior is motivated and has meaning comes from the psychodynamic framework. According to this perspective, behavior arises from internal wishes or needs. Much of what motivates behavior comes from the unconscious.

a, b, and d. These responses do not address the internal forces thought to motivate behavior.

Comprehension/Psychosocial/Analysis

15. *Correct response: b*

Sullivan believed that a child develops a sense of self from the appraisal received from significant others. The mother's increased anxiety levels will be internalized by the infant.

a, c, and d. These theorists place less emphasis on interpersonal aspects of development.

Knowledge/Psychosocial/Analysis

16. *Correct response: a*

Even though the client can return to work, the client persists in thinking of himself or herself as a failure who will be unable to work. According to cognitive theory, negative thoughts, such as these, will keep the client feeling depressed.

b, c, and d. These are not cognitive explanations of depressions.

Application/Psychosocial/Assessment

17. *Correct response: d*

Both negative and positive life changes and developmental events are considered stressful.

a, c, and d. These are correct but incomplete answers.

Knowledge/Psychosocial/Assessment

18. *Correct response: d*

Selye's theory describes how the body responds to stress. There are three stages: the first stage is the alarm reaction; the second is resistance; and the third is exhaustion if the stress continues.

a, b, and c. General adaptation theory does not address these areas.

Knowledge/Physiologic/Assessment

19. *Correct response: d*

The nurse acknowledges the behavior observed and then asks the client to express his or her feelings. This approach will assist the client in becoming aware of anxious feelings.

a. The nurse is offering an interpretation that may or may not be accurate. The nurse is also asking a question that may be answered by a yes or no response.

b. The nurse is intervening before accurately assessing the problem.

c. This statement, which can be answered by a yes or no response, does not encourage the client to focus on anxiety.

Comprehension/Psychosocial/Implementation

20. *Correct response: a*

Flashbacks and nightmares from past experiences are common in post-traumatic stress disorder. Clients with this disorder respond with intense fear to these events.

b and d. The data are insufficient to establish either of these nursing diagnoses.

c. The fear is known in post-traumatic stress disorder and is directly related to the traumatic events precipitating this disorder.

Knowledge/Psychosocial/Analysis (Dx)

21. *Correct response: b*

The fear of having a serious disease is the essential feature of a person diagnosed with hypochondriasis.

a. This may be a symptom of a somatoform disorder but is not the most typical of hypochondriasis.

c and d. These statements could apply to many of the psychiatric disorders.

Knowledge/Psychosocial/Assessment

22. *Correct response: d*

Anxiety is a response to a threat arising from internal or external stimuli.

a, b, and c. These statements are untrue.

Knowledge/Psychosocial/Assessment

23. ***Correct response: a***
Systematic desensitization is a behavioral therapy technique that helps clients with irrational fears and avoidance behavior to face the thing they fear without anxiety.

b. There is no attempt to promote insight with this procedure.

c. The client will not be taught to substitute one fear for another.

d. The client's anxiety may decrease with successful confrontation of irrational fears. However, the purpose of the procedure is specifically related to performing activities that typically are avoided as part of the phobic response.

Application/Psychosocial/Evaluation

24. ***Correct response: c***
The client with obsessive-compulsive behavior uses this behavior to decrease anxiety. The nurse accepts this behavior as the client's attempt to feel secure. When a specific treatment plan is developed, other nursing responses may also be acceptable.

a, c, and d. These are all responses that will increase client anxiety and therefore are not appropriate.

Application/Psychosocial/Implementation

25. ***Correct response: d***
These are all characteristic of generalized anxiety disorder.

a, c, and d. These are not symptoms of generalized anxiety disorder but are related to other psychiatric disorders.

Knowledge/Psychosocial/Assessment

26. ***Correct response: a***
By developing a new personality, the child dissociates from the stress of abuse.

b. In multiple personality, the emerging personality takes full control of the personality. The individual is not usually aware of the other personality.

c. Multiple personality disorder represents a coping problem, not a concentration problem.

d. The new personality is not permanent; rather, the person switches between personalities.

Comprehension/Psychosocial/Analysis

27. ***Correct response: d***
Work history is not as relevant to the sexual problem as are the other areas. The sexual problem can be diagnosed without knowing work history.

a. Physical examination is necessary to determine any physical origins of the problem.

b. Certain medications affect sexual functioning; this is essential information.

c. Sexual history provides needed information about the history of the current problem and the adequacy of past sexual functioning.

Knowledge/Psychosocial/Assessment

28. ***Correct response: a***
The client indicates that she wants to be heterosexual and that she has lesbian feelings. Her conflict needs to be explored so she can identify her sexual orientation.

b. It may or may not be therapeutic to include her parents at this time.

c and d. These criteria are incorrect because the client has not yet identified her sexual orientation.

Analysis/Psychosocial/Evaluation

29. ***Correct response: a***
Intense emotions are easily communicated to others, including the nurse. Self-awareness and support for the nurse is important to avoid countertransference reactions.

b, c, and d. These factors will not help the client learn to modify explosive, intense behavior.

Application/Safe care/Planning

30. ***Correct response: d***
This outcome indicates improvement in behavior patterns typical of antisocial personality disorders.

a, b, and c. These outcomes do not represent positive changes in behaviors.

Comprehension/Safe care/Evaluation

31. ***Correct response: d***

Typically, the client with anorexia nervosa has physical symptoms that are caused by starvation.

a, b, and c. These symptoms are not typical of the physical problems of clients with anorexia nervosa.

Application/Safe care/Assessment

32. ***Correct response: d***

The person with anorexia nervosa usually feels little control over any aspect of life besides eating behavior. Often, parental expectations and standards are quite high and lead to the client's sense of guilt over not measuring up.

a, b, and c. The situation does not provide evidence of criteria for these nursing diagnoses, even though they may be applicable to a client with anorexia nervosa.

Application/Psychosocial/Analysis (Dx)

33. ***Correct response: c***

Inpatient treatment for a client with anorexia nervosa will focus first on establishing a plan for re-feeding the client to combat the effects of self-induced starvation. Behavioral therapy will use a system of rewards and reinforcements to assist re-feeding.

a and d. These implementations may be appropriate at a later time in the treatment program.

b. The nurse needs to assess the client's mealtime behavior continually to evaluate treatment effectiveness.

Application/Psychosocial/Implementation

34. ***Correct response: d***

In psychophysiologic disorders, stress and the response to stress can exacerbate symptoms. Therefore, stress management will help the client reduce physiologic and psychologic responses to stress and increase a sense of control over symptoms.

a. The nurse would not be the medical professional initiating a program of biofeedback, although the nurse may have a role in this intervention.

b and c. These may be areas in which the nurse teaches the clients; however, they will not increase the client's sense of control.

Application/Safe care/Implementation

35. ***Correct response: b***

The nurse should avoid reinforcing any secondary gains the client with a somatoform disorder may get from the physical symptoms.

a. Physical complaints need to be evaluated by the nurse because organic pathology may be possible with this client.

c and d. These would be helpful to the client with a somatoform disorder and would be appropriate nursing care.

Application/Safe care/Planning

36. ***Correct response: a***

One of the essential issues in the family of a client with anorexia nervosa is the issue of control. When the client can make independent decisions and the parents can accept this, family intervention has been successful.

b, c, and d. These responses may occur during the process of therapy, but would not indicate successful outcome. The central family issue of dependence/independence is not addressed in these responses.

Comprehension/Psychosocial/Evaluation

37. ***Correct response: d***

The client with a somatoform disorder displaces anxiety onto physical symptoms. The ability to verbally express anxiety indicates a positive change toward increased health.

a, b, and c. These responses do not indicate any positive change toward increased coping with anxiety.

Knowledge/Psychosocial/Planning

38. ***Correct response: d***

Disregard for established rules of society is the most common characteristic of a client with an antisocial personality disorder.

a, b, and c. These characteristics occur in obsessive-compulsive, schizoid or schizotypal, and dependent personality disorder, respectively.

Comprehension/Psychosocial/Assessment

39. ***Correct response: d***

A matter-of-fact approach and exploration of new ways to relate may assist the client in modifying behavior.

a and b. These responses would be inappropriate because this client is not sincerely attending to the nurse or others.

c. This approach would not elicit a sincere answer or facilitate new behavior.

Analysis/Safe Care/Implementation

40. ***Correct response: b***

Behavioral changes often are subtle in persons with personality disorders.

a and d. These are incorrect statements.

c. This statement could be true, but it would not be the reason for the difficult evaluation.

Comprehension/Psychosocial/Evaluation

41. ***Correct response: c***

Physiologic changes expected with depression include significant decrease or increase in appetite as well as insomnia or hypersomnia.

a, b, and d. These changes are not typical for a client with a diagnosis of major depression.

Application/Psychosocial/Assessment

42. ***Correct response: c***

Direct questioning of the client about suicide is important to determine risk.

a. The client may not bring up this subject for several reasons: guilt regarding suicide; wish not to be discovered; lack of trust in staff.

b. Behavioral cues are important but direct questioning is essential to determine suicide risk.

d. Indirect questions convey to the client that the nurse is not comfortable with the subject of suicide and therefore the client may be reluctant to discuss this.

Application/Safe care/Implementation

43. ***Correct response: a***

Accepting the client's feelings without trying to change them conveys empathy.

b and c. Challenging and denying client's feelings will belittle the client and convey that the nurse does not understand the depth of client's distress.

d. Cheering the client is not possible at this time; improvement will cheer the client.

Comprehension/Psychosocial/Planning

44. ***Correct response: b***

Spending brief periods with the client communicates respect, acceptance, and understanding.

a, c, and d. These approaches would not be helpful at this time.

Application/Safe Care/Implementation

45. ***Correct response: c***

The nurse should take any statements indicating suicidal thoughts seriously and further assess for other risk factors.

a, b, and d. These diagnoses fail to address the seriousness of the client's statement.

Analysis/Safe care/Analysis (Dx)

46. ***Correct response: c***

Flight of ideas occurs when the client's flow of speech is continuous and the client jumps from one topic to another. The client who can speak in coherent sentences shows that concentration has improved and thoughts are no longer racing.

a, b, and d. These outcomes do not relate directly to the stated nursing diagnosis.

Comprehension/Psychosocial/Evaluation

47. ***Correct response: a***

Discharge planning involves specifically delineating the outpatient treatment regimen for the client.

b, c, and d. These plans do not address continued treatment after discharge.

Knowledge/Psychosocial/Planning

48. ***Correct response: c***

This response gives the nurse and the client an opportunity to negotiate on one aspect of the inappropriate behavior. The nurse is including the client in the planning and assisting the client in regulating behavior.

a, b, and d. These responses do not promote client self-esteem and ability to control behavior nor do they offer alternatives for acceptable behavior.

Application/Psychosocial/Implementation

49. ***Correct response: c***

As with many illnesses, a combination of genetic, biologic, and environmental factors is thought to contribute to schizophrenia.

a. This is no longer believed to be the cause—past family research has been deemed inconclusive because no control groups were used.

b and d. These are currently areas of research; however, they are not the sole causes of schizophrenia. It is the combination of various factors that appears to be significant.

Knowledge/Psychosocial/Planning

50. ***Correct response: a***

Sometimes clients do not admit to altered perceptions. The nurse should observe how the client functions in the environment and look for subtle cues about how the client interprets the environment.

b. This answer is not as comprehensive as that given in *a*.

c and d. These responses are not related to the question asked.

Comprehension/Psychosocial/Analysis (Dx)

51. ***Correct response: a***

Under this outcome, goal-specific behaviors that demonstrate realistic interpretation could be listed.

b. Hygiene and grooming skills are not necessarily impaired when a client distorts the environment.

c and d. These could be components of response *a*.

Application/Psychosocial/Planning

52. ***Correct response: c***

Firm, nonpunitive limit-setting and a structured environment are the best approach to a verbally hostile client.

a and b. These measures are too severe, considering that the outbursts are brief and there is no escalation to physical violence.

d. This approach would not be as useful as setting a clear limit on inappropriate behavior, along with a structured, predictable environment.

Application/Safe care/Implementation

53. ***Correct response: a***

The best approach with a withdrawn client is to initiate brief, nondemanding activities on a one-to-one basis. This gives the nurse an opportunity to establish a trusting relationship with the client.

b and c. These approaches will overwhelm a severely withdrawn client.

d. Activities are a therapeutic approach used to help the client reenter reality.

Application/Psychosocial/Implementation

54. ***Correct response: b***

The best approach to delusional ideas is to avoid arguing with them while acknowledging reality. It is also important to respond to the underlying message or affect. In this case, the client is frightened, so the nurse addresses that by saying she believes the client is safe here.

a. This response would be premature. When the client is better, it may be possible to discuss delusions as part of the illness.

c and d. These responses place too much emphasis on the delusions.

Application/Safe care/Implementation

55. ***Correct response: c***

Depersonalization is a feeling of strangeness or unreality about one's own body or body parts.

a. Autism is a focus inward; the individual may create a fantasy world.

b. Ambivalence is having strong opposing emotions about a person or situation.

d. Regression is a defense mechanism whereby the individual returns to an earlier, more comfortable form of behavior.

Knowledge/Psychosocial/Assessment

56. ***Correct response: a***

Alcohol dependence is characterized by an increase in the amount of alcohol consumed, the inability to control consumption, physical complications, and blackouts.

b and d. These are subsumed under alcohol dependence.

c. Blackouts and tolerance are not characteristic of alcohol abuse.

Analysis/Psychosocial/Analysis (Dx)

57. ***Correct response: c***

The statement that drinking occurs because of a nagging spouse is an example of rationalization, justification for the drinking.

a, b, and d. Neither projection, sublimation, nor displacement occurs in this situation.

Comprehension/Psychosocial/Analysis (Dx)

58. ***Correct response: b***

This indicates that the client has stopped using denial and accepts that substance abuse creates personal problems.

a and c. These statements do not indicate acceptance of the fact that substance use causes personal problems.

d. The substance abuser can participate in therapies without giving up the defense mechanism of denial.

Application/Psychosocial/Evaluation

59. ***Correct response: c***

Tolerance is the need for increased amounts of substance to obtain a desired effect. It is one of the characteristics of substance dependence.

a. This is polydrug use.

b. This would be the criteria for substance dependence.

d. This is the phenomenon of withdrawal.

Knowledge/Psychosocial/Assessment

60. ***Correct response: a***

Withdrawal is characterized by CNS excitation when alcohol is abruptly stopped. Vital sign changes occur early, 6 to 12 hours after the last drink.

b and c. These responses do not occur in withdrawal from alcohol.

d. This would occur in intoxication rather than withdrawal.

Application/Psychosocial/Assessment

61. ***Correct response: b***

The nurse's attitudes can impact on the treatment of the client. Negative attitudes can be indirectly communicated and can damage the client's self-esteem.

a and c. Neither of these should be the first intervention, and they should be done only when the nurse can demonstrate respect and a nonjudgmental attitude.

d. This is incorrect as the first intervention, although it may prove helpful for the nurse who lacks information about female addicts.

Application/Safe care/Planning

62. ***Correct response: b***

Babies born to heroin-dependent women are also dependent and need to go through withdrawal.

a, c, and d. There is no evidence to support any of these claims.

Knowledge/Safe care/Planning

63. ***Correct response: d***
Observers are affected by dysfunction in family system and often require help in coping with their emotional responses.
a. Nonvictims are involved passively and can assist in resolving family difficulties.
b. Available data do not support the assumption that nonvictims are more traumatized.
c. This approach supports family alienation and may not be indicated in most cases.
Analysis/Psychosocial/Planning

64. ***Correct response: c***
Difficulty with intrafamilial communication can be explored and altered in therapy in which all family members participate.
a, b, and d. Although dyadic sessions with either the survivor or the abuser (or both) may be indicated to work on individual issues, private therapy is not the most expeditious way of addressing family communications.
Application/Psychosocial/Implementation

65. ***Correct response: a***
Psychodynamic theories identify the need to resolve conflicts associated with history of abuse and impaired impulse control as predisposing factors for abusive behavior.
b. Social learning theory stresses impaired learning resulting from dysfunctional examples.
c and d. These are not factors in psychodynamic theory.
Analysis/Psychosocial/Planning

66. ***Correct response: d***
Socioeconomic status is not a reliable predictor of abuse in the home environment.
a. A safe, supportive environment for abuse survivors is a valuable consideration in this decision.
b. The nurse should identify family strengths and resources available to the client.
c. An abuse victim's trauma can be compounded by feelings of guilt and (unreasonable) responsibility if only the abuser leaves the home environment.
Application/Safe care/Analysis

67. ***Correct response: b***
These would be common behaviors in clients with conduct disorders.
a. These are typical behaviors in a client with attention deficit-hyperactivity disorder.
c and d. These behaviors are typical in schizophrenic and depressive disorders, respectively.
Knowledge/Psychosocial/Assessment

68. ***Correct response: a***
Developmental theory is basic to understanding childhood and adolescent disorders. Deviation from developmental norms is considered significant in diagnosing these disorders.
b, c, and d. Although these theories may be useful to the nurse, they are not essential.
Comprehension/Safe care/Planning

69. ***Correct response: d***
In working with conflicts between parents and children the nurse needs to establish a position of neutrality. This will promote trust and allow the family to negotiate reasonable solutions.
a, b, and c. All of these are appropriate nursing responses and helpful to the entire family.
Application/Psychosocial/Implementation

70. ***Correct response: a***
Deficits in intellectual functioning are among the earliest changes in the cognitive impairment disorder of Alzheimer's disease. Complex tasks, such as balancing a checkbook, confuse the client.
b. This task is relatively simple, relying on automatic functioning. Loss of the ability to accomplish tasks of

daily living, such as using a washing machine, would be expected to occur later in the disease.

c and d. Relating to family members and remembering one's own name would also be expected to occur late in the disease.

Comprehension/Psychosocial/Assessment

71. ***Correct response: b***

Delirium is an acute cognitive impairment with rapid onset, which may be reversible with prompt treatment.

a, c, and d. These statements are incorrect. Dementia is a chronic cognitive impairment that has slow, insidious onset. Treatment is difficult and often the most that can be achieved is to slow the progression of the disorder.

Comprehension/Psychosocial/Assessment

72. ***Correct response: d***

Multiple stimuli increase the client's anxiety level and contribute to emotional lability. Decreasing the stimuli helps to reduce anxiety and direct attention away from the anxiety-producing stimulus.

a, b, and c. These responses all require intellectual processing and would be difficult for the client with Alzheimer's disease.

Application/Safe care/Implementation

73. ***Correct response: b***

A deficiency of the neurotransmitter acetylcholine has been associated with the cerebral nerve cell degeneration characteristic of Alzheimer's disease.

a, c, and d. Although all these substances are neurotransmitters, they have not been associated with the pathophysiology of Alzheimer's disease.

Knowledge/Psychosocial/Planning

74. ***Correct response: c***

The client's daughter is identifying characteristics typical of a caretaker who is becoming overwhelmed with this role. Feelings of stress in relationship with the care receiver as well as depression and possibly anger are related to the long-term role of caretaker.

a and b. Although the family may be experiencing altered processes and ineffective coping, the caregiver is currently identifying self-feelings of being overwhelmed.

d. There is no evidence that the caregiver is socially isolated in this situation.

Comprehension/Psychosocial/Analysis (Dx)

75. ***Correct response: c***

The three factors considered to affect the equilibrium of a person in crisis are perception of the event, situational support, and coping skills.

a, c, and d. These are other factors not necessarily emphasized within the crisis model.

Knowledge/Psychosocial/Assessment

76. ***Correct response: a***

The first stage of grieving consists of shock and disbelief. In this phase, the family tries to realize that their loved one is dead.

b. These actions are more typical of the second phase of grieving.

c and d. These actions typically occur after grief is resolved.

Comprehension/Psychosocial/Assessment

77. ***Correct response: b***

A crisis persisting for more than 3 months usually indicates a more serious problem requiring more help than is given in the typical crisis intervention approach.

a, c, and d. These analyses may or may not be true in this situation; not enough information is given about this situation.

Comprehension/Psychosocial/Analysis

78. ***Correct response: d***

Crisis intervention is based on the idea that a crisis is a disturbance in a steady state. The goal is to help the person return to a previous level of equilibrium in terms of functioning.

a, b, and c. These are not considered the primary outcome of crisis intervention, although they may occur as a side benefit.

Comprehension/Psychosocial/Evaluation

79. *Correct response: b*

The initiation phase is characterized by increased anxiety and uncertainty.

a, c, and d. Group members are more self-reliant in these phases.

Comprehension/Psychosocial/Assessment

80. *Correct response: b*

The use of the pronouns "our" and "we" enhances the sense of the group as a viable unit. The nurse is also clarifying the purpose of the group.

a and c. This response doesn't restrict group spontaneity and it does address group norms.

d. The purpose of group therapy is not to prevent conflict but rather to work on resolving problem areas.

Application/Psychosocial/Implementation

81. *Correct response: a*

As the group progresses into the working phase, group members assume more responsibility for the group. The leader becomes more of a facilitator. Comments about behavior in group are good indicators that the group is active and involved.

b, c, and d. These actions would indicate group progress has not advanced to the working phase.

Analysis/Psychosocial/Evaluation

82. *Correct response: b*

During the termination phase, group members need to evaluate the progress of the group and themselves.

a and d. These actions would fail to handle the issue of termination by denying and avoiding it, respectively.

c. This response would fail to deal with all the issues of termination (ie, both negative and positive experiences are to be reviewed).

Application/Psychosocial/Evaluation

83. *Correct response: b*

The nurse's own feelings and thoughts can have a negative impact on the therapeutic relationship. If the nurse finds that being therapeutic is not possible, then referral of the couple is necessary.

a, c, and d. These responses are inappropriate and reflect the nurse's biases.

Knowledge/Psychosocial/Implementation

84. *Correct response: c*

In good family communication, family members openly encourage clear, direct discussions of issues and feelings. Members identify their feelings and thoughts as important and valued and they are able to initiate discussion.

a. This may not validate that good communication is present. Children may adopt the parental value system in a family where communication is maladaptive.

b. Agreement among family members may not indicate good communication. Members may be enmeshed, in which case individuals are not free to express differences.

d. Parents may feel that they communicate to their children, however, good communication requires feedback. The nurse must further assess whether children can communicate freely to the parents.

Comprehension/Psychosocial/Assessment

85. *Correct response: d*

In a functional family, parents are not expected to agree on all issues and problems. Open discussion of thoughts and feelings is healthy, and parental disagreement in and of itself should not be expected to cause system stress.

a, b, and c. All of these events are life transition occurrences and are expected to increase stress on the family system.

Knowledge/Psychosocial/Assessment

86. *Correct response: a*

The nurse working with families must remain neutral and objective and avoid taking sides. This response will allow the nurse to remain neutral and will also encourage family members to communicate.

b and c. These responses indicate that the nurse has chosen to agree with either the adolescent or the parents on this issue.

d. This response would be avoiding an issue and missing an opportunity to encourage family communication.

Application/Psychosocial/Implementation

87. ***Correct response: b***

These are classic symptoms of dystonia.

a. The specificity of symptoms is more definitive of dystonia than of tension.

c. Parkinsonian symptoms include akinesia or generalized rigidity, drooling, pill-rolling.

d. Toxicity to antipsychotics, which is rare, develops over the course of days. Symptoms are characterized by high fever, muscle rigidity, hypertension, diaphoresis.

Application/Safe care/Analysis

88. ***Correct response: b***

The use of diuretics would cause sodium and water excretion, which would increase risk of toxicity. Clients taking lithium carbonate should be taught to increase their fluid intake and maintain normal intake of sodium.

a, c, and d. There is no information indicating any difficulty with concurrent use of these medications with lithium.

Application/Safe care/Planning

89. ***Correct response: a***

Dry mouth and urine retention indicate that the client is experiencing anticholinergic side effects.

b, c, and d. These are all symptoms of extrapyramidal side effects; they are known as oculogyric crisis, akathisia, and pseudoparkinsonism, respectively.

Application/Safe care/Assessment

90. ***Correct response: d***

Diazepam (Valium) is an anxiolytic agent used to treat anxiety. It does not have any antidepressant activity. The client, if experiencing depression, needs to discuss this new symptom, and the nurse needs to investigate it further.

a. Diazepam is characterized by the potential to become addictive.

b. Abrupt cessation of this drug can precipitate withdrawal symptoms.

c. Diazepam will depress the CNS; when mixed with alcohol or another CNS depressant, the drug can cause severe levels of CNS depression.

Application/Safe care/ Evaluation

91. ***Correct response: c***

Chlorpromazine (Thorazine) can cause a significant hypotensive effect. Blood pressure (lying, sitting, and standing) should be assessed before administering this drug.

a. Although jaundice can be a side effect of this drug (which may cause an elevated bilirubin level), the information in this question does not indicate that the client has had this drug before.

b. Pulse rate can be affected by this drug (which may cause tachycardia). However, blood pressure evaluation would be the essential implementation because postural blood pressure changes can lead to client injury.

d. The drug can cause urine retention, but asking the client to void will not alter this anticholinergic side effect.

Application/Safe care/Implementation

92. ***Correct response: a***

Clozapine (Clozaril), one of the newer, atypical antipsychotic medications, is used to reduce the negative symptoms of schizophrenia (lack of motivation, anergia, impaired social interaction).

b. These are considered positive symptoms of schizophrenia and are more effectively treated with standard neuroleptics (antipsychotics).

c. This drug is not used for clients

who are experiencing these problems.

d. This drug is not an antidepressant and, therefore, would not be used to improve mood, sleep, or appetite problems.

Application/Psychosocial/Evaluation

93. ***Correct response: a***

These foods contain the substance tyramine which, when taken with an MAOI, can precipitate a hypertensive crisis.

b, c, and d. These foods do not contain significant amounts of tyramine and, therefore, are not restricted.

Knowledge/Safe care/Implementation

94. ***Correct response: b***

The onset of action of the tricyclic antidepressant amitriptyline occurs around 2 or 3 weeks after drug therapy begins. Therefore, a client will seldom notice improvement before this time. Continuing to take the drug will be important for this client.

a, c, and d. These responses are not true.

Comprehension/Psychosocial/Analysis

95. ***Correct response: c***

A side effect of imipramine, a tricyclic antidepressant, is urine retention. This may be a problem, especially for an elderly man who may have prostatic enlargement.

a. The drug would have no effect on the client's airway.

b and d. The drug would not predispose the client to infection or loss of fluid volume.

Knowledge/Safe care/Assessment

Index

Page numbers followed by *f* indicate figures; those followed by *t* indicate tabular material; those followed by *d* indicate displays.

M

N

O

P

Q

R

Heritage of China

Heritage of China:

□

Contemporary Perspectives on Chinese Civilization

EDITED BY

Paul S. Ropp

CONTRIBUTORS

T. H. Barrett · Jack L. Dull · Patricia Ebrey
Albert Feuerwerker · David N. Keightley · Stephen Owen
Paul S. Ropp · William T. Rowe · Nathan Sivin
Jonathan Spence · Michael Sullivan · Tu Wei-ming
Karen Turner

UNIVERSITY OF CALIFORNIA PRESS
Berkeley Los Angeles Oxford

University of California Press
Berkeley and Los Angeles, California

University of California Press, Ltd.
Oxford, England

Library of Congress Cataloging-in-Publication Data

Heritage of China : contemporary perspectives on Chinese civilization / edited by Paul S. Ropp ; contributors, T. H. Barrett . . . [et al.].
p. cm.
Includes bibliographical references.
ISBN 0-520-06440-2 (alk. paper).—ISBN 0-520-06441-0 (pbk. : alk. paper)
1. China—Civilization. I. Ropp, Paul S., 1944– . II. Barrett, Timothy Hugh.
DS721.H45 1990
951—dc20 89-37365
CIP

Printed in the United States of America
1 2 3 4 5 6 7 8 9

The paper used in this publication meets the minimum requirements of American National Standard for Information Sciences—Permanence of Paper for Printed Library Materials, ANSI Z39.48-1984. ∞™

CONTENTS

ACKNOWLEDGMENTS

Many people and institutions have supported this volume. At Memphis State University, Assistant Dean of Arts and Sciences H. Delano Black first proposed a public program on Chinese civilization; Dean Jack Wakeley supported our idea of a three-day symposium; Academic Vice President Jerry N. Boone provided generous university funding; and History Chairs Maurice Crouse and Joseph Hawes facilitated the symposium and a whole series of related activities.

In the Memphis community, Betty Goff Cartwright, Emmaline Carrick, Bob Dalton, Larry Harris, and Alice R. M. Hyland provided essential support for the symposium. In addition to some of the authors of this volume, Chun-shu Chang, C. T. Hsia, Daniel Overmyer, Yung Wei, John E. Wills, Jr., and Ying Ruocheng all made valuable contributions to the symposium.

Most important, a generous grant from the National Endowment for the Humanities helped fund the symposium in 1984; in many ways it made this publication possible. Malcolm Richardson of the National Endowment has been a strong source of advice and support at every stage.

At the University of California Press Sheila Levine, Amy Klatzkin, Jay Plano, Lisa Banner, and Lillian Robyn have been indispensable in seeing the manuscript through the slow and painstaking process of publication.

The contributors to this volume have also been helpful and enjoyable collaborators, responding enthusiastically to the challenge facing them, offering essential advice on topics and contributors, and supporting our collective endeavor at every stage. Karen Turner of Holy Cross College has been especially helpful in reading and commenting on several chapters besides her own.

At Clark University Trudy Powers, secretary in the Department of History, has mastered two generations of word-processing systems while working on this project. Ann Gibson of Clark's Cartography Laboratory provided the maps in Appendix 1. Melinda Chan worked on the chronology of Chinese history in Appendix 2, and Tom Massey provided extremely helpful advice on the chronology and the guide to further reading in Appendix 3. Finally, my wife Marjorie, of Clark's Information Resource Center, deserves special thanks for her strong support of a seemingly endless project and for the countless times she rescued me at the computer.

I am grateful to all the above people and institutions for their support, but of course the signed contributors alone are responsible for the views expressed in the following chapters.

INTRODUCTION

Paul S. Ropp

The field of Chinese studies has expanded dramatically in the twentieth century, yet most of the insights generated in this field have been confined to the scholarly community of China specialists. The general public in the United States has become increasingly aware of China as the world's most populous country, as an important factor in American foreign policy, or as a potentially important economic actor on the world stage. But for most Westerners the long record of traditional Chinese civilization still seems a forbiddingly remote and esoteric subject. Our goal in this book is to portray for the general reader or the beginning student of China some of the diverse achievements and distinctive characteristics of traditional Chinese civilization, not for their economic or foreign policy implications but rather as significant elements of our common human experience.

All the chapters in this collection are in some sense comparative. We have tried to use comparisons not to suggest the superiority or inferiority of China or the West but to try to sharpen our understanding of both. For all of us, Chinese and Western alike, studying China becomes a form of self-discovery. In studying any culture comparatively one learns more about the range of possibilities in human experience, including the "roads not taken" in one's own culture. We may start out perceiving another culture's "oddness" but end up coming to see the oddness of our own. Oddness is by definition a culturally relative concept.

For all the dangers and potential crises we face in the late twentieth century, there has never been a more exciting time to study world cultures and world history. It has never been more exciting because it has never been more urgent, and there has never been a time with such an abundance and variety of information and study opportunities available. The study of China's past is just one part of this worldwide endeavor.

Chinese studies are particularly exciting today not only because of China's obvious importance but also because it is still a relatively new field for Westerners to study and because China's historical and archaeological records are so vast. So much is being written in Chinese studies today that one is nearly overwhelmed.

Our purpose in this volume, of course, is not to overwhelm but to stimulate the general reader and the beginning student of China. We hope to suggest some of the varieties of approaches to China's past that are being pursued today, to impart some broad but informed comparative generalizations regarding the main characteristics of Chinese civilization, to suggest important ways that the Chinese and Western experience of civilized life have been similar, different, mutually intertwined, or isolated and distinct, and to give some idea of the intellectual pleasures available in the study of China.

As the world's longest continuous civilization with the longest tradition of record-keeping and collection and with one of the most sophisticated and complex cultures the world has known, China really does deliver on that oft-made promise of modern life: something for everyone. As a contemporary Westerner studying Chinese history, I have always been struck by the ease with which one can be "swallowed up" in China's past. By "swallowed up" I do not mean the hopeless feeling of being buried under mountains of difficult-if-not-impossible-to-read texts (although this happens often enough!) but rather the feeling that one can have, even in the fast-moving contemporary United States, of the relevance and immediacy of China's past. By relevance I refer not to financial or foreign policy gain but to the relevance of understanding others to better understand oneself, of entering into an alien world far enough to feel at home, of appreciating the awe-inspiring achievements and noble ideals of Chinese culture while recognizing and regretting the presence also of injustice, shortcomings, and human frailty, and, perhaps most impressive of all, of observing the spirited perseverance of the Chinese people through the best and worst of times.

As a striking example of Western self-knowledge gained through the comparative study of China, consider a theme that emerges with great regularity in many of the following chapters: comparisons between traditional China and the contemporary West are usually very misleading because they ignore the enormous contrast between traditional and modern ways in the West itself. By comparing China and the West over a span of centuries, it becomes abundantly apparent that contemporary Western ways of living and thinking are of very recent origin. The social and economic systems, artistic and literary values, political structures, and philosophical assumptions that we take for granted in the Western world of the late twentieth century simply did not exist as recently as three or four centuries ago. They did not exist in the West or anywhere else.

Six of our chapters make this argument explicitly. Jack L. Dull notes the relatively recent development of democratic forms of government, even in the West. Nathan Sivin points out both the uniqueness and the relative modernity of the scientific revolution that marked a radical break even with earlier Western scientific traditions. Patricia Ebrey argues that Chinese family patterns parallel those of many other cultures (including the early West), whereas modern Western kinship patterns have diverged sharply from traditional Western patterns in the last few centuries. Albert Feuerwerker and William T. Rowe both point out that the Western European capitalist revolution is the real anomaly in world economic history, not China's "lack" of capitalist development. And I note in my chapter that the modern psychological novel and the intellectual and social prominence of novelists as a group are both uniquely modern phenomena, even in the West. Thus, among other things, the comparative study of China forcefully reminds us how very young our own modern Western culture really is.

Several chapters in our collection explore how China and the West have influenced each other in different areas, but the chapters as a whole suggest that such influences have not been terribly important in either culture. Throughout most of its history China has been relatively isolated from powerful foreign influences. The main exceptions to this have been the rise of Indian-inspired Buddhism after the fall of the Han dynasty and the influence of the West in the twentieth century. In each of these cases China has also transformed the foreign influence profoundly according to Chinese cultural needs and expectations. Both Buddhism and Marxism, for example, were in many ways transformed into very distinctly Chinese forms. Modern Western technology may prove less susceptible to Sinification, but even in this case, if the past is a reliable guide, we should expect to see the continuing resilience and creativity of Chinese culture in adapting foreign influences to meet its own needs and concerns.

China has influenced the West in a variety of important ways but probably not any more fundamentally than the West has influenced China. Nathan Sivin lists a number of Chinese inventions and discoveries that have contributed to the modern world as we know it in the West. Yet many of these developments simply foreshadowed internal Western developments, and, although important, they have probably not been decisive in changing the direction of Western civilization. Many Westerners have been greatly enriched by exposure to Chinese art, Chinese philosophy, and Chinese food, and many have been greatly impressed with China's early genius for complex human organization and the strength and continuity of Chinese culture. But these achievements, great as they are, have not been crucial to the shaping of the modern Western world.

Among the most important legacies of Chinese civilization for the modern world I would include the following: the steady and continuous development of a civilization over many centuries; the relatively peaceful coexistence of different religious traditions on Chinese soil, also over many centuries; the optimistic faith in the human potential for good, both individually and collectively; the strong importance placed on education and the belief in the educability of all people; the ancient Chinese recognition of the mortality of all human institutions; the strong ideals of political unity and social harmony that persisted even through centuries of disunity and turmoil; the profound respect for nature expressed in so much Chinese art and philosophy; and the emphasis in Chinese thought on human morality and historical memory as the main sources of meaning in human existence. These are important legacies, but they are more striking for their contrast with Western traditions than for their influence on the West.

In large part the relative lack of direct mutual influence makes the comparative study of China and the West potentially very fruitful. Because the developments of these two civilizations have been so distinctly different, sometimes parallel but more often divergent, the study of the two in comparison is especially useful in reflecting light into areas that might not otherwise be noticeable or explorable. The many differences between the two serve to caution us against easy assumptions about universal patterns of cause and effect in the development of civilizations. These differences also suggest the importance of human choice in the development of complex societies and remind us that there is more than one effective route to developing complex systems of culture and frameworks of meaning and significance.

Another reason for adopting a comparative approach in these chapters is to make explicit what is often only implicit in Western writings on China. All Western studies of China are in a sense comparative because as Westerners or Western-trained scholars we inevitably bring to the study of China our own (Western-conditioned) concerns and perspectives. The very subject matter of our chapters—government, economics, society, kinship, philosophy, religion, art, literature, and science—reflects the scholarly division of labor and the classifications of knowledge that have evolved in the modern West. As Nathan Sivin notes in his chapter on science, traditional Chinese scholars would have systematized and classified their discussions of their own civilization in quite different ways. By being explicit about our Western approaches and our comparative interests, we hope to avoid the trap of unconsciously evaluating Chinese civilization by contemporary Western values and standards that may not be relevant to the understanding of China's past.

Our comparative perspective in these chapters is primarily confined to China and the West. Comparisons between China and such areas as

South America, Africa, the Middle East, South and Southeast Asia would indeed be illuminating, but none of us felt sufficiently knowledgeable about these other areas to include them in our comparative framework. Even confining ourselves to comparisons between China and the West, some of us have had to move beyond the boundaries of our professional expertise and to risk offending other specialists with our generalizations. We have undertaken such risks quite happily, but for all of us our comparisons had to be limited to those traditions we know best.

In soliciting and editing the chapters for this volume I have asked each contributor to address a general nonspecialist audience and to describe an important aspect of Chinese civilization, keeping in mind the following questions: What are the most important, distinctive, or unique characteristics of Chinese civilization? What have been the most important parallels or contrasts between China and the West? How have China and the West influenced each other in the past? What are the important questions in each major area of Chinese studies? How does a comparative approach help to illuminate the study of China? What are the particular pleasures of studying China?

I purposely did not suggest or recommend particular themes or lines of inquiry to our contributors beyond the stipulation that their chapters have a broad focus, be comparative in some sense, and address a general readership. I wanted the chapters to reflect something of the variety of approaches and views in contemporary Sinological scholarship and not to be skewed in one particular direction by my own interests and preoccupations. As a result, some chapters are more difficult than others, some are more comparative than others, and some are comparative in different ways.

Given our different fields and different perspectives, it is understandable that some conflicting points emerge in these chapters. I cite three examples, and careful readers will doubtless find others. In speaking of Confucianism as an intellectual tradition, Tu Wei-ming emphasizes the importance of cooperation, communal values, and the spiritual quest in the Confucian tradition. Jack L. Dull, as a political historian of China's practice of government, tends to emphasize authoritarian values in the Confucian tradition and in China's political culture as a whole. Karen Turner, by contrast, draws on recent archaeological evidence from the Ch'in–Han era to question stereotypical views of "Chinese despotism" and to note the ways that even the strongest Chinese emperors were limited in their power by a keen sense of historical precedent, by law, and by Confucian advisers.

Given the relative freedom of our contributors in choosing their own themes and approaches, the areas of disagreement between the contributors seem less surprising than the common elements that many of them share. In particular, David N. Keightley's chapter on the origins of

Chinese civilization highlights several themes echoed by a number of the others: the philosophical optimism in early China about the ultimate questions of the nature and purpose of human life; the relatively small interest in tragedy in ancient Chinese art, myth, literature, religion, and philosophy; the deep Chinese concern for order and harmony in society; the strong penchant for bureaucratic organization in the maintenance of social order; and the emphasis on the welfare of human beings as a collectivity rather than as individuals.

Keightley's emphasis on the relative optimism of the early Chinese foreshadows similar observations in several other chapters. Tu Wei-ming portrays Confucius and Confucianism as radically optimistic about the possibility of continual improvement in the human condition. Michael Sullivan, Stephen Owen, and I, discussing Chinese art, poetry, and fiction respectively, all find a relative Chinese disinterest in tragic themes, a strong emphasis on order, balance, and harmony in art, nature, and society, and an optimistic assumption that good art is by definition morally uplifting. Although he does not explicitly emphasize the theme of optimism in his chapter on Chinese Taoism and Buddhism, T. H. Barrett describes two religions that contrast very sharply with the Judeo-Christian tradition, for example, in their relative lack of emphasis on human sin and depravity as being redeemable only by divine intervention. On the more mundane level of politics Jack L. Dull demonstrates the unshakable Chinese confidence, even through long periods of political chaos and disunity, in the cultural continuity of the Chinese tradition and the eventual restoration of political unity, peace, and social harmony.

Keightley is struck by the early Chinese penchant for bureaucratic organization, and this theme is greatly amplified in the chapters by Jack L. Dull and Karen Turner, who deal with Chinese government. In Dull's and Turner's chapters we see the sophistication of early Chinese political thought. The early Confucian and Legalist thinkers displayed a shrewd understanding of collective human behavior (what we now call social psychology), and they shared an overwhelming concern for social order and stability. The political values discussed by Dull and Turner have remained important in guiding and motivating Chinese political leaders into the early twentieth century. The most striking example of an ancient but enduring political ideal is the emphasis, noted in both chapters, on Chinese political and cultural unity. There is an unshakable confidence that unity is best, that periods of disunity, however long, are temporary, and that the only proper aspiration for a Chinese leader is to unify all of China under one rule, from Manchuria to the Burmese border, from Taiwan to Tibet, and from Hong Kong to Mongolia.

In contrasting early Chinese and early Greek assumptions about individuals, the family, and the concept of the hero, Keightley touches again on themes that reverberate through several other chapters. He finds in

China a much greater concern with the welfare of the group and the family; the Greek hero, by contrast, is much more alone in the world, much more autonomous, and much more tragic. In discussing the long and important history of the Chinese family, Patricia Ebrey demonstrates the continuing strength of family-centered ideals and the predominance of the family over the individual throughout Chinese history. In his chapter on art Michael Sullivan notes a definite "impersonality" in an emperor's portrait: the real subject of the painting is the awesome imperial role, not the mere individual who happens to sit on the throne at any given moment. In my own chapter, although I note some exceptions, I see in Chinese fiction less emphasis on individual psychology than in much Western fiction. Tu Wei-ming finds far more individualism in Confucian thought than Keightley does in Shang and Chou dynasty art, yet throughout Tu's chapter we see the strong social consciousness of the major thinkers in the Confucian tradition. For these thinkers individual salvation would be meaningless apart from the welfare of the entire polity and society.

Perhaps the best way to understand the relative Chinese emphasis on group life rather than individual life is not to see it as disinterest in individuals but as an insistence on seeing individuals in their natural context, that is, relating to other individuals. This natural context for the individual extends not only to other human beings but to the whole universe. Tu Wei-ming speaks of an "anthropocosmic vision" in Confucianism that sees all things in the universe as interrelated and mutually interacting. Peace and order begins with self-cultivation, but the purpose of self-cultivation extends far beyond the individual self to the family, the local society, the empire, and finally the cosmos. There is, in Tu's view, a transcendent dimension in Confucianism that unites people, nature, and Heaven and that goes beyond what we today call "secular humanism."

Interestingly enough, what Tu Wei-ming sees as a Confucian concern with social harmony and the cosmic interrelatedness of all things may also be seen in T. H. Barrett's chapter as traits of both the Buddhist and Taoist traditions. Despite the surface differences between Confucian "this-worldliness" and Buddhist "otherworldliness," important strains in both traditions emphasize concrete social practice over abstract theory; and both also emphasize the cosmic consequences of all human action. The Ch'an Buddhist who sees the tao in the performance of mundane tasks is reminiscent of Confucius in viewing the secular as sacred. In other ways Chinese of all faiths shared a belief in the cosmic unity of all things. Consider, for example, the assumed continuity between the living and the dead that is at the heart of the strong tradition of ancestor worship, or the popular assumption that the natural and supernatural realms are merely two aspects of one reality.

The Chinese emphasis on a holistic approach to life is perhaps demonstrated most thoroughly in Nathan Sivin's discussion of Chinese science. In his discussion of Chinese astronomy and astrology Sivin emphasizes the Chinese assumption that people, nature, and the heavens are inseparably interconnected: the regular motions of the heavenly bodies reflect the regular cycles of human life, and irregular heavenly phenomena reflect irregularities in the human world, particularly in the form of the moral shortcomings of the ruler. The close interconnection between people and nature is also evident in Sivin's discussion of geomancy, or siting. In the practice of siting Chinese assumed that whenever making changes in the landscape by building buildings or digging graves people must take care to harmonize with the cosmic forces inherent in the mountains, hills, and rivers of the natural landscape. The goal of humans in such a belief system is to blend harmoniously and nondisruptively with nature, not only to prevent offending the awesome power of the natural world but also to prevent committing an aesthetic offense against the natural beauty of the landscape.

Although the profound sense of humankind's intimate relationship with nature is most closely identified with early Chinese Taoist philosophy, Tu Wei-ming makes clear that Confucius shared this intense appreciation for nature. A strong sense of harmony between people and nature also permeates the landscape paintings discussed by Michael Sullivan and the poetry described by Stephen Owen. In the agricultural poems from the ancient *Book of Songs,* the "founding myth" of Prince Millet, the nature poetry of the recluse T'ao Ch'ien, and Li Po's famous poem on visiting a hermit—all carefully analyzed by Owen—we see across many ages of Chinese poetry an abiding sense of the importance of nature and humankind's closeness to it. It may well be that landscape paintings and nature poetry held their appeal in China because the painters and poets were actually part of a relatively complex, urbanized, and crowded society. Poets and painters sought the solace and peace of nature partly in their imaginations, but in any case they shared a profound respect for nature, and they saw people properly blending with nature as an integral part of nature itself. This belief is a revealing contrast with the Western Judeo-Christian tradition of "man having dominion over nature."

Another striking example of what I have called China's holistic approach to life is seen in Nathan Sivin's discussion of Chinese medicine. By seeing all human organisms in a larger context, Chinese medicine was able to deal with human illness from a very broad and very useful perspective. A diseased organ required treatment of the whole person and not simply the affected organ in isolation. Similarly, a diseased person was perceived not simply as an isolated problem but as a dynamic part of a whole social and biological system. In Sivin's view it was the particular strength of Chinese medicine to see all parts of the human body as interconnected and to see the individual patient in a broad social and biological context.

These Chinese tendencies to see all things as interconnected and to consider phenomena in dynamic systemwide relationships are also evident in the emphasis on the group over the individual in such diverse areas as politics and fiction. Karen Turner illustrates these tendencies in her analysis of law and rulership in early imperial China. Both Turner and Jack L. Dull amply demonstrate that although we might not share the values of such Legalist thinkers as Lord Shang or Han Fei Tzu, we still recognize that their determined focus on the workings of an entire society and their deep insight into the dynamics of collective human behavior allowed them to fashion a remarkably complex, stable, and effective political system.

The Confucian thinkers discussed briefly by Turner, Dull, and Ebrey, and more extensively by Tu, also showed a high degree of sophistication in noting the relative weakness of externally imposed laws in shaping human behavior and contrasting this weakness with the much greater power of the internal controls fostered by such techniques as moral teachings, careful child-rearing, rituals, and habits. In my own chapter on Chinese fiction I also note the Chinese fascination with group dynamics rather than individual psychology. Rather than seeing this emphasis as a shortcoming of Chinese fiction, I suggest that Chinese fiction-writers actually had a very shrewd understanding of the power of social settings, social roles, and expectations in determining the feelings and behavior of individuals. Such an understanding is consistent with the findings of many modern anthropologists and sociologists.

The Chinese understanding of the power of social conditioning is evident in one more theme first raised by David N. Keightley: the importance and effectiveness of ritual in Chinese life. Keightley emphasizes the centrality of ritual in the lives of the Shang rulers, and Tu Wei-ming emphasizes the importance of ritual throughout the long Confucian tradition. Confucians understand the power and importance of good habits in shaping human behavior, but ritual in Chinese culture also goes beyond mere outward form or habitual behavior. Proper rituals properly performed are both satisfying and calming in themselves and are assumed to have beneficial effects for the entire society. The ruler's rituals are perhaps most crucial in maintaining a proper balance between people and Heaven, but every person also has a responsibility to perform proper rituals at the proper time—particularly for births, weddings, and funerals—for the sake of order and harmony throughout society. We have only to look at the magnificent Shang and Chou dynasty ritual bronze vessels, the elaborate tombs of Chinese rulers from all ages, or an ordinary Chinese funeral in Taiwan today in order to see the importance attached to ritual in Chinese culture.

Seven of our chapters (those by Tu, Dull, Ebrey, Feuerwerker, Rowe, Barrett, and myself) deal explicitly with issues of change and continuity over long periods of time. These chapters amply demonstrate the inadequacy of old stereotypes of a "changeless China." And yet, in drawing comparisons with Western history, these chapters also suggest that Chinese traditions have generally seen greater continuity than comparable Western institutions, beliefs, and practices.

The continuity and dominance of the imperial state in China is surely one of the most striking contrasts with the Western experience. The Han dynasty collapse in the early third century A.D. led to several centuries of disunity and the corresponding rise of new religious movements (Buddhism and Taoism), much as the fall of the Roman Empire resulted in centuries of disunity and the rise of Christianity in the West. But beyond these surface similarities the parallels break down rather quickly. A unified empire was never again established in Europe, whereas China was reunified by the Sui dynasty in 589 and managed to maintain imperial unity more or less continuously until 1911. The Christian church in Europe grew strong enough to alter family practices and patterns and, eventually, to rival the power even of Western princes and rulers. Buddhism and Taoism, by contrast, never threatened the resurgent power of the Chinese state from the sixth century onward, and, despite its popularity in the T'ang period, Buddhism never managed to undermine Confucian dominance in politics or society.

Several of our chapters, particularly those by Albert Feuerwerker, William T. Rowe, and myself, emphasize contrasts between China and the West, particularly over the past four or five centuries. Patricia Ebrey and Nathan Sivin discuss developments in Chinese kinship patterns and Chinese science, respectively, over a much longer span of time, but they too are concerned with a question implicit in these other chapters: How does China's experience compare with the experience of the West over a number of centuries? Most of these chapters note that in many ways China was "more advanced" than the West until the fifteenth or sixteenth century of our own era. Its science was more highly developed, its economy more productive, its political life more complex, and its culture more sophisticated. Then came the scientific and industrial revolutions in Western Europe and the relative positions of China and the West were rather suddenly reversed.

Each of these chapters makes very different comparative observations about Chinese and Western experience in the last five centuries, but they also share several important views. All of us see some parallels between Chinese and Western experience over the last five centuries. Like Western Europe in these years, Chinese society was also becoming more urbanized, more complex, economically more developed, and culturally more sophisticated. What was different was the pace of change in China and the West. Change began to occur so rapidly in the West in the eighteenth and nineteenth centuries that China by contrast appeared to be standing still if not moving backward. Rowe, Feuerwerker, and I all argue that in fact China was not standing still at all during this time but was changing, perhaps even more rapidly than through most of its earlier history. Only the unprecedented pace of change in the West made it seem otherwise.

The careful reader of Dull, Feuerwerker, and Rowe will be struck by the contrast from the sixteenth century onward between rapid change in China's economy and society coupled with little change in Chinese political institutions. The relative stability of China's imperial political system certainly also helped form the mistaken Western impression of an unchanging China when Westerners began to go to China in the sixteenth century. In some ways the Chinese state became a victim of its own success: such a balanced equilibrium had been achieved that the need for substantial change or innovation was difficult to perceive.[1] Much suffering in China's modern era has resulted from an inflexible state's inability to cope with rapid social and economic change.

A final point shared by the five chapters on science, society, the family, the economy, and fiction is our conviction that the Chinese experience during the last five centuries is far less unusual or inexplicable than the Western experience. Therefore, all of us reject such questions as "Why did China, with its great scientific traditions, fail to have a scientific revolution? Why did China, with all its economic sophistication, fail to have an industrial revolution? Why did China, with its long and sophisticated literary culture, fail to develop the modern (Western-style) psychological novel?" We reject such questions because they misleadingly imply that Western experience is the norm that other civilizations should have followed. In our view it is the Western experience that is puzzling: the scientific and industrial revolutions were as unique and unprecedented in Western experience as they were in Chinese experience. It is therefore not surprising that these events did not occur in China; what is surprising is that they occurred anywhere at all. This observation is another example of something I noted earlier: the Western study of China ultimately helps us to understand both the Chinese and ourselves.

When Westerners first began studying Chinese civilization (only a few short centuries ago), they naturally began with its philosophical, literary, artistic, and religious traditions. As a result, early Western scholarship tended to reflect the biases and self-images of the Confucian literati, who were the custodians of so many Chinese cultural traditions. In the past

1. The contrast between socioeconomic change and political stagnation in China, with emphasis on the nineteenth century, is noted and discussed in John King Fairbank, *The Great Chinese Revolution: 1800–1985* (New York: Harper & Row, 1986), 48–50.

few decades Western scholars have increasingly turned their attention to non-Confucian traditions and to social, economic, political, and anthropological themes in China's history. Meanwhile, recent archaeological discoveries in China have been nothing short of spectacular in both number and significance. These changes are reflected most clearly in the chapters by David N. Keightley, Jack L. Dull, Karen Turner, Nathan Sivin, Patricia Ebrey, Albert Feuerwerker, and William T. Rowe. Keightley, Turner, and Sivin draw heavily on recent archaeological finds. From different perspectives, Dull, Ebrey, Feuerwerker, and Rowe examine several aspects of the complex relationship between the state, the family, society, and the economy.

China's long tradition of detailed record-keeping over many centuries makes it a particularly inviting subject for social scientists and cultural theorists interested in exploring the fascinating complexities of social and cultural development, historical causation, and change and continuity over several millennia. Large questions of causality in cultural formation and historical development loom over several of these chapters, especially those by Keightley, Ebrey, and Dull. These three, in particular, attempt broad comparative analyses that suggest something of the complexity involved in trying to determine chains of causation in human culture.

David N. Keightley reveals a kind of complex, interlocking, and mutually reinforcing web of beliefs and practices as seen in the Shang and Chou archaeological evidence. Patricia Ebrey shows that changes in family patterns over many centuries were as complicated in China as in the West. Family patterns were influenced by such factors as state policies, legal changes, economic changes, social mobility patterns, relations with neighboring non-Chinese peoples, as well as religious and intellectual developments. Thus, Ebrey strikingly demonstrates that Chinese family patterns can no longer be viewed as simply reflecting the evolving social ideals of the Confucian literati. In tracing the evolution of Chinese forms of government, Jack L. Dull likewise reveals a very complex and changing relationship between state and society throughout Chinese history.

Given the longevity and complexity of Chinese civilization and the rapid growth of Chinese studies over the past three decades, we cannot attempt to be comprehensive in a book this size. Many other themes could legitimately be featured in this kind of work, including geography, material culture, peasant life, popular culture, military organization and values, foreign relations, and the list could go on and on. My choices of topics have been guided by two major concerns: the sufficient development of a field to invite a general survey, and the willingness of qualified contributors to address broad themes for a general audience.

This book, then, is a sampler of some of the varieties of approaches scholars have taken to the study of China's past. We hope this collection might give nonspecialists some sense of the rapidly growing field of Sinology and the insights it can yield. It might serve as a useful supplement to survey textbooks and readers in college courses on traditional Chinese civilization; it might also serve as supplemental reading in more general courses on world history or comparative civilizations. For the general reader unfamiliar with the main outlines of Chinese history, we include a brief chronological table in Appendix 2 and, somewhat more useful, a brief guide to further reading in Appendix 3. To the novice who is completely unfamiliar with traditional Chinese civilization, I strongly recommend one of the general histories listed in Appendix 3—by Charles O. Hucker, Jacques Gernet, Conrad Schirokauer, or the East Asian survey by John Fairbank, Edwin Reischauer, and Albert Craig.

Given the varieties of views on China presented in this book, it is entirely appropriate that the volume begins with Jonathan Spence's chapter, which discusses the enormous range of Western views of China over the past four centuries. Spence implies that Western views of China as often as not reflect Western preconceptions, concerns, and even fantasies as much as the Chinese reality they purport to convey. This assessment is a sobering theme for Western historians of China to contemplate, for we are forcefully reminded that the biases and distortions of past writers are much easier to recognize than are our own. Apart from those rare historians who create works of art, most of us have to admit that our work of necessity can have only a temporary validity. Even the most up-to-date historical scholarship cannot long remain so. But part of the historian's role in both ancient China and the modern West is to challenge subsequent generations to reinterpret the past from the only perspective available to them: the present. If these chapters can stimulate the reader to go beyond them in the exploration of Chinese civilization, they will have served their purpose.

ONE

□

Western Perceptions of China from the Late Sixteenth Century to the Present

Jonathan Spence

If we are unclear today about our feelings for China, we should not worry over much. Westerners have been unclear about China since they first began to live there in any numbers and to write about the country at length. The history of our confusion goes back more than four hundred years: in 1584 the first detailed accounts of China began to appear in the letters home of the Jesuit missionary Matteo Ricci, and Gonzalez de Mendoza's pioneering history appeared a year later. Although Ricci and his other contemporaries were drawing on the preconceptions of earlier generations of travelers to China, the honor of inaugurating a new genre of commentary based on unparalleled firsthand experience nonetheless goes to them.

To the sixteenth-century Westerners China was large, tough, and well-ordered. They never ceased to wonder at the size of the country and the diversity of its products. Few Westerners echoed the hopeful boasts of some early Spaniards—descendants in spirit of the conquistadors—that they could conquer the realm with a few hundred elite troops. The acuter visitors saw that China's cities were walled and those walls were well-patrolled, its armies were huge, and its war junks were numerous and well-armed. They also saw the magistrates' tough approach toward civil disorder, their rigorous control over the civilian population, the terrible savagery of the beatings they were free to inflict on their Chinese subjects, and their control over economic life.

Despite a general view that the first Jesuits were biased in China's favor, I have found no early works in which the dark and light sides did not blend under this early Western gaze. Thus, China's ethical system and the ideal of a mandarinate trained through the Confucian classics, selected by examinations, and posted by an absolute emperor to rule benignly over the peaceful countryside were lyrically described; but the excesses of Buddhist ritual fasting, the magical extravagances of the Taoists, the ever-present evidence of infanticide, the sale of children, and the prevalence of prostitution and male homosexuality were also described. Chinese sophistication in theological debate was noted by many but so was its counterpart of intransigence to the Christian message. To the praise of printing and literati culture in China, which seemed to offer great opportunities for the spread of the Christian missionary message, had to be added the melancholy fact that anti-Christian tracts spread swiftly through the cities and countryside.[1]

The fall of the Ming dynasty in 1644 and the realities of the Manchu conquest thereafter did not lead to greatly changed perceptions. It became easier, of course, to identify with a man like the K'ang-hsi emperor, who ruled from 1661 to 1722, than it had been with the reclusive Wan-li emperor of the Ming, who never saw or spoke to any missionaries or traders during his long reign from 1572 to 1620. K'ang-hsi showed consistent curiosity about the West and even affection for several missionaries until he became worried that they were involved with his son's cabals and also grew aware of the papal pretensions to infallibility in matters of faith and spiritual interpretation. In the writings of the later seventeenth century Jesuits like Bouvet presented K'ang-hsi as a benevolent type of "Sun King" on the model of Louis XIV—not without deliberation, as French funding for the China mission had become a staple for its survival. As Bouvet put it in a letter to King Louis XIV, printed as the preface to his *Histoire de l'empereur de la Chine:*

> The Jesuits, whom Your Majesty sent [to China] some years ago, were astonished to discover at the ends of the earth something that hitherto they had seen only in France: namely, a Prince who, like you, sire, combines a genius that is both sublime and practical with a heart worthy of his empire, who is master of himself and of his subjects and [who is] equally adored by his people and respected by his neighbors. . . . A Prince, in short, uniting in his person most of the great qualities that heroes have, who could be the most accomplished monarch to reign on this earth for a long time were it not that his reign coincided with that of Your Majesty.[2]

But despite such hyperbole, Bouvet's writings, like those of Le Comte who preceded him and Du Halde who followed after, were jammed with

1. For these early works on China see Donald Lach, *Asia in the Making of Europe,* 5 vols. to date (Chicago: University of Chicago Press, 1965–); Pasquale d'Elia, ed., *Fonti Ricciane,* 3 vols. (Rome: Libreria dello Stato, 1942–1949); and Jonathan D. Spence, *The Memory Palace of Matteo Ricci* (New York: Viking, 1984). For Chinese criticisms of the Westerners see John D. Young, *Confucianism and Christianity: The First Encounter* (Hong Kong: Hong Kong University Press, 1983), and Jacques Gernet, *China and the Christian Impact: A Conflict of Cultures* (Cambridge: Cambridge University Press, 1985).

2. J. Bouvet, *Histoire de l'empereur de la Chine* (Paris: 1699; reprint, Tientsin: M. Uytwerf, LaHaye, 1940), 6–7 (my translation).

practical information about Chinese politics and culture. Yet biases also began to appear, especially in the direction of minimizing China's faults so that the tasks of conversion would not appear to be insurmountable. These French writers also dwelt on the ideas that Confucianism somehow presaged the possibilities of a general universal morality and that Chinese written ideographs held within them the hope for a universal language that transcended dialects and geography. Both these facets were to be picked up by the alert philosopher Leibniz, along with the binary mathematical structure that lay behind the arrangements of the sixty-four hexagrams in the *Book of Change* and the hope that China would become a part of a newly internationalized global scientific academy. For a time Leibniz was also intrigued by the figurist position, as it was called, as were other scholars well into the eighteenth century; the figurists, far from being alarmed by the great age and comprehensiveness of the Confucian classics, sought to use the contents of those classics to prove the accuracy of the Biblical chronology, which was beginning to come under serious question. Their work should be seen in the context of what historians of anthropology describe as the last defense of "monogenic" theories of humankind, which trace all humans back to Noah and eventually to Adam. This monogenic view was opposed to the mounting interest in "polygenic" theories, which, by allowing for the multifaceted origins of the human race, made possible the downgrading of segments of the human family and the placing of some humans in a zone of prerationality. Polygenic theories cleared the way for the rise of an allegedly "scientific" justification for racism. By the mid 1730s scholars had begun to do something that would have been literally unthinkable to Ricci: by analyzing the "conic" nature of Chinese heads, they were able to place the Chinese people alongside the Patagonians, the Hottentots, and the American Indians in the category of "homo monstrosus," something fundamentally different from the "homo sapiens" designation that those same scholars claimed for themselves.[3]

The complexity of the story of Western perceptions of China springs in part from the fact that at the very time the Jesuits were falling under political suspicion in Europe, coming under attack from both the lay intelligentsia and the Jansenists and also losing any influence they had once had in China—in other words, during the second quarter of the eighteenth century, at the end of the reign of the Yung-cheng emperor and the beginning of the reign of the Ch'ien-lung emperor—the books

3. Margaret Hodgen, *Early Anthropology in the Sixteenth and Seventeenth Centuries* (Philadelphia: University of Pennsylvania Press, 1964), esp. 413–25; Basil Guy, *The French Image of China before and after Voltaire* (Geneva: Institute et Musee Voltaire, 1963); and David Mungello, *Leibniz and Confucianism: The Search for Accord* (Honolulu: University of Hawaii Press, 1977).

in which they had analyzed China were reaching the peak of their influence. In part this influence was because China was becoming isolationist, restricting trade and travel to a minimum for all foreigners; the Jesuit histories kept their spell because they were firsthand accounts. But in part this influence was also because several French thinkers of the Enlightenment, beginning with Pierre Bayle and continuing through Voltaire, had seized on the data buried in the Jesuit books—especially the reality of an ethically moral Chinese society that was also patently non-Christian—to criticize the role that the Catholic church was playing in the European society of the time. Voltaire praised the Chinese in his writings for their "natural deism." Two examples, *Essai sur les moeurs et l'esprit des nations* and *Orphelin de la Chine,* the first a book of world history and the second a stage play, both completed by 1750, illustrate Voltaire's approach to China: in the first he started the history of civilization with the Chinese state and in the other explained how the stony heart of Genghis Khan was softened by the moral purity of the gentle Chinese.

We must use a real effort of the imagination to understand how great the shock must have been to Voltaire's readers when they saw world history start not with Biblical chronology but with Chinese time. Bouvet's equation was reversed with the defiant opening words of the *Essai,* "The empire of China at that time was vaster than that of Charlemagne." Voltaire went on to praise China's laws: "In other countries the laws are used to punish crimes; in China they do more—they reward virtue." As to Confucius, "his morality is as pure, as stern and at the same time as humane as that of Epictetus," and far from being atheists, the Chinese had their own measured view of the realm of heaven: "The great misunderstanding over Chinese rites sprang from our judging their practices in light of ours: we carry the prejudices that spring from our contentious nature to the ends of the world."[4]

This emphasis on the practical and moral force of the Chinese, their potential for raising the quotient of goodness in the world, was still a matter for serious debate in the late eighteenth century. It was central to the writings of the French physiocrats at the peak of their influence. Lord Macartney took it seriously in his *Journal* as he traveled to China for King George III and the East India Company during 1793 and 1794. Benjamin Franklin bought books on China and debated Chinese social organization; he even contemplated sending commissioners to China so that the "young people" of America could study China's aged laws. Thomas Jefferson reflected on the "natural aristocracy" of the Chinese. As if to encapsulate this tradition of admiration, the wealthy Philadelphia merchant Stephen Girard, putting together a fleet to trade with China in

4. Voltaire, *Essai sur les moeurs et l'esprit des nations* (Paris, 1771), 1:13, 31, 33, and 36.

1795, proudly named the four ships *Voltaire, Rousseau, Montesquieu,* and *Helvetius.*[5]

In fact, had Girard read carefully in Montesquieu and Rousseau, he would have found that they expressed profound reservations about China and about Chinese culture and government. Both writers seem to have picked up strands of disillusion with the Chinese that had been growing alongside the admiration from the beginning of the eighteenth century. For example, hostility to the Chinese is sharp in some of the novels of Defoe and in the memoirs of the formidable English naval commodore George Anson, who visited Canton in the 1740s and found it an awful place, inhabited by a dishonest and craven populace that was controlled by contemptible officials. In the best-selling account of his voyage, published when he returned to a hero's welcome in England after capturing a Spanish galleon, Anson let all his prejudices show: "This much may undoubtedly be asserted," he wrote, "that in artifice, falsehood, and an attachment to all kinds of lucre, many of the Chinese are difficult to be paralleled by any other people; but then the combination of these talents, and the manner in which they are applied in particular emergencies, are often beyond the reach of a foreigner's penetration." The goal of such passages—and there were many others—was to cure other European writers of their "very ridiculous prepossessions." Anson particularly labored to correct the mistaken Western view of Chinese morality.

> But we are told by some of the Missionaries, that though the skill of the Chinese in science is indeed much inferior to that of the Europeans, yet the morality and justice taught and practised by them are most exemplary. And from the description given by some of these good fathers, one should be induced to believe, that the whole Empire was a well-governed affectionate family, where the only contests were, who should exert the most humanity and beneficence. But our preceding relation of the behavior of the Magistrates, Merchants and Tradesmen at Canton sufficiently refutes these jesuitical fictions. And as to their theories of morality, if we may judge from the specimens exhibited in the works of the Missionaries, we shall find them solely material points, instead of discussing the proper criterion of human actions, and regulating the general conduct of mankind to one another, on reasonable and equitable principles.
>
> Indeed, the only pretension of the Chinese to a more refined morality than their neighbors is founded, not on their integrity or beneficence, but

5. In addition to Guy, *French Image of China,* see J. H. Brumfitt, *Voltaire Historia* (Oxford: Oxford University Press, 1958); Lord George Macartney's journal as edited by J. L. Cranmer-Byng, *An Embassy to China: being the journal kept by Lord Macartney during his embassy to the Emperor Ch'ien-lung, 1793–1794* (London: Longmans, 1962); and Jonathan Goldstein, *Philadelphia and the China Trade* (University Park, Pa.: Pennsylvania State University Press, 1978), 35.

solely on the affected evenness of their demeanor, and their constant attention to suppress all symptoms of passion and violence.[6]

These remarks might be dismissed as the mere rumblings of a naval curmudgeon had they not caught a deeper response in France, where the earlier optimism about China was fading. The most solid critique advanced by Montesquieu, which sprang in part from his ongoing interest in geography, climate, and environmentalism, was that there was something awry in China's so-called laws because they inhibited liberty rather than contributing to it and because the Chinese were ruled by fear rather than wisdom. Rousseau, who had quarreled with Voltaire on other matters, also disagreed with Voltaire over China. Rousseau felt that an analysis of Chinese culture proved the correctness of his insight that education could corrupt rather than ennoble manners, that there was a primitive nobility of character that had to be tended if it was to blossom, and that this capacity had atrophied in China. Nicolas Boulanger echoed the same points in his *Oriental Despotism* of 1763. From these perceptions it was not a long way to Condorcet's realization that the Chinese were outside the march of human progress or to Hegel's contentions in the early nineteenth century that China was outside the development of world history, could not partake of the manifestations of the growth of the spirit on earth, and remained forever frozen at an earlier stage of development prior to the growth of the subjectivity and freedom in which Western cultures now rejoiced. Hegel's words are worth pondering, for they demonstrate how rigorously China had now been systematized, how "scientific" the analysis of her backwardness had been made to appear.

In China the Universal Will immediately commands what the Individual is to do, and the latter complies and obeys with proportionate renunciation of reflection and personal independence. If he does not obey, if he thus virtually separates himself from the Substance of his being, inasmuch as this separation is not mediated by a retreat within a personality of his own, the punishment he undergoes does not affect his subjective and internal, but simply his outward existence. The element of subjectivity is therefore as much wanting to this political totality as the latter is on its side altogether destitute of a foundation in the moral disposition of the subject. For the Substance is simply an individual—the Emperor—whose law constitutes all the disposition. Nevertheless, this ignoring of inclination does not imply caprice, which would itself indicate inclination—that is, subjectivity and mobility. Here we have the One Being of the State supremely dominant—

6. Daniel Defoe's critique appears in *The Further Adventures of Robinson Crusoe* (London: W. Taylor, 1719). The quotations are from Richard Walter and Benjamin Robins, comps., *A Voyage around the World in the Years 1704–44 by George Anson* (Oxford: Oxford University Press, 1974), 351–52, 366, 368.

the Substance which, still hard and inflexible, resembles nothing but itself—includes no other element.[7]

There is a good deal of scholarly debate as to exactly what was contributed to Western perceptions of China by the merchants—both European and American—who began to spend long periods of their lives in China as the tributary system sputtered to its end in the late 1820s and 1830s. The record seems mixed: some were entranced, amused, or spoke of the value of their Chinese friendships, but others (like Anson before them) found venality, cruelty, and deceit. But after 1842, when the Chinese armies had been defeated by the British in the Opium War and the country opened to travel, trade, a Western military presence, and evangelization by both Protestant and Catholic missionaries in large numbers, the very obvious weakness of China bred contempt rather than admiration. If there was sympathy, it was for the individual Chinese poor rather than for the country as a whole, its government, its ethical system, or its art.

Whatever sincere admiration both Americans and Europeans had for Chinese decoration in the eighteenth century, the period of "chinoiserie" when they eagerly bought Chinese furnishings, porcelain, wallpaper, and silks, faded in the ebullient hard-driving world of the early industrial revolution and the railway age. The world of rococo faded in the glare of Victorian self-esteem. One can pick up many traces of waning Western interest, from the gently dismissive comments of Goethe to his faithful companion Eckermann that the symbol for Chinese culture is the lightness of wicker furniture or the comments of Charles Dickens's Mr. Pickwick on the impossibilities of a meaningful Chinese morality down to Ralph Waldo Emerson's analysis of fatalism and withdrawal and his contrast of these with the freedom and dynamism he now ascribed to the West. China would have to be "regenerated" by the West, Emerson wrote, if it is to enter the modern world; it had been the "playground of the world's childhood" but now would have to be forced to grow up. Karl Marx concurred in his early writings that touched on China's problems. It would be a long time before China saw the words "liberté, égalité, fraternité" inscribed on the Great Wall, he wrote; indeed, Western imperialism and colonization would have a positive role in the Chinese case as they battered down the barriers of isolation that made China a holdout against the spread of capitalism across the world. For it was only when that spread had been completed that the emergence of a new socialist consciousness would become a meaningful possibility.[8]

7. G. W. F. Hegel, *Lectures on the Philosophy of History,* trans. J. Sibree (New York: Dover, 1956) 120–21 and Guy, *French Image of China.*

8. For background references see Stuart Creighton Miller, *The Unwelcome Immigrant: The American Image of China, 1785–1882* (Berkeley: University of California Press, 1969),

In the later nineteenth century, except for missionaries still able to be moved by Chinese poverty or the ravages of opium addiction, China was a political problem that was far away and out of mind to most Europeans. After 1849, however, Americans no longer had the luxury of not thinking about China: they had to face the new and startling problems of rising Chinese immigration into the western United States. As the number of Chinese immigrants rose into the tens of thousands and made its presence felt in the building of the western railroads, in the mines, and in the market gardening and fishing industries, the newly perceived threat of a cheap labor force undercutting the gains of the European immigrants became a potent political issue. A racist rhetoric of loathing and fear, with talk of "mongolization," tainted blood, and disease, became a part of political electioneering. Discriminatory legislation in housing, workplace, and school became commonplace. Chinese were killed by mobs in California and Wyoming. Their strangeness to European immigrants and their perceived desire to return to their ancestral land rather than to settle and build a better United States were invoked against them, along with the appalling conditions of their "China towns," which local legislation had so cruelly helped to create and perpetuate. The melancholy story of restrictive immigration laws against the Chinese—restrictions levied then at no other foreign nationals—is one facet of late-nineteenth-century history that must simply be confronted; China was circumscribed by the immigration treaties of 1882 and 1892 and then, after the trauma and the very real horror of the Boxer risings in 1900, by the final passage of the Exclusion Act of 1904.[9]

We should not be surprised to find that fictional works echoed or even helped to trigger events in the real world. By the 1890s a new genre of anti-Chinese writings had spread into the popular marketplace in the United States. Novels now played on fears of a Chinese amphibious attack on the coasts of California or, more fearsomely, postulated an alliance of the Chinese in the United States with American Indians and Blacks for the purpose of destroying the white population of the continent. Chinatowns became perfect settings for stories of lust, deception, and intrigue. I was amused to discover that in one of these novels, pub-

---

and Mary G. Mason, *Western Concepts of China and the Chinese, 1840–1876* (New York: Seeman, 1939). For other specific examples see Charles Dickens, *The Pickwick Papers* (London: Chapman and Hall, 1837), 414; Johann Peter Eckermann, *Conversations of Goethe with Eckermann* (New York: Dutton, 1930), 164; F. I. Carpenter, ed., *Emerson and Asia* (Cambridge: Harvard University Press, 1930), 37, 239; and Dona Torr, ed., *Marx on China, 1853–1860* (London: Lawrence and Wishart, 1951).

9. For an introduction to the huge literature on this subject see Michael Hunt, *The Making of a Special Relationship: The United States and China to 1914* (New York: Columbia University Press, 1984).

lished in 1900, the fiendish crime king of a "tong" syndicate is a Chinese Yale graduate whose racial "shortcomings" obviously transcend the powers of his East Coast Ivy League education to change his nature; but all is not lost for white America because the villain is destroyed by a Yale classmate just before he can bring his awful plans to fruition. It was a short jump from this kind of thing to the fuller plans of Fu Manchu for world domination and to his constant frustration at the hands of his white nemesis.[10]

In the post-Boxer Chinese world of the Open Door, the collapsing Ch'ing dynasty, the fledgling republic, the warlord period, and the Kuomintang-Communist civil war, Westerners would probably not seek to glean much wisdom from China. Of course, with events such as the First World War, the Bolshevik revolution, the Great Depression, and the rise of Nazism, Westerners could hardly congratulate themselves that all was well in their own cultures. And yet, interestingly, the early twentieth century saw the development of a major interest in Chinese studies on the part of Westerners. The pioneering nineteenth-century efforts of James Legge, Thomas Wade, W. A. P. Martin, and S. Wells Williams were followed by the remarkable achievements of Edouard Chavannes and Otto Franke in classical historiography, Arthur Waley in poetry, Osvald Siren in the history of art, H. B. Morse in diplomatic history, and Kenneth Scott Latourette in mission history. Most of us writing in this volume have intellectual debts to this particular congerie of scholars, and it is hard not to see the dedication of so much of their intellectual energy to China early in this century as being a mark of respect for China's past intellectual richness. (There were of course some mischievous and cautionary frauds like Edmund Backhouse, but surely he remains an anomaly.)[11]

My sample list of major scholars, given in the preceding paragraph, contains a Swede, a Frenchman, a German, an Englishman, and an American, indicating that by the twentieth century the history of Western perceptions of China must be approached in an international context. Perhaps this internationalization was because of the telegraph and the growth of daily newspapers that used foreign correspondents, perhaps it was because of changes in the world publishing industry, or perhaps it was because of the prevalence of self-selected (or politically induced) exile in each other's Western countries. But the twentieth cen-

10. See William F. Wu, *The Yellow Peril: Chinese Americans in American Fiction, 1850–1940* (Hamden, Conn.: Archon Books, 1982).

11. A good background to the growth of this Sinological tradition is Arthur F. Wright's "The Study of Chinese Civilization," *Journal of the History of Ideas* 21 (1960). On Backhouse, see Hugh R. Trevor-Roper, *Hermit of Peking: The Hidden Life of Sir Edmund Backhouse* (New York: Knopf, 1977).

tury has seen such a proliferation of the modes in which perceptions of China are expressed that I have to abandon chronology and assess these modes in broad categories if I am to make any sense of what has been happening.

Such a detailed overview can be built on the accurate, but perhaps limiting, focus of Harold Isaacs's influential *Scratches on Our Minds.*[12] Isaacs broke the American perception of China down into the following periods: "benevolence" from 1905 to 1937, "admiration" from 1937 to 1944, "disenchantment" from 1944 to 1949, and "hostility" through the 1950s. This schema makes good sense in describing American reactions to the Kuomintang years, the war of resistance to Japan, the civil war, and the Communist victory. During this period, for the first time, American attitudes were being molded by comprehensive and deliberate political forces—from Henry Luce's *Time-Life* efforts to influence American views of China to the McCarthyites and the Committee of One Million and their attempts to scare Americans out of sympathy for the mainland. I might add that if I were to update Isaacs's schema, I would postulate a period of "reawakened curiosity" from 1970 to 1974, of "guileless fascination" from 1974 to 1979, and of "renewed skepticism" from 1979 through the 1980s. The future will doubtless hold other shifts.

Rather than repeating or expanding on Isaacs's formulations for the twentieth century, which would require a survey of all modern histories and political reportage on China, I instead focus briefly on how the most influential purveyors of perceptions in fictional form (which must include films and television in addition to books) have chosen to present the relationships of their protagonists to the Chinese themselves.

The most obvious mode of representation is to focus on the Chinese in China. This approach is, of course, the stuff of most political and historical analysis, and it has produced interesting fictional results. The most influential example has been Pearl Buck's view of the suffering of China's peasants in their own parched and battered landscape (most famously in *The Good Earth*).[13] Her oddly archaic language sought to root China's contemporary experiences in a timeless zone that has been at the center of so many Western views of China—including Montesquieu's and Hegel's. But other writers drew other lessons from their Chinese actors in Chinese settings. In Judge Dee, Robert van Gulik created a

12. Harold Isaacs, *Scratches on Our Minds: Western Images of China and India* (New York: John Day, 1958), reprinted as *Images of Asia* (New York: Harper Torchbooks, 1972), and as *Scratches on Our Minds* (White Plains, NY: Sharpe, 1980); the 1980 edition published by Isaacs contains a new preface. Isaacs's periodization is outlined on p. 71 (same pagination in all editions).

13. Pearl Buck, *The Good Earth* (New York: John Day, 1931). An excellent evaluation of Pearl Buck is given by Michael Hunt, "Pearl Buck: Popular Expert on China," *Modern China* 3 (1977): 33–63.

symbol of shrewdness and integrity; the judge more than compensated for the harshness of his times. In the Kai Lung stories Ernest Bramah created a hilarious parody of "Confucian" rectitude by trading on every nuance of over-blown Chinese vocabulary.[14] In recent years new genres of anti–Cultural Revolution fiction have emerged, ranging from the subtleties of Chen Jo-hsi's stories in *The Execution of Mayor Yin* to the derring-do of *The Coldest Winter of Peking*.[15]

This approach to China should be separated from the very different one that places Western protagonists on Chinese soil with the goal of reaching the Western reader with greater immediacy. (Of course there is a paradox at work here because the "immediacy" for the Western reader is inevitably once removed from the "reality" of the Chinese psyche.) Such books share at one level the opportunities for reportage caught by many talented Western visitors, including Edgar Snow in *Red Star over China,* Graham Peck in *Two Kinds of Time,* and more recently Simon Leys in *Chinese Shadows* and Vera Schwarcz in *Long Road Home*.[16] The novel and the film, in contrast with reportage, can highlight their central figures and bring the drama into sharper focus: one thinks especially of John Hersey's eager young American engineer sizing up the opportunities for transforming the Yangtze for hydroelectric purposes in *A Single Pebble,*[17] the kidnapped heroine trying to make up her mind about China's war in the film *The Bitter Tea of General Yen,* or the success that James Clavell and Robert S. Elegant had in linking the worlds of Hong Kong and China in either *Taipan* or *Dynasty*.[18] The most magical work in this mode is the novel by the art historian Victor Segalen titled *René Leys*. Segalen's creation of a brilliant European linguist and decadent illuminates the fading grandeur and internal corruption of the Manchu Court.[19] Most books focusing on the Westerner in China end up making him or her appear isolated and frustrated and increase our sense of

14. See, for example, Ernest Bramah, *The Celestial Omnibus: Collected Tales of Kai Lung* (1940; reprint, Chester Springs, Pa.: Dufour, 1987) and *Kai Lung beneath the Mulberry Tree* (1940; reprint, Salem, N.H.: Ayer, 1978). See also van Gulik's Judge Dee stories, which are available in paperback editions by Scribner's, Dover, and The University of Chicago Press.

15. Hsia Chih-yen [pseud.], *The Coldest Winter of Peking: A Novel from Inside China,* trans. Liang-lao Dee (New York: Doubleday, 1978). See also *The Execution of Mayor Yin* (Bloomington: Indiana University Press, 1978).

16. Edgar Snow, *Red Star over China* (New York: Random House, 1938); Graham Peck, *Two Kinds of Time* (Boston: Houghton Mifflin, 1950); Simon Leys, *Chinese Shadows* (New York: Viking, 1977); and Vera Schwarcz, *Long Road Home: A China Journal* (New Haven: Yale University Press, 1984).

17. John Hersey, *A Single Pebble* (New York: Knopf, 1956).

18. James Clavell, *Taipan* (New York: Delacorte, 1983), and Robert S. Elegant, *Dynasty* (New York: Fawcett, 1982).

19. Victor Segalen, *René Leys* (Paris: Gallimard, 1971).

being unable to bridge the gap between "us" and "them." John Hersey's intriguing 1985 novel *The Call* shows the continuity of this theme.[20]

What then of the changes wrought when we transport a lone Chinese into the Western setting? In this case we seek the possibilities for an assimilation of the Chinese that we deny to ourselves. Charlie Chan, bumbling but usually successful, is the reassuring obverse of Fu Manchu because we are ultimately confident of his deference to the whites around him. The kung fu masters, those lonely, peripatetic heroes, fit safely into the mystique of white Western gunfighters rather than into the crowded, unsettling image of the Chinatown. In its way their intense loneliness is as reassuring as deference because it is firmly rooted in a moralistic code that supports Western society. Similar isolated figures can be placed in Europe or in the ambiguous zones of Malaysia, Singapore, and Hong Kong, as Paul Scott, James Farrell, and Han Suyin have done so well.[21] But the potential to use an individual Chinese figure so as to shock the Western reader into illumination comes best from a Chinese writer of power living in the United States and writing about Chinese values: witness the success of Maxine Hong Kingston and the angry, tongue-tied yet articulate central narrator of *The Woman Warrior*.[22] In this work Western white civilization gets transposed into the world of demons and ghosts that haunted her own parents.

I have been speaking of works that are in different ways about China and designed to affect our perceptions. But books set in China do not have to be about China: China can also be a device, a foil, as Voltaire knew. Thus, some of the most famous books set in China are not really about China but are about the author's own politics and should be read and treated as such. I think of two works by André Malraux, *The Conquerors* and *Man's Fate,* in which careful reading shows how rarely the Chinese appear as major actors in the story and how all the statements *about* them are made by other mouths.[23] This is true to an even more obvious extent in Bertolt Brecht's *Good Woman of Setzuan,* in which China is a backdrop with little precise significance.[24] Those who believe that Brecht had some deeper realistic purpose for setting his story in China's huge, fertile, landlocked Western province in the warlord period may have that belief laid to rest by the fact that Brecht, at the time he was

20. John Hersey, *The Call* (New York: Knopf, 1985).

21. See Paul Scott, *The Chinese Love Pavilion* (London: Eyre and Spottiswood, 1960), reprinted in the United States as *The Love Pavilion* (New York: Carroll and Graf, 1985); James G. Farrell, *Singapore Grip* (New York: Carroll and Graf, 1986); and Han Suyin [pseud.], *A Many Splendoured Thing* (London: J. Cape, 1952).

22. Maxine Hong Kingston, *The Woman Warrior* (New York: Knopf, 1976).

23. See André Malraux, *Man's Fate,* trans. Haakon M. Chevalier (New York: Modern Library, 1965) and *The Conquerors,* trans. Stephen Becker (New York: Grove Press, 1977).

24. Bertolt Brecht, *Good Woman of Setzuan* (New York: Grove Press, 1966).

writing, thought Szechwan was a town. Kafka's China, too, is totally cerebral even though exquisitely described. It is a world for phantom explorations of loneliness and time. (These explorations may be seen most vividly in his short story "The Great Wall of China.")[25]

Another extraordinary example of a work that uses China as a device is J. G. Ballard's 1984 novel *Empire of the Sun.* Set in the Japanese civilian internment camp in Lunghua, near Shanghai, during World War II, the novel is mainly a profound and brilliant meditation on suffering and will. The mutual tragedies of the Western internees and the Japanese pilots at the adjacent airfield are seen through the eyes of a starving child, Jim, but the Chinese people appear offstage for the most part, as mobs or as silent, dying figures. Near death in an old football stadium where the Japanese transferred their prisoners and their loot, "Jim lay without moving, as the fires from the burning oil depots at Hongkew played across the stands, lighting the doors of the looted refrigerators, the radiator grilles of the white Cadillacs and the lamps of the plaster nymphs in the box of the Generalissimo." This is a world of nightmare, although it is also a country dominated by the Yangtze, "that vast river barely large enough to draw all the dead of China through its mouth."[26]

Ultimately, the images fade even further away from China, perhaps the outer limit being when those studying China are used by a given author to present his feelings for other things. Fine books though they are, Western readers will gain little insight about *China* as a civilization from Joseph Knecht and his search for the tao in Herman Hesse's *Glass Bead Game* and even less from the crazed and broken China scholar Peter Kien, who burns his house, his Chinese library, and himself in the final immolation that is the climax of Elias Canetti's *Auto da fe.*[27] Despite the apparent particularity of China in these works, here the universalization of human life has become complete.

Such ambiguous or bleak images, however, in no way imply that Westerners will not continue to seek to find themselves through China and to inch toward understanding its remarkable people and their culture. Whatever their limitations, it is not adequate to view the majority of these divergent views as solely reflecting the biases within Western culture or a patronizing and exploitative attitude toward Eastern civilizations. Edward Said, who emphasizes the "cognitive imperialism" of Western scholars in his influential and passionate book *Orientalism* leaves out

25. Franz Kafka, "The Great Wall of China," *Selected Short Stories of Franz Kafka,* trans. Willa and Edwin Muir (New York: Modern Library, 1952), 129–47.

26. J. G. Ballard, *Empire of the Sun* (New York: Simon & Schuster, 1984), 211, 228.

27. Canetti's novel, for which he later received the Nobel Prize in Literature, was first published in 1935 in German as *Die Blendung. Auto da fe* was the title he used in England, though an early U.S. edition was titled *Tower of Babel.* See *Auto da fe* (New York: Farrar, Straus & Giroux, 1984).

too much of the story.[28] There have been so many twists and turns along the way to depicting China during the last four hundred years that no such broad generalizations can hold. And that is as it should be. No one is easy to understand. And the more blurred and multifaceted our perceptions of China become, the closer we may be to that most elusive thing: the truth.

28. Edward W. Said, *Orientalism* (New York: Pantheon Books, 1978).

TWO

□

Early Civilization in China: Reflections on How It Became Chinese

David N. Keightley

If we are to understand how the culture of China differs from that of other great civilizations, two fundamental and related questions need to be addressed: How did China become Chinese and how do we define "Chineseness"? Answers to these questions not only aid our understanding of the origins of Chinese culture but also, by implication and contrast, throw light on how Western values and social organization developed differently.

Before pursuing these questions, three prefatory comments are in order. First, only in broad, comparative treatments such as this one are generalizations about "Chinese culture" permitted. Even for the early period, we need to remember that there were many versions of Chinese culture that varied with time, place, and social level; I hardly do justice to all of them in this chapter. In particular, I focus less on the explicit philosophical tradition represented by such early thinkers as Confucius and more on the religious, social, aesthetic, and political practices of the Neolithic to the early Bronze Age from which these philosophers drew their assumptions and values.

Second, it must be stressed that my concerns as a historian are explanatory, not judgmental. I emphasize this point because on occasion I describe early China as having "lacked" certain features present in my Mesopotamian and Greek "touchstone cultures." But this negative ter-

One version of this essay was given at Stanford University on 18 November 1986. I have done my best to take account of the valuable criticism offered by many colleagues, who are not, of course, responsible for my errors. In particular I should like to thank David Johnson, Thomas Metzger, David Nivison, Jeffrey Riegel, Betsey Scheiner, Irwin Scheiner, Raphael Sealey, David Ulansey, Richard Webster, and Yeh Wen-hsin for their careful reading of an earlier draft.

minology is contrastive, not pejorative; as we see by the end, it is in no sense meant to imply that such features ought to have been present.

Third, I should like to call attention to the word "reflections" in my subtitle, for it serves a double function. Our visions of early Chinese (or Greek, or Mesopotamian) culture are partly and inevitably a product of the later culture's own conceptions of what its past was or ought to have been. The values of the present, generated by the past, reflect back on that past; fact is seen as value, and value in turn affects what facts are seen. Accordingly, the present chapter does not simply express my reflections on how the Chinese became Chinese. It also in part reflects how the later elite Chinese, on their reflection—represented by the editing and promoting of certain texts and quasi-historical scenarios—thought that they became Chinese. The discrepancies that arise between these later idealizing reflections and earlier unedited reality are the continuing concern of the professional historian. It is one of the functions of this chapter to place those concerns in a wider context.

THE HERO AND SOCIETY

Heroic Action: Its Representation and Consequences

Because cultures are man-made and serve to define man's conception of himself, it is helpful in considering the question of what it means to be "Chinese" to start by comparing the conception of man as hero in ancient China with analogous conceptions in Classical Greece (fifth to fourth century B.C.), a culture that has contributed so much to our Western understanding of the human condition. The legend of Achilles and the Amazon queen, for example, which was popular in both Greek and Roman cultures, expresses strategic views about the individual and society that would have been entirely foreign to Chinese contemporaries.[1]

If we consider the legend of Achilles and the Amazon queen as treated by the Penthesileia Painter on a kylix vase from ca. 460 B.C. (figure 2.1), we note a variety of characteristic features. The two protagonists are heroic in size, seeming to burst the confines of the bowl. Achilles is virtually naked. And the representation is characterized by the particularity of both its subject and its artist: we can identify the two figures, Achilles and Penthesileia, and we can identify, at least as an artist if not by name, the individual who made the vase. Most important, there is the ironic tale itself. At the moment when Achilles plunges his sword into the breast of his swooning victim, their eyes cross—and he falls in love! That moment of dramatic and fatal pathos is the one the artist has captured.[2] The

1. For an introduction to the legend, see Emily Vermeule, *Aspects of Death in Early Greek Art and Poetry* (Berkeley: University of California Press, 1979), 158–59.

2. For an introduction to the artistic representations of this story see J. J. Pollitt, *Art and Experience in Classical Greece* (Cambridge: Cambridge University Press, 1972), 20–22.

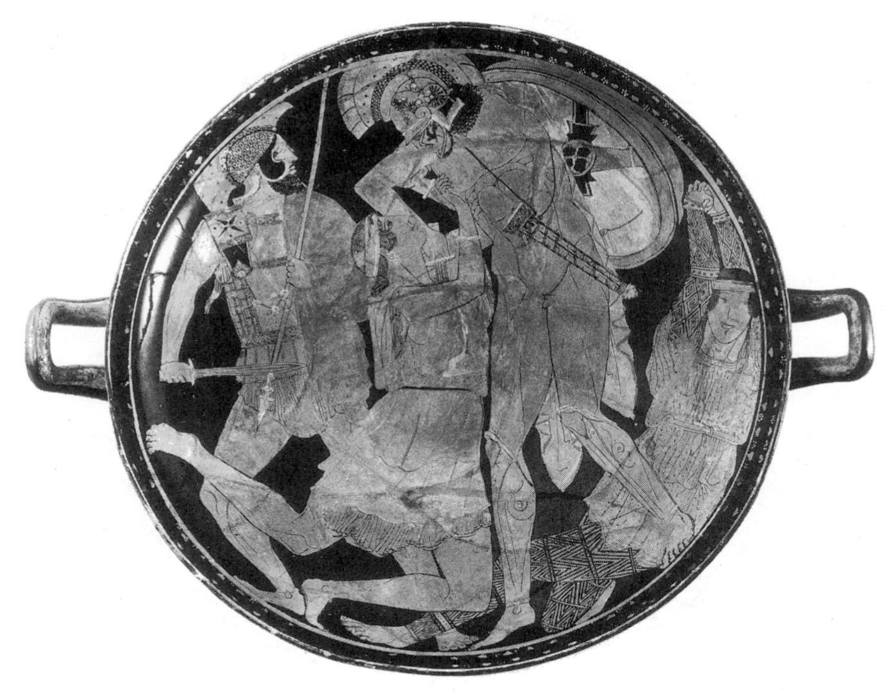

Figure 2.1. Kylix by the Penthesileia Painter. Munich, Antikensammlung. Photograph: Hirmer Fotoarchiv München.

painting and the legend express in powerful, individual, and supposedly historical terms one of the major assumptions of the classical tradition in the West, namely, that the human condition is tragic and poignant, that the best and most heroic deeds may lead to unwished-for consequences, and that even heroic virtue must be its own reward. People live in a quirky, unpredictable, and ironic world that is by no means responsive to human values and desires.

The decoration found on an Eastern Chou Chinese bronze *hu* vase from about the same period (figure 2.2) is strikingly different. Instead of individuals we are presented with stereotypical silhouettes, all of whom wear the uniform of their fellows. We do not know the names of any of the people represented. We do not know the names of any of the people involved in casting the vessel. We do not even know with any assurance the meaning of the actions depicted (see figure 2.2 caption). Whatever their precise iconographic coherence—which may have involved some generalized depiction of rituals and martial skills—the overwhelming impression conveyed by these tableaux is one of contemporaneous, regimented, mass activity, whether in peace or war; even the birds appear to be flying in formation. The individuals portrayed, small and

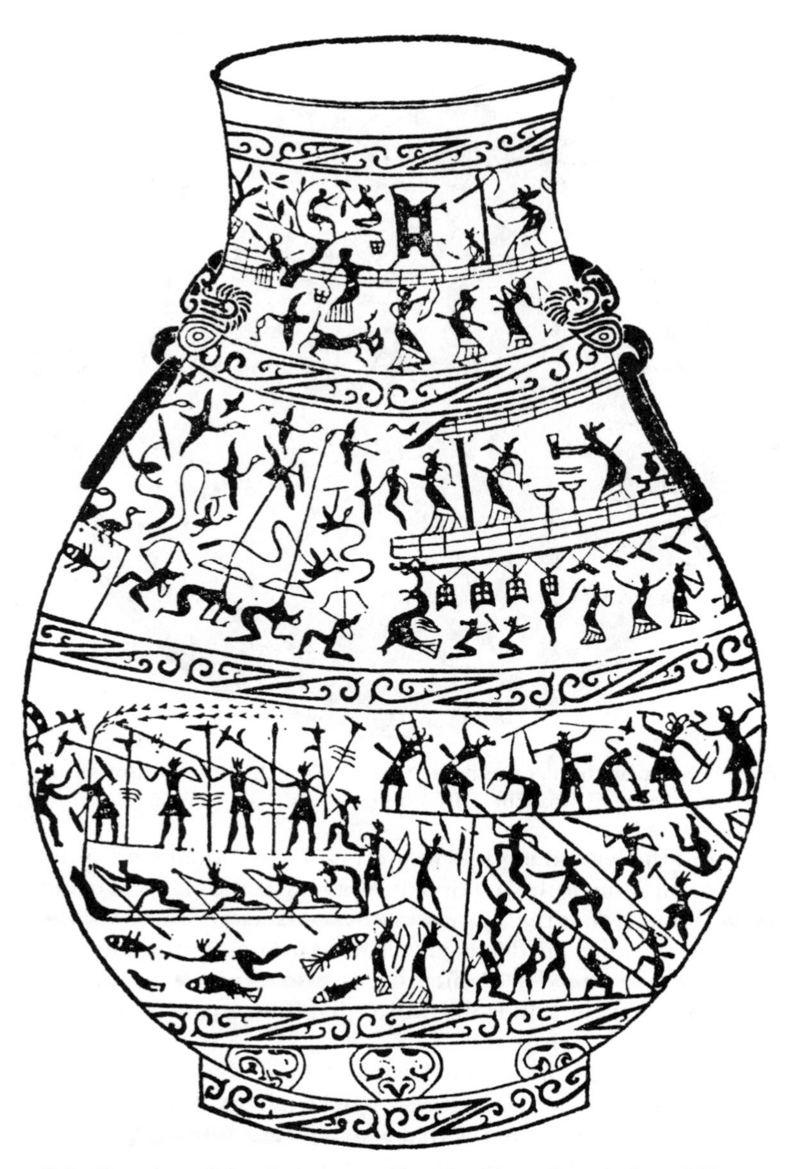

Figure 2.2. Drawing of the decor on an Eastern Chou (late sixth to fifth century B.C.) *hu* wine vase from Chengtu, Szechwan. From *Wen-wu* 1977.11:86. Moving up the vessel, we see: *bottom register,* a battle by land and sea; *middle register, clockwise from bottom left,* archers shooting at birds, a banquet scene, a bell-and-chime orchestra; *top register,* more archery (*in the bottom half*), the plucking of mulberry branches (perhaps for the making of bows), an archery contest. At least three examples of bronze *hu* decorated with these kinds of scenes have been found. See Jenny F. So, "The Inlaid Bronzes of the Warring States Period," in *The Great Bronze Age of China,* ed. Wen Fong (New York: Metropolitan Museum and Knopf, 1980), 316, and Esther Jacobson, "The Structure of Narrative in Early Chinese Pictorial Vessels," *Representations* 8 (Fall 1984): 77–80.

anonymous, have been subordinated by an equally anonymous master designer to a larger order.

This Chinese vase expresses the ideals of organization that were being applied with increasing effectiveness during the period of the Warring States (453–221 B.C.), a period when men fought less for individual honor, as Achilles had done, and more for the survival of the state. Aesthetic concerns were focused on the general, the social, and the nonheroic rather than on the particular, the individual, and the heroic. This stereotyping, this bureaucratization of experience, is implicit not only in the decor of the Chinese bronze—for somebody was presumably overseeing these soldiers and orchestra players—but also in its manufacture—for somebody had surely directed the numerous artisans involved in the industrial-scale casting of the vessel. Once again, this contrasts sharply with the practices of the Greeks, who both admired the individual and who organized their workshops around a series of acts performed by single craftsmen.

The Hands of the Hero: Dirty or Clean?

The role of hero and protagonist was radically different in the two cultures. Achilles acts for himself. He feels the thrust of the blade as it pierces his opponent's breast; he is directly responsible; he has "dirty hands." The analogous Chinese vision of the hero, at least by the time of the Eastern Chou, was radically different. Ssu-ma Ch'ien, for example, the "Herodotus of China," who wrote at the start of the first century B.C., presents five Chou and Ch'in case histories in a chapter entitled "Biographies of the Assassin-Retainers."[3] The leitmotif is that of a statesman who has an enemy he wishes to dispatch. Rather than undertaking the task himself, as Achilles would have done, the Chinese protagonist relies on the charisma of his elevated social and political position to engage an assassin. The assassin, in turn, attempts to perform the deed (with results fatal to himself in four of the five cases), not for monetary gain but to requite the overwhelming social honor the lord had conferred by deigning to entrust him with the task.

The genesis of such characteristic social obligations is a theme to which I return later. Here I simply note that the lord delegates what, in the Greek case, would have been the heroic, the personal, and thus the tragic, task. His hands are clean; they are not on the sword; he is not even near when the deed is undertaken. A bureaucratic chain of command protects the initiator from the shock and consequences of his deeds. The lord is not the hero; he has become an administrator. The hero, in these cases, does not act for himself; he is a delegate. There is a

3. Burton Watson, trans., *Records of the Historian: Chapters from the "Shih Chi" of Ssu-ma Ch'ien* (New York: Columbia University Press, 1969), 45–67.

division between the lord's original motivation for the deed and the protagonist's heroic execution of it.

Ambiguity and Optimism

The pedagogical role of the hero (or the heroine—the role of gender in such matters would be worth exploring) in the two cultures also differed. The heroes of the Greeks often served only as tragic, negative examples; few Greeks would wish to imitate Achilles by killing the woman he loved (or imitate Oedipus by killing his father, Orestes by killing his mother, or Antigone by killing herself—the examples are numerous). And when Greeks in their hubris acted in the arbitrary and passionate ways of the gods, they met disaster. Achilles would have loved Penthesileia, but he killed her; he did love Patroclus, but his arrogance as he sulked in his tent led to Patroclus's death.

In early China, by contrast, heroes were heroes precisely because they were models worthy of emulation; the universe of moral action, at least as it was represented in the accounts of myth and history, was untrammeled by ambiguities. The basic, optimistic assumption of the *Tso chuan*, the massive semihistorical chronicle compiled in the fourth century B.C., was that the virtuous man would be rewarded here and now—by promotions, honors, and status. Cause and effect in the universe were rigorously fair; the moral prospered, the wicked did not. The subversive thought that the best intentions might lead to chaos and regret—not, as in the cases of Confucius or Ch'ü Yuan, because those in power were too unenlightened to employ them, but because there was something flawed in the human condition itself—was rarely dramatized (see the discussion of theodicy below).[4]

One could multiply many instances of this early, uncomplicated Chinese view of man as a social being, embedded in and defined by the obligations and rewards of a hierarchical, ethical, bureaucratic system. The large-scale recruitment of labor by a centralized bureaucratic elite (as suggested by figure 2.2), the members of which, as Mencius (ca. 372–289 B.C.) pointed out, labor with their minds rather than their hands, may be discerned in the Chinese record from at least the early Bronze Age, if not earlier (see the discussion of Neolithic burials below). Eastern Chou states were builders of major public works, particularly city walls and the long, defensive walls that eventually culminated in the building of the Great Wall at the end of the third century B.C. The massive recruitment of labor was idealized in semihistorical accounts in which the

4. The only direct expression of this subversive thought in early China appears in Ssu-ma Ch'ien's "Biography of Po Yi and Shu Ch'i" (in Watson, *Records*, 11–15), in which the historian is sorely troubled by virtuous actions that are unrewarded and unrecognized. On Confucius's philosophical equanimity in a world where perfection is not possible, see Benjamin I. Schwartz, *The World of Thought in Ancient China* (Cambridge: Harvard University Press, 1985), 80–81.

people, both elites and masses, had cheerfully flocked to serve virtuous rulers, often dynasty founders, who had won their allegiance not by coercion but by exemplary government. Virtue was again rewarded, in this instance by the loyal service of others.

Such optimistic faith in the comprehensibility and benevolence of the universe, which runs through the classical texts and which was explicitly articulated in the view of Mencius that man's nature is basically good, can be related to what Thomas A. Metzger has termed the fundamental "epistemological optimism" of early Chinese philosophy. This optimism may be defined as the willingness to accept large, roughly defined moral ideas—like "benevolence" or "righteousness"—as reliable, universal, and objective; Metzger contrasts this with the kind of pessimistic epistemology represented by Descartes's "clear and distinct ideas."[5] Optimism about man's lot helps to explain the lack of interest in dramatic detail found in early Chinese texts (discussed below). It also helps explain the Chinese distrust of laws and constitutions, the traditional preference for *jen-chih,* "government by men," rather than for *fa-chih,* "government by laws."

Later I consider the sources of this confidence, but it was surely such "radical world optimism,"[6] such trust in one's leader as a moral *chün-tzu,* or "noble man," and the optimistic assumption—by the recruiters, if not always by the recruits—that such voluntary and nonproblematic state service was natural and proper that helps to explain the Chinese readiness to trust great leaders, whether Emperor Wu of the Han or Mao Tse-tung of the People's Republic. This optimism also helps to explain the lack of safeguards against the power of the state that has characterized Chinese government for at least two thousand years. If leaders are good—and if the good is unambiguous—who needs to be protected against them? Achilles, his hand on the sword, his act regretted as it is committed, represents a more somber vision. To the Greeks, the hero might not be bad, but he might be fundamentally and tragically mistaken. To the Chinese, a hero, by definition, was good; his mistakes, if he made any, were likely to be tactical in nature. His intent was free from error and regret.

THE NEOLITHIC TO BRONZE AGE TRANSITION

I now turn to the evolution of Chinese culture in the Neolithic and early Bronze Ages, with particular attention to such subjects as individualism (or

5. Thomas A. Metzger, "Some Ancient Roots of Ancient Chinese Thought: This-worldliness, Epistemological Optimism, Doctrinality, and the Emergence of Reflexivity in the Eastern Chou," *Early China* 11–12 (1985–1987): 66–72.

6. The phrase is Max Weber's. See Max Weber, *The Religion of China,* trans. Hans H. Gerth, with an introduction by C. K. Yang (New York: Free Press, 1951), xxx, 212, 227–28, 235.

its absence), ritual and decorum, bureaucratic control, dependency and obligation, and metaphysical optimism. The Neolithic is of fundamental importance because of the remarkable continuity of post-Neolithic cultural development in China. It is probably truer for China than for most parts of the world that as the Neolithic twig was bent the modern tree has inclined.

Neolithic cultures in China flourished during the Postglacial Climatic Optimum, when it is probable that temperatures were some two to four degrees Celsius warmer than they are today and rainfall, in at least the Middle Yangtze and north China, was more abundant. The development of early Chinese culture must be understood in the context of these relatively beneficent natural conditions.

Socially, the transition from the Neolithic to the Bronze Age in China, as elsewhere in the world, witnessed the evolution of urban forms, the genesis of the state, the institutionalization of exploitation and servitude, the validation of characteristic forms of sacrifice, and the systematic articulation of religious beliefs. Spiritually and psychologically, this transition witnessed the development of a temperament and mentality that found certain worldviews and cosmological assumptions natural and comfortable, involving, in particular, the willing acceptance of hierarchy, filiality, and obedience.

In the realm of religion, the Neolithic and Bronze Age cultures of the Near East, Greece, and East Asia—to say nothing of those of Egypt and India—developed belief systems and institutions that dealt in different ways with the one certainty that faces us all: eventual death. Death can, paradoxically, be a lively topic, for from Neolithic times onward the way people have treated death and the dead has been deeply expressive of, and has had a significant impact on, the way they have treated the living.

Neolithic China

Archaeological evidence provides considerable reason for thinking that distinctions between rich and poor, male and female, and the powerful and the weak were emerging in China by the fourth and third millennia B.C. Not only did grave goods become more abundant, but the general egalitarianism of the early Neolithic burials was replaced by marked discrepancies in energy input, wealth, and ritual care in later burials (figure 2.3). Similarly, certain houses and certain village areas begin to reveal differentiation in the goods available to the living. The presence of grave goods—which, although finely made, were generally items of daily life—presumably indicates a belief in some kind of postmortem existence.

The burial, particularly in Eastern sites, of superbly made polished stone and jade tools, such as axes and spades, whose edges reveal no traces of use, also indicates that status differentiation was prolonged beyond the grave. These objects suggest that certain members of the so-

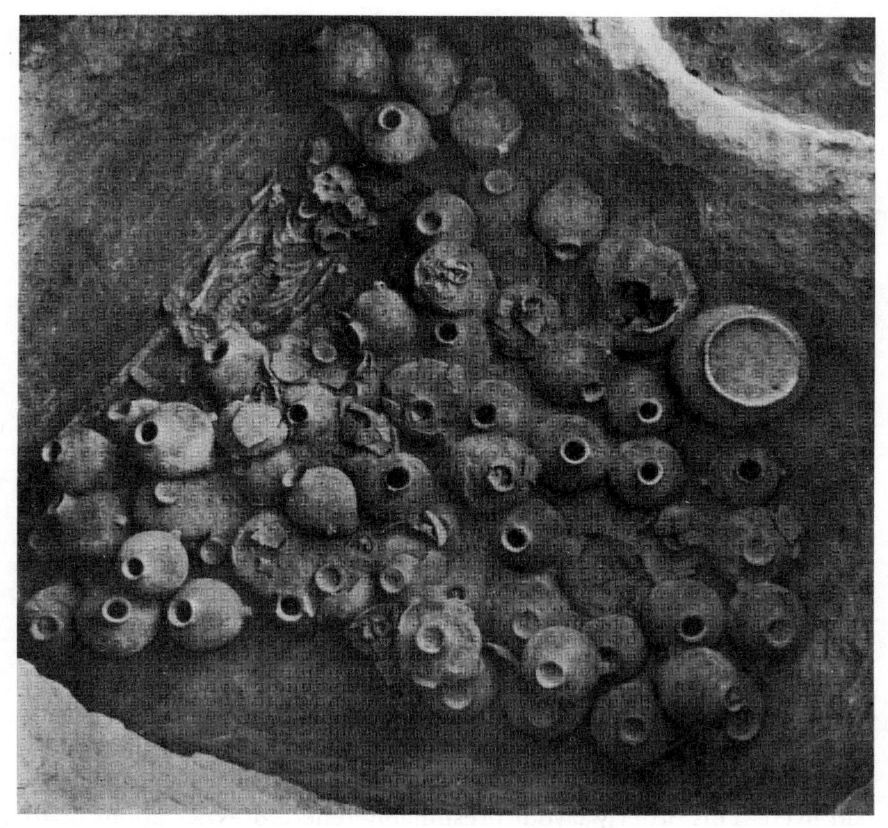

Figure 2.3. A Late Neolithic supine-extended burial with abundant grave goods at Liu-wan, eastern Tsinghai. From *K'ao-ku* 1976.6, plate 2.

ciety had been the possessors of symbolic, rather than working, tools—emblems of the owner's power to control the labor of others, both in this life and in the next. There were already by about the mid fourth millennium B.C. some people in China whose hands were not as "dirty" as those of others.

The Late Neolithic saw the emergence of scapulimancy and plastromancy, methods of divination in which the scapulas of animals (usually cattle) or the plastrons of turtles were scorched or burnt, the diviner interpreting the resulting cracks to foretell good or ill fortune. The presence of some of these "oracle bones" in cemetery areas suggests that the living, by cracking oracle bones, were attempting to communicate with the dead. One may assume that a consistently successful diviner would have acquired increased political authority, an authority supported by his powerful kin, both living and dead.

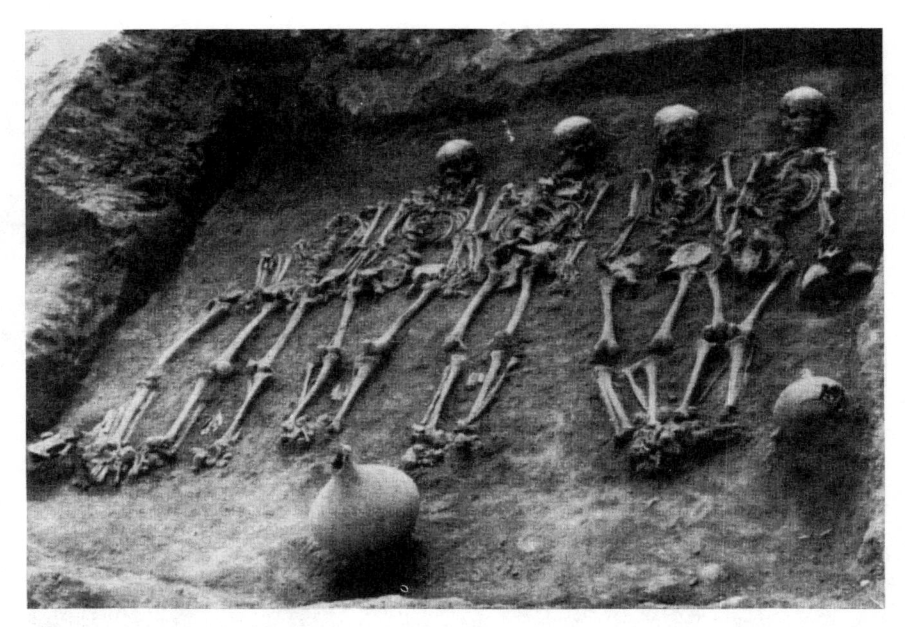

Figure 2.4. Secondary burials in grave M441 at Yuan-chün-miao, Shensi. From *Yuan-chün-miao Yang-shao mu-ti* (Peking: Wen-wu Ch'u-pan-she, 1983), plate 33.

The Neolithic Chinese treated their dead with remarkable and characteristic assiduity. Corpses were buried in orderly rows, oriented to certain compass directions depending on the area of China in which they had lived. This orderly layout presumably reflected expectations of social order among the living. The corpses were also generally buried in the supine-extended position (see figure 2.3), a practice that required more labor for the digging of the burial pit than, for instance, a flex burial. The log construction of coffin chambers in certain Eastern burials, particularly at the Ta-wen-k'ou site in Shantung, or of tomb ramps in the northwest is a further indication of the labor expended on mortuary concerns.

The practice of collective secondary burial, which, although never dominant, flourished in the Central Plains and the Northwest during the fifth millennium, is particularly revealing. The cleaning away of the flesh and the careful reburial of the bones—frequently arranged in the standard supine-extended posture of the primary burials, and with skulls oriented to the prevailing local direction (figure 2.4)—implies the ability to mobilize labor resources for the collective reinterment of up to seventy or eighty skeletons in one pit. It also implies that the dead must have been kept alive in the minds of their survivors during the period of months, if not years, between primary and secondary burial.

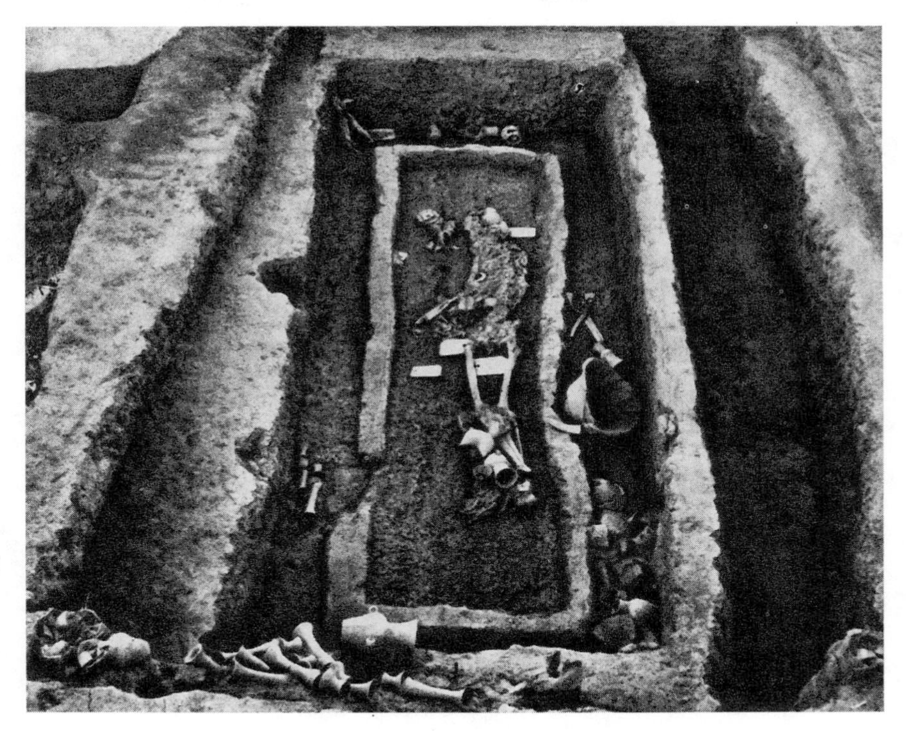

Figure 2.5. Grave M25 at Ta-wen-k'ou, Shantung. The eight tall *pei* goblets at the bottom of the picture had been placed in the earth fill and had presumably been used in a farewell ritual. From *Ta-wen-k'ou: Hsin-shih-ch'i shih-tai mu-tsang fa-chueh pao-kao* (Peking: Wen-wu Ch'u-pan-she, 1974), plate 13.3.

Other mortuary rituals were employed. The placement of some of the jars and goblets in Neolithic burials, for example, suggests the existence of farewell libations by mourners as the grave was being filled in (figure 2.5); the precarious, tall-stemmed black goblets of the East (figure 2.6)—whose fine, eggshell-thin construction itself suggests some special ritual function—may have been used for the consumption of millet wine at the time of interment.

One of the most remarkable of all Neolithic burials is M3 at the Liang-chu culture site of Ssu-tun in Kiangsu (ca. 2500 B.C.; figure 2.7), which gives ample evidence of ritual activity: the corpse had been placed atop ten jade *pi* disks that had been burned; the body had then been surrounded by a variety of jade and stone tools and ornaments, including a perimeter of twenty-seven jade *ts'ung* tubes; and five of the twenty-four jade *pi* in the burial had been deliberately broken in two and placed in different parts of the grave. Given the difficulty of working with jade, a material that has been described as "sublimely impractical," the presence

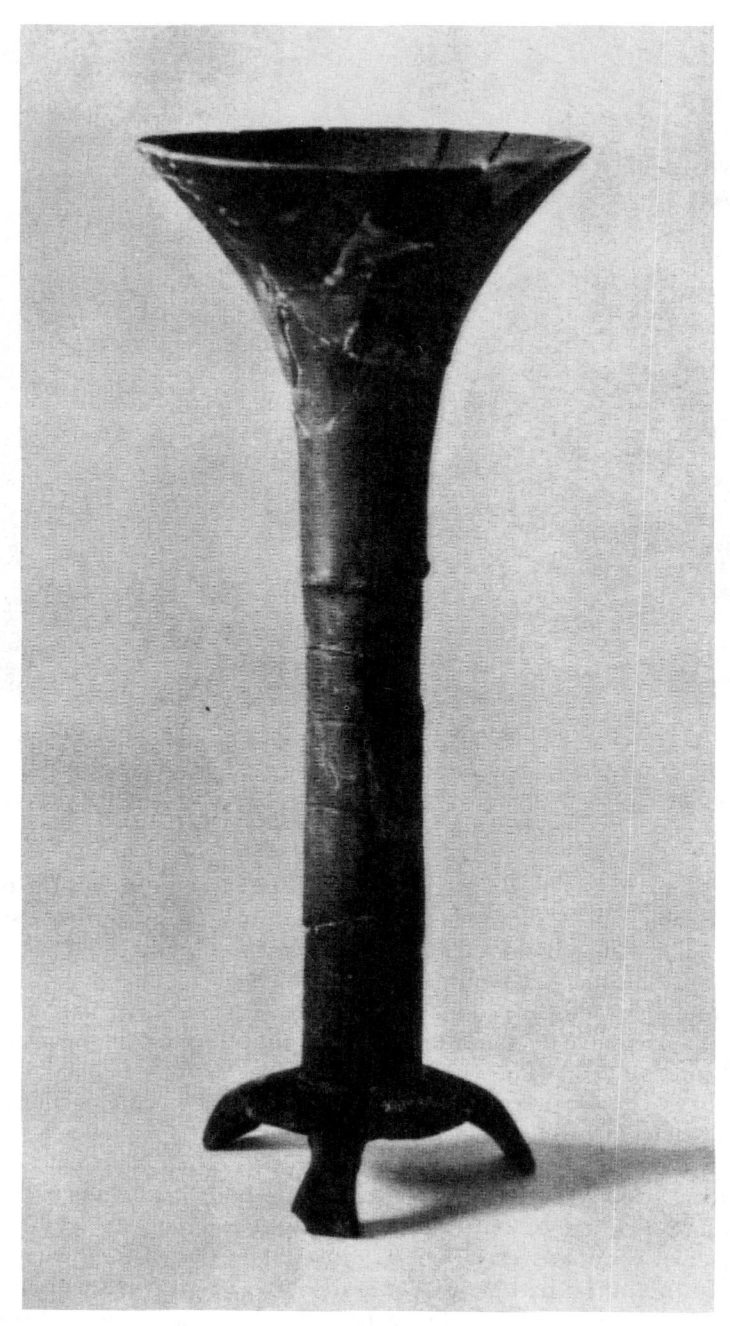

Figure 2.6. *Pei* goblet from P'i hsien, Kiangsu. From *Chiang-su sheng ch'u-t'u wen-wu hsuan-chi* (Peking: Wen-wu Ch'u-pan-she, 1963), no. 43.

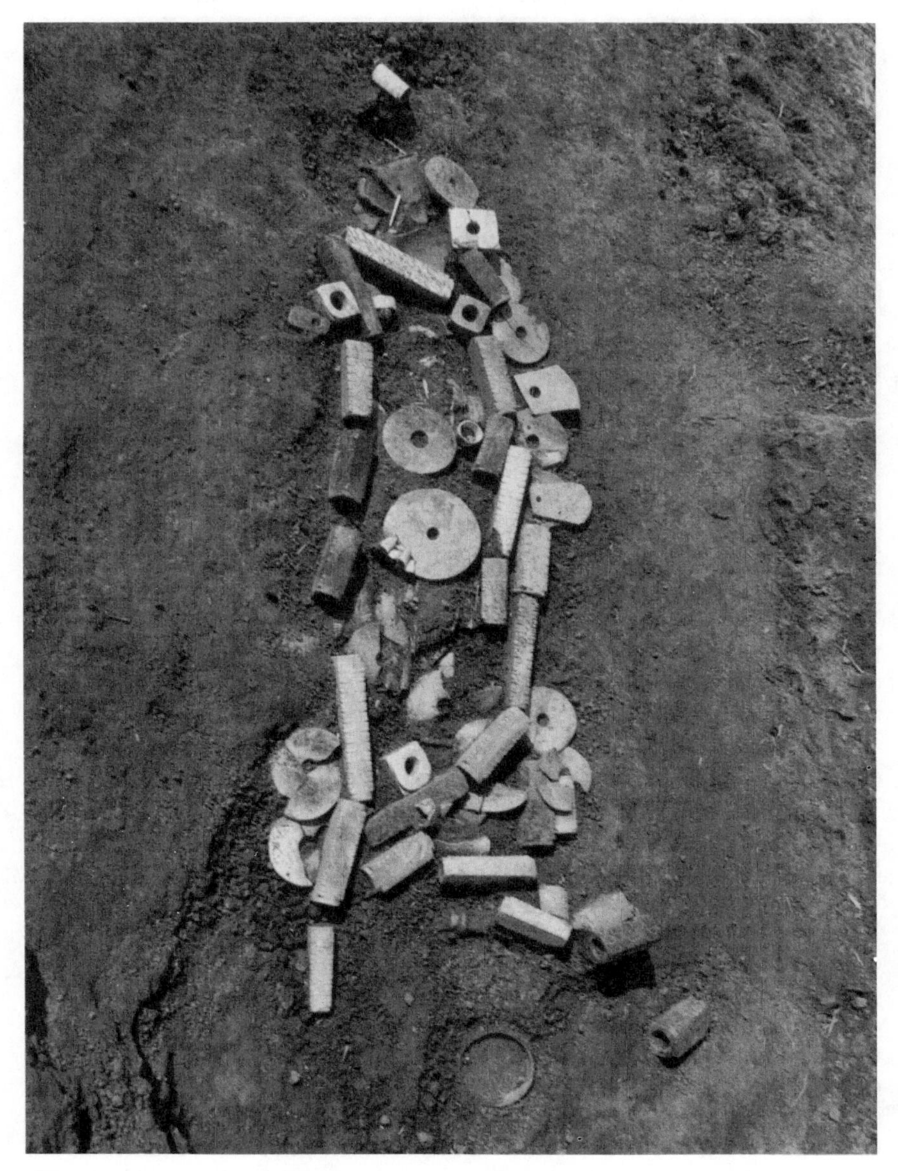

Figure 2.7. Grave M3 at Ssu-tun, Kiangsu. The corpse is "shrouded in jade." From *K'ao-ku* 1984.2, plate 2.

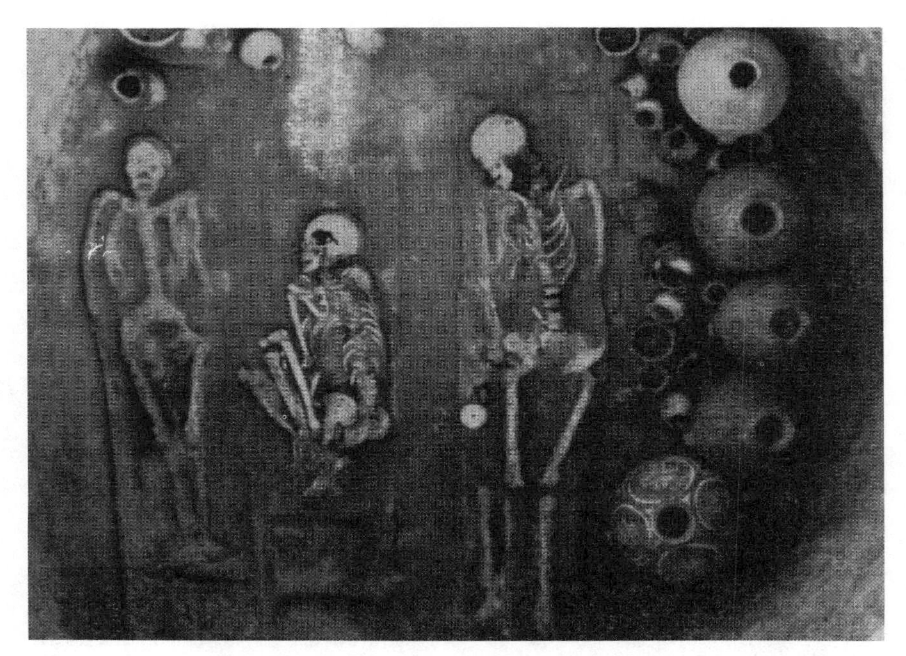

Figure 2.8. Grave M327 at Liu-wan, eastern Tsinghai. The central corpse, buried in a flex position, is thought to have accompanied the other two corpses in death. From *Wen-wu* 1976.1 : 75, figure 11.

of large numbers of finely carved jade *pi* and *ts'ung* in other Lower Yangtze burials of the third millennium—they have never been found in the housing remains—is further indication of the way in which the labors of the living were exploited for the service of the dead.

Some burials also contained victims: animal and, occasionally, human. Human sacrifice was not widespread in the Neolithic, but there is evidence—both in a Yang-shao burial at P'u-yang in northern Honan (end of the fifth millennium?) and in Ma-ch'ang and Ch'i-chia burials in eastern Tsinghai and western Kansu (toward the end of the third millennium)—that a small number of people were accompanying others in death, further evidence of the kinds of payments the living were constrained to offer the dead (figure 2.8). The presence of an occasional tool by the side of the victim indicates, at least in the later sites, that a servant in this life was to continue as a servant in the next life. Ties of obligation and servitude were so strong that they persisted after death.

Bronze Age China

By the Late Shang period (ca. 1200–1045 B.C.), represented by the archaeological finds at Hsiao-t'un, near Anyang in the northern Honan

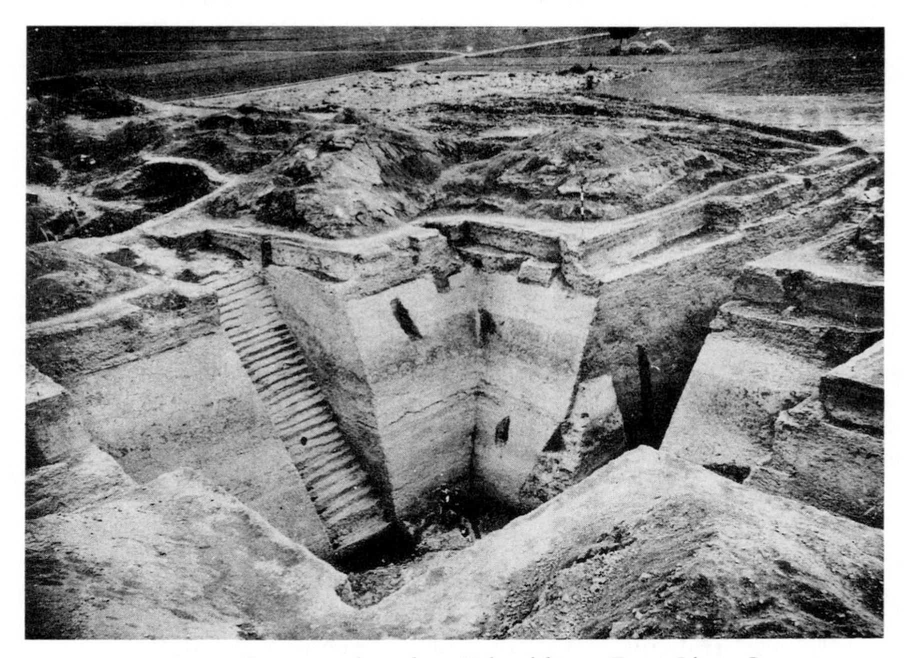

Figure 2.9. A Late Shang royal tomb at Hsi-pei-kang. From Liang Ssu-yung and Kao Ch'ü-hsun, *Hou-chia-chuang 1002-hao ta mu* (Taipei: Academia Sinica, Institute of History and Philology, 1965), plate 3.

panhandle, increasing stratification and the institutionalization of power were both represented and reinforced by a highly developed cult of the dead. The oracle-bone inscriptions reveal that the dead were worshiped as ancestors according to an increasingly precise ritual schedule. Neolithic mortuary traditions were amplified but not radically altered.

With regard to grave goods, for example, the unrifled burial known as M5—which has been linked to Fu Hao, a consort or royal woman associated with the powerful king Wu Ting (ca. 1200–1181 B.C.)—contained over sixteen hundred grave goods, including 468 bronzes whose total weight was over one and one-half tons. Extrapolation from this relatively small burial suggests that the contents of the looted tombs in the royal cemetery at Hsi-pei-kang, across the river to the northwest of Hsiao-t'un, would have been even more impressive. The tombs were veritable underground storehouses of the finest products that Shang civilization could create; these great cruciform, ramped pits, up to forty-two feet deep (figure 2.9) and equipped with beamed, room-sized grave chambers up to nine feet high, were monuments to the affection and obligation that linked living descendants to dead parents.

Such tombs are eloquent proof of the intensity with which the mortuary cult both exploited and stimulated the labors of the community. The digging and refilling (with rammed earth) of such a pit alone, quite apart from the labor involved in furnishing it with the wooden chamber, coffin, and costly grave goods like bronzes and jades, would have taken one hundred men well over two hundred days to complete. The continual draining of wealth to provide goods for the dead was the early Chinese equivalent of conspicuous consumption and planned obsolescence; it stimulated the productive powers of craftsmen and laborers by expropriating the fruit of their efforts in a culturally rational manner. A system of exchange was evidently involved. Motivated by spiritualized kinship ties, mortuary taxes on the immediate wealth of the living served to guarantee the future prosperity of their descendants.

The number of human victims associated with the Shang royal burials is impressive, as it was undoubtedly intended to be. It may be estimated that some of the royal four-ramp tombs would have claimed the lives of over three hundred sacrificial victims and accompaniers-in-death and that, over the course of the approximately one hundred and fifty years in which it was in use, some five thousand victims may have been buried in the Hsi-pei-kang burial complex; these figures, which do not include some ten thousand human sacrifices recorded in divinations about the regular ancestral cult, represent a rate of about thirty-three victims a year, or 550 per king. The mortuary victims were drawn from a cross section of Shang society: elite accompaniers-in-death, placed near the king and buried whole, sometimes with their own coffins, grave goods, and even accompaniers-in-death; guards, buried whole with their weapons; and prisoners of war, the most numerous group, generally young males, decapitated or dismembered and buried in the earth fill, in the ramps, or in adjacent sacrificial pits. This last group, the sacrificial victims, outnumbered the accompaniers-in-death by a ratio of about twenty to one.

Similar large-scale immolations were not unknown in Mesopotamia—for example, in the royal cemetery of Ur, where from three to seventy-four attendants accompanied the ruler—but there the custom was short-lived and virtually unrecorded in texts. Human sacrifice was rarely practiced in the Greek Bronze Age.[7] More significantly, there is virtually no evidence of accompanying-in-death. Elite Greeks were not linked to each other by ties of obligation and dependency that bound them in death as they had presumably been bound in life. In China, by contrast,

7. That Achilles, in book 23 of the *Iliad,* put "twelve radiant sons of Troy" to the sword at the funeral of Patroclus was more a sign of his fury than common custom. (The quotes from the *Iliad* and the *Odyssey* in this chapter are taken from the translations of Robert Fitzgerald, which are published by Doubleday.)

the custom was practiced for a far longer period, continuing to a significant degree in the burials of local rulers and even emperors down to the Ch'in–Han period and beyond, with the number of victims varying from a few to over a hundred.

The oracle-bone inscriptions—with their records of systematic offerings to dead kings, whose own powers and abilities to intercede with Ti, the Lord on High, extended to such fundamental areas as weather, climate, and victory in battle—reveal the central, institutionalized role that ancestor worship played in the workings of the Shang state. This power accorded to dead fathers and grandfathers suggests, accordingly, that Shang lineages were strong and that kinship affiliation, reinforced by religious sanctification, was a powerful force for allegiance and motivation. It may be supposed that Shang ancestor worship, which promoted the dead to higher levels of authority and impersonality with the passage of generations, encouraged the genesis of hierarchical, protobureaucratic conceptions and that it enhanced the value of these conceptions as more secular forms of government replaced the Bronze Age theocracy.

Ancestor Worship and Its Consequences

The Late Shang state emerged by building upon and institutionalizing, rather than opposing, the ties of affection, obligation, and dependency indicated by the mortuary practices of the Neolithic. The close fit between dynastic and religious power that resulted had at least three significant consequences.

First, it meant that there was no independent priesthood that might serve as an alternative locus of power or criticism; the king, as lineage head, was his own priest. The heads of all powerful lineages had access to the independent and friendly religious power of their own ancestors without the mediation of other religious specialists. Second, it meant that the way in which the values of kinship obligation, ancestor worship, and dynastic service reinforced one another led to an enduring unitary conception of the state as a religio-familial-political institution that could embrace, ideally, all aspects of one's allegiance, leaving little ideological ground vacant as a base for dissent. Given the totality of the Chinese state, it is no wonder that the only Eastern Chou "oppositionists" who left much of an intellectual mark, the Taoists of the Chuang Tzu school, had to reject conceptions of service and hierarchy. Confucius and his followers could certainly lament contemporary realities, but they were essentially meliorists working within the value system rather than radical critics of the system itself. It is also no wonder that rebels against the state were frequently to appeal to the vast world of popular nature powers, gods, and Buddhist saviors, who stood outside the normative politico-religious structure of the lineage. Third, it meant that the Chinese humanism of the Eastern Chou, represented by such great social thinkers as Confucius, Mencius, and Hsun Tzu, did not see any opposition between secular and religious values and was able, in Fingarette's striking phrase, to treat "the secular as sacred."[8] The humanism that resulted, therefore, was based on social and kin relations sanctified by religious assumptions. Ritual and hierarchical expectations were applied to all aspects of a monistic cosmos; just as there had been no opposition between king (or lineage head) and priest, so there was no tension between the counterclaims of god and man, between a Zeus and a Prometheus. The optimism of the Chinese tradition, which has already been noted, can be understood as both producing and being reinforced by this fundamental sense of harmonious collaboration. There was, once again, no sense of immanent moral paradox or conflict.

DEATH AND THE BIRTH OF CIVILIZATION

Next I attempt to integrate early Chinese mortuary practices with other aspects of the culture, considering how the meaning of one set of customs may be more richly understood when seen in the context of others, how one set of assumptions about the human condition was reinforced by, and would have reinforced, others.

Death and Continuity

Shang burial customs helped to define what it was to be a ruler (or a retainer). The wealth, the dependents, and the victims accompanying the king into the next world demonstrated that his superior status (and the inferior status of his retainers) would be unchanged after death. This view of death as a continuity rather than a new beginning had already been implied by the grave goods and mortuary customs of the Chinese Neolithic. Death offered none of the escape, none of the psychic mobility offered by the mystery religions of the Near East or by Christianity itself with its vision of a redemptive death and rebirth as "in Abraham's bosom." In early China death provided an effective opportunity for survivors to validate the central values of the culture. No dead Chinese king would have been permitted the lament made by Achilles in book 11 of the *Iliad*—"Better, I say, to break sod as a farm hand/for some country man, on iron rations,/than lord it over all the exhausted dead"—for such an admission would have undermined the respect and obedience owed to the dead elites and thus to their living descendants. Once a king, always a king; death could not change that.

8. Herbert Fingarette, *Confucius: The Secular as Sacred* (New York: Harper, 1972). Anyone reading this provocative book should also read the detailed critique provided in Schwartz, *The World of Thought in Ancient China.*

Death as Unproblematic

One striking feature of the early Chinese written record is its view of death as unproblematic. Death was simply not the issue it was for the ancient Mesopotamians or the ancient Greeks. Nowhere, for example, in the ancient Chinese record does one find the mythical claim, found in Mesopotamian texts, that death existed prior to the creation of both the universe and man. Nowhere does one find the angry and anguished voice of a Gilgamesh, horrified by the death of Enkidu and by Enkidu's depressing account of the life to come:

> the house where one who goes in never comes out again,
> the road that, if one takes it, one never comes back,
> the house that, if one lives there, one never sees light,
> the place where they live on dust, their food is mud.
> . . . .
> My body, that gave your heart joy to touch,
> vermin eat it up like old clothes.
> My body, that gave your heart joy to touch,
> Is filled with dirt.[9]

There is no ancient Chinese myth, like that of the Garden of Eden, that accounts for the "invention" of death or that treats death as some flaw in the divine plan. There are no visits to, or descriptions of, the realm of the dead that would compare with the descriptions we have of the Netherworld for the Mesopotamians or of Hades for the Greeks. Nowhere do we find the epic concerns of the *Iliad* and *Odyssey,* which focus on the manner of death, the ritual treatment of the dead, and the unhappy fate of the shades after death and which express so powerfully the tragic (once again the word recurs) poignancy that death confers on the human condition. Nowhere do we find a philosophical discourse, like Plato's *Phaedo,* that is devoted to the nature of death and the soul.[10] The very silence of the Chinese texts about such matters suggests a remarkable Chinese ability to emphasize life over death. Ancestor worship and the endurance of the lineage served to render the loss of the individual more palatable. Indeed, these practices would have served to promote, as they were promoted by, a conception of the individual and his role quite different from that held by the Mesopotamians and Greeks.

9. John Gardner and John Maier, trans., *Gilgamesh: Translated from the Sin-leqi-unninni Version* (New York: Knopf, 1984), tablet vii, column iv, tablet xii, column iv, 178, 265.

10. The ripostes and anecdotes about death found in the *Chuang Tzu* merely confirm this point. Chuang Tzu is arguing for a nonhuman view of death precisely because he is arguing for a nonhuman view of life. He is, in these passages, less concerned about death itself than with the institutions and values that the civilized Chinese had developed to deal with it. Unlike Plato, he deals with death as a social problem, not a philosophical one, because, in his view, society itself is the problem. His cheerful acceptance of death might well have filled Plato with envy.

Morality and the Absence of Theodicy

The great mythic themes in China were not dying and death but social order and social morality; there is no Chinese equivalent to the heroic and adversarial universe of Gilgamesh or Inanna, Achilles or Hector. One is impressed and attracted by the general harmony that pervades the relations of the Chinese to their gods. For example, although there had been a flood, dimly described, its main function was to provide the sage emperor Yü with a sphere for his labors in political geography, delineating the borders for the various regions of China. The famous saying, recorded in the *Tso chuan,* "But for Yü we should have been fishes," pays tribute to his having made the world habitable; the myth does not address the issue of why the flood occurred. There is, in fact, a characteristic lack of theodicy in early Chinese culture, its fundamental optimism seeming to render unnecessary any explanations for the presence of evil.

There was no sense in early Chinese mythology that the gods were malevolent, that they resented human success, that they might conspire to destroy man, or that man was becoming too numerous and too tiresome, themes that are all present in Mesopotamian and Greek myth and in the Old Testament. Just as there was no Prometheus, neither was there any Zeus. Given this lack of divine animus, of immanent man-god hostility, it was natural that death in China should not have been regarded as an affront to mortals to the degree that it was in Mesopotamia and Greece; rather, it was part of the inevitable and harmonious order. In a kin-based society where the royal ancestors were in Heaven, there was little discord between god and men. There was little need, in short, for a Chinese Gilgamesh or a Chinese Job, asking why a man who has done no wrong should die or suffer. The issue, when it did arise, as in the cases of Po Yi and Shu Ch'i (note 4, this chapter) or of Confucius himself, who was shunned by the rulers of his age, was usually conceived in terms of employment, reward, and recognition rather than suffering or destruction. Even in his moving letter to Jen An in which the great historian Ssu-ma Ch'ien, who had been punished by Emperor Wu of the Han, laments his castration, his regrets are characteristically couched not in terms of his own loss but in terms of his having failed to serve the emperor and his colleagues effectively.[11]

Death, the Individual, and the Supernatural

Attitudes toward death depend on cultural conceptions of what has been lost. Just as the bitter reactions to death in the cases of the *Gilgamesh* and

11. The letter is translated in Burton Watson, *Ssu-ma Ch'ien: Grand Historian of China* (New York: Columbia University Press, 1958), 57–67.

the Greek epics, for example, may be related to strong conceptions of personal roles in the two cultures, so may the quieter, more accepting responses of the early Chinese, who were less anguished metaphysically by death, be related to their deemphasis on individual heroic action.

The lack of emphasis on the individual may also be seen in the realm of the supernatural. By contrast with the Mesopotamians and Greeks, for whom misfortune and defeat stemmed from the harassment and disorderly interference of individual gods like Enki and Ishtar or Zeus and Aphrodite, the Shang Chinese presumably would have explained such events in terms of improper sacrifices and dissatisfied ancestors. Those ancestors would have been mollified not by the particularistic pleas of humans or by erratic interventions and divine favoritism but by ordered sacrifices whose efficacy was tested in advance through divination and offered in accordance with the status of the ancestors responsible. Given this protobureaucratic attitude toward the supernatural, it was entirely natural that death itself would also be treated in a more matter-of-fact, more impersonal manner.

The Chinese of the Western Chou, whose Mandate of Heaven doctrine moralized the political culture, explained misfortunes and defeats in terms of immoral behavior; some thinkers of the Eastern Chou, by contrast, adopted the impersonal cycles of *yin-yang* and "five-phase" theory. No matter which of these explanations one turns to, the Shang and Chou elites lived in a more ordered, more "rational" world of large, general forces that implemented the will of hierarchically ordered ancestors or "Heaven," on the one hand, or that were incarnated in natural cycles, on the other. By contrast to the Mesopotamian or Greek deities, Chinese ancestral spirits were remarkably depersonalized, a point to which I return later.

Origins and Eschatology

The absence of origins myths until relatively late in the Chinese record was also surely related to conceptions of life and death. I would suggest that conceptions of creation ex nihilo are related to and stimulated by a radical, nihilistic view of death itself. Cultures that are less anxious about eschatology, such as that of ancient China, are less likely to be concerned about their origins; cultures that are more worried about final destinations, such as those of Mesopotamia and Greece, are more likely to devote attention to the question of whence they came. The Greek concern with questions of origins, "first causes," and "first principles" is well known. In China, where identity was conceived as biological and social, the question of origins was often one of genealogy and history. A hierarchy of ancestors leading back to a dimly perceived founding ancestor or ancestress was answer enough because it satisfied the kinds of questions that were being asked.

Critical Distance

The "openness" of Greek society, which was coming into existence during the Archaic period (ca. 760–479 B.C.), has been called "its most precious single legacy," serving to encourage both "the intellectual speculations of the few and individual freedom among the many."[12] The characteristic Greek readiness to question and complain about the human condition—whether that questioning was religious, metaphysical, or political—may be related to the marked difference that distinguished mortals from immortals in Greek legend. This distance allowed the Greeks to take a stance more critical than that permitted a Chinese worshiping his ancestors, who were merely ex-humans, not radically different beings.[13] A strong, hierarchical, lineage system does not encourage children to criticize parents or descendants to criticize spiritualized ancestors; it also does not encourage the pursuit of radical innovations. I would not deny that, as Nathan Sivin notes in Chapter 7 of this volume and as Joseph Needham's extensive work has revealed,[14] Chinese craftsmen and technologists have been among the most inventive in the world. The point is, however, that such innovators were generally not rewarded with or stimulated by commensurate social prestige.

For the early Chinese, as for their imperial descendants, it was the past that was normative. The Greeks, like most traditional cultures, certainly revered the past; yet they succeeded in a situation that M. I. Finley has referred to as one of "compulsory originality" in producing a series of unprecedented cultural innovations.[15] The past was accorded greater respect by the Chinese because the past was, through the lineage, the integrated source of biological, religious, and political identity. This great respect helps explain the lesser emphasis placed on individual creativity and innovation; emulation of dead ancestors was all the originality required. Such an environment encouraged what might almost be called a spirit of "compulsory unoriginality." Once again we encounter the strength of the lineage in early Chinese culture—already seen in the mortuary evidence and the cult of ancestor worship—as one of its most

12. Anthony Snodgrass, *Archaic Greece: The Age of Experiment* (Berkeley: University of California Press, 1980), 161.

13. See Vermeule, *Aspects of Death,* 125, on the way in which the epic permitted the Greeks to laugh at and even despise their gods. Jasper Griffin has made a related point. For the Greeks the "world makes less sense through moral self-examination"—which would have been the Chinese approach—"than through recognition of the gulf that separates mortal men from the serene superiority and shining gaze of the immortal gods" ("From Killer to Thinker," *New York Review of Books* 32, no. 11 [27 June 1985]: 32).

14. Joseph Needham, *Science and Civilisation in China,* 7 vols. projected (Cambridge: Cambridge University Press, 1954–).

15. M. I. Finley, *The Ancient Greeks: An Introduction to Their Life and Thought* (New York: Viking, 1964), 23.

distinctive features. It is no accident that the greatest innovations in early statecraft and social theory appeared in the Warring States period (453–221 B.C.) of the "hundred schools," the age when the great aristocratic lineages of the Spring and Autumn period (721–479 B.C.) were disappearing from the scene.

AESTHETICS AND STYLE

Ingrainedness

Characteristically, there is no visual image or even textual description of any early Chinese ruler or deity to compare with the images and descriptions of particular rulers, heroes, and gods we have from Mesopotamia and Greece. There is no Chinese equivalent to the bronze head, which may depict King Sargon the Great, no Chinese version of a heroic, life-size, naked bronze Poseidon. In the Neolithic, the Shang, and the Western Chou the iconographic tradition was, with few exceptions, profoundly nonnaturalistic. Gombrich's formula, "making comes before matching,"[16] was not only true of the designs painted on Chinese Neolithic pots but continued to be true until relatively late in the Bronze Age. Whatever the so-called monster masks on the Shang and Chou bronzes (see, for example, figure 11.3 in Chapter 11) represented—and it is by no means clear that they were intended to "match" any natural animal—they were primarily magico-aesthetic expressions of design, symmetry, and an almost dictatorial order.

This concern with general order rather than particular description—manifested in the early aesthetics, social rituals, and philosophy of early China—may also be seen, to return to one of our earlier themes, in representations of death. No early Chinese text provides vivid, unflinching details like the worm crawling out of the dead Enkidu's nose in the *Gilgamesh* or the brains bursting from a mortal thrust and running along the spearhead in book 17 of the *Iliad.* The relative unconcern with material details can be seen as a further expression of the "epistemological optimism" referred to earlier, the willingness to embrace ideas that were more dependent on social custom and general category than on rigorous analysis and precise description.

Both aesthetically and socially, the Chinese did not manifest what has been called "the Greeks' personifying instinct," that instinct that rendered Greek myths so rich in personalities and thus so un-Chinese.[17] Indeed, if one word had to be used to describe early Chinese aesthetic, and

16. E. H. Gombrich, *Art and Illusion: A Study in the Psychology of Pictorial Representation* (Oxford: Phaidon, 1977), 99.

17. L. R. Farnell, *Greek Hero Cults and Ideas of Immortality* (Oxford: Oxford University Press, 1921), 359.

even philosophical, expression, I would suggest "ingrainedness." By ingrainedness I mean the willingness to concentrate on the symbolic meaning of an event, usually moral or emotional and frequently expressive of some normative order, rather than to express, or derive comfort or insight from, its existential qualities for their own sake. Such ingrainedness has nothing to do with abstractions or with the ideal forms of Plato's dialogues. It is in the Chinese case entirely immanent. The patterns, symbols, messages, rules, and so on are entirely within reality; they do not transcend reality metaphysically but merely render its existential details of minor importance. As Girardot has written of Chinese myths,

> Mythic materials and themes have entered into Chinese literature as a series of extremely abstract, and essentially static, models for organizing and evaluating human life.
>
> Mythic themes in early Chinese literature, in other words, often seem to be reduced to their inner "logical" code or implicit cosmological structure of binary *yin-yang* classification.[18]

Chinese ingrainedness, then, stands in sharp contrast to the passionate Archaic Greek attention to individual detail for its own existential sake, the recognition of the quirky, ironic, indifferent, nonsymbolic, existential, nonessential nature of reality, the "outgazing bent of mind that sees things exactly, each for itself, and seems innocent of the idea that thought discerps and colors reality." These traits are absent in the early Chinese texts that have come down to us. John Finley has referred to this Archaic Greek attitude as that of "the Heroic Mind"; his account is worth quoting in full for the contrasting light it throws on the Chinese evidence.

> When in the sixth book of the *Iliad* Hector briefly returns to Troy . . . and meets his wife and infant son at the gate and reaches out to take the boy in his arms, the child draws back frightened at his father's bronze armor and helmet with horsehair crest; whereupon Hector laughs, takes off the helmet, and lays it all-shining on the ground. In so deeply felt a scene surely no one but Homer would have paused to note that helmet still shining beside the human figures. It is as if in whatever circumstances it too keeps its particular being, which does not change because people are sad or happy but remains what it is, one of the innumerable fixed entities that comprise the world. Similarly in the heroic poems ships remain swift,

18. Norman J. Girardot, "Behaving Cosmogonically in Early Taoism," in *Cosmogony and Ethical Order: New Studies in Comparative Ethics,* ed. Robin W. Lovin and Frank E. Reynolds (Chicago: University of Chicago Press, 1986), 71. Girardot also refers to Sarah Allan's judgment (*The Heir and the Sage: Dynastic Legend in Early China* [San Francisco: Chinese Materials Center, 1981], 18) that "in using myth in political and philosophical argumentation, the Chinese writer operated at a higher level of abstraction and with greater self-consciousness than is normally associated with mythical thought. He did not narrate legend but abstracted from it."

> bronze sharp, the sky starry, rivers eddying. Though heroes fight and die, everything in the outflung world keeps its fit and native character.[19]

There are no comparable scenes, no "shining helmets," in early Chinese literature. Even in the *Book of Songs* (*Shih ching*), where early Chinese lyricism is most prominent, the general supersedes the particular, and nature is pregnant with allegorical or symbolic meaning, usually moral. There are love poems but no great lovers. Nature is not independent but participates in man's moral and emotional cosmology; its role is to express human concerns. To put the matter another way, early Chinese texts, like early Chinese bronze designs, reveal marks of what, to a Greek artist, would have seemed like severe editing, in which particular detail had been sacrificed to abstract order. Either there never was a Chinese equivalent of the Heroic Mind or it has left no reflection; in either case the contrast with the Classical Greeks, who were so deeply inspired by the epics of the Archaic period, is significant.

The Heroic Mind is superficially reminiscent of the epistemological optimism of the early Chinese thinkers. Both forms of thinking reveal unquestioning acceptance. The differences, however, are fundamental. First, the Heroic Mind accepts existence without question; the epistemologically optimistic mind, by contrast, accepts ideas and formulations. Second, the Heroic Mind in Finley's analysis yields by the Classical Age, to what he calls the "theoretical mind" and then the "rational mind"; what we may call the "metaphysical optimism" of Homer is replaced by the "epistemological pessimism" of Plato. No such radical evolution was to take place in China, whose thinkers were to remain consistently satisfied with their epistemological optimism, an optimism they would characteristically reassert in the eventual Confucian response to Buddhism's nihilistic metaphysics. This lack of change, this satisfaction with early, and hence ancestral, cultural forms, is a theme to which I return.

Metaphysical and Technological Correlates

Although Plato's concern with ideal forms, which is so radically un-Chinese in its metaphysical assumptions about a separate, nonimmanent realm of perfection, is alien to the Homeric view of reality, one can nevertheless note the way in which it derives from the Homeric emphasis on individual particulars, objects, and persons. When, for example, Plato employs metaphors of the workshop in discussing such matters, it

19. John H. Finley, Jr., *Four Stages of Greek Thought* (Stanford: Stanford University Press, 1966), 3, 4, 28. Similar observations about Homer's style in the *Odyssey* may be found in "Odysseus' Scar," the opening chapter of Erich Auerbach's *Mimesis: The Representation of Reality in Western Literature* (Princeton: Princeton University Press, 1953).

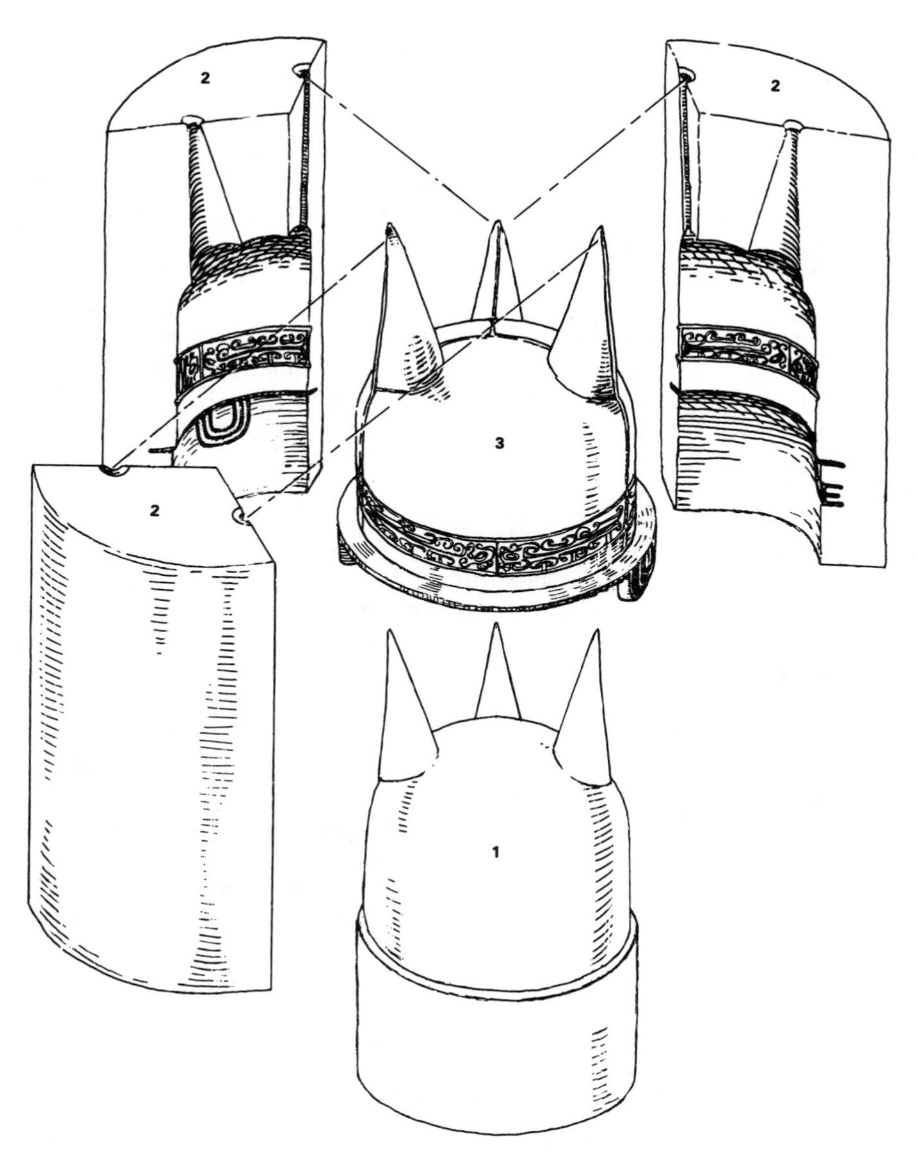

Figure 2.10. Schematic drawing of the piece-mold casting assembly used to cast a Middle Shang tripod: (1) core, (2) mold sections, (3) completed bronze vessel. From Wen Fong, ed., *The Great Bronze Age of China: An Exhibition from the People's Republic of China* (New York: Metropolitan Museum and Knopf, 1980), 72. Drawing by Phyllis Ward.

is the shoemaker's inability to make individual and identical shoes each time, his inability to match the ideal conception of a shoe, that concerns him. Bronze-working in classical Greece would have manifested the same troubling variance; each wrought object—such as Achilles' sword—would have been made singly and thus differently by a smith, hammering and beating it into an approximation of the ideal form. Chinese piece-mold bronze casting, by contrast, permitted no such individual variation. The technological process, involving ceramic molds placed around a central core, guaranteed that when molten bronze was poured into the space between the mold and the slightly pared down or shrunken core, the initial clay model would be duplicated virtually exactly (figure 2.10).[20] This duplication of models is analogous, in the technical realm, to the emulation of heroes and ancestors referred to earlier, just as the Greek techniques of smithy bronze production are analogous to the Greek emphasis on the individual hero.

Given this context, it is fitting that the problem of variance, of the failure to match an abstract ideal, did not occur to the early Chinese as a major theoretical problem, as opposed to a practical one. They assumed that individuals were identified and valued in terms of the human roles they played within the kinship group. "There is good government," said Confucius, "when the father is a father and the son a son" (*Analects* 12.11). They also assumed, with characteristic optimism, that people were educable to the good and were capable of performing those roles adequately; their epistemological optimism did not require them to define or analyze those roles, such as that of father and son, with the rigor and precision that a Plato, more pessimistic about the human capacity to know and understand, would have demanded.

The Absence of Drama

The central importance of dramatic performances in the Athens of the fifth century B.C., acted in theatrical competitions before audiences of some fourteen thousand citizens and challenging and lampooning some of the most cherished values of the state while being supported in part by public funds, needs no comment here; the absence of such an artistic and political form in China is another feature that separates the two cultures.

The absence of dramatic confrontation may also be discerned in other areas of Chinese expression. I have already noted, for example, the lack of narrative tension in the pictorial representations on the Eastern Chou

20. For a brief introduction to piece-mold casting and its aesthetic consequences see Robert W. Bagley, "The Beginnings of the Bronze Age: The Erlitou Culture Period," in *The Great Bronze Age of China: An Exhibition from the People's Republic of China,* ed. Wen Fong (New York: Metropolitan Museum and Knopf, 1980), 70–73.

hu vases (see figure 2.2). In the realm of expository prose one of the striking differences between the writings of the early Chinese philosophers and Plato is the particularism with which Plato incarnates his arguments, describing the time, the place, and the persons to give dramatic force to Socrates' conversations. Confucius's sayings, by contrast, are usually divorced from the emotional hurly-burly of debate with keenly delineated individuals on particular historical occasions. There is little dramatic tension in early Chinese philosophical texts comparable to the "tense liveliness," the "dialectical friction," of Plato's dialogues.[21] This successful incarnation of the general in the particular characterizes Greek art, philosophy, and conceptions of the immortals. In China, by contrast, in art, philosophy, and religion the individual is submerged in more general concerns.

This absence of dramatic tension in both philosophy and art relates to the Chinese concern with ritualized social hierarchy that we see emerging as early as the oracle-bone inscriptions of the Shang and that becomes fully developed in the classical ritual texts of the Eastern Chou and Han. The Chinese *li* were canons of status-based, role-related social decorum, reciprocity, and ethical consideration that operated in the religious, social, and political spheres; they implied by their very nature that basic social questions had already been resolved in favor of a patriarchal status quo. The ideals of social behavior were known: "Let the father be a father, the son a son"; the only point at issue—so well exemplified by the early Han in the esoteric moral catechisms of the *Kung-yang* (late Chou) and *Ku-liang* (early Han?) commentaries to the *Spring and Autumn Annals,* supposedly composed by Confucius—was how to fit particular cases to general rules.

Such a socio-moral taxonomy, eventually articulated in the doctrine of the "rectification of terms" (*cheng-ming*), is both impersonal and undramatic. Assuming that a familial-style commitment to shared values is preferable to a society of adversarial relationships, the promoters of the *li* manifested a cast of mind that was uninterested in logical argument designed to change opinions; they preferred instead to appeal in set-position speeches to the authority of hallowed books and traditions.

Art and Ancestor Worship

Chinese aesthetic and even philosophical uninterest in particular detail may also be related to ancestor worship. As Fortes notes, "The ancient

21. The phrases are those of Alvin W. Gouldner, *Enter Plato: Classical Greece and the Origins of Social Theory* (New York: Basic Books, 1965), 361, 385. Even in the *Chuang Tzu,* A. C. Graham notes the rarity of "genuine debates" in which "spokesmen of moralism . . . and of worldliness . . . are allowed their say before being defeated" (*Chuang-tzu: The Seven Inner Chapters and Other Writings from the Book "Chuang-tzu"* [London: Allen & Unwin, 1981], 234).

Greeks appear to have had elaborate cults concerned with beliefs about ghosts and shades, but no true ancestor cult." He emphasizes that "ancestor worship is a representation or extension of the authority component in the jural relations of successive generations; it is not a duplication, in a supernatural idiom, of the total complex" of kin or other relationships. Ancestor worship, in short, does not simply involve belief in the dead; it involves belief about the dead, who are conceived in a certain way.[22]

Following this line of thought, I propose that an inverse relationship exists between an emphasis on hierarchical roles of authority, whether for the living or the dead, and the vagueness with which the afterlife is conceived. The cultures that depict the afterworld, or even this one, with some attention to specific detail may not need, or may do so precisely because they do not have, a well-defined social hierarchy or ancestral cult. When the authority of the elders and ancestors functions well in this world, there is less need to depict the environs of the next. This suggestion—which may be related to the earlier discussion of the impersonality of the dead—would also help explain the well-known fact that, although there are many mythic personages alluded to in ancient China, there is little evidence of a sustained, anecdotal mythology.[23] In this view there would have been no need in China for the precision of event and personality that we associate with the art and mythology of Mesopotamia and Greece; the "mythological issues," as it were, would have already been resolved by the invention of the ancestors, who were ancestors precisely because they were not comprehensive or detailed representations of personality and social role. The Mesopotamian and Greek concern in both religion and art with personality, social role, and the chaos of unstructured, adversarial existence was replaced in China, if it had ever been present, by a generalized concern with harmonious order and design and with ingrained and symbolic meanings.

Harmony and Moral Chauvinism

The emphasis on harmony in early Chinese art, literary expression, and philosophy—a corollary to the absence of critical and dramatic tension—may also be related to the deep-seated moral and epistemological optimism and confidence already noted. This optimism and confidence

22. Meyer Fortes, "Some Reflections on Ancestor Worship in Africa," in *African Systems of Thought,* ed. M. Fortes and G. Dieterlen (London: Oxford University Press, 1965), 125, 133.

23. Derk Bodde, "Myths of Ancient China," in *Mythologies of the Ancient World,* ed. Samuel Noah Kramer (Garden City, N.Y.: Doubleday Anchor, 1961), 369–70; Bodde notes that "the gods of ancient China . . . appear very rarely or not at all in art, and are commonly described so vaguely or briefly in the texts that their personality, and sometimes even their sex, remains uncertain."

could only—and here I speak as a child of the Western tradition—have been achieved by glossing over, frequently by generalizing and classifying, those sharp, awkward, and frequently nonharmonious details that caught the attention of the Greek artist or philosopher.

One of the characteristic and non-Chinese features of the *Iliad,* for instance, is that the audience hears, and has its sympathies engaged by, both sides of the story, within the walls of Troy as well as without. Similarly, neither Creon in *Antigone* nor Oedipus in Sophocles' trilogy is presented as an unsympathetic or unremittingly evil figure. This ambiguity about what and who is right lies at the essence of the tragic vision; our sympathies are not, should not, and cannot all be on one side.

Greek epics derive much of their complexity and dramatic tension from the frank recognition that unresolvable conflicts exist in the world, that choices are frequently made not between good and evil but between two goods. By contrast, no early Chinese writings—with, as is so frequently the case, the possible exception of the *Chuang-tzu*—take a similarly detached and complex view of the human condition. There is no passage in early Chinese literature analogous to Antigones' wrenching cry, "Ah Creon, Creon, / Which of us can say what the gods hold wicked?"; the epistemological optimists of China thought that they could say. The vanquished were simply categorized as "ingrainedly" immoral and their point of view was never presented as worthy of consideration, dramatically or historically. From the *Book of Documents* (*Shu ching*) through *Mencius* and beyond, last rulers of dynasties were by definition bad and those who overthrew them, whom we should unquestioningly trust, were by definition good; there was no sense of a "loyal opposition" as even conceivable, let alone desirable or human. There are few Trojans in early Chinese literature; generally, there are only Achaeans, only victors.[24]

RELIGION, LINEAGE, CITY, AND TRADE

Ancestor Worship: The Strategic Custom

To the extent that it is possible to speak of one strategic custom or institution in the mix of early China's cultural variables—strategic because

24. Even in Ssu-ma Ch'ien's detailed portrayal of Hsiang Yü—the great antagonist of Liu Pang, who eventually founded the Han dynasty—there was little tragic about his defeat, which, if we take the Grand Historian at his word, was entirely justified: "It was hardly surprising that the feudal lords revolted against him. He boasted and made a show of his own achievements. He was obstinate in his own opinions and did not abide by established ways. . . . 'It is Heaven,' he declared, 'which has destroyed me. . . .' Was he not indeed deluded!" (Watson, *Records,* 104). Even if Ssu-ma Ch'ien is being ironic here, he in no way portrays Hsiang Yü with the kind of sympathetic and dramatic detail that Homer accords Hector. Although Hsiang Yü's flawed character brings destruction, the destruction is not tragic because his character is not presented as admirable.

of its pervasive ability to sanctify all other aspects of life and to legitimate and reinforce the lineage—it would seem to be ancestor worship and its social and political corollaries involving hierarchy, ritual deference, obedience, and reciprocity. At some point, probably still in the Neolithic, the commemoration of the dead—a feature common to many early cultures, including the Greek and Mesopotamian—probably became more orderly and articulated in China, taking on an ideological and juridical power of its own. The values of this new ancestor worship would have been intimately related to, and could not have been generated without, the existence of strong lineages. The traditional Chinese ideal of the extended family in which several generations were to live under one roof is only practicable when family members are trained to value group harmony above personal independence. Indoctrination in the value of *hsiao* (filiality or obedience), whose roots can be discerned in the sacrifices made by the Shang kings, if not in the offerings placed in Neolithic burials (see figures 2.3 and 2.5), provided just such a training and socialization. Forming part of a rich vocabulary of familial and religious dependence and obligation in which even rulers would refer to themselves as a "small child," presumably still under the eye of their dead parents, *hsiao* was precisely not the kind of lineage virtue that would have been validated by the independence and unpredictability of the Mesopotamian and Greek gods and heroes.

In addition to its impact on mortuary practices and its validation of filiality, ancestor worship had important demographic consequences. To the extent that a cult of the ancestors requires the procreation of cultists to continue the sacrifices, the eschatology of death in early China encouraged population growth in a significant way. This sanctification of posterity, and especially of male progeny, is a constant theme in the bronze inscriptions of the Western Chou, many of which end with a prayer such as, "For a myriad years, may sons of sons, grandsons of grandsons, long treasure and use (this vessel)." The multiplication of progeny recurs as a theme in the *Book of Songs* (*Shih ching*) and is given its most articulate emphasis in Mencius's famous dictum that nothing is more unfilial than to fail to produce descendants. The supreme obligation to one's ancestors was to become an ancestor oneself.

The considerable demands of the ancestral cult, visible in the grave goods of both the Neolithic and the Bronze Ages, also served to stimulate the production of material wealth. In social rather than economic terms, however, the order being "revitalized" by Chinese mortuary cults was the lineage, the power of senior kin over junior kin, and the conservative and ascriptive ties of affection, obligation, and exploitation that were stronger than life itself.

Belief in ancestors had additional consequences. Although there is no doubt that the Shang and Chou Chinese worshiped nature powers or spirits—rivers, mountains, and fertility figures like Hou Chi (Prince Millet), the legendary ancestor of the Chou—the argument that these spirits had originally been local deities, the ancestors of particular tribes, has much to recommend it.[25] Similarly, there is some evidence that Shang Ti, the Lord on High, may have once been a progenitor of the Shang royal lineage. And it is clear that the Chou ruler came to regard himself as the T'ien Tzu, "Son of Heaven." Even though the biological relationships are murky in many of these cases, the general conception of man's relationship to the spirits of the universe was implicitly genealogical. Rulers were thought to have a special, quasi-familial relationship to the supreme deity; man was the offspring of the spirits, ancestral and otherwise. Accordingly, there was no sense of a radical difference between spirits and humans. The spiritual universe was unitary and man's relationship to that universe relied less on personal observation and exploration and more on participation in the social groups that were the primary focus of religious feeling.

The Ancient Chinese City

Despite its ability to focus and accentuate cultural values, religion is not an independent variable. Because religion operates within society and is a product of society, we cannot ignore the environment and the economic context that produced the Chinese form of lineage dominance. The ancient Chinese city is instructive in this regard because it differed significantly from the city found in Mesopotamia or Classical Greece. Not only was it visually and aesthetically different, being built largely of rammed earth, timber, thatch, and tile rather than of stone, but its political composition was different too. Early Chinese cities may be regarded as politico-religious embodiments of lineage and dynastic power, centered on a palace-temple complex and existing primarily to serve the needs of the ruling elites whose ancestors were worshiped there. These settlements were characterized by a regulated layout and unitary power structure in which merchants and artisans, subordinate to the elite lineages, played a relatively minor political role.

In Mesopotamia, by contrast, the sprawling cities grew by accretion and housed large and diverse populations. Secular power and religious power were clearly distinguished and often in opposition; the palace was confronted by countervailing sources of authority as represented by the temple, the military, private wealth, and merchants. Lineages, in particular, do not seem to have played the significant political role they did in China; the character of Mesopotamian urbanism appears to have "dissolved" the social and religious strength of the kinship units.

Ancient Chinese cities stand in even sharper contrast to those of Clas-

25. See David N. Keightley, "Akatsuka Kiyoshi and the Culture of Early China: A Study in Historical Method," *Harvard Journal of Asiatic Studies* 42 (1982): 294–99.

sical Greece. Greek cities were characterized by their variety of changing political forms, such as tyranny, oligarchy, and democracy, their emphasis on overseas colonization and commerce and the consequent exposure to the challenge of other cultural traditions, their reliance on "citizens," who had both rights and duties in the state, their emerging conception of equality before the law, their dependence on legal and economic slave-labor and the corollary discovery of personal freedom. In Athens the lack of any permanent officialdom, the preference for direct citizen participation in government—once more the reliance on "dirty hands"—rather than on representation and bureaucracy, is particularly notable. The Eastern Chou analogues of the Greek citizens, the *kuo-jen*, "people of the state" (the state being conceived primarily as the walled capital itself), may have had certain privileges, but they appear to have had no separate corporate or legal existence.

Notable also is the absence in China—so puzzling to Marxists inspired by the Greek case—of the *stasis*, or social conflict, between "the few" and "the many" that was a characteristic feature of the Greek city states. The rare urban upheavals recorded in the *Tso chuan* involved factional struggles among the noble lineages and their supporters; they did not involve class interests and were not fought over economic issues.[26]

This nonpluralistic Chinese urbanism helps to explain why the shift from kin-based to class-structured society that is associated with the rise of states in general seems to have taken place less completely in traditional China, where the government at both the dynastic and bureaucratic level continued to be marked by its familial nature in terms of both ideology and personnel. Despite the remarkable commercial activity that characterized many cities of post-Sung China—Marco Polo, for example, was astonished by their size and wealth—merchants in China did not achieve the kind of political, legal, and economic independence that they did in the West. This is a distinction of fundamental importance whose deep and ancient roots are partly to be found in a political system that gave kinship ties and their political extensions priority over commercial and legal ones.

THE ULTIMATE QUESTION

The ultimate question is, Why did early China develop in these particular ways? Why did its values and cultural style differ from those of the ancient Near East or ancient Greece? Speculation is tempting.

26. See, for example, the struggles in the state of Wei in 470 B.C. (James Legge, trans., *The Chinese Classics,* vol. 5, *The Ch'un Ts'ew with the Tso Chuen* [Oxford: Oxford University Press, 1872], 856–57); the palace workers, of relatively high status themselves, provided the manpower, not the motivation, for the revolt of the great officers. Their role is in some ways analogous to that of the assassin-retainers discussed earlier.

First, the great abundance of Neolithic sites in China suggests greater population density than in Mesopotamia and Greece, even at this early date. If this impression is confirmed by subsequent excavations and by statistical analysis, we may conclude that Chinese experience would have been more "peopled" and that such "peopling" is congruent with a less individualistic, more group-oriented social ethic.

Second, one can speculate that the Chinese environment, which encouraged such population growth, together with the population growth itself, helped to set the basic mood of the culture. If one can relate the trusting and self-confident mood of the ancient Egyptians to the benevolence of the Nile valley, and the pessimism and anxiety of the ancient Mesopotamians or ancient Greeks to the comparative harshness and uncertainty of their environment, then one may argue that the comparatively favorable Neolithic climate in China would have encouraged a characteristic optimism about the human condition. The agrarian nature of the civilization also suggests that the characteristic dependence on superiors was related to the inability to move away from coercive leaders once one's labor had been invested in clearing the land and rendering it fertile.

Third, the nonpluralistic nature of early Chinese culture is a trait of great significance for which we should try to account. I have noted the relatively undifferentiated character of the early cities. We may further note the lack of significant foreign invasions and the absence of any pluralistic national traditions; the challenging linguistic and cultural contrast that the markedly different Sumerian and Akkadian traditions presented to the inhabitants of early Mesopotamia, for example, was simply not present for the early Chinese literati. Also, to the degree that the trading activities of merchants and the value placed on them in Mesopotamia and Greece can be explained by their relatively resource-poor hinterlands, then private merchants would have been less powerful in China because they would have been less needed. In this case geography may have played a role. Because the major rivers in north and central China—the Yellow, the Huai, and the Yangtze—flow from west to east rather than along a north-south axis, trade, to the extent that it followed the river valleys, would have generally been between regions in the same latitude whose crops and other natural products would have been similar; the distinctive ecogeographical zones in China are those of north and south, not east and west.

In this view the market economy would not have had the strategic value in China that it had in other parts of the world. A significant proportion of Chinese trade in early historical times, in fact, seems to have been tribute trade—reciprocal or redistributive in character, political in function, and dealing in high-cost, luxury items reserved for the elites, who controlled the merchants by sumptuary regulations and by co-opting them as necessary into the administrative bureaucracy.[27] The lack of an inland sea like the Mediterranean, the absence of rocky shores and good harbors along much of the north and central China coast, the absence of major trading partners across the China Sea to provide cultural as well as economic stimuli, and the presence of deserts and mountains separating north China from Central Asia, would have further encouraged the noncommercial, agrarian bias of the early Chinese city and state and the self-confidence of its isolated, indigenous culture.

These considerations, which are basically geographic, suggest that characteristically Chinese formulations of property and legal status would have developed in a culture where economic power was primarily agrarian power. Although there is no early evidence to support Karl Wittfogel's view of an agromanagerial despotism running the state's essential water-control works, one can nevertheless see that wealth in the early state would have depended less on control of land—there was probably a surplus—and more on control of a labor force that could clear that land and make it productive. Social control—originally motivated and legitimated by religious and kinship ties—rather than technological or military control, would have been the key to political success. Access to lineage support, ancestral power, and divinatory reassurance would have been more important and more inheritable than mere claims on unpeopled, and thus unworkable, property. The problem, as revealed by King Hui of Liang near the start of the *Mencius* (1.A.3) in a conversation that is purported to have occurred ca. 320 B.C., was how to attract people to serve a ruler and his state: "I do not find that there is any prince who exerts his mind as I do. And yet the people of the neighboring kingdoms do not decrease, nor do my people increase. How is this?" This problem was one of the major concerns of the Eastern Chou philosophers. It is worth recalling that the kind of bronze-casting industry that the Shang elites patronized and that expressed both their military and their religious power had depended on the ability to mobilize labor on a large industrial scale.[28] These early patterns of behavior and legitimation subsequently made possible the larger water-control projects of imperial times; it was not the projects that created the patterns.

27. These speculations need to be treated with caution for at least two reasons. First, the traditional Confucian bias against trade has meant that commercial activity has not been well recorded in the early texts. Second, the kinds of archaeological techniques that would enable us to "finger-print" the sources of pots and jades, for example, have not yet been applied to the Chinese evidence. For both reasons the commercial role of early cities in China and the kinds of exchange networks that linked them to one another and to other regions of China still remain to be explored.

28. Ursula Martius Franklin, "The Beginnings of Metallurgy in China: A Comparative Approach," in *The Great Bronze Age of China: A Symposium*, ed. George Kuwayama (Los Angeles: Los Angeles County Museum of Art, 1983), 94–99.

Speculations of this sort encourage us to seek for still earlier, more "ecological," more geopolitical, more material explanations for the origins of Chinese culture. They do not, however, satisfactorily explain why early Chinese culture took the precise forms that it did. That question, in fact, unless we narrow its scope, is unanswerable because cultures are to a large extent self-producing, the products of a virtually infinite combination of interacting factors. Many of these factors are mental and many of them are unidentifiable in the archaeological or early historical record. To put the matter another way, with the exception of the most basic precultural factors, such as climate and geography, which can only provide the most general of answers, there is nothing but dependent variables. It is truer to what we understand of cultural development—and truer, perhaps, to Chinese than to traditional Western approaches to explanation—to think in terms of the gradual coevolution of many factors rather than of a few prime movers.[29]

Because we cannot explain "everything," universal laws of development with a specificity sufficient to explain the genesis of Chinese, or any other, culture must elude us. Nevertheless, we can, as I have attempted to do, suggest some significant and characteristic features of early Chinese culture whose interrelationships were strong and whose subsequent influence on the civilization of imperial China was large.

CONCLUSION

What then do we mean by "Chinese" from the Neolithic to the early imperial age in the Han? Impressionistic though any attempt to define a worldview or cultural style must be, it may be suggested that "Chinese" referred in part to a cultural tradition permeated by the following features (listed, on the basis of the above discussion, in no order of causal priority):

1. Hierarchical social distinctions—as revealed by opulent Late Neolithic burials (see figures 2.3 and 2.7), by the high status of the Bronze Age elites both in this life and in the next, and by the human sacrifices demanded, both in blood and in obligation, by those elites.
2. Massive mobilization of labor—as revealed by the early Bronze Age city walls, the royal Shang tombs (see figure 2.9), the industrial

29. On the correlative or "organismic" Chinese view of the world in which "conceptions are not subsumed under one another, but placed side by side in a *pattern*, and things influence one another not by acts of mechanical causation, but by a kind of 'inductance,'" see Joseph Needham, with the research assistance of Wang Ling, *Science and Civilisation in China*, vol. 2, *History of Scientific Thought* (Cambridge: Cambridge University Press, 1956), 280–81.

scale of Shang bronze-casting (see figure 2.10), and the large-scale public works, such as the long walls and tombs of imperial times.
3. An emphasis on the group rather than the individual—expressed in the impersonality and generality of artistic and literary representation (see figure 2.2) and generated and validated by a religion of ancestor worship that stressed the continuity of the lineage and defined the individual in terms of his role and status in the system of sacrifice and descent.
4. An emphasis on ritual in all dimensions of life—seen in Neolithic mortuary cults (see figures 2.5 and 2.7), in the emphasis on ritual practice revealed by the oracle-bone inscriptions of the Shang, and in the classical cult treatises of the Eastern Chou and Han.
5. An emphasis on formal boundaries and models—as revealed by the constraints involved in rammed-earth construction, by the use of molds in Neolithic ceramic technology and in the bronze technology that evolved from it (see figure 2.10), by the dictatorial design system of the bronze decor (see figure 11.3), by the use of models in both bronze technology and social philosophy, and by the great stress on social discipline and order in ethics and cosmology.
6. An ethic of service, obligation, and emulation—consider the burials of accompaniers-in-death and human victims in Neolithic (see figure 2.8) and Shang times, the elevation of sage emperors and culture heroes who were generally administrators rather than actors, the motivations of Ssu-ma Ch'ien's assassin-retainers, and the obligations and unquestioning confidence that the princely man might engender. The endurance of this ethic is dramatically expressed by the army of some seven thousand life-sized terracotta soldiers, buried ca. 210 B.C., proud and confident as they accompanied the First Emperor of China in death (figure 2.11).
7. Little sense of tragedy or irony—witness the evident belief, well developed even in the Neolithic, in the continuity of some form of life after death. Witness, too, the general success and uncomplicated goodness of legendary heroes and the understanding of human action as straightforward in its consequences. Confucian optimism about the human condition was maintained even in the face of Confucius's own failure to obtain the political successes that he needed to justify his mission. The optimism, both moral and epistemological, was a matter of deep faith rather than of shallow experience.

This list is by no means exhaustive, but I am proposing that particular features such as these, combined in the ways I have described, help to define what we mean by Chinese for the early period. It must be stressed that other scholars could well emphasize different features of

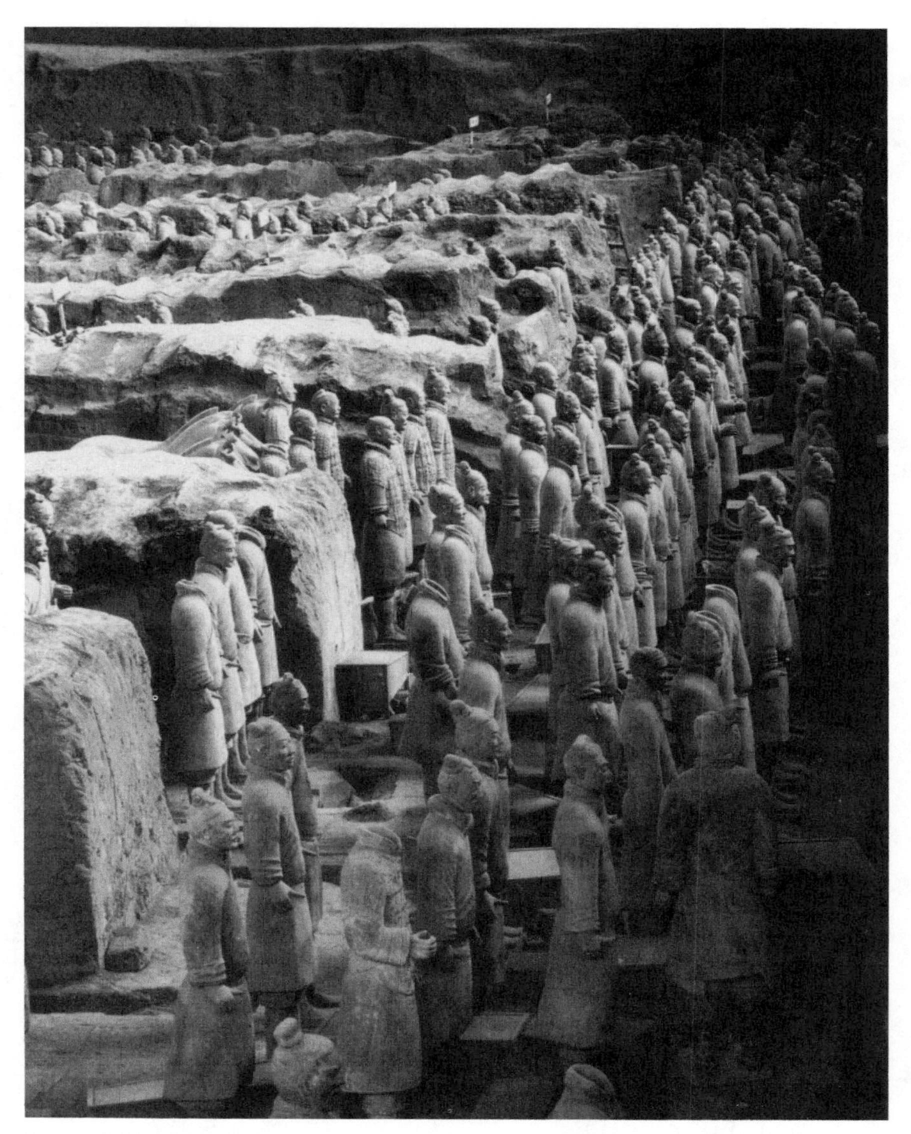

Figure 2.11. Part of the seven-thousand-man army of terra-cotta figures buried with the First Emperor of China, ca. 210 B.C. From *Ch'in Shih Huang ling ping-ma yung* (Peking: Wen-wu Ch'u-pan-she, 1983), no. 7.

the culture—such as the influence of millet and rice agriculture, the acceptance of a monistic cosmology, the influence of a logographic writing system, the nature of early historiography, the role of shamanism, and Confucian conceptions of benevolence and good government. As I indicated at the start, I do not focus on the Eastern Chou philosophers not only because they have already been studied extensively by Western scholars[30] but also because my main concerns are "prephilosophical"; I attempt to relate legend, history, aesthetics, and political practice to the culture of the Neolithic-to-Bronze-Age transition. My analysis, accordingly, is neither definitive nor comprehensive; it does not propose to explain "everything."

Furthermore, in making cultural comparisons, we should generally think in terms of emphasis or nuance, not absolute distinctions. I do not claim that the ancient Chinese had no sense of individual heroism, that no leader ever did things for himself, that death was not a source of terror, that the early Chinese ignored details, or that merchants played no role. But if one imagines a series of axes on which individualism, personal involvement, attention to detail, anguish at the death of loved ones, service to the group, and so on could be plotted, one would find that the Chinese responses differed to a significant degree from those of other seminal civilizations.

Finally—to return to a caution raised at the start of this chapter—I would remark that the very nature of cultural comparison, which involves moving from the familiar culture to the unfamiliar one, results in a rhetoric that seems critical of the "target" culture, which is described as deficient in certain features. But should such features have been present? Is what has been called the Greek "lust to annihilate" attractive?[31] Are gods who masquerade as swans to rape their victims? Are sons who overthrow their fathers? What we may regard as the good and the bad features of any culture are inextricably linked. All great civilizations have their costs as well as their benefits, and it would be instructive—indeed, it is essential if full cultural understanding is to be achieved—to rewrite this chapter from the Chinese point of view, stressing and seeking to explain all the features that early Greek culture, for example, lacked. The most notable of these would surely include the emphasis that many early Chinese thinkers placed on altruism, benevolence, social harmony, and a concern with human relations rather than abstract principles.

The cultural traditions established in the Neolithic and the Bronze

30. The most recent comprehensive study is that of Schwartz, *The World of Thought in Ancient China*.

31. Eli Sagan, *The Lust to Annihilate: A Psychoanalytic Study of Violence in Ancient Greek Culture* (New York: Psychohistory Press, 1979).

Ages of China were ancestral to all that followed, continuing to exert their influence down to recent, if not contemporary, times. It could be argued—as the discussion about the extensive ramifications of ancestor worship has suggested—that the Chinese were relatively slow to desacrilize their world. Ancient social practices tied to the lineage continued to be attended with powerful religious qualities throughout imperial times. A major question—in our own case as well as that of the Chinese—is to what degree will the older, deeply seated traditions help or hinder the search for new solutions? Recent claims that "traditional Chinese cultural values may be conducive to the economic life typical of the modern epoch" suggest that the answer is by no means a foregone conclusion.[32] The combative individualism of the West may yet prove more costly than the harmonious social humanism of China. To address a question such as this, surely, is one of the reasons we study history and why it is important to understand the past as clearly as we can. As Ssu-ma Ch'ien wrote some two thousand years ago, "He who does not forget the past is master of the present." When we consider George Santayana's more negative formulation that "those who forget the past are condemned to repeat it," Ssu-ma Ch'ien was the more optimistic. But that would have been characteristic. And how appropriate that his should have been a confidence in the virtues of the past.

32. John C. H. Fei, "The Success of Chinese Culture as Economic Nutrient . . . ," *Free China Review* 36, no. 7 (July 1986):43.

THREE

□

The Evolution of Government in China

Jack L. Dull

Americans, perhaps more than people of other nations, need to remind themselves from time to time that democracy is not the natural political condition of humankind. Even in the West, democracy is relatively new. In the premodern West, and in the rest of the world as well, authoritarian patterns of government in which the governed have little peaceful input into the political process have been common. Government in traditional China was (and in many respects still is) highly authoritarian. If popular participation is the measure of the desirable government, then Chinese governments are not likely to fare very well. But if the success of any government or institution is judged by its ability to sustain itself over long periods of time, then many governments in Chinese history were remarkably successful.

Attention is often drawn to the imperial bureaucracy created by the First Emperor of the Ch'in dynasty in 221 B.C. because, in its general outline, the government that he imposed on China persisted down to the overthrow of the Ch'ing dynasty in 1911. This generalization requires two kinds of qualification. First, the Chinese political system experienced continuity only in the most general aspects of its institutional structures. Second, even if the government had been unchanging, it did not operate in an unchanging social, economic, or intellectual milieu. In other words, despite a high degree of structural continuity, the Chinese government functioned very differently at different times as society underwent profound changes over the last two thousand years.

I posit a four-stage periodization in the evolution of premodern Chinese governments. The earliest stage extended from the dimly limned beginnings of the Shang state to the creation of the first empire; its predominant characteristic was patrimonialism. The second stage was a meritocracy that ended after four hundred years in the third century

A.D. The third stage was an aristocracy that dominated the government of China until the tenth century. The final period of the premodern era is commonly designated as gentry government. In the twentieth century governments in China have been nominally committed to some form of democracy, but none has been either willing to create or successful in creating this kind of government, even though efforts along those lines are ongoing and repeatedly requested or demanded. The fourfold division of the premodern period—patrimonial, meritocratic, aristocratic, and gentry (the definitions of these terms follow)—draws attention not only to the structure of the government but also to the nature of the society within which the government operated and the principal means by which men entered government service.

REGIMES OF PATRIMONIAL DOMINATION

Although the government of the Shang dynasty (traditional dates: 1766–1122 B.C.) is not yet well understood, historians and archaeologists using oracle-bone inscriptions and other sparse data have been able to sketch a picture of government in this early period.[1]

The Shang ruler conceived of himself as utterly without peer. He referred to himself as "I, The One Man" or "I, The Unique One." There was little or no sense of shared power; he governed all, he dominated all, and all official acts were conducted in his name. He seems to have operated on the assumption that he could command the obedience of everyone in the realm. He governed Shang China as a powerful father figure who looked on everyone else as a member of his family and therefore as under his control. This kind of personal domination by a single figure in part warrants the term "patrimonial" in reference to the Shang state.

The Shang world was divided into zones. At the core was the Shang capital (which was moved repeatedly during the dynasty) and its immediate environs, which was under the direct control of the Shang ruler and his appointees. The second zone, surrounding the first, was in the hands of administrators appointed by the Shang ruler. These administrators bore titles that we might refer to as protobureaucratic or protofeudal. The third zone was likewise in the hands of royal appointees, but, unlike those in the first two zones, they seem to have been most concerned with defending the Shang realm from its enemies.[2] The fourth

1. For a general study of the Shang period see Kwang-chih Chang, *Shang Civilization* (New Haven: Yale University Press, 1980). For a discussion of the materials on which historians of the Shang depend see the beautiful volume by David N. Keightley, *Sources of Shang History: The Oracle-Bone Inscriptions of Bronze Age China* (Berkeley: University of California Press, 1978).

2. For analytical purposes we may speak of civil and military officials, but it is important to bear in mind that such a sharp distinction would have been foreign to the Shang ruler.

zone included the enemies of the Shang, some of whom were under tribal chieftains, who were given titles on offering allegiance to the Shang throne.

The highest official was the equivalent of chancellor and several are known by name. The founder of the Shang dynasty relied heavily on his chancellor, I Yin, who was of such importance in Shang history that he received offerings in the same manner as the deceased Shang rulers. Beneath him were various clerical officials and scribes as well as diviners. Agricultural officials, referred to on the oracle bones, operated in the core area and perhaps in the second zone.

Local administration was in the hands of members of the Shang ruling house. In other words, the administrative structure was essentially familial, including fictive relatives, that is, men who were not members of the ruling family but who were treated as such (in-laws provide the model). These officials were expected to obey the king for the simple reason that he was the head of the patrimonial family.

The titles held by the king's servitors are a mixture of both feudal and bureaucratic elements, many of which recur in later periods in Chinese history. Most titles show little standardization and little functional specificity. Instead, relatives of the king were instructed to perform certain tasks. Proximity to the king was probably more important than the title, bureaucratic or feudal, that a person held.

Military operations were not necessarily under the command of military officials. The king's relatives who administered pieces of territory were in effect rulers of petty states within the Shang realm. When Shang territory was under attack the king had the rulers of these statelets call up men for military duty. We have evidence that at least one of the rulers of a small state was a Shang queen who was able to call up a large number of fighting men to assist the king in a campaign. Troops were organized around war chariots that served as mobile command posts. The king himself did not have to rely on conscription. Under his direct control were large militarylike units of people who ordinarily engaged in agriculture and other assigned tasks. The king had only to mobilize these people for military purposes. In the succeeding Chou dynasty, the military power of the rulers was distinctly different. What is most significant about the Shang military situation was that the king did not maintain a standing army; he was dependent on the continued allegiance of his family members, who summoned and commanded the troops.

Throughout Chinese history the means of access to office have been closely related to the nature of the society in a given period. In the Shang dynasty the basic structure of the society was along lineage lines. Accord-

---

Indeed, throughout Chinese history there was not a professional military (although there were of course people who spent their entire lives in the military).

ing to funerary evidence, there were considerable variations in wealth and presumably in power within lineages.[3] Thus, the fault lines in this society were not horizontal, separating class from class, but vertical, separating lineage from lineage. At the local level the heads of lineages were the administrators of their lineages and perhaps other local people; in some cases such lineage heads would have been rulers of petty states. Ranking members of the lineages also served in the royal administrative structure.

In the Shang belief system political activities were not consciously separated from all other activities, for the secular and the sacred realms were undifferentiated. The Shang ruler divined frequently about the weather, crops, hunts, sons, and other matters. The recipients of offerings included a complex pantheon of gods and spirits, but most important were his powerful ancestors; he appealed to these ancestors to intercede with the gods on his behalf and on behalf of the rulers of the small statelets within his realm. Thus, as David N. Keightley makes clear (see Chapter 2), ancestor worship bonded the sociopolitical system into a whole; when the king approached his ancestors he was also appealing to the ancestors, albeit more distant ancestors, of many of the lineage heads of his realm. And of course all would have known that it was only a matter of time until the king himself entered the ranks of those ancestors, who were powerful intermediaries between the secular and the sacred realms; in Shang thinking, however, the living and the dead did not occupy two worlds but rather shared one ontological continuum.

The Chou dynasty is historically divided into the Western Chou (traditional dates: 1122–771 B.C.) and the Eastern Chou (770–256 B.C.), indicating a move of the capital and a drastic reduction of the power of the Chou house in the eighth century B.C. During the earlier period the basic social and political organization of life seems to have differed little from that of the Shang dynasty.[4] The Chou founders apportioned their newly conquered territory among over one hundred lineages, most of which were related or treated as if they were related to the Chou house. The heads of these lineages were the governors of their areas; they held such feudal-sounding titles as duke and marquis, depending on the size and importance of their pieces of territory. In many cases they were also obligated to serve at the Chou court, where they would hold an official position in addition to the feudallike title.

The major institutional change introduced during the Chou was that the king claimed a near monopoly of military power. For the first several hundred years the Chou kings maintained sizable forces in both the

3. Yang Hsi-chang, "The Shang Dynasty Cemetery System," in *Studies in Shang Archaeology*, ed. K. C. Chang (New Haven: Yale University Press, 1986).

4. On the Western Chou see Herrlee G. Creel, *The Origins of Statecraft in China*, vol. 1, *The Western Chou Empire* (Chicago: University of Chicago Press, 1970).

western and eastern parts of their empire. Initially, the rulers of the statelets were probably allowed to maintain little more than a local peace-keeping force, but by the end of the Western Chou period the king's armies were in decline and the military forces within the emerging states were becoming larger and more numerous.

The dual responsibilities of the heads of the petty states to their own states and to the Chou court were to contribute to the weakening of the Chou regime, for these heads found themselves more concerned with administering their own territories than with aiding the Chou king in the administration of his. Because of population growth and new lands that had been brought under cultivation by the latter part of the Western Chou period, the petty states in many cases became powerful states that could challenge and engulf their smaller neighbors. Rulers of such states were not inclined to turn their backs on their own states and people.

The founders of the Chou dynasty, particularly the Duke of Chou, are credited with a major development in political thought, namely, the creation of the idea of the Mandate of Heaven (*T'ien-ming,* which can also be translated as the Mandate of God). Faced with the problem of explaining the overthrow of the Shang dynasty, the Chou founders asserted that Heaven had withdrawn the mandate to rule from the Shang house; the grounds for the withdrawal of the mandate had been the inability of the last Shang ruler to govern in a manner that was pleasing to Heaven. Hence, went the argument, the mandate was retracted from the Shang and granted to the Chou. A part of the argument was that the Shang had succeeded its predecessor, the Hsia dynasty, on exactly the same basis. The Chou charges gave rise to the idea of the bad last emperor—the one who brings about the loss of his dynasty. This idea was to become a common feature of Chinese political culture and could be used by officials who would caution their rulers to behave or face the prospect of the loss of the mandate and the end of the dynasty.

The ruler soon bore a new title that was based on the legitimating concept of the Mandate of Heaven: the Son of Heaven. The term was not taken in the literal sense to mean that the Chou king was descended from Heaven and therefore divine, but it did convey the idea that the king had been chosen by Heaven. Just as lineage heads were patrimonially responsible to the Chou king, so too was he responsible, as a son, to Heaven, who could withdraw the mandate and confer it on a more deserving, that is, a more morally responsible, ruling house.

The Chou period is sometimes referred to as feudal, but whether one has the Western Chou or the Eastern Chou in mind, the designation is not applicable. To be sure, the Chou king parceled out people and pieces of territory to real and fictive family members for them to govern, but at that point the similarity to Western feudalism ends. Three characteristics of Western feudalism highlight the differences. First, the relationship between a lord and his vassals in the West was a legal one in which the two parties were equals before the law; the notion of a legally binding contract between equals was not present in the Chou period, nor was it to become a feature of later Chinese law. Second, at the base of the pyramid of Western feudalism was the mounted knight; above him was a lord who might be at the same time lord over that knight but vassal to a higher lord. The process of subinfeudation by which this vassalic pyramid was built, although not totally unknown in China at this time, was not common. The Chou king himself created most of the small states. The leaders of those states owed family loyalty, not a legally defined obligation, to the king, not to some intermediate lord. Third, the primary function of the Western knight was to fight for his lord; in Chou China there were simply no knights. Hence, the most fundamental building block of European feudalism is missing in China. Indeed, in the Western Chou period there was no cavalry.

By the early eighth century B.C. the Chou house was losing its grip on the empire. The Chou king often could not control his armies, which were weakened anyway. His dukes and other rulers of the component states of the empire were unwilling to continue to serve in his administration and he had to rely on lesser lords over whom he could exercise his declining power. The rulers of the petty states, however, were increasingly wealthy and powerful. Foreign invaders, probably aided by disaffected Chou nobles, brought an end to the Western Chou in 771 B.C.; the Chou house continued to exist for over five hundred years, but it was not able to command obedience among the nobles nor to regain its former position. Chou China then entered a prolonged period of competition among the states that was to end in the unification of China by the Ch'in dynasty in 221 B.C.

Profoundly important political and social changes occurred during this half millennium, changes that were to have permanent consequences for subsequent Chinese history.[5] First, as states disappeared, their ruling elites were cast adrift and could offer their services to other states; these developments tended to weaken familial ties as the principal criterion for appointments to governmental and military positions. Second, within some individual states ruling families were supplanted by families of their ministers, and ministerial families also fell victim to their upwardly mobile inferiors. Third, the development of private ownership of land and growing urban markets facilitated social mobility in other parts of the society. This wrenching social disequilibrium provides the immediate background to the thinkers of the time; Confucius and others sought to prescribe the steps that would restore a peaceful equi-

5. Hsu Cho-yun, *Ancient China in Transition* (Stanford: Stanford University Press, 1965).

librium to the age. And in the political realm patrimonial values, so long a feature of early China, declined and were replaced by meritocratic values, which were to characterize Chinese life for about four centuries. This keenly competitive age nurtured the ruler's demand for people with proven ability. What had been merely protobureaucratic features of an earlier age now blossomed into an imperial bureaucracy.

Between the seventh and third centuries B.C. four noteworthy developments occurred in the sphere of political institutions. First, because the powerless Chou kings were no longer able to mobilize and command the rulers within the empire against such common threats as foreign tribesmen and other states, the institution of the hegemon developed to meet this need. The hegemon was the powerful leader of a league of states organized under an oath to take common action against a commonly perceived threat. Because state power was difficult to sustain over long periods of time, hegemony shifted from state to state, at one time even being held by the ruler of the large southern state of Ch'u, against whom the first league had been organized. By approximately 400 B.C. this institution no longer existed, but its memory was to persist into the present because the hegemon became the symbol of the ruler who commanded by brute force as opposed to the Confucian ideal of the king who governed by moral suasion.

Second, local level administrative units were created so that the increasingly powerful rulers could maintain direct political control over newly conquered lands instead of turning them over to potentially competing lineages. First *hsien* (translated as prefecture or county for early periods in Chinese history and as district for the late imperial period) and then *chün* (commanderies) were created, with the prefectures becoming subordinate to the commanderies. The rulers appointed local-level administrators to these positions to hold office at the pleasure of the ruler; these new institutions were important in enhancing the power of the rulers in the period.

Third, by 334 B.C. rulers of two of the formerly petty states arrogated to themselves the title "king"; rulers of other states soon followed. These acts of self-aggrandizement are significant in revealing the low esteem in which the now powerless Chou king was held, for until the fourth century B.C. only the Chou ruler held the title of king.

These developments culminated in 221 B.C. when the king of Ch'in completed the conquest of the last remaining opposing state and inaugurated the imperial bureaucratic system. However, patrimonial ideas continued to exist. For example, later emperors never thought of themselves as supreme bureaucrats; they were more often guided by patrimonial values. Furthermore, most of the Confucian classics were written or compiled in the preimperial period; thus, students of Confucianism continued to absorb patrimonial ideas long after the creation of the imperial bureaucracy. Throughout subsequent Chinese history there was to be a tension between the patrimonial ruler, on the one hand, and his bureaucratic staff, on the other hand.

MERITOCRATIC CHINA

The brevity of the Ch'in dynasty in no way indicates its historical importance because the Ch'in empire symbolizes a culmination of many of the changes that had been building for the preceding five hundred years.[6] Because it lasted for only fifteen years, the details of its governmental organization and operation are lost to us, but it is probably safe to assume that many of the practices of the succeeding Han dynasty were direct continuations from the Ch'in period. Therefore, I leave the detailed discussion of meritocratic government and society to the Han period.

The founder of the Ch'in created a new title for himself: *huang-ti*. Older titles, such as king, did not adequately reflect the glory deserved by the new centralized bureaucratic empire. *Huang-ti,* usually translated as emperor, was to remain until 1911 as one of the major designations of the occupant of the Chinese throne. *Huang* means "august" and *ti* means "emperor." But *ti* also meant god; the emperor did not think of himself as a theocrat, but the term suggests the awesome majesty of the Chinese ruler. There were no codified or legal restraints on the emperor. He was the legislator of the realm, the chief executive of the empire, and the highest judge in cases of appeal. He was, in theory at least, above the law. In practice, of course, as Karen Turner emphasizes in her chapter on law in this volume (see Chapter 4), he was dependent on his officials for much of his knowledge about his empire, and they could appeal to historical precedent as well as to reason to persuade him to avoid or to undertake actions.

The central government of the Ch'in regime consisted of a chancellor (*ch'eng-hsiang*), an imperial secretary (*yü-shih ta-fu*), and a grand commandant (*t'ai-wei*). The chancellor was the head of the bureaucracy and assisted the emperor in all activities. The imperial secretary was responsible for issuing orders from the throne and was a close assistant to the chancellor. In later periods the same Chinese term was used to refer to the censorate but in the early period of Chinese imperial history the censorial functions were not well developed. The grand commandant was not a regularly filled position; as the title suggests, it was concerned with military operations.

Beneath this triumvirate were the "nine ministers" (*chiu-ch'ing*), who

6. The best history of the Ch'in is now Derk Bodde, "The State and Empire of Ch'in," in *The Cambridge History of China,* vol. 1, *The Ch'in and Han Empires, 221 B.C.–A.D. 220,* ed. Denis Twitchett and Michael Loewe (Cambridge: Cambridge University Press, 1986).

were charged with various functions ranging from the ceremonial to central government revenues. What is probably most significant about these offices is the extent to which their names preserve patrimonial attitudes. Most of the names derive from the household staff of the patrimonial ruler as opposed to a process of bureaucratic rationalization—a process that was to develop over the following centuries.

At the local level (which in the Chinese context means anything that is not a part of the central government) the Ch'in regime built on earlier trends common to many of the states of the preimperial period by dividing the realm into commanderies (*chün*) that were subdivided into prefectures (*hsien*). For each of the thirty-six (later forty-two) Ch'in commanderies three officials were appointed by or with the approval of the throne: an administrator (*shou*) responsible for administering all affairs of the commandery; an oversight official (*chien yü-shih*), who made sure that the administrator was carrying out imperial policies; and a commandant (*wei*) who served as a chief of police and who was responsible for conducting the military training of conscripts. At the prefectural level were three imperial appointees with essentially the same division of responsibilities, except that there was an assistant prefect (*hsien-ch'eng*) instead of an oversight official. The law of avoidance (which definitely existed in the Han period and probably during the Ch'in as well) prevented an imperial appointee from serving in his own jurisdiction. The commandery and prefectural officials were thus "outsiders," but their clerical staffs, whom we can refer to as subbureaucratic because they did not hold imperial appointments, were all locally hired. The local prefect (*ling*) guided and relied on these subbureaucrats for such essential basic functions as conducting the census, collecting and forwarding taxes in both kind and money, maintaining roads and bridges, administering justice, and so on.

The protofeudal elements of earlier eras were not preserved in this bureaucratic empire. In later Confucian-inspired historiography, the First Emperor was condemned for destroying these lineage-based institutions, and the obliteration of the old kingdoms was a contributing factor in the downfall of the Ch'in because loyalty to these kingdoms remained strong throughout the brief Ch'in dynasty.

The Han dynasty, after an extended civil war, dated its founding to 206 B.C. It was to last over four hundred years, but is customarily treated as existing in two parts: the Former (or Western) Han, lasting until A.D. 9, and the Later (or Eastern) Han, extending from A.D. 25 to 220.[7] The period between the two parts saw a very short dynasty, the Hsin, founded

7. On the Han period see *The Cambridge History of China,* vol. 1. On government in the Han see also Hans Bielenstein, *The Bureaucracy of Han Times* (Cambridge: Cambridge University Press, 1980).

by Wang Mang, who is traditionally treated as a usurper; although he attempted some fascinating political and social reforms, Wang's efforts will not be treated here. The Han dynasty, as the first long-lasting imperial bureaucratic empire, has often been idealized in Chinese thinking, and its successes were instrumental in firmly implanting many of the practices of imperial Chinese political history.

The Han emperor was not fundamentally different from his Ch'in predecessor, except that, as a result of a slowly growing Confucian influence, he was also referred to as the Son of Heaven. His empire was, however, distinctly different. The Han founder, acknowledging the continuing loyalties to the old kingdoms and being faced with powerful generals who had to be suitably rewarded, created or recognized the preimperial kingdoms. About half the empire was thus placed in the hands of autonomous kings. During the course of the next half century, however, severe actions were taken against these kings. First, all kings who were not members of the imperial family were eliminated; then the remaining kings were deprived of their autonomy. The kingdoms came to be governed by imperial appointees as the rough equivalents of the commanderies, even though the kingdoms were usually smaller than the commanderies had been. Marquisates were also founded and granted to particularly meritorious officials and military officers. Both kingdoms and marquisates were inheritable; they accorded prestige and income to their recipients. In preserving kingdoms and marquisates within an otherwise bureaucratic empire the Han rejected certain Ch'in political attitudes and restored some of the old traditional Chou institutions. But by eliminating all power from the kingdoms, the Han rulers indicated their preference for an empire ruled fully from the imperial throne.

As in the Ch'in dynasty, at the peak of the bureaucracy was a triumvirate, often referred to collectively as the three ducal ministers, consisting of the chancellor, the imperial secretary, and the grand commandant. Several significant changes occurred in these offices during the course of the Han. First, imperial distrust of the great power that was concentrated in the hands of the chancellor meant that at times there were experiments with a left and right chancellor in order to dilute the concentration of power. Toward the end of the Former Han period, under Confucian influence, the chancellor's responsibilities were nominally shared among the three ducal ministers. Because the position of grand commandant was irregularly filled, it came to be a position to which male members of the consort families could be appointed without having to work their way up through the normal bureaucratic ranks. Thus, power, particularly in the Later Han period, tended to flow to that office. Additionally, emperors who were determined to rule as well as to reign sought to circumvent the regular bureaucracy by creating a private secretarial staff known as masters of writing (*shang-shu*). The position of the head of the masters of writing was often concurrently held by the grand commandant, thus further consolidating power in his hands.

The nine highest ministers, the next layer in the central administration, were a continuation of the Ch'in system, even though there were some changes in the names of some of the offices. Improvements in functional specificity may be seen in the development of bureaus. Although the early history of these bureaus is rather murky, by the beginning of the Later Han they had become well established. Significantly, they were under the grand commandant; they did not supplant the nine ministries, but tended to take over their functions.

At the local level the *chün-hsien* (commandery-prefecture) system of the Ch'in was nominally replaced by the *chün-kuo* (commandery-kingdom) system. But, as I observed earlier, the kingdoms lost all power and the local-level institutions of the Han were in practical terms no different from the Ch'in. Within the commandery there was one notable exception: the censorial function of the second official in each commandery was dropped and that position was converted into an assistant to the commandery administrator (see the later section on oversight at the local level). By the end of the Former Han dynasty there were approximately one hundred commanderies (including kingdoms) and approximately fifteen hundred prefectures (including their administrative equivalents: marquisates).

Over the course of the dynasty important developments occurred at two administrative levels: between the commanderies and the central government and within both the commanderies and the prefectures. The basic problem for the Han central government was one of surveillance: how was it to keep tabs on what was going on in the commanderies? Initially, commissioners (*shih*) were sent out from the capital on an ad hoc basis, but in 106 B.C. the court divided the realm into thirteen regions (*pu*) over each of which was placed a regional inspector (*tz'u-shih*). This inspector was charged with a censorial role vis-à-vis the commanderies; he was also supposed to pay attention to powerful families that sometimes dominated the local scene. By the end of the Former Han the regional inspectors had accumulated sufficient administrative power that they were formally recognized as administrative officials, and the office name changed to provincial shepherds (*chou-mu*). Throughout most of the Later Han the earlier institution (regional inspectors) was maintained, but in both the early and the later stages of that period, when there was an urgent demand for powerful local military commanders, the provincial shepherds were restored. The growth of such large and powerful centers was a contributing factor to the eventual breakup and destruction of the Han empire.

Another important development took place within the commanderies and prefectures when their amorphous clerical staffs gave way to highly structured bureaus. A host of bureaus dealing with personnel, justice, taxation, transportation, ritual, postal, and other matters had come into existence by the end of the Former Han dynasty. Within each bureau a clearly defined system of positions, ranging from bureau heads to clerks and factotums, also emerged. This precisely articulated set of subbureaucratic positions was intimately associated with the system whereby men were recruited for service in the imperial bureaucracy.

The recruitment system of the Han, unlike the later and much more famous civil service examination system, was based essentially on recommendation. Ranking officials were ordered to recommend a specified number of men for bureaucratic service. Those chosen often came from the commandery or prefectural bureaus. At the local level young men customarily started their careers in the subbureaucratic clerical positions, moved on to become heads of increasingly important local bureaus, and would then be recommended to the central government under such rubrics as "abundantly talented" (*mao-ts'ai*) or "filial and incorrupt" (*hsiao-lien*). The historical significance of this recruitment process is clarified by noting that from the Sung dynasty on men spent years and sometimes decades studying the Confucian classics in order to prepare themselves for government service, whereas in the Han period comparable aspirants to bureaucratic careers were in effect serving an apprenticeship in the lower reaches of the imperial order. At the point where the state and society met in the Han period the average person having contact with local units dealt with men who hoped that by establishing their merit they could move on to higher positions; by the Ming and Ch'ing periods the average person having contact with local units had to deal with men who were usually seen as déclassé: the infamous runners. Although we have neither the yardstick nor the data to measure governmental quality, I would suggest that Han local administration was of a higher quality than that of later periods in Chinese history. Han subbureaucratic officials hoped by establishing their merit as officials to be promoted to regular bureaucratic positions; late imperial subbureaucrats knew such upward mobility was impossible and sought, often through unscrupulous and corrupt behavior, to exact as much as possible from the populace.

The foregoing structures and recruitment procedures were based on the assumption that merit was individually established through direct experience; those who worked their way up to the imperial bureaucracy and further upward within that bureaucracy were clearly part of a meritocracy. Such was the ideal, but by the Later Han period the system was being undercut by the growth of local powerful families.[8] Such families

8. On Han society see Ch'ü T'ung-tsu, *Han Social Structure*, ed. Jack L. Dull (Seattle: University of Washington Press, 1972).

were able to dominate the local subbureaucracies and thus assure themselves of recommendations to the imperial bureaucracy. A recruitment system that was designed to draw on individual merit was being dominated by powerful social forces that the state could not control.

ARISTOCRATIC CHINA

Chinese historians of the post-Han period do not agree on the use of the term aristocratic to refer to China in the period from the fall of the Han to the end of the T'ang (A.D. 906).[9] Nevertheless I use the term here in order to draw attention to the marked shift in social values that distinguishes this period from the earlier meritocratic age. This period may be divided into two parts. The first, beginning in A.D. 220 with the demise of the Han and the division of China into three kingdoms, lasted until 589 when China was reunified under the Sui dynasty (China was briefly reunified in 265 by the Chin, but because that empire lasted only about a generation, I do not single it out for attention here). This span of three centuries is often referred to as the Period of Disunion. The Sui was not able to sustain itself, and in 618 it was supplanted by the T'ang (618–906)—another great age in Chinese history and an age when Chinese models of government, law, and ideology permanently influenced developments in Korea and Japan. Although the first part of the aristocratic age witnessed the conquest of north China by non-Chinese and semi-sinified rulers early in the fourth century and although the Chinese regimes in the south were chronically weak, there were important developments in the nature of the government of China during this period.

The emperorship existed in markedly different circumstances in the north and the south during the Period of Disunion. Northern rulers were foreign conquerors who imposed themselves on the population, but despite their non-Chinese origins the general trend was toward the sinification of the rulers and their regimes. Rulers in the south imposed themselves on an indigenous Chinese elite with whom they had to collaborate. In general, the rulers of the south were never as able as their northern counterparts to mobilize the resources of the society. Hence, it is not surprising that the reunification of China came from the north where the state was able to resecure an adequate tax base and to create the requisite military might.

The aristocratic age saw a reflourishing of many patrimonial values,

9. The titles of the following two works suggest the differences regarding the nature of society in this period: David G. Johnson, *The Medieval Chinese Oligarchy* (Boulder, Colo.: Westview Press, 1977) and Patricia Buckley Ebrey, *The Aristocratic Families of Early Imperial China: A Case Study of the Po-ling Ts'ui Family* (Cambridge: Cambridge University Press, 1978).

for example, in the creation of powerful kingdoms ruled by members of the imperial family of the Chin dynasty (265–316) and in the social values of the elite such as arranged marriages, but despite such reversions to an earlier age the process of bureaucratization also went forward. This process is clearly seen in the evolution of the administrative arm of the central administration. The office of masters of writing (*shang-shu*), originally designed to serve as the Han emperor's private secretariat, slowly developed administrative powers and by the beginning of the Period of Disunion was transformed from an imperial secretariat into the central executive branch of the bureaucracy. Thereafter it is customarily referred to as the Department of Affairs of State (*shang-shu-sheng*). The nine high ministers of the Han, their names continuing to echo patrimonial thinking, persisted but as a rule without significant power and frequently only to provide sinecures. Within the Department of Affairs of State bureaus were replaced with boards, varying in number but finally settling down to six. The six boards (*liu-pu*) thereafter varied in number and importance but continued to exist into the twentieth century, when, as part of late Ch'ing reforms, they were converted into Western-style ministries.

At the local level the three-tiered system of provinces, commanderies, and prefectures persisted with two notable characteristics. First, provincial governors often exercised considerable military power. The age demanded major military commitments not only because of the nature of domestic politics but also because of the intermittent attempts to reunify China. Hence, there was a high level of militarization at the local level as well as in the higher levels of the state. Second, the throne responded to powerful local forces by dividing them and, at the same time, assuring that numerous positions were available for political patronage. The consequence of these policies was a bizarre proliferation of local-level units. By the early sixth century the thirteen regions/provinces of the Han had swollen to 113, commanderies had increased over sixfold to at least 683, and prefectures, which had numbered about fifteen hundred in the entire Han empire, reached 1,474 in the small southern state of Ch'i (479–501) alone. Before the end of the Period of Disunion, strong efforts in both the north and the south led to great reductions in the number of these various units; the Sui dynasty at one point simply eliminated all commanderies.

Recruitment during the Period of Disunion was based on two contradictory principles: ascription and merit. The civil wars and social chaos that accompanied the breakup of the Han empire thoroughly disrupted the normal system of recommendation for office. As a remedy, the government of the Ts'ao-Wei dynasty created a system whereby people who were not in their home areas could be recommended for office on the basis of indirect judgments. The key office charged with making recommendations was that of rectifier (*chung-cheng,* also translated literally as "the Impartial and Just"). Rectifiers operated at all levels of government. In theory they were supposed to judge the capabilities of men for office and recommend them. In fact, shortly after its creation in 220 the office came to be used by the elite to perpetuate itself; judgments were based on the status rank ranging from one—the highest—to nine of the elite families to which the potential officials belonged. One's entry-level position in the bureaucracy was correlated with one's social-status rank. Aristocrats did not take low governmental positions and the socially inferior did not enter high bureaucratic posts. The aristocracy dominated the upper levels of the bureaucracy throughout the Period of Disunion and throughout the T'ang dynasty.

Many government offices were not among the nine ranked grades of officialdom (similar to G.S. ratings in the U.S. civil service); these positions came to be referred to as "outside the current" (*liu-wai*) of officialdom, and they too were ranked. People in the various bureaus at the local- and the central-government level continued to serve in a meritocratic manner, undergoing a Han-style apprenticeship and then entering the positions designated as "outside the current." The dividing line between aristocratic and nonaristocratic (the so-called cold gate or poor scholar) families was not as sharp as this bifurcation would suggest. First, in theory nonaristocratic families could move up and, although not common, some did. Second, aristocratic families were socially ranked, but their rankings could change depending on their political and administrative skills. Nevertheless, the throne, particularly in the southern regimes, could not confer aristocratic status on anyone born outside the aristocracy, no matter what the value of his service.

An imperial bureaucratic regime is fundamentally incompatible with an aristocracy. It is to the emperor's advantage to have as much choice as possible in the selection of his officials, but an entrenched aristocracy in which social status is established independent of the throne precludes that free choice on the part of the ruler. Hence, there was an imperial urge to circumvent, if not eliminate, the aristocracy. Southern rulers thus turned more and more to those "outside the current" for the discharge of governmental functions—a process made easier by the unwillingness of many aristocrats to dirty their hands in administrative tasks. In the north decisive, but not fatal, action was taken against the aristocracy when the nine-grade social rank system was officially abolished in 583. The step was important but did not eliminate the aristocracy as a class.

The Sui dynasty (589–617) reunified China but was not able to sustain itself. It proved, as the Ch'in had done earlier, the feasibility of empire and left a legacy not only of political unification but also of geographic unity, particularly as seen in the canal system that joined the grain-rich south to the north for the first time in over three centuries. Had its rulers not wavered in their commitment to an ideology (Buddhist impulses sometimes prevailed over Confucianism) and had they not engaged in costly wars of expansion and construction projects, it might have prevailed. Because the T'ang administrative system was far more enduring and because it perpetuated most Sui practices, I move directly to the T'ang period.

The T'ang dynasty (618–907), although in many ways consciously modeled on the Han, constitutes a major transitional era in Chinese history.[10] Intellectually, Taoism was honored, in part because the T'ang ruling house claimed descent from Lao Tzu, but after Emperor Hsuan-tsung's unsuccessful attempt to create a Taoist orthodoxy, intellectual inspiration from Taoism was not a potent political factor. Buddhism, which well into the T'ang had inspired many thinkers, was by the end of the dynasty a comforting religion but devoid of the philosophical excitement of earlier periods. These developments left much of the field of intellectual endeavor to a resurgent Confucianism. Confucianism had been state orthodoxy from the beginning of the dynasty, but initially it had not created much excitement. Socially, in the beginning of the period the aristocracy dominated both the political and the social scene, but by the beginning of the Sung dynasty in 960 the aristocracy was no longer of much significance. The T'ang government underwent, and perhaps more important consolidated, changes that were to strengthen the bureaucratic elements within the imperial structure.

The longevity of the T'ang proved once again the practicality of an empire that was extensive in both geographic scope and temporal duration. Never again was China to be as divided as it had been during the pre-Sui period. The emperor exercised power effectively (at least for the first half of the T'ang) through an elaborate bureaucracy that covered a vast area. And yet the historian senses that imperial power was not as firmly exercised or as heavy-handed as it was to become in later periods in Chinese history; the continued existence of the aristocracy probably precluded these later developments, which were to make the power of the throne truly awesome.

The highest level of the central administration of the T'ang consisted of three major bodies: the Department of Affairs of State, the Department of the Secretariat (*chung-shu-sheng*), and the Department of the Chancellery (*men-hsia-sheng*). The Department of Affairs of State was the key administrative agency in the central government; under it were the six boards separated along specific functional lines. The secretariat

10. *The Cambridge History of China,* vol. 3, *Sui and T'ang China, 589–906, Part 1,* ed. Denis Twitchett (Cambridge: Cambridge University Press, 1979), provides a fine political history of the Sui and T'ang periods.

had evolved along the same lines as the Department of Affairs of State. In the Han there had been a corps of palace writers who during the Period of Disunion were slowly and intermittently transformed into an administrative agency that at times overlapped with the Department of Affairs of State; in the T'ang the secretariat took the form of a body that was responsible for issuing orders from the throne. The chancellery likewise had its roots among the Han advisers to the emperor, and during the Period of Disunion it sometimes competed with the chancellery. By the T'ang its position had become routinized as the agency that passed judgment on policy formulations coming out of the secretariat. These three agencies were known collectively as the three departments (*san-sheng*). Their directors (*ling*) and vice directors (*p'u-yeh*) served as a collegial body in advising the emperor. The normal routing for a policy decision was that the secretariat put the decision in final form, the chancellery reviewed it (and recommended changes in it if necessary), and the Department of Affairs of State, on receipt of the order, distributed it to one of the six boards for execution.

Other central administrative positions included the nine courts (*chiu-ssu*) and five directorates (*wu-chien*). The nine courts were perpetuations of the nine highest ministers of the Han period; seven of them were directly and exclusively concerned with the emperor's person and his ritual functions. The other two courts exercised supervisory functions over justice and granaries. The older patrimonial functions in the hands of the courts were clearly separated from the bureaucratic functions performed by the six boards.

The most important of the five directorates was responsible for the high-level schools located in the capitals (others dealt with imperial factories, waterways, armaments, and palace buildings). The top-ranked school was open only to the sons of high-ranking officials and holders of noble ranks; the second-ranked school was open to middle-ranking officials' sons and the third-ranked allowed entrance by sons of low-ranking officials and some commoners. Clearly, the schools were designed to perpetuate the influence of established families.

Local administration in the T'ang dynasty continued the familiar two-tiered system. China was divided into about 350 prefectures (*chou*), which were equivalent to Han commanderies, and approximately 1,500 districts, which were equivalent to Han prefectures; these numbers must be left as approximations because they fluctuated with the size of the empire and with political considerations. As in the past, imperially appointed officials were in charge of each of these units and, as in the past, subbureaucratic staff members were locally hired and eligible to move up into regular bureaucratic offices. There was, however, a major difference between the Han and the T'ang with regard to the subbureaucratic officials: the examination system effectively deprived them of Han-style upward mobility into the higher levels of regular officialdom. This T'ang practice can be traced to the aristocracy and the "outside the current" appointment and hiring practices that I noted in the Period of Disunion. This slowly emerging trend was to continue in later periods of Chinese history.

Faced with the problem of the surveillance of the prefectural and district officials, the T'ang government at first relied on ad hoc commissioners sent from the capital to supervise a variety of activities. After the first century of the T'ang (that is, in 706) the empire was divided into ten circuits (*tao*) with a commissioner (*shih*) in charge of each. In the frontier areas military commanders simultaneously became military commissioners (*chieh-tu-shih*) and circuit commissioners. Later, in order to suppress the An Lu-shan Rebellion (755–763) more and more circuit commissioners were made concurrent military commissioners. In the aftermath of the rebellion the throne worked for decades, without full success, to recover control over the military commissioners who controlled the appointments of prefectural and district officials and who also controlled tax receipts within their circuits. These military commissioners (also called military governors) were instrumental in the ultimate destruction of the T'ang empire.

China's renowned examination system was significantly developed in the T'ang period. When the Sui government announced the abolition of the nine-grade rank system, it also initiated an examination system. The institution was not entirely new, but the Sui and the T'ang differed from earlier practices in that the examinations took on a much greater importance. Recommendation was still a prerequisite for examination participation, but a recommendation was now based less on one's proven administrative abilities than on one's literary gifts.

The slow evolution of the examination system as the principal means of recruitment is demonstrated in an institutional change that occurred in 736. At that time oversight of the examinations was moved from the board of personnel to the board of ritual. This move clearly signified that the old practice of selection on the basis of subbureaucratic experience was at an end; long years of study of the classics and the honing of literary skills now replaced practical training and bureaucratic experience as the means to a successful career.

GENTRY CHINA

The Sung dynasty (960–1279) may be taken as the beginning of a distinct stage in Chinese history (without suggesting abrupt changes in the society). By this time, the aristocracy was largely gone; many aristocratic families had been wiped out in the latter part of the T'ang and in the period of warfare before the founding of the Sung. Furthermore, a provincial elite had been slowly growing in the last half of the T'ang, thereby changing the societal characteristics of T'ang China. The availability of printed texts facilitated less expensive mastery of the Confucian classics and probably contributed to literacy on a much wider scale than had been the case in earlier periods. The level of wealth in the society was far higher than it had been in the T'ang because the economic center of gravity had shifted to the richly endowed lands of the Yangtze valley. There were also important changes in all levels of government.[11]

Sung dynasty emperors were more powerful than their predecessors, and the emperor now adopted a more remote and formal pose; the relative informality in the earlier relationship between the ruler and his ministers now gave way to a distant relationship based on the exchange of formal documents. The ruler no longer had to face a socially autonomous aristocracy; the examination system was now the primary means of determining political, and therefore social, status. Changes in political institutions eliminated the military commissioners cum warlords, who had threatened many pre-Sung emperors. Confucianism began to stress different values, particularly those that demanded obedience of one's superiors. Finally, the continuing presence of powerful states on the northern frontier of the Sung, which created military tensions and at times led to major wars, may have strengthened Sung authoritarian tendencies, as suggested by a slogan from this period, "Expel the barbarians; honor the emperor."

The Sung regime created the most complex administrative structure and system of official designations of any imperial Chinese government. Accordingly, its treatment is even more condensed than the treatment of other periods.

In the central administration the three departments were continued from the T'ang, but they often enjoyed little more than a nominal existence. Real power was in the hands of the grand councillors, who might concurrently hold a position in one of the three departments and one or more other designations. As a rule there were two grand councillors (*tsai-hsiang*) and a fluctuating number of vice councillors (*fu-hsiang*); hence, the total number of grand and vice councillors at any one time varied from five to nine. They supervised the administration and served as the principal advisers to the emperor. The councillors had a sizable staff, whose most important members were Hanlin academicians (*han-lin hsüeh-shih*). This title had originated in the T'ang as a private drafting and revising office for the emperor and by late T'ang times the academicians became palace councillors. In the Sung the academicians had be-

11. E. A. Kracke, Jr., *Civil Service in Early Sung China, 960–1067* (Cambridge: Harvard University Press, 1953). This book is the most useful work on the Sung government, even though its coverage is temporally limited.

come sufficiently bureaucratized that they were recognized as holders of substantive positions.

One of the hallmarks of the Sung administration (and continuing into later periods) was a high degree of functional specificity. At the central government level it is seen in the finance commission (*san-ssu*), which for the first century of the Sung took over the functions of the board of revenue and two other of the six boards, thus concentrating fiscal matters in the commission's hands. After the first century these responsibilities were returned to the standard boards. There was a parallel development in the creation of a bureau of military affairs (*shu-mi-yüan*), headed by a commissioner (*shih*) who was directly responsible to the emperor. The commission and the bureau tended to weaken the powers of the grand councillors (although occasionally grand councillors served concurrently in these commissioner positions). This division between the civil and the military does not indicate professionalization (the military commissioner was usually a civil official), but it demonstrates the throne's concern about keeping military and fiscal matters out of the hands of the same, potentially dangerous, person.

In 1080 major reforms, carried out under the impetus of conservative bureaucrats, diminished the role of the fiscal commissioner and restored the now familiar six boards. The boards were nominally under the Department of Affairs of State, but that office tended to be absorbed by the grand councillors; hence the six boards (and their subordinate bureaus) were directly overseen by the highest organ of government. The nine courts, still principally concerned with imperial activities, also continued from the T'ang. The directorates, of which the Directorate of Education, in charge of the national university, was the most important, likewise continued from the T'ang. However, the rising importance of the examination system reduced the role of that institution and its students were no longer the "sons of the state."

Although local administrative units bore a close resemblance to their pre-Sung antecedents, there were also some significant differences. As a rule, in the early Sung appointments were not made to the roughly three hundred positions of prefect and the approximately fifteen hundred positions of district magistrate; instead, all officials held central government positions and were dispatched to manage the affairs of prefectures and districts. Such personnel practices were common in the first century of the Sung and contributed to the bewildering array of titles and offices that an official might hold at any one time. These practices were designed to convince all officials that they were part of the central administration, serving directly under the emperor. Imperial distrust of the prefects led to the practice of sending other officials, also with positions in the central government, to spy on the prefect and to report on his administration or maladministration. These controller-generals (*t'ung-p'an*), as they were formally known, had to countersign every order issued by the official who was actually the prefect. After the first century of the Sung, these controller-generals were transformed into assistant prefects.

The quality of the government that the average commoner could expect deteriorated further during the Sung. Many of the subbureaucratic functionaries were now conscripted to serve without pay. In fact, often they were financially abused and had to make up deficiencies from their own resources at the end of their service periods. Faced with that prospect, many tried to avoid service or, failing that, to cover their own costs by leaning on the taxpaying peasants. Thus, government agents who confronted the general populace were, by this time, strikingly different from the apprentice officials of the Han period.

The major institutional reform at the local level in the Sung was the result of still another attempt to sandwich a supervisory or surveillance unit between the central government and the prefectures. This reform may be cited as a clear case in which Chinese officials actually learned from history. Certainly the Han and the T'ang experiences with provinces that managed to accumulate great military and economic power was a potent lesson in how not to build political institutions. The Sung solution to the problem, already suggested by the T'ang creation of fiscal commissioners, was to establish commissioners for military, fiscal, judicial, and supply functions. Sung China was divided into ten circuits (*lu*, later increased to twenty-six but reduced to sixteen after the loss of north China) with a fiscal and a judicial commissioner (*shih*) for each circuit. The geographical areas under the military and supply commissioners did not necessarily correspond with the boundaries of the regular circuits. This kind of functional division made it impossible for a single official to consolidate various powers in one office; the throne was thereby made more secure.

The institutionalization of the examination system is generally treated as a major achievement of the Sung period. Building on earlier developments, the Sung government refined the system into a three-stage process. The lowest level examinations were given at the prefectural level; those who passed then went on to the metropolitan examination in the capital. Finally, those who passed at that level were given a palace examination, sometimes administered by the emperor himself. The examinations were held on a three-year cycle that became standard in subsequent Chinese history. The most prestigious degree was that of Presented Scholar of which, on average, about six hundred were conferred every three years. Although the prerequisites for taking the prefectural examinations are not known, the scholarly consensus is that the Sung examinations were more open than any pre-Sung recruitment system.

The historical significance of the examination is at least threefold. First, it allowed upward social mobility for those who could afford to educate themselves or their sons. The advent of printing was undoubtedly a contributing factor in such social mobility. Second, it freed the throne from dependence on an aristocracy and conferred on the throne, through its examiners, the power to elevate those of modest social origins. Third, the examination system created the gentry. The full sociopolitical significance of the gentry was not to emerge until the Ming and Ch'ing periods, but even in the Sung period the examination system set off people in the society by officially recognizing them as successes in the intensely competitive examinations. Successful examinees, even those who passed only the lowest level, secured for themselves elite status. Their educations may have been paid for only because their fathers were wealthy farmers or landlords, but their status derived from their successes in the examination process.

At its greatest geographic extent the Sung dynasty never controlled as much territory as had the T'ang empire. From the beginning of the dynasty northwest China was in the hands of the Hsi-Hsia state and part of northeast China was controlled by the Liao dynasty. By 1125 all of north China was lost to the semisinified Chin dynasty, and in 1279 the Mongols completed the conquest of all of China. For want of space, I make no comments on the governments of these regimes; I note only one factor because of its importance to Ming T'ai-tsu (r. 1368–1398), the founder of the Ming dynasty (1368–1644). T'ai-tsu was convinced that the Mongol rulers of the Yuan dynasty (1279–1367) had been too lax; consequently, many of his efforts were devoted to making sure that China was stringently governed and that the ruler would participate directly in meeting that goal.

The Ming dynasty was more autocratic than even the later Manchu conquerors of China, whose Ch'ing dynasty ruled China from 1644 until 1911.[12] The differences between the two dynasties were more in tone and style than in institutional substance. Although introducing some changes from Ming government, the Manchus maintained a regime that was markedly similar to the Ming. Because of these similarities, the following paragraphs treat the Ming and Ch'ing together, only noting the ways in which the last dynasty deviated from the practices of its predecessor.[13]

The higher levels of autocracy were facilitated by several factors. First, Neo-Confucianism, which was the state orthodoxy under both the

12. Charles O. Hucker, *The Ming Dynasty: Its Origins and Evolving Institutions* (Ann Arbor: University of Michigan Center for Chinese Studies, 1978), and idem, *The Traditional Chinese State in Ming Times* (Tucson: University of Arizona Press, 1961).

13. There is no major modern study of the Ch'ing government. Hsieh Pao-chao, *The Government of China (1644–1911)* (Baltimore: Johns Hopkins University Press, 1925), is very dated and must be used with care. Local administration is covered in Ch'ü T'ung-tsu, *Local Government in China under the Ch'ing* (Cambridge: Harvard University Press, 1962) and James R. Watt, *The District Magistrate in Late Imperial China* (New York: Columbia University Press, 1972).

Chinese rulers of the Ming dynasty and the Manchu rulers of the Ch'ing, placed much more stress on authoritarian relationships within the family, the society, and the state than did any earlier form of Confucianism. Second, institutional changes made possible much more strict control of all levels of the bureaucracy. Third, although the role of the gentry was much enhanced in the last two dynasties, it was a role that required the gentry to work closely with the imperial bureaucracy. In effect, there was a partnership between the social elite and the bureaucratic elite, or, to be more precise, we might say that a partnership existed between those members of the gentry in office and those members of the gentry not in office.

Ming T'ai-tsu left more of an imprint on the Chinese imperial institution than did most of his predecessors. He was well aware that the practices he established would be binding on his descendants, and he accordingly issued numerous decrees, orders, and laws. His aims were to overcome the perceived laxity of the Mongol administration of China and to control rigorously both the administrative structure and the society. He also sought to recreate Chinese society, particularly with regard to morality and social behavior, according to Neo-Confucian prescriptions.

The highest level of the central administration, the Grand Secretariat (*nei-ko*), did not take final form until late in the fifteenth century. Ming T'ai-tsu had a deep distrust of high-level officials, a distrust that led him to abolish the secretariat that he had continued from the Yuan and earlier dynasties. He fractured central bureaucratic authority into the hands of the six ministries and five coequal military commissions (*wu-chün tu-tu-fu*). When he was faced with the difficult task of dealing with numerous governmental agencies, he turned to the Hanlin academicians for assistance. The Grand Secretariat, which was composed of low-ranking Hanlin academicians, who were customarily also given titles of nominal offices that had no real power, came out of this reliance on the academicians. The imperial aim was clearly to avoid the concentration of power in the hands of the old-style secretariat, to say nothing of the even greater power that had belonged to the chancellor of the Han dynasty.

The grand secretaries were in an uncomfortable political situation. Although their actual positions were quite low, their proximity to the emperor meant that they were the superiors of most members of the bureaucracy. Furthermore, their normal route to office was through the Hanlin and other academies, not upward through the bureaucracy; hence, many officials looked on them not as part of the regular governmental apparatus but as minions of the emperor. Finally, they often found themselves working closely with other members of the inner court, particularly the increasingly important eunuchs. The grand secretaries were treated with suspicion by willful emperors and oftentimes with contempt by members of officialdom.

In the Chinese political context the grand secretaries can be seen as a recurrent reminder of the deeply felt patrimonial values that marked the early nature of the institution of the ruler. Throughout imperial Chinese history, rulers sought to avoid bureaucratizing their own position; the presence of the grand secretaries and such pre-Ming equivalents as the Han dynasty masters of writing demonstrate the rulers' determination along these lines. Over time, however, the repeated bureaucratization of these low-level, secretarial-advising positions indicates that whereas the rulers may have been successful so far as their own position was concerned, they could not prevent the bureaucratization process from occurring even in the case of their close advisers.

The transition of the Ming grand secretaries from an "inner court" advisory role to an "outer court" administrative role was not complete until 1730, well into the Ch'ing dynasty. The emperor then turned to the Council of State (*chün-chi-ch'u*) for autonomous advice. The council consisted of five members, two Chinese and two Manchus, and was usually headed by another Manchu. As a rule, members of the council concurrently held substantive positions as ranking members on one of the six boards. Their importance derived from their daily meetings with the emperor at which policy decisions were reached and orders issued.

The presence of both Chinese and Manchus on the Council of State reveals that the Manchu leadership learned from the historical experience of the Yuan dynasty that sharing power with the Chinese produced better government and more amicable social relations. There was thus a doubling of central government positions in order to accommodate officials from both ethnic groups. At lower levels, however, Chinese numerically dominated the administrative structure.

The paramount administrative organs in both the Ming and the Ch'ing dynasties were the six boards. Aside from joint Chinese-Manchu membership, there was a high degree of continuity from the Ming to the Ch'ing. The Manchus added the equivalent of a seventh board, called the Court of Colonial Affairs (*li-fan-yuan*), which testifies to the greater geographic extent of the Ch'ing empire. This court was responsible for conducting foreign relations between the Ch'ing government and Mongol tribes, Tibet, Russia, and the oasis states of Central Asia. In 1861, in an institutional change dictated by Westerners, this court was transformed into a Western-style foreign office.

Censorial and closely related remonstrance functions have a long and checkered history in imperial China.[14] A tripartite approach to the general problem helps to clarify some issues, but there is still much work to be done on these institutions. Remonstrance, the generic term referring

14. Charles O. Hucker, *The Censorial System in Ming China* (Stanford: Stanford University Press, 1966), is the only book-length study of the censorate. See also the works cited in nn. 6, 7 and 10.

to advising the emperor that he is wrong, was a constant concern of officials and was deeply embedded in Confucian thought. In view of the absence of any institutionalized restraints on imperial power, emperors had to be convinced that they were dependent on the wisdom and guidance of their Confucian officials (as opposed to the kinds of advice that they might receive from consort family members, eunuchs, and others). From the Period of Disunion through the Sung period remonstrance officials were attached to the chancellery and to the secretariat. A major change occurred in the Ming when remonstrance functions were primarily assigned to the censorate and there was no remonstrance body as such. The Ch'ing continued this institutional practice.

Remonstrance officials and remonstrating censors often found themselves putting their careers and even their lives in jeopardy when they held positions that were in opposition to those of the emperor. Thus, the formal disappearance of the remonstrant officials may be seen as victories for both the throne and members of officialdom: the throne because it no longer had to tolerate men whose responsibility it was to make the emperor look bad; officialdom because its members would no longer be charged with duties that often took great courage and that could be devastating to those who carried them out.

The other two parts of these oversight activities are central and local censorial responsibilities. The concept of a well articulated censorate did not emerge until the Sui and, particularly, the T'ang dynasties. In the T'ang the censorate (*yü-shih-t'ai*) was exclusively concerned with oversight and surveillance of all levels of the administration. With few exceptions this arrangement was continued into the Ming until the 1382 reforms, when the investigating censors (*chien-ch'a yü-shih*), although still nominally under the censorate, were in fact placed under the direct control of the emperor. The 110 investigating censors were organized along provincial lines but were regularly dispatched on missions whose geographic extent was not necessarily the same as the provincial boundaries. In addition, each of the six ministries had an office of scrutiny existing independently of the censorate. The Ch'ing emperors placed the six offices of scrutiny under the censorate, thereby eliminating any remaining remonstrance function. The Ming period saw the apogee of censorial powers, which is not surprising considering the extent to which autocracy was developed in that period.

Local-level surveillance proved to be the most difficult for the emperor to maintain. In the Ch'in–Han period and again in the Sung, local surveillance officials were transformed into assistants of the men over whom they were supposed to maintain surveillance. Similarly, in both the Han and the T'ang regional inspectors were converted into high-level administrators with major fiscal, personnel, and military powers, further blurring the line between oversight and administration. Resolution of this problem was achieved in the Ming and Ch'ing period with the creation of provinces and subprovincial agencies with authority over the district magistrate.

The borders of the provinces were outlined in the Yuan dynasty, took definite shape in the Ming, and became substantive administrative units in the Ch'ing. Early in the Ming three officials were appointed for each province: a provincial administration commissioner (*ch'eng-hsuan pu-cheng shih ssu*), a provincial surveillance commissioner (*t'i-hsing an-ch'a shih ssu*), and a regional military commissioner (*tu chih-hui shih ssu*). To coordinate the civil aspects of this structure, grand coordinators (*hsun-fu*) were sent out. They lacked staff members and were dispatched on duty assignments merely as coordinators. In the Ch'ing the coordinators were replaced by regular provincial governors holding substantive positions but still lacking an administrative staff. The military counterpart of the provincial governor in the Ming was the supreme commander (*tsung-tu*), who might coordinate military matters over a larger area than a single province. The Ming coordinators and the Ch'ing governors usually served concurrently as censors; thus, they held broad impeachment powers. The Ch'ing created a supraprovincial post: the governor-general. The occupants of this post had been regional military commanders during the Ming. Each governor-general had two or three provinces under his direction. In the cases of six of the nine governors-general, they were also governors of one of their provinces (three provinces did not have governors-general). The governors and governors-general were carefully chosen by the emperor himself. The majority of provincial and lower-level positions were held by Chinese. Unlike the situation in the central government, where Manchus held many important posts, there was no ethnic sharing at the local level.

In the Ming and the Ch'ing many provincial-level commissioners were of great importance. The administration commissioner (*pu-cheng-shih*) was overwhelmingly concerned with fiscal matters. The surveillance commissioner (*an-ch'a-shih*), who exercised censorial functions over all officials in the province, was also concerned with the administration of justice. The education commissioner (*t'i-tu hsueh-cheng*), based in the capital, supervised the schools of a province and certified candidates for the civil service examinations. Functional specificity by imperial appointees thus reached a new and higher level.

Provinces were divided into circuits as early as the Ming, and these territorial subdivisions were sustained in the Ch'ing (there were eighty-nine circuits in the mid eighteenth century). Below the circuit there was a three-tiered structure consisting of prefectures, departments, and districts (the numbers of these units in the late Ming were, respectively, 159, 234, and 1,144; the same figures for the Ch'ing in 1812 were 182,

214, and 1,293). The pyramid is not quite as neat as this wording suggests; some departments had no subordinate districts, and some districts were administered directly by prefectures. Furthermore, in the Ch'ing in some particularly important strategic and fiscal areas a subprefecture was added between the prefectures and the departments, and was often directly subordinate to the provincial office. The districts and, in some cases, departments were the only units in direct contact with the general population; all others were designed to supervise, audit, impeach, and direct their lower units. What is perhaps most striking in a comparison of these arrangements with those of the Han is the complexity of the structure above the district and the relatively small number of districts.

There was a marked degree of specialization at all levels except that of the district. From the circuits down to the departments and even some districts, special units were created to focus on such activities as water control, transportation, fiscal matters, and the salt trade. Overlapping duties were probably common only with regard to censorial obligations. The whole operation of government at the local level was finely tuned. Only at the level of the district magistrate was one official responsible for the manifold operations of administering justice, collecting taxes, controlling water, transporting grain, overseeing schools, participating in ritual activities, and so on.

Given this structure and the constant oversight, one might assume that corruption was exceptionally rare, but in fact this was not the case. In a society in which there are extreme scarcities, in which some people have money but little political power, in which others have political power but little money, and in which the idea of the rule of law is poorly developed—in short, in most of the premodern world—one has to expect corruption. Bribery and corruption were common throughout Chinese history and so long as it was kept below a vaguely understood but never precisely delimited threshold, it was tolerated.

The multiple layers of government between the district and the province probably served a useful social role in providing places for those who had passed the examinations. The proliferation of offices at the local level during the Period of Disunion provides a historical parallel for such a speculation. During the Ming and the Ch'ing the pass rate for the provincial-level examination was about 1 percent; for the metropolitan examination, it was about 2.5 percent. Passing the provincial-level examination allowed entry into relatively low positions, such as that of district magistrate. The layers of government above the district thus accommodated large numbers of men who otherwise would not have been able to find positions. This discussion is not meant to suggest that the supradistrict positions were sinecures but only that these positions required staffing by men who benefited by imperial patronage and who simultaneously made sure that the imperial will was carried out at the local level.

The relatively small number of districts in the Ch'ing period stands in striking contrast to the figures for earlier periods in Chinese history, and the contrast is even more striking when we note that the population of the Ch'ing was about six times larger than it had been in the Han. In contrast to most previous eras, during the Ch'ing fewer district magistrates were responsible for a vastly larger population. Who gained by such an arrangement? One possible and very likely answer is the gentry. Because district magistrates were fully occupied in dispensing justice, collecting taxes, and discharging other specified obligations, many local activities were thus left to the nonofficial gentry (I return to this point later). Despite its autocratic nature, the government of the Ming and Ch'ing dynasties was a mutually beneficial arrangement in which the emperor was secure on his throne and the gentry enjoyed considerable latitude on the local scene.

The renowned Chinese civil service examination system came into its own in the Ming and the Ch'ing dynasties after a millennium of evolution. All local governments, from the prefecture down to and including the district, were required to maintain Confucian schools with set quotas of students. Entry into the schools required considerable preparation, and many entry examinations had to be passed. Those students who earned the title of licentiate (*sheng-yuan*)—not by graduation but by passing the examination for that degree—could not enter office, but the degree conferred social status, recognizable by the garments one was authorized to wear, certain legal privileges, and a government stipend that made continued study possible. Most important, the licentiate degree allowed the student to sit for the provincial examination. The provincial graduate could enter government service, but his chances of reaching high office with that degree were quite limited. The 2 to 3 percent who passed the metropolitan examination then participated in a palace examination, which few failed. Those who succeeded at the metropolitan level were assured of rapid entry into high positions in the capital or the provinces.

There were exceptions to this pattern that can be no more than noted in passing. As a general rule throughout Chinese history, the sons (and sometimes other relatives as well) of the highest officials were able to enter officialdom without passing examinations or to avoid part of the examination process. When the state was particularly short of funds it sold titles such as licentiate degrees or positions in the national university or positions in officialdom. Furthermore, special examinations were occasionally given to allow truly outstanding scholars to enter officialdom without going through the full examination process. Finally, the examinations given to the Manchus and to their Mongol allies were less demanding than those given to the Chinese applicants. Nevertheless, Chinese occupied the vast majority of governmental positions.

The examination process created the social elite, the gentry. Some members of the gentry were also members of officialdom, but the vast majority of degree-holders, to say nothing of the aspirants to that sociopolitical status, were not serving officials. Nevertheless, the gentry played important roles in the political life of the Ming and Ch'ing periods. There were countless activities at the local level that the overburdened district magistrate had neither the time nor the energy to conduct. These activities included maintaining Confucian schools and Buddhist temples, undertaking famine relief, guiding construction of irrigation projects, and settling local disputes. Members of the gentry were called on to perform these and other functions that in an earlier age would have been the responsibility of local officialdom.[15]

Over the long course of Chinese history a reasonably satisfactory symbiotic relationship emerged between the imperial state and the social elite. This relationship, which reached its highest stage of development in the Ch'ing, can be highlighted by comparing the Han and the Ch'ing situations. At the beginning of the Han a powerful local elite was seen as a potential threat to the throne and various actions were taken to weaken that elite. Han Confucianism expressed grave concerns about the nature of imperial power, and the paramount issue in Han Confucianism was how to deal with the newly created imperial regime. By the latter part of the Han the local elite had come to dominate the subbureaucratic positions; it had, in effect, decided that cooptation should supplant confrontation. This shift in the political scales, leading to the post-Han aristocracy, left imperial power weakened until the advent and refinement of the examination system. By the Ch'ing period the imperial system was so well accepted that members of the social elite competed with each other through the examination system for degrees that served as the only entrée into officialdom and that provided imperial validation of elite status. The emperor, no longer threatened by rival social forces, could make his will felt through a complex, multitiered political structure. The members of the gentry found rewarding positions in this structure and at the same time realized that its very nature at the local

15. The standard works on the gentry are Ho Ping-ti, *The Ladder of Success in Imperial China: Aspects of Social Mobility, 1368–1911* (New York: Wiley, 1962); Chang Chung-li, *The Chinese Gentry: Studies on Their Role in Nineteenth Century Chinese Society* (Seattle: University of Washington Press, 1955); and idem, *The Income of the Chinese Gentry* (Seattle: University of Washington Press, 1962). For a much broader study of Ch'ing society see Susan Naquin and Evelyn S. Rawski, *Chinese Society in the Eighteenth Century* (New Haven: Yale University Press, 1987).

level left them with a fair amount of latitude. Barring major catastrophes that might throw the entire arrangement into violent disequilibrium, both sides benefited.

CONCLUSION

I conclude with several broad generalizations on traditional Chinese government. In particular, I draw attention to three topics: (1) imperial power, (2) the control of the bureaucracy, and (3) the nature of various recruitment systems within a changing social milieu.

The power of the emperor was clearly not a constant in Chinese history. Entrenched social forces such as the powerful families of the Later Han and the aristocracy of the post-Han through T'ang periods acted as a brake on imperial power. Even in the Sung period, when the aristocracy was no longer politically present, Chinese emperors sought to woo the elite. By the Ming the situation had changed drastically in favor of the emperor, who was sometimes brutal and always demanding in asserting his superiority. The Manchus learned from the excesses of their Chinese predecessors, particularly the abuse of imperial power by unchecked eunuchs, and sustained or improved the imperial bureaucratic mechanism while softening the imperial image. Thus, the throne continually adjusted to changing social patterns and in the long run managed to strengthen itself at the expense of the various elites. The paramount constant in the history of the imperial institution is that it always managed to hold itself above the bureaucracy; its patrimonial roots continued to be nurtured by Confucianism (and vice versa).

One of the ways that the throne augmented its power was by discovering means to exercise better control over the component parts of the imperial bureaucracy. This ongoing trend manifested itself in the intricate ways that officials were made responsible for specific functions. This functional specialization had two consequences. First, the more precise definition of functions led to higher quality work, with the result that the throne could be assured that duties were being efficiently discharged. In early periods broad areas of responsibility necessarily caused some prioritizing, which diminished the attention given to certain concerns. With increasing reliance on commissioners for taxes, transportation, education, and other functions, the throne was better able to establish priorities, and the officials were given less flexibility. Second, functional specificity was also a means to limit power. In the Han and the T'ang periods the disastrous consequences of the consolidation of military, fiscal, and personnel power by regional inspectors and governors-general were painful lessons for the throne that were avoided in the Sung and later periods. With fiscal power in the hands of one official, judicial power in the hands of another, and military power in the hands of a third, post-T'ang rulers worried much less about their own officials tearing their empires apart.

From the perspective of the emperor Chinese social structure should be determined by the throne; minimally, the emperor should be able to dictate the terms according to which one entered the social elite, which should have been indistinguishable from the political elite. In the imperial period the throne was able to do this during two long temporal spans, but it did so each time on distinctly different grounds. The throne proved incapable of acting as a gatekeeper to high social status for almost a millennium, from the latter part of the Han through the T'ang, when the aristocracy managed to determine its own membership. In the throne's two periods of success it relied, first, on administrative merit and, later, on scholarly merit. In the first period, which was the Han ideal and which had its origins about three centuries before the founding of the Han in 206 B.C., merit established in subbureaucratic positions was the principal means of entry into higher governmental positions and social esteem. In the post-T'ang period once the examination system was in place, merit was not administrative but scholarly. Whereas the Han model allowed the cultivation of administrative expertise through practice, the later model required years, sometimes decades, of study of the Confucian classics and the honing of the literary arts. In both cases the throne determined the nature of the recruitment mechanism and by creating intense competition assured itself that it would not be dependent on autonomous social elements. Although Chinese social structure was far more complex than this approach suggests, the examination system assured the well educated (and the wealthy who could afford to educate their sons) that they had access to the process that might grant them superior political and social status. Clearly, most would not achieve success in the higher-level examinations, but the hope of success at even the lowest level meant that these people had a vested interest in preserving the system. These vested interests eased imperial worries about social forces beyond imperial control.

FOUR

□

Sage Kings and Laws in the Chinese and Greek Traditions

Karen Turner

The central importance that political philosophers in early China assigned to law as a means to curb the arbitrary, personal element in rulership is often overlooked in assessments of Chinese political culture and government. New materials on early Chinese law, unknown until the archaeological excavations of the past two decades, are now stimulating us to reexamine concepts of law in some of the most important texts that were produced in the formative years of the Chinese political system, the sixth through the second centuries B.C.

In order to highlight Chinese ideas about the proper role of law in government, I propose to look at how certain influential early Chinese and Greek political writers treated the problem of balancing the rule of man with the rule of law. The dilemma is not only ancient but, judging from the wealth of recent writing on the topic, timeless as well.[1]

THE PROBLEM

We cannot apply modern standards when we discuss the rule of law in any ancient society because the formal apparatus of the rule of law—an

Note on translations used in this essay: Passages from Greek and Latin texts are taken from standard translations, which I have cited in the notes. For Chinese materials I have in all cases referred to the original text, but I have included in the notes selected translations.

1. See a recent survey of the issue in the Western tradition in Dean J. Spader, "Rule of Law v. Rule of Man: The Search for the Golden Zigzag between Conflicting Fundamental Values," *Journal of Criminal Justice* 12, no. 4 (1984): 379–94. For Chinese speculations on this topic in modern times, see Hsiao Kung-ch'uan, *A History of Chinese Political Thought,* trans. F. W. Mote (Princeton: Princeton University Press, 1979). Professor Hsiao, writing in the 1940s, declares that a true, Western-style rule of law never developed in classical China and that this flaw hindered democratic reforms in the modern period. More recently the Chinese press has been filled with articles advocating rule of law. See as but one example in English, "The rule of law," *China Daily,* June 29, 1985.

independent judicial system free of executive pressure and political taint—is a relatively recent phenomenon in the West. But the heart of the quandary of finding a workable relationship between the certainty of law and the flexibility offered by good leadership has remained remarkably constant over time. The rule of man allows for creative decisions based on the discretionary judgments of enlightened individuals who can often preserve the spirit of the law better than a system devoted to a rigid attention to rules. The rule of law, however, ideally protects the ruled from the whims of their rulers, who are subordinated to the laws and charged with overseeing the fair and consistent administration of the enacted laws of the state.

In the period surveyed here, the first millennium B.C., an epoch in world history when a few extraordinarily creative thinkers scrutinized their past more objectively than ever before, the alternatives were murky indeed.[2] No matter what their history or their hopes for the future, these thinkers seemed all too keenly aware that genuinely wise and just rulers appear only rarely. Yet fragile political and legal institutions often failed to preserve order, and charismatic personal leadership seemed at times to promise the only refuge from anarchy. On the whole, however, I have found that some of the most important classical Chinese writers who directly address the problem of law and leadership are just as concerned as their Western counterparts with the question of whether a government of laws can offer more stability in the long run than rule based on the personal abilities of a monarch and his ministers.[3]

Detecting a common respect for law in seminal Chinese and Greek thinkers is surprising because modern observers point to major differences in legal traditions and institutions when explaining the evolution of divergent political systems in China and the West.[4] Law in the West has been associated at various times with divinity, the limitation of kingly power, institutions created to protect the God-given rights of individuals, and in modern times, with the efforts of legal specialists to resolve

2. In his study of thought in early China, Benjamin Schwartz refers to the concept of an "axial age," first proposed by Karl Jaspers, as one reference point for comparing Chinese and Western thought. Any student interested in comparative ideas should refer to this important study. See Benjamin Schwartz, *The World of Thought in Ancient China* (Cambridge: Harvard University Press, 1985).

3. The term "rule of law" is laden with historical and theoretical implications and has carried different meanings at different times in the European legal tradition. See Franz Neumann, *The Democratic and the Authoritarian State: Essays in Political and Legal Theory* (Glencoe, Ill.: Free Press, 1957), for one view of some of the issues and their historical roots.

4. A recent article by William Alford takes issue with one argument that China was unable, by virtue of shared assumptions in its classical traditions, to even conceive of the rule of law in the Western sense. See William P. Alford, "The Inscrutable Occidental? Implications of Roberto Unger's Uses and Abuses of the Chinese Past," *Texas Law Review* 64 (1986): 915–72.

conflicts fairly and justly. Despite changes in meaning and function over time, law has been viewed generally as a positive force in the West. St. Thomas Aquinas, for example, celebrated divine law as the ultimate standard for judging worldly authority, but he also respected the laws issued by the state to maintain order. His definition of law as "an ordinance of reason for the common good, made by him who has care of the community, and promulgated" still rings true to those of us imbued with Western values.[5]

By contrast, China's dominant tradition held that law was not the gift of the gods but the product of barbarian tribes whose culture developed outside the pale of the civilized world. Even today, the standard textbook view of Chinese history describes law in China as a simple administrative tool used by the ruler and his magistrates to control an unruly populace. The Legalist statesmen, who wrote most forcefully about the importance of positive laws, are blamed for formulating a theory and practice of law that placed the ruler above the laws, which he and his officials could formulate at will, without regard for morality and custom. The Confucians, who celebrated the efficacy of ritual and benevolent personal leadership, seem by contrast rather simple-minded idealists with no understanding or appreciation of the need for law. Both depictions are too narrow, but historical reasons explain how these skewed perceptions of the classical tradition came about.

Although the Confucians were no less eager to shape political life, the Legalist officials were better positioned to implement their political ideas. The state of Ch'in became the center for Legalist reforms, which enjoyed some local success but could not be so easily imposed in other states after the king of Ch'in attempted to extend his laws and institutions over the whole of China when he conquered the warring kingdoms in 221 B.C. The demise of the Ch'in empire after less than two decades was one of the most influential failures in Chinese history; it bolstered the Confucianists' contention that education and moral leadership preserved social order better in the long run than laws and formal institutions. For the Confucians the very existence of written, fixed laws had always signaled a failure because in their view it was only when good men lost their power to influence society that laws would be needed at all. In Confucian political theory, published laws did not bring order but encouraged chaos because they could be manipulated so much easier than traditional notions of right behavior.

Confucian disapproval of legalistic trends and the lessons learned from the failure of the Ch'in imperial state had a profound impact on China's intellectual and political history. The founder of the Western

5. Thomas Aquinas, *Summa Theologica,* trans. Fathers of the Dominican Province, Part 2, 1st part, query 90, article 4; reprinted in The Great Books of the Western World series, Vol. 20 (Chicago: Encyclopedia Britannica, 1952), 208.

Han dynasty, which succeeded the Ch'in, tried to pacify his new subjects by promising above all to simplify and mitigate the Ch'in laws. Indeed, from Han times into the twentieth century, the Ch'in dynasty's harsh government by law has been castigated by Confucian historians and philosophers (whose views dominated interpretations of history) as both deeply immoral and disastrously ineffective.[6] Yet laws proliferated and continued to serve as the backbone of the Chinese empire throughout the two thousand years of its existence.

MATERIALS AND METHODS

Our vision of ancient political theory is inevitably colored by the texts we read and the questions we ask of them. Out of a very rich tradition in both China and the West I have focused on a few classical works that address directly the issue of the role of law in government. I also use selected new materials from China that inspire fresh interpretations of old questions. My own expertise and interests are centered on the early Chinese case, and the Greek examples are used more to illuminate Chinese themes than to provide a genuinely comparative assessment.[7] Yet stepping outside the Chinese tradition offers certain advantages for the study of Chinese legal history.

The stereotypical view of Chinese political culture presents both the Legalists and the Confucians as proponents of rule of man: the Legalists because they placed the ruler above the law, and the Confucians because they preferred governance by sage kings rather than laws. But when compared with the thinking of Plato and Aristotle on the subject of laws, Chinese thinkers of both persuasions seem more inclined to support government by law than unfettered rulership by man. The Legalists separated the interests of the ruler from the well-being of the state and aimed to protect the state from irresponsible leadership at the top with laws to circumscribe the ruler's activities. The Confucians hoped for the rule of sage kings, but they understood all too well how rarely such exemplary men had appeared in history.[8] Their mission focused on convincing contemporary rulers to abide by the models, or Laws, set forth

6. Western historians have tended to agree. See, for example, the assessment of the Ch'in government in Frederick W. Mote, *Intellectual Foundations of China* (New York: Knopf, 1971).

7. The benefits of comparing classical China with Greece are noted in Jean-Pierre Vernant, *Myth and Society in Ancient Greece* (Atlantic Highlands, N.J.: Humanities Press, 1980), 71–91. In Jerome Frank, *Courts on Trial: Myth and Reality in American Justice* (Princeton: Princeton University Press, 1949), 378–84, the author describes how the Chinese and Greek legal systems resembled each other in their common disdain for litigation and their preference for arbitration.

8. I have deliberately used "men" or "man" in this essay when it seems clear that the thinkers whose works I am describing eliminated women from consideration as participants in government, even though women often exercised informal political influence.

by a very select group of ancient model-rulers in the interest of preserving a social environment that would encourage the moral development of all humans. Although it would be inaccurate to claim that Chinese and Greek writers held similar views on all aspects of government, in general Chinese political theorists are more in sympathy with Aristotle's government of laws than with Plato's ideal of rule by man.

In the texts that take up the issue of law, we glimpse the pessimistic side of Chinese writers, their doubts that government could be so simple or humankind so perfectible that laws would not be necessary. Given the strong warnings against arbitrary interference in government that permeate so many texts, it seems that by the beginning of the Warring States period (403–221 B.C.) many thinkers realized that the personal character of what Jack L. Dull calls a "patrimonial" form of ruling (see Chapter 3) had brought only chaos to the world. We can better understand their arguments against arbitrary rulers and in favor of accountability if we recognize that classical political theorists wrote in an age when the excesses of local despots muted any hope for peace and prosperity. What seems to have most troubled thinkers in China's classical era was not whether laws were necessary in government but how to find reliable Laws for guiding political and social life in a time of great change.

How we interpret any writer's position on law depends a great deal on how we define law. In the texts I have used, the Chinese graph, *fa,* usually translated as "punitive law" or "positive law," actually covers a range of meanings, from the broadest sense of a model or standard, a rule or regulation, to the narrower meaning of an ordinance governing punishments, just as the word "law" in English conjures up images as weighty as the Law of God and as mundane as the laws of the road.[9] In many early Chinese texts law seems to carry more than one meaning at once because the laws governing punishments ideally sprang from models derived either from the natural world or from the practices of the ancient sage kings. As I shall show later, Chinese rulers were responsible for seeing that the positive laws enacted by the state did not offend higher notions of Law. Confucian thinkers would have approved of the statement of Han Ch'eng-ti (r. 32–7 B.C.): "The aim must be to conform with the laws of antiquity."[10]

My own analysis of law in early China has been shaped by the histories

9. To clarify the difference between enacted, positive laws and Law as a higher standard that guides the creation of these laws, I have distinguished the former as "law" and the latter as "Law" when appropriate. At times, however, these meanings are ambiguous.

10. This is in *Han-shu* (Peking: Chung-hua, 1962), Chüan 23, p. 1103. For a translation of Chüan 23, see A. F. P. Hulsewe, *Remnants of Han Law,* vol. 1 (Leiden: E. J. Brill, 1955). Other chapters of the *Han-shu* are translated in Burton Watson, trans., *Courtier and Commoner in Ancient China: Selections from the History of the Former Han by Pan Ku* (New York: Columbia University Press, 1974), and in Homer H. Dubs, trans., *The History of the Former Han Dynasty by Pan Ku,* 3 vols. (London: Kegan Paul, 1938–1955).

of the period and by recently discovered texts. Most important for legal philosophy is the *Ching-fa*, a series of writings transcribed on silk found in a Han dynasty tomb at Ma-wang-tui, Hunan province, in 1973–1974. The nine short treatises that are called *Ching-fa* by modern scholars describe Law as emanating from the tao, which the anonymous author, probably writing just before the Ch'in unification in 221 B.C., presents as an abstract, universal, and timeless principle of nature.[11] Law in these treatises is described as a standard, which the ruler cannot alter or abrogate, for guiding and judging the most important activities of government. A comparison of the *Ching-fa* with other second- and third-century Chinese texts demonstrates that many of its notions about law are shared, albeit not so unequivocally presented, by other writers.

More practical information about law in the administration of the Ch'in empire comes from the guidelines for officials inscribed on bamboo slips discovered at Shui-hu-ti in 1975. In these documents, found in the grave of a Ch'in local official, we see that the Ch'in imperial state did indeed attempt to prescribe legal formulas to cover the most intimate aspects of its subjects' lives. But these writings also show that Ch'in officials were themselves bound by a rigid code that circumscribed capricious decisions. These new materials, along with works in the transmitted tradition, demonstrate that in some documents law, not the will of the ruler or his officials, ideally guided government in early China.

THE ROLE OF LAW IN GOVERNMENT

In ancient Athens the reflections of Plato and Aristotle on the best form of government seem relatively dispassionate when compared with the early Confucian and Legalist writings in China. These Greek thinkers witnessed the rise and fall of different types of governments, and their assessments of the relative merits of monarchy, oligarchy, and democracy were based on experienced observation. A centralized monarchy existed in southern and central Greece in the late Bronze Age, but after it disintegrated large-scale political union was not again espoused as an ultimate goal.[12] By the sixth century B.C. the focus of the Greeks remained deliberately centered on the small city-state as the ideal setting for universal citizen participation in political life.

From the earliest times, however, Chinese writers seem to have assumed that a unified empire under one ruler offered the only viable structure to bring order. And Chinese thinkers above all valued order as the aim of politics. By the time of Mencius (371–289 B.C.), most Chinese

11. For a survey of available opinions on dating, authorship, and the major ideas in these texts, see Tu Wei-ming, "The Thought of Huang-Lao: A Reflection on the Lao Tzu and Huang Ti Texts in the Silk Manuscripts of Ma-Wang-Tui," *Journal of Asian Studies* 39, no. 1 (Nov. 1979): 95–110.

12. See Anthony Andrewes, *The Greeks* (New York: Knopf, 1967), 21–57.

thinkers had lost their faith in the ability of the entrenched hereditary rulers to transcend their narrow territorial loyalties in the interest of peace. In the meritocracy of morality that emerged out of China's classical age, kings were no more immune from censure than their ministers. We find no parallel in China with Plato's eloquent argument that the sage ruler could act as a law unto himself. Chinese writers aimed above all to warn and advise the ruler of the dire consequences of violating the prescriptions that defined good kingship. Despite deep differences between the Confucians and the Legalists over the purposes and proper forms of government, both schools agreed the ruler was bound by a set of norms that constituted a Law transcending his own will and the immediate needs of the state.

Like their Greek counterparts, the Chinese writers I shall examine lived in troubled times. Confucius (551–479 B.C.) observed the decline of the hereditary nobility and the rise of new men who could govern by dint of talent rather than by right of birth, but he still held hopes that the *li,* the ritual prescriptions that bound the old nobility, could be extended to define proper behavior for all classes. Mencius, his spiritual successor, upheld Confucius's optimistic conviction that the standards of the past can guide the present. Neither Confucius nor Mencius placed much emphasis on punitive laws beyond a reluctant acknowledgment that they were a necessary sanction for those who refused to be educated in morality. Confident that the quality of the leader affected the character of his people, these early Confucian writings reveal far more interest in the methods of the early sage kings, methods that would form an overarching Law for later kings, than in the enacted, positive laws of the state.

Their rivals, the Legalist reformers, who often operated in the highest levels of government, attempted to replace time-honored customs with strict laws, but they understood that customs must be kept in mind when making laws. Their goal was to formulate clear, public laws that would apply to everyone in the state, including the ruler. Resistance to Legalist ideas was fierce, and many of these reformers paid dearly for their efforts to tamper with the past. Lord Shang (d. 338 B.C.), prime minister of the state of Ch'in, guided his state to preeminence with practical administrative techniques based on the assumption that the state was primary and the people's welfare secondary; but he was executed by an ungrateful ruler. Han Fei Tzu (ca. 280–233 B.C.), the Legalist nobleman who refined Shang Yang's pragmatic methods a century later, has been compared with Machiavelli for his hardheaded approach to political life. His stance as a radical reformer and his reputation as a brilliant strategist made him so potentially dangerous that he was forced into suicide by his master.

From a comparative standpoint, Plato (ca. 428–348 B.C.) was more idealistic than the Legalists but equally radical for his willingness both to view the state as a construct and to assess the tradition according to how well it could bolster the state. In Plato's idealized political order, all citizens followed well-defined and permanent roles; it was the job of the philosopher king to be wise and moderate and if he cultivated these virtues, it would follow that he would be just. For Plato, justice was assured if every human filled an appointed role in the state and order rested not on laws but on a common acceptance of the rightness of this order as a governing principle in all social relationships.[13]

A strong emphasis on the importance of maintaining proper boundaries so that no individual usurped the privileges and duties of others, was in China most strongly argued by the Legalists. But in contrast with Plato, the more bureaucratic-minded Chinese thinkers stressed that social roles should be determined by ability rather than formal knowledge available only to a few individuals. On the issue of the need for strict and written laws, Plato would have differed with the Legalists, because he saw law as a hindrance to the free play of a good ruler who could better use his talents to adjust laws to new circumstances if he remained free of binding standards. "Law," according to Plato, "does not perfectly comprehend what is noblest and most just for all and therefore cannot enforce what is best."[14] Plato recognized the threat of tyranny, however, and in his later work, *Laws,* admitted that Law could be effective for distinguishing good and evil governments and for preventing despotism.

Plato's famous pupil Aristotle (384–322 B.C.) was a pragmatist who examined and categorized political organizations. His writings form a practical handbook of statecraft in the same spirit as the texts from the "hundred schools" in early China. Like most Chinese thinkers, Aristotle was more concerned with the actual workings of political organizations rather than with their theoretical underpinnings, and like them, he did not simply respond to his world but prescribed how it ought to be. Aristotle accepted the human condition as inevitably complex, fragmented by competing demands and loyalties and marked by an interplay between luck and rational choice that could weaken the resolve of the best of men.[15]

Aristotle's views on the importance of laws in government may well stem from this concern with the fragility of the good man. He shared the

13. See Ernest Barker, *Greek Political Theory* (London: University Paperbacks, 1960), 204.

14. In *Statesman,* para. 254. See *The Dialogues of Plato,* trans. Benjamin Jowett; reprinted in The Great Books of the Western World series, vol. 7.

15. As Margaret C. Nussbaum argues in her brilliant study *The Fragility of Goodness: Luck and Ethics in Greek Tragedy and Philosophy* (Cambridge: Cambridge University Press, 1986), Aristotle, in stark contrast with Plato, "wants to investigate and in some way to preserve as true the idea that luck is a serious influence in the good life, that the good life is vulnerable and can be disrupted by catastrophe" (322).

early Confucian assumption that punitive laws would not be necessary in an ideal world but acknowledged that laws were of fundamental importance for ensuring order. He emphasized as well that a higher Law must serve as the foundation of the state, and like Confucian writers, he held that the state existed not for its own sake but to provide a sound environment for its citizens.[16] Aristotle did not share Plato's conviction that the highest good, the source of all values, rested in the intellect of the sage ruler, whose talents would cement the citizens of the state in a peaceful and productive coexistence. But Aristotle, like Plato, wavered about the role of law in government when he acknowledged that an exceptionally sage man could at times act above the law. And Aristotle had little respect for written laws unless they were founded in timeless, just principles that transcended human creation.

In China early Confucian writers hoped for the appearance of sages who would emulate the good kings of old and who would be guided by ritual and the counsel of educated men like themselves. Such sage kings would naturally govern more effectively and more humanely than fixed laws and impersonal political institutions. The Confucians believed that education through the powerful example of moral rulership ultimately offered a more lasting chance of creating order than laws that could be exploited once they were made public and no longer tied to ethical concerns. But neither Confucius nor Mencius argued for a society without punitive laws for the ruled and higher Laws for the ruler. A balance was needed, as Mencius stated: "Virtue alone is not sufficient for the exercise of good government; laws alone cannot carry themselves to perfection."[17] While Mencius believed that a virtuous ruler could keep order by the sheer force of his goodness in his own time, he knew that these personal qualities would not survive to lead future generations: the good king's laws and institutions would guide his successors. Thus, the laws of the earliest-known rulers, the sage kings, would for later generations be elevated to the status of Law.

THE OLD LAWS

For Aristotle, the old laws were the best laws, and justice could prevail only when the state's laws were guided by a Law that had its origins in what had always been right. Positive laws were necessary for the use of the magistrates who were charged with supervising the implementation of the laws and checking transgressors, according to Aristotle. Positive

16. See Alexander D'Entreves, *The Notion of the State: An Introduction to Political Theory* (Oxford: Oxford University Press, 1967), for a useful analysis of Aristotle's views of law in government.

17. *Mencius,* Book 4, part 1, chap. 1. See James Legge, trans., *The Chinese Classics,* vol. 2, *The Works of Mencius* (1893–1895; reprint, Hong Kong: Hong Kong University Press, 1960).

laws fixed boundaries, defined privileges and responsibilities, encouraged good habits, and therefore supported orderly government.

The creation of the city-state founded on laws that bound all its citizens had taken shape at least two centuries before Aristotle's time. A written law code that began to place in the hands of the state matters of punishment that had formerly remained private was set forth around 620 B.C. by Drakon. Like the first written codes in China, Drakon's laws on homicide were considered unduly severe. Legal reforms that aimed to temper aristocratic economic power followed under the guidance of the great reformer, Solon (fl. 594 B.C.).[18] But as some of the great tragedies reveal, customary obligations still at times seriously conflicted with civic duties defined by laws. Aristotle, who firmly believed that the city-state provided mankind with the best possible environment, also recognized the tension between customs so revered that they seemed only natural and the laws of the state. In his *Rhetoric* Aristotle cites the scene in which the playwright Sophocles (496–406 B.C.) has Antigone violate her ruler's edict forbidding burial of her dead brother in Athenian soil. Antigone's refusal to accede to the wishes of the king sprang from principles higher than the will of the ruler or the needs of the state, for there were more sacred Laws: "Not of today or yesterday they are, but live eternal. None can date their birth."[19]

In their devotion to the "eternal yesterday" as the source of all values and precedents for political behavior, the Confucians of China's fourth and fifth centuries B.C. had a good deal in common with Aristotle. For them, as for Aristotle, the king was not ideally a creator of new laws and institutions but a guardian of all that was held dear from the past. Of the idealized founder of the Chou dynasty, who had lived five centuries before him, Confucius said: "The Chou [kings] carefully attended to the weights and measures, examined the [existing] laws and regulations . . . and its government spread throughout the world."[20] Confucian thinkers appreciated the problems of knowing the past accurately, but to them it still seemed a more trustworthy guide than the myriad of demands and the inevitable shortsightedness of the present. For them, the laws of the state should reinforce and never collide with the old Law that governed kinship relationships and ritual obligations.

Confucius's view of the golden age focused on the early Chou; Mencius drew on a more complex tradition for his models of good govern-

18. See Douglas M. MacDowell, *The Law in Classical Athens* (Ithaca: Cornell University Press, 1978), 41–43.

19. *Rhetoric*, trans. W. Rhys Roberts, Book 1, chap. 15 (I have altered punctuation here), in *The Works of Aristotle*, reprinted in The Great Books of the Western World series, vol. 9. I have consulted this edition for all of Aristotle's works. *The Politics* is translated by Benjamin Jowett.

20. *Analects*, Book 20, chap. 1. See James Legge, trans., *The Chinese Classics*, vol. 1, *The Confucian Analects*.

ment. He believed that the best Law had already been revealed in the past: "Never has one fallen into error who followed the Law of the ancient kings" (*Mencius* 4.1.1). For Mencius the laws of the former kings operated as a set of prescriptions for ruling that took on the status of a sacred Law. The scriptural sources of this Law were not philosophical treatises, but the oldest books—*The Book of Songs, The Book of Documents,* and the *Spring and Autumn Annals*—which preserved records of the activities of the early kings. And these texts contained a clear message: the ruler's duty to uphold the Law was weighty; if he failed in it he no longer deserved to be called a king, but became in the famous words of Mencius, a "robber," a "ruffian" who can legitimately be removed from office (*Mencius* 1.2.8).

Aristotle too argued that a ruler who offended the old ways could no longer be recognized as a true king but instead became a tyrant. He seems more realistic than Mencius, however, for he tacitly conceded that the general interest might be better served if the tyrant disguised his true nature rather than provoke rebellion with flagrantly offensive behavior. Aristotle listed tyranny—which he defined as lawless, self-interested one-man rule rather than the more preferable rule by elite participation—as one possible form of government, albeit a degraded one. Aristotle acknowledged that government by laws must ultimately be administered by men and that whoever held authority must of necessity act as legislator. But he was obliged to make laws that were just and timeless, laws that could guide future generations. In *Politics* Aristotle clearly states, "And the rule of the law . . . is preferable to that of any individual. On the same principle, even if it be better for certain individuals to govern, they should be made only guardians and ministers of the law" (*Politics* 3.16).

Aristotle's political theory, like that of the Confucians, reveals a wary attitude toward change, which always carries the risk of instability and unforeseen problems. In Chinese legal history the conservative outlook dominated political writings and we find great reluctance to sanction changes in the laws. The *Kuan Tzu,* an eclectic text with sections on law that were probably produced in the late Warring States period, warns the ruler that he must never alter the laws out of affection for his people, for "the laws should be honored more than the people."[21]

THE REFORMERS

A willingness to sponsor change distinguished legal reformers, usually Legalists, from Confucian political theorists in China. The Legalist view

21. Chap. 6, p. 7a. (*Ssu-pu pei-yao* ed.) See Allyn Rickett, trans., *Kuan-tzu: A Repository of Early Chinese Thought,* vol. 1 (Hong Kong: Hong Kong University Press, 1965), and a recent translation of additional chapters by the same author, *Guanzi: Political, Economic, and Philosophical Essays from Early China,* vol. 1 (Princeton: Princeton University Press, 1985).

of law developed as an alternative response to Confucian political theory and was formulated by men generally more immersed in the pragmatic business of concentrating power in the state than in guarding the interests of society. Lord Shang, for example, has been remembered as the creator of the ruthless brand of statecraft that would eventually give the state of Ch'in the edge over other states in their competition to unify China under one ruler. On the issue of the need for standards to control the human passions of the ruler and his magistrates, Lord Shang's concerns parallel those of Aristotle as they are recorded in *Politics:* "Passion perverts the minds of rulers, even when they are the best of men. The law is reason unaffected by desire" (*Politics* 3.16). In Lord Shang's view, rulers unfortunately do not generally display unusual virtue, wisdom, or courage.[22]

Lord Shang argued that a strong state was the goal of politics, and the subordination of the ruler to law but one step in placing the state above the interests of any individual. For Lord Shang laws provided the means to transcend the personal limitations of most rulers. Laws also ensured that good government would not die with the king: "Sages cannot transfer to others the personality and nature that is inherent in them; only through law can this be accomplished" (*Shang-chün-shu* 3.3b). For these reasons, Lord Shang advised the ruler to change the laws already in existence only with great care because they possessed a force and a continuity that no single ruler could achieve.

What was the source of the law in Lord Shang's view? Unlike the Confucians, who portrayed the early kings as the passive transmitters of the laws of their predecessors, Lord Shang presented them as lawgivers: "The sage's way of organizing a country is not to imitate antiquity or to conform to the immediate present but to govern in accordance with the important needs of the times and to make laws that take customs into account" (*Shang-chün-shu* 3.2a). In this passage, Lord Shang assigned the sages the important role of creating laws, but he warned that new laws would not work unless they did not obviously offend the people. Lord Shang called on the past to legitimate the ruler as a lawmaker; but like the Confucians, he interpreted the past to serve his own ends. The Confucians presented the ancient sage rulers as transmitters of law. Lord Shang portrayed them as active legislators.

Lord Shang has been singled out since Han times as the primary culprit responsible for advocating a ruthless theory of punitive law that would ultimately be used by the state of Ch'in to destroy not only the territorial kings but the culture of the past as well. That his policies were radical in his own day can be seen from the debate that they provoked at

22. *Shang-chün-shu,* Chap. 4, p. 9a. I have used *Shang-chün-shu chieh-ku* (Ch'engtu, 1935). For a complete translation, see J. J. L. Duyvendak, trans., *The Book of Lord Shang* (London: Probsthain, 1928).

the court of Duke Hsiao of Ch'in in 359 B.C. over the wisdom of changing the laws.[23] Duke Hsiao was well aware of the dangers involved in reforming the old laws of Ch'in: "I intend to alter the laws so as to ensure an orderly government and to reform the rites so as to teach the people. But I am afraid that the world will criticize me." The kind of censure that would indeed be leveled at him was expressed by one of his ministers, Kan Lung: "I have heard it said that . . . a wise man achieves good government without altering the laws. . . . Now if your highness alters the laws without adhering to the old customs of the Ch'in state and reforms the rites in order to teach the people, I am afraid the world will criticize you and I wish that you would reflect soberly."

Lord Shang argued for reform on the grounds that so varied and complex a past could not serve the present: "The emperors and kings [of antiquity] did not copy one another, so what rites should we follow?" He agreed that the habits of the people should be understood before changing the laws, and he appealed to the past to argue that reform should offer rewards for the people: "I have heard that when the enlightened princes of antiquity established laws, the people were not wicked . . . because these laws were clear and benefited the people."

But he warned the ruler not to listen to the multitude or to the scholars who would try to befuddle him. The law, not his advisers, facilitated clear thinking and timely activity. In another passage, we learn that Lord Shang implied that although the ruler could make laws, he was also bound by them: "An enlightened ruler is cautious with regard to the laws and regulations. He does not heed speech that is not centered in the law, and he does not exalt actions or perform deeds that are not centered in the law" (*Shang-chün-shu* 5.7b). Throughout his writings Lord Shang placed clear priority on a state that could be run with order and efficiency, not on a regime that catered to the whims of the ruler. For him the ruler was neither superior to the laws nor unhampered by them—but was both a source of Law and the servant of the best of the existing laws. Lord Shang shared the insight of the Greeks and the Confucians that fixed, rigid laws could hinder reform. And he did not, despite frequent claims to the contrary, portray the ideal ruler as a capricious despot arbitrarily issuing laws for his own ends.

What then was so radical about Lord Shang's thought? After all, he was more concerned with evaluating the content of the tradition than dismissing it wholesale. But like Plato he believed that tolerating the old myths without reflection inhibited any hope of adjusting government to the circumstances of the day. A modern interpreter of Plato's theory of the state describes this aspect of Plato's philosophy, radical in its own time, in terms that could well apply to Lord Shang's stance toward tradi-

23. This debate is recorded in *Shang-chün-shu,* 1.1a–2b. See Duyvendak, 167–75, for a full account in English.

tion: "[Plato] declared that to build our moral and political life upon tradition meant to build on shifting sands. Whoever trusts in the mere power of tradition, whoever proceeds only by practice and routine, says Plato in his *Phaedrus,* acts like a blind man who has to grope his way. . . . He must have a lodestar—a guiding principle of his thought and his actions. Tradition cannot play this role—for it is blind itself."[24]

The most balanced and sophisticated approach to the problem of the rule of man or the rule of law is found in the writing of Hsun Tzu (298–238 B.C.), a Confucian thinker who produced Legalist students. Hsun Tzu shared Aristotle's concern for the actual workings of government at the lower levels, a reflection perhaps of his service as a county magistrate late in life. His writing displays little of the optimistic faith of the earlier Confucians in the goodness of humankind. But like Plato, Hsun Tzu ultimately leaned toward the ruler as the linchpin of a smoothly run government because he believed that the circumstances generated by human beings were too diverse to be anticipated by fixed laws. If a law existed to cover a situation, it should be applied, according to Hsun Tzu, and if not, an analogous one should be cited. The ruler, who acted as an interpreter of the laws out of necessity, must be tutored to fulfill his charge responsibly and the people must be educated to respond to his laws properly, Hsun Tzu stressed, for no matter how free from opinion the laws may be, in the end they must be interpreted by men. But he by no means advocated that the ruler have free rein in his activities. "Laws cannot stand alone . . . for when they are implemented by the [right] person, they survive, but if neglected, they disappear. . . . Law is the basis of good government, but the superior man is the basis of law."[25]

Hsun Tzu's most famous student, Han Fei Tzu, the Legalists' major political theorist, is linked more closely in his thinking about law with Lord Shang than with his teacher. He was far more cynical than Hsun Tzu about the efficacy of rule by man and stated that even the sage kings could not govern autonomously: "Only with laws and techniques could they oversee and implement the correct way."[26] He pointed out as well that laws worked only if the ruler had the power to enforce them. Lord

24. This interpretation of Plato's thought is from Ernst Cassirer, *The Myth of the State* (New Haven: Yale University Press, 1946), 72–73.

25. *Hsun-tzu,* Chap. 8, p. 1a. (*Ssu-pu pei-yao* ed.) For a translation of Hsun-tzu's works, see Homer H. Dubs, trans., *The Works of Hsüntze* (London: Probsthain, 1928), and Burton Watson, trans., *Hsun Tzu: Basic Writings* (New York: Columbia University Press, 1963). A more recent scholarly translation is also available: John Knoblock, *Xunzi: A Translation and Study of the Complete Works,* vol. 1, books 1–6 (Stanford: Stanford University Press, 1988).

26. *Han Fei-tzu,* Chap. 8, p. 480 (*Han Fei-tzu chi-shih,* 2 vols. [Shanghai: Chung-hua, 1958]). For a complete translation of Han Fei Tzu's works, see W. K. Liao, trans., *The Complete Works of Han Fei Tzu,* 2 vols. (London: Probsthain, 1959). See also Schwartz, *The World of Thought in Ancient China,* 321–49, for an important view of the Legalists in comparative perspective.

Shang had focused his attention on the role of the ruler as legislator, but Han Fei Tzu shared Aristotle's concern with actually administering the laws and controlling the magistrates. Well aware of the need to set up public standards to replace personal, arbitrary guidelines, Han Fei Tzu stated that no one, not even the ruler, could adhere to private standards once the laws were established. Yet in other passages of his manual on statecraft he manipulates the tradition to present the ancient sage kings as accountable neither to their own past nor to fixed standards; he does this in order to sanction the contemporary ruler's right to create laws. Han Fei Tzu's world was a more violent, uncertain one than Lord Shang's, and he was an even more ruthless pragmatist. More than any of the writers we have surveyed, Han Fei Tzu comes closest to justifying the ruler as a free agent in running the state. Nonetheless, he by no means advocated that positive laws should be created by whim, nor did he legitimate the ruler's right to disregard the laws.

THE CASE FOR CLEAR LAWS

Han Fei Tzu's arguments for clarity in law and certainty in punishments echo those of Lord Shang. For Lord Shang clear laws could be applied and understood universally, unlike customary laws, which had grown out of more particular experiences. Just as he believed that truly talented rulers were scarce indeed, so too he held that most people had only a limited understanding of the actual mechanics of government and could be reached only if the laws were clear, simple, and unambiguous: "Laws should not be made so that only the intelligent ones can understand them. . . . Therefore when the sages created laws, they made them clear and easy to understand" (*Shang-chün-shu* 5.14a). Han Fei Tzu compared the laws to a mirror that would only properly reflect reality when clear and stationary. If like an immobile reflection in a mirror, the laws remained clear, the people could see for themselves how to obey them. If the laws were muddied with contradictions, they would lose their guiding function. In his opinion, knowledge of the laws should neither be the exclusive domain of the legal officials nor the special province of the scholars. Like Lord Shang, Han Fei Tzu considered clear, public laws absolutely essential for order, and he warned the ruler that neglecting to clarify the laws would seriously weaken his position.[27]

That centrally sponsored codification of laws would accompany the drive toward a unified empire seems logical according to Max Weber's

27. Eric Havelock, *The Greek Concept of Justice: From Its Shadow in Homer to Its Substance in Plato* (Cambridge: Harvard University Press, 1978), offers a most interesting and relevant discussion of why metaphors of vision, such as clarity, became important as written documents began to replace the oral tradition in Greece.

writings on law in the early modern West. Clear, public laws served the interests of rulers who desired unity and order and bureaucrats who hoped for broader opportunities for employment: "Legal uniformity renders possible employment of every official throughout the entire area of the realm [with the result that] career choices are, of course, better than where every official is bound to the area of his origin by his ignorance of the laws of any other part of the realm. While thus the bourgeois classes seek after 'certainty' in the administration of justice, officialdom is generally interested in 'clarity' and 'orderliness' of the law."[28] Weber's theories offer the historian of China a comparative context for assessing the arguments for the importance of clear laws and predictable punishments in a period of statebuilding.

In China the writers who argued for clarity and certainty stated that these ideals could be applied only if the standard for measuring authority came from a source that was unattached to the customs or the historical figures of any particular historical time. When Han Fei Tzu recounted his vision of Lord Shang's methods of legal reform, he pointed out that only after the *Book of Poetry* and the *Book of History,* the oldest and most cherished repositories of the ways of the ancient kings, were destroyed could the laws and ordinances be made clear (*Han Fei-tzu* 4.239). But if the past could no longer serve as a useful model, a different and more abstract principle for measuring government had to be found. After about 300 B.C. in China for some thinkers this ultimate principle became the tao, which is most often simply translated as "the Way." The concept of tao is usually connected with the Taoist school, particularly with Lao Tzu, a mysterious figure who supposedly lived about the same time as Confucius. Lao Tzu's writings take up kingship only incidentally and do not discuss law; the king is but one element in a universe that is ordered not by human institutions but by passive alignment with the workings of the natural world—which are but one expression of the tao. The Taoist notion of kingship rejected worldly wisdom and intellectual ability, preferring instead a nonactive king, a man who has absorbed the power of the natural world so that his presence could enrich all the creatures of the earth.

In time the tao took on more pragmatic meanings. Han Fei Tzu described tao as a useful model for ruling because it was at once unified and the source of all things. But the text that presents one of the most systematic arguments for the tao as a practical guide to the art of ruling is one that is new to us, the *Ching-fa*. "The tao gives birth to the Law," the author begins, "and Law is what marks success and failure. Used as a

28. Max Weber, *Economy and Society: An Outline of Interpretive Sociology,* trans. and ed. Guenther Roth and Claus Wittich (Berkeley: University of California Press, 1978), 2:847–48.

marker it clarifies what is crooked from what is straight." The anonymous author goes on to describe the tao as a timeless, universal, impartial standard and the Law it generates as a reliable guide for the hard decisions that fall to any ruler: when to begin a military campaign and when to wait until conditions are suitable, when to punish the people and when to show lenience, how to obtain clear, trustworthy information from subordinates, and how to organize subordinates according to their abilities. The ruler who conquers a territory and attempts to establish a government is clearly the target for this author, who advises the ruler to preserve the existing laws and issue commands for labor and military service only after gaining the people's trust and learning of their customs and habits. A great portion of the *Ching-fa* concerns the eternal problem of using force lawfully, distinguishing between a just war and a useless slaughter and differentiating appropriate punishments from personal vendettas. The text warns the ruler who makes arbitrary decisions to punish and to make war that he will himself be destroyed by force. And only by following laws founded in the tao can he understand the boundaries between just and unjust actions. The *Ching-fa*'s ideas are consistent with other works that were in circulation in early imperial times, but we have no way of knowing whether it actually ever reached an imperial audience.[29]

LAW AND NATURE

The concept of tao has no exact counterpart in Western thinking. Although tao serves as a source for all things, including Law, it is not a divinity.[30] Rather, tao serves as a valuable standard precisely because it is a mechanistic principle of nature free of the fickle personality traits of an anthropomorphic deity. The tao cannot be influenced, manipulated, changed, or disturbed in its regular patterns. The monarch who patterns himself on this natural principle can oversee the world with clarity and wisdom while remaining above its vicissitudes and temptations. Such a ruler governs with predictability and justness.

The tao is unified and universal. Therefore the laws that emanate from it apply to all peoples, regardless of their local customs and traditions. Such a basis for law could serve well the ruler who not only strove to create a unified empire but who also understood the need to establish a government that would be viewed as legitimate by the people he con-

29. I discuss the theory of law in the *Ching-fa* and the importance of the text for legal history in more detail in Karen Turner, "The Theory of Law in the *Ching-fa*," *Early China*, no. 14, forthcoming.

30. See Leo Chang and Hsiao-po Wang, *The Philosophical Foundations of Han Fei's Political Theory*, Monographs of the Society for Asian and Comparative Philosophy, no. 7 (Honolulu: University of Hawaii Press, 1986), for Han Fei's concept of tao and why it is not comparable with Western notions of *logos*.

quered. Despite the many unanswered questions about this intriguing text, the *Ching-fa* is important because it establishes a connection between ethics, law, and coercion. It differs from Confucian writings by preferring Law based on nature rather than on the practices of the sage rulers and from the Legalists by placing the welfare of the people above the needs of the state. However, its vision of a universal community of humankind subject to common values and constraints is not unique. The Legalists advocated universal laws and punishments, and the Confucians based their belief in the transforming power of education and exemplary leadership on the presumption that all humans operate within a common moral dimension.

By contrast, classical Greek thought was more exclusive at heart. Plato and Aristotle framed their political theory in terms of the right of individual citizens to take an active role in running the state; but their citizenry was limited to freemen alone, and they rationalized slavery as natural and right.[31] In ancient China slaves were categorized differently from freemen in the legal codes when determining the severity of punishments, but their status as slaves was not legally permanent. In the extraordinarily fluid society of Ch'in and Han times, when a swinebreeder could become a Grand Secretary, so too anyone could fall into slavery as the result of punishment for crime, capture in war, or decline into poverty.[32] Most important, slavery was not justified by the philosophers as a rightful and natural condition, nor were slaves described as creatures permanently beyond the reach of moral influence.

In his writing on natural law Aristotle refuted earlier ideas that laws were merely conventional creations with no uniform thread or link with natural or ethical standards. But most modern writers agree that a political theory that placed all humankind within the same moral and legal universe was articulated in Greece only after Alexander's empire brought the Greeks into direct contact with the cultures of the East. Some thinkers of the Stoic school who flourished in Greece after the death of Aristotle in 322 B.C., refined a theory in which natural law became a source for enacted law, a bond linking all humankind that transcended the particularism of Aristotle's thinking with its disdain for the barbarian and its acceptance of slavery.[33] The most famous spokesman for natural law theories was not a Greek, but Cicero (106–43 B.C.), a Roman jurist and or-

31. See Vernant, *Myth and Society in Ancient Greece,* p. 82, on the psychological and social importance of slavery.

32. See C. Martin Wilbur, *Slavery in China during the Former Han Dynasty, 206 B.C.–A.D. 25* (New York: Russell & Russell, 1943). Donald Munro discusses differences in Chinese and Greek concepts of equality in *The Concept of Man in Early China* (Stanford: Stanford University Press, 1969), 18–21, 178–82.

33. See C. E. Robinson, *Hellas: A Short History of Ancient Greece* (Boston: Beacon Press, 1948), for a very readable discussion of Greek thought and the Stoics.

ator. Cicero is interesting for our purposes because his description of the basic character of natural law has much in common with the *Ching-fa*'s notion of the law of nature. Natural law, according to Cicero is a "true law . . . of universal application, unchanging and everlasting; it summons to duty by its commands, and averts from wrong-doing by its prohibitions. . . . It is a sin to try to alter this law . . . or to abolish it."[34] Perhaps the most important tenet of the natural law of the Stoics was that all humans are equal before it, allied by a bond that could not be severed by artificially created institutions or misfortune.

Although in China and the West, natural law served as a measure to transcend territorial laws during periods of unification, the ultimate purpose served by natural law was different. For the Stoics, as for early medieval European thinkers, natural law served as one yardstick to gauge the reasonableness of the institutions of the state, including its laws and punishments. In time in the West, natural law would be linked with the natural rights of humans vis-à-vis the state.[35] But the early Chinese thinkers did not separate the natural world from the social and political realms; for them all actions in one sphere resonate in the other. Natural law in ancient China existed not as a principle available to all humans to measure the justness of the state's commands and laws but as a guide that would allow the enlightened ruler to determine how to use force correctly, that is, in a manner that would cancel out the evil and disruptive effects of deviance on behalf of all society.

THE CLASSICAL LEGACY

In the West, Stoic thought became even more important after the Roman empire claimed the territories once linked by Alexander, in part because these ideas were so compatible with a large ethnically diverse empire. As Charles H. McIlwain points out in his study of the political theory of the Middle Ages: "The Stoic doctrine of the brotherhood of man and the citizenship of the world was not ill-suited to a state that seemed destined to bring all races within its political control."[36] Roman government had at times been unstable and despotic; but Rome's legal tradition was never rejected. On the contrary, in the early Middle Ages,

34. *The Republic,* Book 3, chap. 22. See *De Re Publica, De Legibus,* trans. Clinton W. Keyes (Cambridge: Loeb Classical Library, Harvard University Press, 1928), 211.

35. Although natural law might seem to be a positive force as I have described it here, some legal theorists argue that it has at times been used for evil purposes. For a short introduction to the problem see A. P. d'Entreves, *Natural Law: An Introduction to Legal Philosophy* (London: Hutchinson's University Library, 1951), and John Finnis, *Natural Law and Natural Rights* (Oxford: Clarendon Press, 1980).

36. Charles H. McIlwain, *The Growth of Political Thought in the West: From the Greeks to the End of the Middle Ages* (New York: Macmillan, 1932), 106.

many a tribal king was proud to link his laws with the charisma of Rome long after the empire had dissolved in the West. Rome transmitted to the Middle Ages a concept of universal law, the ideal of a unity of humankind (which would be amplified and spread by Christianity), and a legal system that emphasized rights of property and contract—legal ideas that remain viable.

The actual influence of natural law and its relation to positive law in the West is open to debate.[37] But the conviction that enacted law must not offend what is reasonable and natural still governs Western assessments of law. And although some modern legal theorists support Plato's argument that true justice might be better preserved by exceptionally good and wise judges than by the straightjacket of laws, Aristotle's commitment to a government of laws and not of men has endured as a basic tenet of rule of law in the West.

Assessing the actual influence of early philosophy on Chinese institutions is difficult because of the deep traditional prejudice against the Ch'in empire and its laws, even though, like the Roman empire, the Ch'in imperial state created a unified political structure that would encourage the spread of classical ideas. If we remember, however, that law existed above all to ensure the correct administration of punishments and if we look at materials produced in Ch'in and Han times rather than at later interpretations, we can see that some practices in the early imperial period are consonant with classical political theory.

Some thinkers argued for clear laws based on unchanging natural principles that would be implemented by fair-minded officials. Although we have no evidence that Ch'in or Han emperors actually referred to natural law based on the tao when making decisions, we do find several instances from the *Records of the Historian,* written by Ssu-ma Ch'ien about a century after the founding of the Han dynasty, that some rulers took seriously their charge to clarify the laws. Ssu-ma Ch'ien tells us that the First Emperor of Ch'in advertised himself on stone tablets erected to convince the newly conquered peoples of the east of his good intentions as a "clarifier of laws," a king who would "abolish ambiguities."[38] But the Ch'in dynasty earned the animosity of early Han statesmen for failing to keep its promise to clarify and simplify the laws and to control the magistrates. One Han official observed that the Ch'in bureaucracy allowed

37. Alan Watson, *The Making of the Civil Law* (Cambridge: Harvard University Press, 1981), traces the ways that the natural law theories preserved in Roman law, particularly Justinian's *Corpus juris civilis,* influenced Western interpretations of law.

38. *Shih-chi* (Peking: Chung-hua, 1959), Chap. 6, p. 245. For a translation of portions of this text, see Burton Watson, trans., *Records of the Grand Historian of China: Translated from the Shih chi of Ssu-ma Ch'ien,* 2 vols. (New York: Columbia University Press, 1961), and Yang Hsien-yi and Gladys Yang, trans., *Selections from Records of the Historian* (Peking: Foreign Languages Press, 1979).

officials to take "advantage of the many confusing laws to bolster their own authority . . . and to make life and death decisions according to their own wanton lights" (*Han-shu* 49.2296).

Han opinions of Ch'in and its laws are ambivalent: we find awe that it was able to fulfill the hopes of the philosophers by bringing union and peace to the world mixed with fear of the kind of tyranny possible with a strong monarchy and dismay at the oppressive costs of maintaining the institutional machinery of empire. It is difficult to evaluate Ch'in because our primary source has been the historian, Ssu-ma Ch'ien, who was mutilated at the orders of the Han Emperor Wu (141–87 B.C.), a monarch whom he immortalized as a tyrant second only to the First Emperor of the Ch'in dynasty. But important external evidence indicates that the Ch'in government had at least attempted to implement punishments consistently. The writings inscribed on bamboo from Shui-hu-ti include documents that provide a working Ch'in local official with detailed procedures for investigating cases and deciding punishments, examples of enacted laws with explanations, and an essay that dictates how a good official should conduct himself. Also discovered in this cache were sets of rules that applied to reporting local disasters to the center, sending and receiving documents properly, and conducting and recording criminal investigations. Sample cases provide guidelines for determining punishments appropriate for different crimes. For example, one case describes a fight between two women that resulted in a miscarriage for one. The official in charge of the investigation determined a proper punishment only after learning whether the fight had in fact precipitated the miscarriage and the age of the fetus at the time of death. Another sample case states that parents could kill a deformed baby at birth without fear of punishment, but infanticide for less compelling reasons constituted a criminal offense.[39]

These materials demonstrate that the Ch'in state assumed the right to interfere in the most intimate affairs of its subjects' lives and that it was concerned above all with protecting human and material resources for its own uses. But they also reveal that the officials who represented the central government were expected to carry out their duties honestly, fairly, and efficiently. The Ch'in official buried in the Shui-hu-ti tomb died armed with a manual that outlined the qualities the state had expected of him: a clear knowledge of the laws, wide-ranging competence, honesty, and public-spiritedness. He was warned that punishment awaited the lazy, the boastful, and the arbitrary official. These documents are not

39. The Shui-hu-ti laws are translated and discussed by A. F. P. Hulsewe, *Remnants of Ch'in Law* (Leiden: Brill, 1985), and by Robin D. S. Yates and Katrina C. D. McLeod, "Forms of Ch'in Law: An Annotated Translation of the *Feng-chen shih*," *Harvard Journal of Asiatic Studies* 41 (1981): 111–63.

simply theoretical tracts bespeaking hopes and ideals but rather working rules for functionaries. They add an important dimension to our understanding of what the Ch'in state expected of its magistrates. Han and Ch'in official law focused on matching crimes with appropriate punishments, for just as the philosophers had warned, only if punishments were determined carefully and appropriately could the human and natural worlds be kept in harmony.

We cannot ignore, however, the many instances in the histories that reveal how deeply the people hated Ch'in's harsh punishments and its interference in their daily lives. Perhaps the Ch'in empire's greatest mistake was implementing too hastily its own territorial laws in new areas, which undoubtedly had developed laws suited to particular local practices. Han rulers attempted to avoid the mistakes of Ch'in, and although its legal and bureaucratic institutions remained virtually intact in Han government, the histories show us how carefully Han monarchs cloaked their activities in traditional guise to avoid unfavorable comparisons with the First Emperor's interventionist style of ruling. The conservative side of classical political theory, which warned against disturbing the status quo and advocated preserving the old laws, seems to have been followed in Han times. Laws needed to be adjusted to changing circumstances, but emperors personally avoided this critically important task, concentrating instead on issuing amnesties—sometimes on a large scale—to pardon criminals already sentenced.[40] They assigned the dangerous task of legal reform to their high officials, many of whom paid with their lives for meddling with the laws. For example, one Han minister, Ch'ao Ts'o, not only redefined the laws at the emperor's request but made new laws as well. Like many other legal reformers, he was eventually executed. Ssu-ma Ch'ien left no doubt about the cause of Ch'ao Ts'o's demise when he ended his biography with a warning to all innovators: "Changing what is old, confusing what has always been, will bring disaster if not death" (*Shih-chi* 101.2748).

Many times we find the emperors and their officials consulting the oldest books for advice in making legal decisions. Despite the disdain for the past expressed by such Legalist thinkers as Han Fei Tzu, by Han times working legal officials were usually well versed in the texts that would form the heart of the Confucian canon because these records offered written guidance for making difficult legal decisions. They could be used too as cautionary tales. History sobered Chinese monarchs, and their officials never tired of relating the tales of earlier kings who had provoked catastrophes for neglecting their duties and misusing the re-

40. For a useful study of the importance of amnesties see Brian McKnight, *The Quality of Mercy: Amnesties and Traditional Chinese Justice* (Honolulu: University of Hawaii Press, 1981).

sources of the state. More than one Han official told the emperor to his face that the ruler who abused the trust placed in his office would be brought down by violence.

Did Confucian arguments in favor of abiding by the old laws of the former kings have any influence on Han monarchs? The historians mention several instances in which members of the imperial clan were said to be subject to the old laws. One interesting case concerns Emperor Wu and describes him in a manner most surprising for so famous a tyrant. When he was forced to sentence to death his nephew, his dead sister's son, Emperor Wu "wept and sighed" in front of his court as he pronounced his judgment. Why did Emperor Wu perform his duty even when it affected his own clan? As it is recorded, he said: "Our laws and regulations were created by the former emperors. If I should do violence to their laws just because of my sister, how could I face the ancestral temple of Kao-tsu?" (*Han-shu* 65.2852). Possibly, the emperor had reason to welcome a chance to eliminate a male rival and simply used clan laws to justify his decision. But he dared not present the sentence as a purely personal one. And it just might have been that this willful ruler was in fact cowed by the prospect of offending the old laws of his ancestors.

CONCLUSION

In the classical traditions of China and the West we find a respect for law coexisting with a recognition that undue attachment to the fixed laws can inhibit effective government. In general, early Chinese thinkers seem more concerned with peace and harmony than with the rights of individuals to participate fully in governing. Although the Greeks considered in more depth the many possible forms of government and how laws and institutions might be mixed with the authority of educated citizens, the Chinese from the beginnings of their history assumed that the ideal order rested on a large-scale inclusive system that unified all people under one ruler. And because kingship was always considered the best means to order the world in China, political theorists refined their thinking about the qualities of a good king to a degree not matched in the West until the early Middle Ages, when kingship became accepted as the normal form of governing.

Many of the Western writings that aimed to delineate the role of kings, particularly in the Germanic kingdoms in the early Middle Ages, sound familiar to students of Chinese history. As one scholar of kingship and law in early medieval Europe states, "The deeply-rooted Germanic idea of law was that of the good, old law, unenacted and unwritten, residing in the common sense of justice, the sum total of all the subjective rights of individuals. The king's right to rule was but his private right, a mere parcel of the law itself."[41] Even when laws had to be made, they were supposedly made with the old laws in mind. An edict issued by a seventh-century Lombard King reads: "We have established by inquiring into and recalling to mind the ancient laws of our ancestors which have not been written."[42] This notion of law comes very close to the esteem for the old laws that the Confucians expressed in China. Similarly, Isidore of Seville (d. A.D. 636), a Spanish bishop and adviser to the Visigothic rulers, stated that kings must abide by law and defined kingship in terms that sound remarkably Confucian: "A king is king through his ruling, and he does not rule who does not correct. Therefore the title of king is held by proper administration, by wrongdoing it is lost."[43] By the eleventh century in Europe, we find the case for rebellion against a bad king articulated in language as uncompromising as that of Mencius. As the Saxon monk Manegold put it, a king who acts incompetently is little more than a "swineherd" who has neglected his charge, and he should be dismissed and punished even more severely because his responsibilities are so much weightier.[44]

Despite some important similarities in their early traditions, by the early modern period, the institutional aspects of monarchy and its relation to law took shape very differently in China and the West. The reasons are complex, and I can only suggest a few here. For one, a genuine feudal system, in which the king is inserted into an elaborate and specifically defined network of property rights and obligations to his vassals, never took hold in China. Perhaps this is one reason that, despite the efforts of Chinese reformers in the late nineteenth and early twentieth centuries, a formal constitution that spelled out and separated the rights and duties of the king in relation to his subjects never came to fruition. Most important, in China the elites, who interpreted the law and reprimanded the ruler when he stepped beyond the bounds of righteousness, always remained ultimately tied to the monarchy for their right to participate in government. No separate organization emerged in China to challenge institutionally the authority of the monarchs. There was no powerful religious body like the Church, with its own spiritual leader, rituals for legitimating kingship, laws, legal experts, courts, and sanctions to offer alternatives to Chinese imperial law.

We find in traditional Chinese government certain creative tensions. The Legalists lost their campaign to apply the laws equally, but the Confucian bureaucrats who judged cases had to work with a detailed legal

41. See Fritz Kern, *Kingship and Law in the Middle Ages* (New York: Harper Torchbooks, 1956), xx.

42. Cited in Charles H. McIlwain, *The Growth of Political Thought in the West,* 173.

43. Ibid.

44. In John B. Morrall, *Political Thought in Medieval Times* (New York: Harper Torchbooks, 1958), 37–38.

code that contained precedents for judging punishments and carrying out routine administration. After the Han dynasty, the law became more overtly "Confucianized"; as a result, the relationship between the individuals in a case mattered more than the nature of the crime itself. A father would not be seriously punished for deliberately killing his son, for example, but a son could be severely punished for accidentally bringing harm to his father. The laws supported Confucian definitions of proper roles within the family and the government.[45]

Although the Chinese monarchy became stronger after the Sung dynasty, as Jack L. Dull points out (see Chapter 3), we find examples of later rulers who did operate carefully when deciding when and how to use force. One example of the lasting power of the tradition of responsible kingship that emerged out of China's classical period can be seen in the musings of the K'ang-hsi emperor (r. 1662–1722) over the distasteful business of giving a final verdict on the death sentences sent to him for ratification: "Though naturally I could not go through every case in detail, I nevertheless got in the habit of reading through the lists in the palace each year, checking the name and registration and status of each man condemned to death, and the reason for which the death penalty had been given. Then I would check through the list again with the Grand Secretaries and their staff . . . and we would decide who might be spared."[46] Personal responsibility for life and death decisions was but one of the ruler's duties, but it was considered one of the most important; by the Ch'ing period these expectations were so clearly defined that any monarch, whatever his ethnic origins, could play his role well—if he chose to.

The common understanding that the monarch could lose his support if he abused his privilege was a destabilizing factor because it implied that his authority was conditional, but the tradition of warning the king with examples from history clearly set forth what was expected of him. As we have seen, Chinese political theory took shape in an age of disorder created by local despots and no practical thinker could afford to rationalize a government based purely on the instincts of a philosopher-king.

When comparing a concept as complicated as law in two very different cultures, we must be careful to notice differences as well as similarities. The particular problems that confronted Chinese philosopher-statesmen in the early years of state-building and the reservoir of myth and history at their disposal to resolve them were uniquely Chinese. In ancient

45. See Ch'ü T'ung-tsu, *Law and Society in Traditional China* (Paris and The Hague: Mouton, 1961) for a classic discussion of the development of Chinese law.

46. Jonathan Spence, *Emperor of China: Self Portrait of K'ang hsi* (New York: Knopf, 1974), 32–33.

China there were no courts, no lawyers, no institutions to judge and to punish a ruler who violated the laws of his community. But the classical era in China did produce a rich body of writings that warned the monarch who made decisions arbitrarily, without respect for Law, that he no longer deserved the support of the community. And what Max Weber termed "psychic coercion," that is, the fear of ostracism by the community, had an impact on some Chinese monarchs. The historical writings reveal many instances when the ruler heeded his officials' warnings that the cherished ideals of kingship must take precedence over the will of individual kings, especially in matters of war and punishment. The remarkable longevity of the Chinese imperial system owes a great deal to the definitions of responsible rulership that emerged in the formative period of the imperial state. Good government in China ultimately rested on a flexible balance between the certainty of law and the discretion of rulers and their worthy ministers.

FIVE

□

The Confucian Tradition in Chinese History

Tu Wei-ming

Confucianism, a generic Western term that has no counterpart in Chinese, is a worldview, a social ethic, a political ideology, a scholarly tradition, and a way of life.[1] Although Confucianism is often grouped together with Buddhism, Christianity, Hinduism, Islam, Judaism, and Taoism as a major historical religion, it is not an organized religion. Yet it has exerted profound influence on East Asian political culture as well as East Asian spiritual life. Both in theory and practice Confucianism has made an indelible mark on the governments, societies, educational practices, and family life of East Asia. It is an exaggeration to characterize traditional Chinese life and culture as "Confucian," but for well over two thousand years Confucian ethical values have served as a source of inspiration as well as the court of appeal for human interaction at all levels—individual, communal, and national—in the Sinic world.

Confucianism was not an organized missionary tradition, but by the first century B.C. it had spread to those East Asian countries that were under the influence of Chinese literate culture. In the centuries following the Confucian revival of Sung times (A.D. 960–1279), Confucianism was embraced in Chosŏn dynasty Korea beginning in the fifteenth century and in Tokugawa Japan beginning in the seventeenth century. Prior to the arrival of the Western powers in East Asia in the mid nineteenth century the Confucian persuasion was so predominant in the art of governance, the form and conduct of elite education, and the moral dis-

1. The adjective "Confucian" derives from "Confucius," the Latinization of K'ung Futzu, or Master K'ung. The term "Confucianism" was coined in Europe only in the eighteenth century. It is used, not entirely accurately, to translate the Chinese term *ju-chia,* which literally means "family of scholars," signifying a genealogy, a school, or a tradition of learning. Please note that my citations from the *Analects* are given by book and verse number and thus are the same for any edition.

course of the populace that China, Korea, and Japan were all distinctively "Confucian" states. In Southeast Asia Vietnam and Singapore were also influenced by Confucianism.

In this chapter I attempt to outline the development of the Confucian tradition in China from the time of Confucius down to recent times. In Chapter 2 of this volume David N. Keightley gives an account of Shang and Chou dynasty values that provides a useful background for this review of Confucianism. Confucius had a profound faith in the cumulative culture of the past. He saw himself as a "transmitter" rather than a "creator." The fact that traditional ways had declined by his own time did not in his view diminish their great potential for innovation in the future. Thus, the history of Confucianism is in many ways a history of the continual quest for the rediscovery, revitalization, and adaptation of the living traditions of the Chou dynasty.

Although it is a daunting task to try to describe an intellectual tradition as long, varied, and rich as Confucianism in one chapter, I propose to do so not by offering a comprehensive historical narrative but by reflecting on the highlights of the tradition from a modern perspective. I pay particular attention to what I see as the core values of the Confucian tradition as shaped by Confucius, Mencius, and Hsun Tzu in classical times, by the Han dynasty synthesis of Tung Chung-shu, by the Confucian revivalists of the T'ang and Sung dynasties (culminating in the achievements of Chu Hsi), and finally by further elaborations in Ming and Ch'ing times. Throughout this chapter I try to give a sense of the spirit of the Confucian tradition and the impact of its values on Chinese life.

THE LIFE OF CONFUCIUS

Considering Confucius's tremendous importance, his life seems starkly undramatic, or as a Chinese expression has it, "plain and real." The plainness and reality of Confucius's life, however, illustrate his humanity not as a revealed truth but as an expression of self-cultivation, the ability of human effort to persevere in the endless but ennobling tasks of self-improvement and humanitarian service. The faith in the possibility that ordinary human beings can become awe-inspiring sages and worthies is deeply rooted in the Confucian heritage and the insistence that human beings are teachable, improvable, and perfectible through personal and communal endeavor is typically Confucian.

Confucius was born in 551 B.C. in Ch'ü-fu in the small feudal state of Lu (in modern Shantung province), which was noted for its preservation of the traditions of ritual and music of the Chou civilization. Confucius's ancestors were probably members of the aristocracy who had become virtual poverty-stricken commoners by the time of his birth. His father died when Confucius was only three years old. Instructed first by his mother, Confucius distinguished himself as an indefatigable learner in his teens. He recalled toward the end of his life that his heart was set on learning at fifteen (2.4, that is, book 2, chapter 4 of the *Analects*).

Confucius served in minor government posts managing stables and keeping books for granaries before he married a woman of similar background when he was nineteen. He may already have acquired a reputation as a multitalented scholar at an early age. Confucius's mastery of the six arts—ritual, music, archery, charioteering, calligraphy, and arithmetic—and his familiarity with the classical traditions, notably poetry and history, enabled him to start a brilliant teaching career in his thirties.

Confucius is known as the first private teacher in China, for he was instrumental in establishing the art of teaching as a vocation, indeed as a way of life. Before Confucius aristocratic families hired tutors to educate their sons and government officials instructed their subordinates in the necessary techniques, but he was the first person to devote his whole life to learning and teaching for the purpose of transforming and improving society.

For Confucius the primary function of education is to provide the proper way of training noblemen (*chün-tzu*), a process that involves constant self-improvement and continuous social interaction. Although he emphatically noted (14.25) that learning is "for the sake of the self" and that the end of learning is self-realization, he found public service a natural consequence of true education. Confucius confronted learned hermits who challenged the validity of his desire to serve the world; he resisted the temptation to "herd with birds and animals" (18.6), to live apart from the human community, and opted to try to transform the world from within. For decades Confucius was actively involved in the political arena wishing to put his humanist ideas into practice through governmental channels.

In his late forties and early fifties Confucius served first as a magistrate, then as an assistant minister of public works, and eventually as minister of justice in the state of Lu. But his political career was short-lived. At fifty-six, when he realized that his superiors were uninterested in his policies, he left the state of Lu in an attempt to find another feudal state in which to render his service. Despite his political frustration he was accompanied by a growing circle of students during this self-imposed exile of almost thirteen years. His reputation as a man of vision and mission spread. At the age of sixty-seven, he returned home to teach and to preserve his cherished classical traditions by writing and editing. He died in 479 B.C. at the age of seventy-three. According to the *Records of the Historian* seventy-two of his students mastered the "six arts," and three thousand people claimed to be his followers.

THE *ANALECTS* AS THE EMBODIMENT OF CONFUCIAN IDEAS

The *Analects* (*Lun-yü*), the most revered sacred text in the Confucian tradition, was probably compiled by the second generation of Confucius's disciples.[2] Based primarily on the master's sayings, which were preserved in both oral and written transmissions, the *Analects* captures the Confucian spirit in form and content in the same way that the Platonic dialogues underscore the Socratic pedagogy. The purpose in compiling this digest of Confucius's statements seems not to have been to present an argument or to record an event but to offer an invitation to its readers to take part in an ongoing conversation. Dialogue is used to show Confucius in thought and action, not as an isolated individual, but as a center of human relationships.

Confucius's life as a student and teacher exemplified the Confucian idea that education is a ceaseless process of self-realization. When one of his students reportedly had difficulty describing him, Confucius came to his aid: "Why did you not simply say something to this effect: he is the sort of man who forgets to eat when he engages himself in vigorous pursuit of learning, who is so full of joy that he forgets his worries, and who does not notice that old age is coming on?" (7.18).

The community that Confucius created through his inspiring personality was a scholarly fellowship of like-minded men of different ages and different backgrounds from different states. They were attracted to Confucius because they shared his vision and in varying degrees took part in his mission to bring moral order to an increasingly fragmented polity. This mission was difficult and even dangerous. The master himself suffered from joblessness, homelessness, starvation, and, occasionally, life-threatening violence. Yet, his faith in the survivability of the culture that he cherished and the workability of the approach to teaching that he propounded was so steadfast that he convinced his followers as well as himself that Heaven was on their side. When Confucius's life was threatened in K'uang, he said: "Since the death of King Wen [founder of the Chou dynasty], does not the mission of culture (*wen*) rest here in me? If Heaven intends this culture to be destroyed, those who come after me will not be able to have any part of it. If Heaven does not intend this culture to be destroyed, then what can the men of K'uang do to me?" (9.5).

This expression of self-confidence may give the impression that there was presumptuousness in Confucius's self-image. However, Confucius made it explicit that he was far from attaining sagehood and that all he really excelled in was "love of learning" (5.28). In this sense Confucius

2. For a good translation of the *Analects* see D. C. Lau, trans. *The Analects* (Harmondsworth: Penguin, 1979).

was neither a prophet with privileged access to the divine nor a philosopher who has already seen the truth, but a teacher of humanity who is an advanced fellow traveler on the way to self-realization.

As a teacher of humanity, Confucius stated his ambition in terms of human care: "To bring comfort to the old, to have trust in friends, and to cherish the young" (5.26). Confucius's vision of the way to develop a moral community began with a holistic reflection on the human condition. Instead of dwelling on abstract ideas, such as the state of nature, Confucius sought to understand the actual situation of a given time and use this understanding as a point of departure. His aim was to restore trust in government and to transform society into a moral community by cultivating a sense of human caring in politics and society. To achieve this aim, the creation of a scholarly community, the fellowship of *chün-tzu* (noblemen), was essential. In the words of Confucius's disciple, Tseng Tzu, the true nobleman "must be broad-minded and resolute, for his burden is heavy and his road is long. He takes humanity as his burden. Is that not heavy? Only with death does his road come to an end. Is that not long?" (8.7). However, the fellowship of *chün-tzu*, as moral vanguards of society, did not seek to establish a radically different order. Its mission was to reformulate and revitalize those institutions that were believed to have maintained social solidarity and enabled people to live in harmony and prosperity for centuries.

An obvious example of such an institution is the family. The role and function of the family was related in the *Analects* when Confucius was asked why he did not take part in government. He responded (2.21) by citing a passage from an ancient classic, the *Book of Documents*, "Simply by being a good son and friendly to his brothers a man can exert an influence upon government!" This passage shows that what one does in the confines of one's private home is politically significant. This position is predicated on the Confucian conviction that the self-cultivation of each person is the root of social order and that social order is the basis for political stability and universal peace. The assertion that family ethics are politically efficacious must be seen in the context of the Confucian conception of politics as "rectification" (*cheng*). In this conception rulers are supposed to govern by moral leadership and exemplary teaching rather than by force. The government's responsibility is not only to provide food and security but also to educate the people. Law and punishment are the minimum requirements for order; but social harmony can only be attained by virtue, which is achieved through ritual performance. To perform ritual is to take part in a communal act to promote mutual understanding.

One of the fundamental Confucian values that ensures the integrity of ritual performance is filial piety. Confucius believed that filial piety was the first step toward moral excellence. He seemed to contend that the way to enhance personal dignity and identity is not to alienate ourselves from our family but to cultivate our genuine feelings for our parents. To learn to embody the family in our minds and hearts is to enable ourselves to move beyond self-centeredness or, to borrow from modern psychology, to transform the enclosed private ego into an open self. Indeed, the cardinal Confucian virtue, *jen* (humanity), is the result of self-cultivation. The first test for our self-cultivation is our ability to establish meaningful relationships with our family members. Filial piety does not demand unconditional submissiveness to parental authority; rather it demands recognition of and reverence for our source of life.

The purpose of filial piety, as the Greeks would have it, is "human flourishing" for both parent and child. Confucians see it as an essential way of learning to be human. They are fond of applying the family metaphor to the community, the country, and the universe. They prefer to address the emperor as the Son of Heaven, the king as ruler-father, and the magistrate as the "father-mother official" because they assume that implicit in the family-centered nomenclature is a political vision. When Confucius responded that taking care of family affairs is itself active participation in politics, he made it clear that family ethics are not merely a private, personal concern. Rather, family ethics make possible the realization of the public good.

In response to a question from his favorite disciple, Yen Hui, Confucius defined humanity as "conquer yourself and return to ritual" (12.1). This interplay between inner spiritual self-transformation (the master is said to have freed himself from four things: "opinionatedness, dogmatism, obstinacy, and egoism" [9.4]) and social participation enabled Confucius to be "loyal" (*chung*) to himself and "considerate" (*shu*) of others (4.15). Understandably, the Confucian golden rule is "Do not do unto others what you would not want others to do unto you" (15.23). Confucius's legacy, laden with profound ethical implications, is captured by his "plain and real" appreciation that learning to be human is a communal enterprise: "A man of humanity, wishing to establish himself, also establishes others, and wishing to enlarge himself, also enlarges others. The ability to take as analogy what is near at hand can be called the method of humanity" (6.28).

THE FORMATION OF THE CLASSICAL CONFUCIAN TRADITION

Although some of Confucius's disciples may have generated a great deal of enthusiasm among their own students, it was not at all clear at the time that the Confucian tradition was to emerge as the most powerful persuasion in Chinese history. Judging from the historical situation a century after Confucius's death, the disintegration of the Chou "feudal" ritual system and the rise of powerful hegemonic states clearly showed that the Confucian attempt to moralize politics was not working and that wealth and power had the greatest impact. The most influential thinkers of this era were the early Taoist hermits, who left the mundane world in order to seek self-preservation and spiritual sanctuary in nature, and the proto-Legalists ("realists"), who played the dangerous game of assisting ambitious kings to gain wealth and power so that the proto-Legalists could influence the political process. The Taoists and the Legalists were setting the intellectual agenda. The Confucians refused to be identified with the interests of the newly emerging elites because their social consciousness impelled them to condemn rule by force. They were in a dilemma. They wanted to be actively involved in politics but they could not accept the status quo as a legitimate arena in which authority and power were exercised. In short, they were in the world but not of the world; they could not leave the world, nor could they effectively change it.

Mencius: The Paradigmatic Confucian Intellectual

Mencius (371–289 B.C.) is known as a self-styled transmitter of the Confucian way.[3] Educated first by his mother and then allegedly by a student of Confucius's grandson, Mencius was a brilliant social critic, moral philosopher, and political activist. He argued that cultivating a class of scholar-officials who would not be directly involved in agriculture, industry, and commerce was vital to the well-being of the state. In his sophisticated argument against the physiocrats (those who advocated the supremacy of agriculture) he employed the idea of the "division of labor" to defend those who "labor with their minds" and observed that "service" is as important as "productivity." To Mencius, Confucians serve the vital interests of the state as scholars not by becoming bureaucratic functionaries but by assuming the responsibility of teaching the ruling minority the art of "humane government" (*jen-cheng*) and the kingly way (*wang-tao*). In his dealing with feudal lords Mencius conducted himself not only as a political adviser but also as a teacher of kings. He explicitly stated that a true or noble man (*chün-tzu*) cannot be corrupted by wealth, subdued by power, or affected by poverty.

To articulate the relationship between Confucian moral idealism and the concrete social and political realities of his time, Mencius criticized the pervading ideologies of Mo Tzu's collectivism and Yang Chu's individualism as impractical. Mo Tzu advocated "universal love," but Mencius contended that the result of the Mohist admonition to treat a stranger as intimately as one would treat one's own father would be to treat one's own father as indifferently as one would treat a stranger. Yang Chu, however, advocated the primacy of the self. Mencius contended that ex-

3. For a good translation of the book of *Mencius* see D. C. Lau, trans., *Mencius* (Harmondsworth: Penguin, 1970).

cessive attention to self-interest leads to political disorder. He argued that in Mohist collectivism "fatherhood" cannot be maintained and that in Yang Chu's individualism "kingship" cannot be established.

Mencius's strategy for social reform was to change the language of profit, self-interest, wealth, and power into a moral discourse with emphasis on rightness, public-spiritedness, welfare, and exemplary authority. However, Mencius did not argue against profit. Rather, he instructed the feudal lords to opt for the benefit that would sustain their own profit, self-interest, wealth, and power in a long-term perspective. He urged them to look beyond the horizon of their palaces and to cultivate a common bond with their ministers, officers, clerks, and the seemingly undifferentiated masses. Only then, he contended, would they be able to maintain their own livelihood. He encouraged them to extend their benevolence and warned them that this was crucial for the protection of their own families.

Mencius's appeal to that which is common to all people as a mechanism of government was predicated on his strong "populist" sense that the people are more important than the state, that the state is more important than the king, and that the ruler who does not act in accordance with the kingly way is unfit. In an apt application of the Confucian principle of the "rectification of names," Mencius concluded that an unfit ruler should be criticized, rehabilitated, or, as the last result, deposed. Because "Heaven sees as the people see; Heaven hears as the people hear," in severe cases revolution (literally, "to change the Mandate") is not only justifiable, it is a moral imperative (5A.5, that is, chapter 5 in part A of book 5 in *Mencius*).

Mencius's "populist" conception of politics is predicated on his philosophical vision that human beings are perfectible through self-effort and that human nature is good. Although he acknowledged biological and environmental factors in shaping the human condition, he insisted that we become moral simply by willing to be so. According to Mencius the reason that "willing" entails a transformative moral act is that our nature's propensity to be good is automatically activated whenever we decide to bring it to our conscious attention. As an illustration, Mencius built his idea of the humane government on the assertion that every human being is capable of commiseration: "No man is devoid of a heart sensitive to the suffering of others. Such a sensitive heart was possessed by the former kings and manifested itself in humane government. With such a sensitive heart behind humane government, it was as easy to rule the world as rolling it on your palm" (2A.6). Mencius observed that each human being is endowed with four feelings: commiseration, shame, modesty, and a sense of right and wrong. As a fire starting up or a wellspring coming through, these feelings serve as the bases for cultivating the four cardinal virtues: humanity, rightness, ritual, and wisdom. Mencius's message is that we become moral not because we are told we must be good but because our deepest nature spontaneously expresses itself as goodness.

Mencius taught that we all have the inner spiritual resources to deepen our self-awareness and broaden our networks of communal participation. Biological and environmental constraints notwithstanding, we always have the freedom and the ability to refine and enlarge our Heaven-endowed nobility (our "great body"). Mencius's idea of degrees of excellence in character building vividly illustrates this continuous refinement and enlargement of our selfhood:

> He who commands our liking is called good (*shan*).
> He who is sincere with himself is called true (*hsin*).
> He who is sufficient and real is called beautiful (*mei*).
> He whose sufficiency and reality shine forth is called great (*ta*).
> He whose greatness transforms itself is called sagely (*sheng*).
> He whose sageliness is beyond our comprehension is called spiritual (*shen*). (7B.25)

Furthermore, Mencius asserted that if we fully realize the potential within our hearts, we will understand our nature; and by understanding our nature we will know Heaven. This profound faith in the human capacity for self-knowledge and for understanding Heaven by tapping spiritual resources from within enabled Mencius to add an "anthropocosmic" dimension to the Confucian project. In this Mencian perspective, learning to be fully human entails the cultivation of human sensitivity to embody the whole universe as one's lived experience: "All the ten thousand things are there in me. There is no greater joy for me than to find, on self-examination, that I am true to myself. Try your best to treat others as you would wish to be treated yourself, and you will find that this is the shortest way to humanity" (7A.4). The Confucian nobleman, as envisioned by Mencius, is an exemplary teacher, a political leader, a spiritual thinker, and a prophetic intellectual.

Hsun Tzu: The Transmitter of Confucian Scholarship

If Mencius brought Confucian moral idealism to fruition, Hsun Tzu (fl. 298–238 B.C.) conscientiously transformed the Confucian project into a realistic and systematic inquiry on the human condition, with special reference to ritual and authority.[4] Widely acknowledged as the most eminent of the notable scholars who congregated in Chi-hsia, the capital of the wealthy and powerful Ch'i state in the mid third century B.C., Hsun Tzu distinguished himself in erudition, logic, empiricism, practical-mindedness, and argumentation. His critique of the "twelve philoso-

4. Burton Watson, trans., *Hsun Tzu: Basic Writings* (New York: Columbia University Press, 1963).

phers" gave an overview of the intellectual scene of his time. His penetrating insight into the shortcomings of virtually all the major currents of thought propounded by his fellow thinkers helped to establish the Confucian school as a forceful political and social persuasion. His principal adversary, however, was Mencius, and he vigorously attacked as naive moral optimism Mencius's view that human nature is good.

True to the Confucian (and, for that matter, the Mencian) spirit, Hsun Tzu underscored the centrality of self-cultivation. He outlined the process of Confucian education, from nobleman to sage, as a ceaseless endeavor to accumulate knowledge, skills, insight, and wisdom. He believed that unless social constraints are well articulated, humans are prone to make excessive demands to satisfy their passions. As a result, social solidarity, the precondition for human flourishing, is undermined. The most serious flaw in the Mencian commitment to the goodness of human nature is the practical consequence of neglecting the necessity of ritual and authority for the well-being of society. By stressing that human nature is evil, Hsun Tzu singled out the cognitive function of the mind (human rationality) as the basis for morality. We become moral by voluntarily harnessing our desires and passions to act in accordance with societal norms. This harnessing may be alien to our nature, but it can be perceived by our mind as necessary for both survival and well-being.

Like Mencius, Hsun Tzu believed in the perfectibility of all human beings through self-cultivation, in humanity and rightness as cardinal virtues, in humane government as the kingly way, in social harmony, and in education, but his view of how these goals could actually be reached was diametrically opposed to Mencius's. The Confucian project, as shaped by Hsun Tzu, defines learning as socialization. The authority provided by the ancient sages and worthies, the classical tradition, the ancestral religious rituals, the conventional norms, the teachers, the governmental rules and regulations, and the political officers are all important for transforming human nature. A cultured person is by definition a fully socialized participant in the human community who has for the public good successfully sublimated his instinctual demands. Hsun Tzu's tough-minded stance on law, order, authority, and ritual seems precariously close to the Legalists', whose policy of social conformism was designed exclusively for the benefit of the ruler. His insistence on objective standards of behavior may have contributed ideologically to the rise of authoritarianism, which culminated in the dictatorship of the Ch'in (221–206 B.C.). Two of the most influential Legalists, the theoretician Han Fei Tzu (d. 233 B.C.) from the state of Han and the Ch'in minister Li Ssu (d. 208 B.C.), were his pupils. Yet Hsun Tzu was instrumental in the continuation of the Confucian project as a scholarly enterprise. His naturalistic interpretation of Heaven, his sophisticated understanding of culture, his insightful observations on the epistemological aspect of the mind and the social function of language, his emphasis on moral reasoning and the art of argumentation, his belief in progress, and his interest in political institutions so significantly enriched the Confucian heritage that for more than three centuries he was revered by the Confucians as the paradigmatic scholar.

The Confucianization of Politics

The short-lived dictatorship of the Ch'in marked the brief triumph of Legalism, but in the early years of the Western Han (206 B.C.–A.D. 9) the Legalist practices of absolute power for the emperor, the complete subjugation of the peripheral states to the central government, the total uniformity of thought, and the ruthless enforcement of law was modified by the Taoist practice of reconciliation and noninterference. This practice is commonly known in history as the Huang-Lao method, referring to the art of rulership attributed to the Yellow Emperor (Huang Ti) and the mysterious "founder" of Taoism Lao Tzu. A few Confucian thinkers such as Lu Chia and Chia I made important policy recommendations, but before the emergence of Tung Chung-shu (ca. 179–ca. 104 B.C.) the Confucian persuasion was not particularly influential. However, the gradual Confucianization of Han politics must have begun soon after the founding of the dynasty. The decisions of the founding fathers, including those who helped the First Emperor gain the empire, to allow the reinstitution of the feudal system and of the First Emperor to implement an elaborate court ritual opened up the basic structure of Han government to Confucian influence. The imperial decision to redress the cultural damage done in the book-burning fiasco of the Ch'in dynasty by retrieving the lost classics through an extensive search and oral transmission indicated a concerted effort to make the Confucian tradition an integral part of the emerging political culture.

By the reign of Emperor Wu (the Martial Emperor, 141–87 B.C.), who acted in some ways as a Legalist despot,[5] the Confucian persuasion was deeply entrenched in the central bureaucracy through many ideas, institutions, and practices: the clear separation of the court and the government with the government often under the leadership of a scholarly prime minister, the process of recruiting officials through the dual mechanism of recommendation and selection, the conception of social structure as family-centered, the agriculture-based economy, and the state sponsorship of education. Confucian ideas were also firmly established in the legal system as ritual became increasingly important in governing behavior, defining social relationships, and adjudicating civil disputes. Yet it was not until the prime minister Kung-sun Hung (d. 121 B.C.) had persuaded Emperor Wu to announce formally that the *ju* school alone

5. See Karen Turner's discussion of the Emperor Wu in Chapter 4 of this volume.

would receive state sponsorship that Confucianism became the officially recognized imperial ideology and state cult.

As a result, the Confucian classics became the core curriculum for all levels of education. In 136 B.C. Emperor Wu set up at court five Erudites of the Five Classics and in 124 B.C. assigned fifty official students to study with them, thus creating a de facto imperial university. By 50 B.C. the student enrollment at the university had grown to three thousand, and by A.D. 1 one hundred men a year were entering government service through the examinations administered by the state. In short, those with a Confucian education began to staff the bureaucracy. In A.D. 58 all government schools were required to make sacrifices to Confucius, and in A.D. 175 the court had the approved version of the classics, which had been determined by scholarly conferences and research teams under imperial auspices over several decades, carved on large stone tablets. These steles were erected at the capital and are today well preserved in the national museum in Sian. This act of committing to permanence and to public display the precise content of the sacred texts symbolizes the completion of the formation of the classical Confucian tradition.

The Five Classics

The concrete manifestation of the coming of age of the Confucian tradition is the compilation of the Five Classics.[6] By including both pre-Confucian texts, the *Book of Documents* and the *Book of Poetry,* and contemporary Ch'in–Han material, such as certain portions of the *Book of Rites,* it seems that the project to establish the core curriculum for Confucian education was an ecumenical one. The Five Classics can be described in terms of five visions: metaphysical, political, poetic, social, and historical. The metaphysical vision, represented by the *Book of Change* (*I ching*), combines divinatory art with numerological technique and ethical insight. According to the philosophy of change the cosmos is a great transformation occasioned by the constant interaction of two complementary as well as conflicting vital energies, *yin* and *yang*. The universe, which resulted from this great transformation, always exhibits organismic unity and dynamism. The profound persons, inspired by the harmony and creativity of the universe, must emulate the highest ideal of the "unity of humanity and Heaven" through ceaseless self-exertion.

The political vision, represented by the *Book of Documents* (*Shu ching*), addresses the kingly way in terms of the ethical foundation for a humane government. The legendary Three Emperors (Yao, Shun, and Yü) all

6. Excerpts from the Five Classics are translated in Wing-tsit Chan, *A Source Book in Chinese Philosophy* (Princeton: Princeton University Press, 1963), and in William Theodore de Bary, Wing-tsit Chan, and Burton Watson, comps., *Sources of Chinese Tradition,* vol. 1 (New York: Columbia University Press, 1960).

ruled by virtue. Their sagacity, filial piety, and work ethic enabled them to create a political culture based on responsibility and trust. Through exemplary teaching they encouraged the people to enter into a "covenant" with them so that social harmony could be achieved without punishment or coercion. Even in the Three Dynasties (Hsia, Shang, and Chou), moral authority in the form of ritualized power was sufficient to maintain political order. Humankind, from the undifferentiated masses to the enlightened people, the nobility, and the sage-king, formed an organic unity as an integral part of the great cosmic transformation. Politics means "rectification" and the purpose of the government is not only to provide food and maintain order but also to educate and mold the people into moral subjects.

The poetic vision, represented by the *Book of Songs* (*Shih ching*), underscores the Confucian belief in common human feelings. The majority of the verses express emotions and sentiments of persons and communities from all echelons of society on a variety of occasions. The internal resonance, the basic rhythm, of the poetic world characterized by the *Book of Songs* is mutual responsiveness. The tone as a whole is honest rather than earnest and evocative rather than expressive.

The social vision, represented by the *Book of Rites* (*Li chi*), defines society not as an adversarial system based on contractual relations but as a community of trust based on social responsibility. The society organized by the four functional occupations—scholar, farmer, artisan, and merchant—is, in the true sense of the word, a cooperative. As a contributing member of the cooperative, each person is obligated to recognize the existence of others and to serve the public good. According to the principle of the rectification of names, it is the king's duty to act kingly and the father's duty to act fatherly. If the king or father fails to behave properly, he cannot expect his minister or son to act in accordance with ritual. A chapter in the *Book of Rites* titled the "Great Learning" specifies, "From the Son of Heaven to the commoner, all must regard self-cultivation as the root." This pervasive "duty-consciousness" features prominently in all Confucian literature on ritual.

The historical vision, represented by the *Spring and Autumn Annals* (*Ch'un-ch'iu*), emphasizes the significance of collective memory for communal self-identification. Historical consciousness is a defining characteristic of Confucian thought. By defining himself as a transmitter and a lover of antiquity, Confucius made explicit his belief that a sense of history is not only desirable but necessary for self-knowledge. Confucius's emphasis on the importance of history was in a way his reappropriation of ancient Sinic wisdom: reanimating the old is the best way to attain the new. Confucius may not have authored the *Spring and Autumn Annals,* but it seems likely that he made moral judgments about political events that occurred in China from the eighth century to the fifth century B.C. In his political criticism he assumed a godlike role in evaluating politics by assigning ultimate praise and blame in history to the most powerful and influential political actors of the period. This practice not only inspired the innovative style of the Grand Historian, Ssu-ma Ch'ien (d. ca. 85 B.C.), but also was widely employed by others writing dynastic histories in imperial China.

The Five Classics, as five visions—metaphysical, political, poetic, social, and historical—provide a holistic context for the development of Confucian scholarship as a comprehensive inquiry in the humanities.

Tung Chung-shu: The Confucian Visionary

Like Ssu-ma Ch'ien, Tung Chung-shu (ca. 179–ca. 104 B.C.) took the *Spring and Autumn Annals* absolutely seriously. However, his own work, *Luxuriant Gems of the Spring and Autumn Annals,* is far from being a book of historical judgment. Rather, it is a metaphysical treatise in the spirit of the *Book of Change.* Tung was extraordinarily dedicated to learning; he is said to have been so absorbed in his studies that for three years he did not even glance at the garden in front of him. And he was known for his strong commitment to moral idealism. One of his often-quoted dicta is "rectifying rightness without scheming for profit; enlightening the way without calculating efficaciousness." Combining this strong idealism with an eclectic love of learning, Tung was instrumental in developing a characteristically Han interpretation of the Confucian project.

Despite Emperor Wu's pronouncement that Confucianism alone would receive imperial sponsorship, Taoists, yin-yang cosmologists, Mohists, Legalists, shamanists, healers, magicians, geomancers, and others all contributed to the cosmological thinking of the Han cultural elite. Tung himself was a beneficiary of this intellectual syncretism; he freely tapped the spiritual resources of his time in formulating his own worldview. His theory of the correspondence between man and nature is predicated on an organismic vision in which all modalities of being are interconnected in a complex network of relationships. The moral to draw from this metaphysics of interrelatedness is that human actions have cosmic consequences.

Whether or not the theory of the "five phases" (metal, wood, water, fire, and earth) should be attributed to Tung, his inquiries on the correspondence of man and the numerical categories of Heaven, his research on the sympathetic activation of things of the same kind, and his studies of cardinal Confucian values such as humanity, rightness, ritual, wisdom, and trustworthiness enabled him to develop an elaborate worldview that integrated Confucian ethics with a naturalistic cosmology. What Tung accomplished was not merely a theological justification for the emperor as the Son of Heaven. Rather, his theory of mutual responsiveness between Heaven and humankind provided Confucian scholars with a higher law to judge the conduct of the ruler. His rhetoric of "portents of catastrophes and anomalies," which specified that floods, droughts, earthquakes, comets, eclipses, and even benign but unusual natural phenomena such as "growing beards on women" are celestial signs warning against the ruler's wicked deeds, later acted as an effective deterrent to the whims and excesses of the monarchs. Tung offered the Confucian intellectuals an interpretive power that had far-reaching political implications.

Tung's mode of thought reflects the scholarly penchant for prognostication, divination, and numerological speculation that was prevalent during his time. Known as adherents of the "New Text" school for their arguments based on the reconstructed classical texts written in the "new" script of the Han, these scholars were intensely interested in exploring the "subtle words and great meanings" of the classics in order to influence politics. The usurpation of Wang Mang (A.D. 9–23) was in part occasioned by the demand of the Confucian literati that a change in the Mandate of Heaven was inevitable at that time.

Despite Tung's immense popularity his worldview was not universally accepted by Han Confucian scholars. A reaction in favor of a more rational and moralistic approach to the Confucian classics, known as the "Old Text" school, had already set in before the fall of the Western Han. Yang Hsiung (ca. 53 B.C.–A.D. 18), in his *Model Sayings,* a collection of moralistic aphorisms in the style of the *Analects,* and the *Classic of the Great Mystery,* a cosmological speculation in the style of the *Book of Change,* presented an alternative worldview. This school, claiming its own recensions of authentic classical texts—allegedly rediscovered during the Han period and written in an "old" script before the Ch'in unification—was widely accepted in the Eastern Han (A.D. 25–220). As the institutions of the Erudites and the imperial university expanded in the Eastern Han, the study of the classics became more refined and elaborate. Confucian scholasticism, like its counterparts in Talmudic and Biblical studies, became too professionalized to remain a vital intellectual force.

Yet Confucian ethics exerted great influence on government, schools, and society at large. By the end of the Han as many as thirty thousand students attended the imperial university. All public schools throughout the land offered regular sacrifices to Confucius, many temples were built in his honor, and he virtually became the patron saint of education. The imperial courts continued to honor Confucius from age to age; a Confucian temple eventually stood in every one of imperial China's two thousand counties. As a result, teachers, together with Heaven, earth, the emperor, and parents, came to be the most respected authorities in traditional China.

Confucian Ethics in the Taoist and Buddhist Context

Incompetent rulership, faction-ridden bureaucracy, a mismanaged tax structure, and the domination of the eunuchs toward the end of the Eastern Han first prompted widespread protests by the students of the imperial university. The court's high-handed decision to imprison and kill thousands of them and their official sympathizers in A.D. 169 may have put a temporary stop to the intellectual revolt, but a downward economic spiral made the peasant's life unbearable. Peasant rebellions, led by Confucian scholars as well as Taoist religious leaders of faith-healing sects, combined with open insurrections by the military, brought down the Han dynasty and thus put an end to the first Chinese empire. With the breakdown of the imperial Han system, not unlike the decline and fall of the Roman Empire, nomads invaded from the north. The northern China plains became a battleground, despoiled and controlled by rival nomadic tribes, and a succession of states was established in the south. This period of disunity, from the early third century to the late sixth century, marked the decline of Confucianism, the upsurge of Neo-Taoism, and the spread of Buddhism.

As T. H. Barrett notes in Chapter 6 in this volume, the growing Taoist and Buddhist influences among the cultural elite and the populace in general did not mean that the Confucian tradition had disappeared. In fact, Confucian ethics had by then become virtually inseparable from the moral fabric of Chinese society. Confucius continued to be universally honored as the paradigmatic sage. The outstanding Taoist thinker Wang Pi (226–249) argued that by not speculating on the nature of the tao Confucius had demonstrated an experiential understanding of it superior to that of Lao Tzu. The Confucian classics remained the foundation of all literate culture, and sophisticated commentaries were produced throughout the age. Confucian values continued to dominate in such political institutions as the central bureaucracy, the recruitment of officials, and local governance. Also, the political forms of life were distinctively Confucian. When a conquering dynasty adopted a Sinicization policy, notably in the case of the Northern Wei (386–534), it was by and large Confucian in character. In the south systematic attempts were made to strengthen family ties by establishing clan rules, genealogical trees, and ancestral rituals that were all based on Confucian ethics.

The reunification of China by the Sui (581–618) and the restoration of lasting peace and prosperity by the T'ang (618–907) gave a powerful stimulus to the revival of Confucian learning. The publication of a definitive official edition of the Five Classics with elaborate commentaries and subcommentaries and the implementation of Confucian rituals at all levels of government, including the compilation of the famous T'ang legal code, were two outstanding examples of Confucianism in practice. An examination system based on literary competence was established for governmental positions. It made the mastery of the Confucian classics a prerequisite for political success and was therefore perhaps the single most important institutional innovation in defining elite culture in Confucian terms.

Nevertheless, the intellectual and spiritual scene of the T'ang was dominated by Buddhism and, to a lesser degree, Taoism. The philosophical originality of the dynasty was mainly represented by monk-scholars such as Chi-tsang (549–623), Hsuan-tsang (596–664), and Chih-i (538–597). An unintended consequence in the development of Confucian thought in this context was the prominent rise of some of the metaphysically significant Confucian texts, notably the *Doctrine of the Mean* (*Chung-yung*) and the *Great Commentary on the Book of Change* (*I-chuan*), which appealed to some Buddhist and Taoist thinkers. A sign of a possible Confucian turn in the T'ang was Li Ao's (d. ca. 844) essay on "Returning to Nature," which foreshadowed some salient features of Sung (960–1279) Confucian thought. However, the most influential precursor of a Confucian revival was Han Yü (768–824). A great essayist, he attacked Buddhism with telling effectiveness from the perspectives of social ethics and cultural identity. He discussed and provoked interest in the question of what actually constitutes the Confucian way. The issue of *tao-t'ung*, the transmission of the way or the authentic method to repossess the way, has stimulated much discussion in the Confucian tradition from the eleventh century to the present.

THE CONFUCIAN REVIVAL

The Buddhist conquest of China and the Chinese transformation of Buddhism, a process that involved the introduction, domestication, growth, and appropriation of a distinctly Indian form of spirituality, lasted for at least six centuries. Because Buddhist ideas were introduced to China via Taoist categories and because the Taoist religion benefited from modeling itself on Buddhist institutions and practices, the spiritual dynamics prevalent in medieval China were characterized by Buddhist and Taoist values. Against this background the reemergence of Confucianism as the leading intellectual force involved both a creative response to the Buddhist and Taoist challenge and an imaginative reappropriation of classical Confucian insights. Furthermore, after the collapse of the T'ang dynasty, the grave threats to the survival of Chinese culture from the Khitans, the Jurchens, and later the Mongols prompted the literati to protect their common heritage by deepening their communal critical self-awareness. To enrich their personal knowledge as well as to preserve China as a civilization and state, they explored the symbolic and spiritual resources that made Confucianism a living tradition.

The Sung Masters

The Sung dynasty (960–1279) was militarily weak and covered much less area than the T'ang, but its cultural splendor and economic prosperity were unprecedented in human history. The Sung commercial revolution produced social patterns that included flourishing markets, densely populated urban centers, elaborate communication networks, theatrical performances, literary groups, and popular religions that remained in many ways unchanged into the nineteenth century. Technological advances in agriculture, textiles, lacquer, porcelain, printing, maritime trade, and weaponry demonstrated that China excelled in not only the fine arts but also the natural sciences. The decline of the aristocracy, the widespread availability of printed books, the democratization of education, and the full implementation of the examination system led to the formation of the gentry, a new social class noted for its literary proficiency, social consciousness, and political participation. The outstanding members of this class, such as the classicists Hu Yuan (993–1059) and Sun Fu (992–1057), the reformers Fan Chung-yen (989–1052) and Wang An-shih (1021–1086), the writer-officials Ou-yang Hsiu (1007–1072) and Su Shih (1036–1101), and the statesman-historian Ssu-ma Kuang (1018–1086), contributed to the revival of the Confucian persuasion in education, politics, literature, and history. Collectively, their works were the basis of the development of the literatus style, a way of life informed by Confucian ethics.

Nevertheless, the Confucian revival, which is usually understood in traditional historiography as the establishment of the lineage of the "learning of the tao" (*tao-hsueh*), is traced through a line of thinkers from Chou Tun-i (1017–1073) to Shao Yung (1011–1077), Chang Tsai (1020–1077), Ch'eng Hao (1032–1085), Ch'eng I (1033–1107), and finally to the great synthesizer Chu Hsi (1130–1200). These thinkers developed an inclusive humanist vision that integrated personal self-cultivation with social ethics and moral metaphysics in a holistic philosophy of life. In the eyes of the Sung literati this new philosophy authentically reanimated the classical Confucian insights and successfully applied them to the concerns of their own age.

Chou Tun-i ingeniously articulated the relationship between the "great transformation" of the cosmos and the moral development of the person. In his metaphysics humanity, as the recipient of the highest excellence from Heaven, is itself a center of "anthropocosmic" creativity. He developed this all-embracing humanism by a thought-provoking interpretation of the Taoist diagram of the great ultimate (*t'ai-chi*). Shao Yung further elaborated on the metaphysical basis of human affairs, insisting that a disinterested numerological mode of analysis was most appropriate for understanding the "supreme principles governing the world." Chang Tsai, however, focused his attention on the omnipresence of "vital energy" (*ch'i*). He also advocated the oneness of principle (*li*), comparable to the idea of natural law, and the multiplicity of its manifestations as the principle expresses itself through the vital energy. As an article of faith, he pronounced in the opening lines of the *Western Inscription:* "Heaven is my father and earth is my mother, and even a small being like myself finds a central abode in their midst. Therefore, that which fills the universe I regard as my body and that which directs the universe I consider as my nature. All people are my brothers and sisters, and all things are my companion."

These themes of mutuality between Heaven and humankind, spiritual kinship between all people, and harmony between humankind and nature were brought to fruition in Ch'eng Hao's definition of humankind as "forming one body with all things." To him the presence of the Heavenly principle (*T'ien-li*) in all things, including human nature, enables the human mind to purify itself in a spirit of reverence. Ch'eng I, following his brother's lead, formulated the famous dictum: "Self-cultivation requires reverence; the extension of knowledge consists in the investigation of things." However, by making special reference to the "investigation of things" (*ko-wu*), he raised doubts about the appropriateness of focusing exclusively on the inner illumination of the mind in Confucian self-cultivation, as his brother seemed to have done. The learning of the mind as advocated by Ch'eng Hao and the investigation of things as advocated by Ch'eng I became two distinct modes of thought in Sung Confucianism.[7]

Chu Hsi, who followed Ch'eng I's school of principle with emphasis on "the investigation of things" and implicitly rejected Ch'eng Hao's school of mind, developed a pattern of interpreting and transmitting the Confucian way that for centuries defined the Confucian project not only for Chinese believers but also for Koreans and Japanese.[8] If, as quite a few scholars have argued, Confucianism is a distinct form of East Asian spirituality, it is the Confucianism shaped by Chu Hsi. Master Chu virtually reconstituted the Confucian tradition, giving it new meaning, new structure, and new texture. He was more than a synthesizer; through conscientious appropriation and systematic interpretation he created a

7. On the philosophy of the Ch'eng brothers see A. C. Graham, *Two Chinese Philosophers: Ch'eng Ming-tao and Ch'eng Yi-ch'uan* (London: Lund Humphries, 1958).

8. Chu Hsi is well represented in the anthologies listed in n. 6. In addition, see Wing-tsit Chan, trans., *Reflections on Things at Hand: The Neo-Confucian Anthology Compiled by Chu Hsi and Lu Tsu-ch'ien* (New York: Columbia University Press, 1967). Important studies of Chu Hsi include Wing-tsit Chan, ed., *Chu Hsi and Neo-Confucianism* (Honolulu: University Press of Hawaii, 1986), and Daniel Gardner, *Chu Hsi and the Ta-hsueh: Neo-Confucian Reflection on the Confucian Canon* (Cambridge: Council on East Asian Studies, Harvard University, 1986).

new Confucianism, known as Neo-Confucianism in the West but often referred to as "the Learning of the Principle" (*Li-hsueh*) in modern China.

The *Doctrine of the Mean* and the *Great Learning,* originally two chapters in the *Book of Rites,* had become independent treatises and, together with the *Analects* and *Mencius,* had been included in the core curriculum of Confucian education centuries before Chu Hsi's birth. However, Master Chu put these works in a particular sequence (namely, the *Great Learning,* the *Analects, Mencius,* and the *Doctrine of the Mean*) and synthesized their commentaries, interpreting them as a coherent humanistic vision and calling them the Four Books. Master Chu fundamentally restructured the priority of the Confucian textual tradition by placing the Four Books above the Five Classics. From the fourteenth century on, the Four Books became the central texts for both primary education and civil service examinations in traditional China. Thus, they have exerted far greater influence on Chinese life and thought in the last six hundred years than any other works.

As an interpreter and transmitter of the Confucian way, Chu Hsi identified the early Sung masters who rightly belonged to the authentic lineage of Confucius and Mencius, both because they were his own spiritual fathers and because they were true bearers of the sagely teaching. His judgments, later widely accepted by governments in East Asia, were based principally on philosophical insight. Chou Tun-i, Chang Tsai, and the Ch'eng brothers—the select four—were Chu Hsi's cultural heroes. Shao Yung and Ssu-ma Kuang were originally on this august list, but Chu Hsi apparently changed his mind, perhaps because of Shao's excessive metaphysical speculation and Ssu-ma's obsession with historical facts.

Until Chu Hsi's time the Confucian thinking of the Sung masters was characterized by a few fruitfully ambiguous concepts, notably the great ultimate, principle, vital energy, nature, mind, and humanity. Master Chu defined the process of the "investigation of things" as a rigorous discipline of the mind that probes the underlying principle in things so that its vital energy can be transformed and humanity enlightened. Accordingly, he recommended a twofold method of study: to cultivate a sense of reverence and to pursue extensive knowledge. This combination of morality and wisdom made his pedagogy an inclusive approach to humanist education. Book reading, quiet sitting, ritual practice, physical exercise, calligraphy, arithmetic, and empirical observation all have a place in his pedagogical program. Chu Hsi reestablished the White Deer Grotto in present-day Kiangsi as an academy. It became the intellectual center of his age and provided an instructional model for all schools in East Asia for generations to come.

Chu Hsi was considered the preeminent Confucian scholar in Sung China, but his interpretation of the Confucian way was seriously challenged by his contemporary, Lu Hsiang-shan (Chiu-yuan, 1139–1193).

Claiming that he appropriated the true wisdom of Confucian teaching by reading Mencius, Lu criticized Chu Hsi's theory of the "investigation of things" as a form of fragmented and ineffective empiricism. Instead, Lu advocated a return to Mencian moral idealism by insisting that the establishment of the "great body" is the primary precondition for self-realization. To Lu, the learning of the mind as a quest for self-knowledge provided the basis on which the investigation of things assumed its proper significance. Lu's face-to-face confrontation with Master Chu in their famous meeting at the Goose Lake Temple in 1175 further convinced him that the Confucian project as Chu Hsi had shaped it was not Mencian. Although Lu's challenge remained a minority position for some time, his learning of the mind later became a major intellectual force in Ming China (1368–1644) and Tokugawa Japan (1600–1867).

Confucian Learning in the Chin, Yuan, Ming, and Ch'ing Dynasties

For approximately 150 years, from the time the Sung court moved its capital to the south in 1127 until the Mongol conquest in 1279, northern China was ruled by three conquest dynasties, the Liao (916–1125), the Hsi-hsia (990–1227), and the Chin (1115–1234). Although the bureaucracies and political cultures of both the Liao and the Hsi-hsia were under Confucian influence, no discernible intellectual developments helped to further the Confucian tradition. But the situation in the Jurchen Chin dynasty was entirely different. Despite the paucity of information about the Confucian renaissance in the Southern Sung, the Chin scholar-officials continued the classical, artistic, literary, and historiographic traditions of the north and developed a richly textured cultural form of their own.

The Mongols reunited China in 1279, and the intellectual dynamism of the south profoundly affected the northern style of scholarship. The harsh treatment that scholars received under the Yuan (Mongol) dynasty (1271–1368) seriously damaged the well-being of the scholarly community and the prestige of the scholar-official class. Nevertheless, outstanding Confucian thinkers emerged during this period. Some opted to withdraw from the world and to purify themselves so that they could repossess the way for the future; others decided to engage in politics to put their teaching into practice.

Hsu Heng (1209–1281) took the practical approach. Appointed by Khubilai, the Great Khan in Marco Polo's *Description of the World,* as the president of the imperial academy and respected as the leading scholar in the court, Hsu conscientiously and meticulously introduced Chu Hsi's teaching to the Mongols. He assumed personal responsibility for educating the sons of Mongol nobility to become qualified teachers of the Confucian classics. His erudition and skills in medicine, legal affairs, irrigation, military science, arithmetic, and astronomy enabled him to function as an informed adviser to the conquest dynasty. He set the tone for the eventual success of the Confucianization of the Yuan bureaucracy. In fact, the Yuan court was the first to officially adopt the Four Books as the basis of the civil service examination, a practice that was to be religiously observed until 1905. Thanks to Hsu Heng, Chu Hsi's teaching prevailed in the Mongol conquest, but the shape of the Confucian project envisioned by Master Chu was significantly simplified.

The hermit-scholar Liu Yin (1249–1293), however, allegedly refused Khubilai's summons in order to maintain the dignity of the Confucian way. To him, education was for self-realization. Loyal to the Chin culture in which he was reared and faithful to the Confucian way that he had learned from the Sung masters, Liu Yin rigorously applied philological methods to classical studies and strongly advocated the importance of history. True to Chu Hsi's spirit, Liu endorsed the idea of the investigation of things and put a great deal of emphasis on the learning of the mind. Liu Yin's contemporary, Wu Cheng (1249–1333), further developed the learning of the mind. Wu Cheng fully acknowledged the contribution of Lu Hsiang-shan to the Confucian tradition, even though as an admirer of Hsu Heng Wu considered himself a follower of Chu Hsi. Wu assigned himself the challenging task of harmonizing the difference between Chu and Lu. As a result, he reoriented Chu's balanced approach to morality and wisdom to accommodate Lu's existential concern for self-knowledge. This harmonization prepared the way for the revival of Lu's learning of the mind in the Ming (1368–1644).

The thought of the first outstanding Ming Confucian scholar, Hsueh Hsuan (1389–1464), revealed a turn toward moral subjectivity. Although a devoted follower of Chu Hsi, Hsueh's *Records of Reading* shows that he considered the cultivation of "mind and nature" to be particularly important. Two other early Ming scholars, Wu Yü-pi (1391–1469) and Ch'en Hsien-chang (1428–1500), defined the meaning of a Confucian education for those who studied the classics: a Confucian education was not simply a means of preparing for examinations; it was also a learning of the "body and mind."

Wang Yang-ming (1472–1529), the most influential Confucian thinker after Chu Hsi, took up where Wu and Ch'en left off.[9] Wang Yang-ming allied himself with Lu Hsiang-shan's learning of the mind, which was critical of the excessive attention to philological details that was characteristic of Chu Hsi's followers. He advocated the precept of "uniting thought and action." By focusing on the transformative power of the

9. On Wang Yang-ming see Wing-tsit Chan, trans., *Instructions for Practical Living and Other Neo-Confucian Writings by Wang Yang-ming* (New York: Columbia University Press, 1963); Julia Ching, *To Acquire Wisdom: The Way of Wang Yang-ming* (New York: Columbia University Press, 1976); and Tu Wei-ming, *Neo-Confucian Thought in Action: Wang Yang-ming's Youth* (Berkeley: University of California Press, 1976).

will, he inspired a whole generation of Confucian students to return to the moral idealism of Mencius. His own personal example of combining teaching with bureaucratic routine, administrative responsibility, and leadership in military campaigns demonstrated that he was a man of deeds. Yet, despite his competence in practical affairs, his primary concern was moral education, which he felt had to be grounded on the "original substance" of the mind. He later identified this term as the "good conscience" (*liang-chih*), a primordial existential moral awareness that every human being possesses. He further suggested that good conscience is the Heavenly principle and that it underlies all things, from the highest forms of spirituality to grass, wood, bricks, and stone. Because the universe consists of vital energy informed by good conscience, it is a dynamic process rather than a static structure. Human beings must learn to regard Heaven, earth, and the myriad things as one body by extending their good conscience to embrace an ever-expanding network of relationships.

Wang Yang-ming's "dynamic idealism," as Wing-tsit Chan characterizes it,[10] set the Confucian agenda for several generations in China. His followers, such as the conscientious communitarian Wang Chi (1497–1582), who devoted his long life to building a community of the like-minded, and the radical individualist Li Chih (1527–1602), who proposed to reduce all human relationships to friendship, broadened the Confucian project to accommodate a variety of life-styles.[11]

Among Wang's critics, Liu Tsung-chou (1578–1645) was the most brilliant. His *Human Schemata* (*Jen-p'u*) offers a rigorous phenomenological description of human mistakes as a corrective to Wang Yang-ming's moral optimism. Liu's student Huang Tsung-hsi (1610–1695) compiled a comprehensive biographical history of Ming Confucian scholars based on Liu's writings. One of Huang's contemporaries, Ku Yen-wu (1613–1682), was also a critic of Wang Yang-ming. He excelled in studies of political institutions, ancient phonology, and classical philology. Although Ku was well known in his time and honored as the patron saint of evidential learning in the eighteenth century, his contemporary Wang Fu-chih (1619–1692) was discovered two hundred years later to have been one of the most sophisticated original minds in the history of Confucian thought. His extensive writings on metaphysics, history, and the classics made him one of the most thorough critics of Wang Yang-ming and his followers.

10. Wing-tsit Chan, trans. and comp., *A Source Book in Chinese Philosophy* (Princeton: Princeton University Press, 1973), p. 654.

11. For an anthology of essays on Ming thought as expressed in literature, drama, and philosophy see William Theodore de Bary, ed., *Self and Society in Ming Thought* (New York: Columbia University Press, 1970).

The Confucianization of Chinese society reached its apex during the Ch'ing (1644–1912) when China was again ruled by a conquest (Manchu) dynasty. The Ch'ing emperors outshone their counterparts in the Ming in presenting themselves as exemplars of Confucian kingship. They consciously and ingeniously transformed Confucian teaching into a political ideology, indeed a mechanism of symbolic control. Jealously guarding their imperial prerogatives as the ultimate interpreters of Confucian truth, they substantially undermined the ability of the scholars to transmit the Confucian way by imposing harsh measures on them, such as a literary inquisition. Understandably, Ku Yen-wu's classical scholarship, which was politically neutral, rather than his insights on political reform inspired the eighteenth-century evidential scholars.[12] Tai Chen (1724–1777), the most philosophically minded philologist among the evidential scholars, couched his brilliant critique of Sung learning in his commentary on "the meanings of terms in the *Book of Mencius.*" Tai Chen was one of the eminent scholars appointed by the Ch'ien-lung emperor in 1773 to compile a library of imperial manuscripts. This massive scholarly undertaking, *The Complete Library of the Four Treasures,* represented the Manchu court's goal to give a comprehensive account of all the important works of the four branches of learning in Confucian culture: the classics, history, philosophy, and literature. The project comprised more than thirty-six thousand volumes, with comments on about 10,230 titles; it employed as many as fifteen thousand copyists and lasted for twenty years. Ch'ien-lung and the learned scholars around him may have enclosed their cultural heritage in a definitive form, but the Confucian tradition was yet to encounter its most serious threat.

Modern Transformation

At the time of the Opium War (1839–1842), East Asian societies had been Confucianized for centuries. The continuous growth of Mahayana Buddhism throughout Asia and the presence of Taoism in China, shamanism in Korea, and Shintoism in Japan did not undermine the power of the Confucian persuasion in government, education, family rituals, and social ethics. In fact, Buddhist monks were often messengers of Confucian values, and the coexistence of Confucianism with Taoism, shamanism, and Shintoism was characteristic of the syncretic East Asian religious life. The impact of the West, however, which has essentially compressed the effects of the Mongol military conquest and the millennium-long Buddhist influence into one generation, has so fundamentally un-

12. For a study of Ch'ing evidential scholarship see Benjamin Elman, *From Philosophy to Philology: Intellectual and Social Aspects of Change in Late Imperial China* (Cambridge: Harvard University Press, 1984).

dermined Confucian roots in East Asia that scholars and others debate whether Confucianism can remain a viable tradition in the contemporary era.

Despite the gradual erosion of Chinese intellectuals' faith in the viability of Confucian culture in the modern era, the modern Chinese intelligentsia has maintained unacknowledged, sometimes unconscious, continuities with the Confucian tradition at every level of life: behavior, attitude, belief, and commitment. Indeed, Confucianism is still an integral part of the "psycho-cultural construct" of the contemporary Chinese intellectual as well as the Chinese peasant; it remains a defining characteristic of the Chinese mentality.

The rise of Japan and the other newly industrialized Asian countries (South Korea, Taiwan, Hong Kong, and Singapore) as the most dynamic examples of sustained economic development since World War II has generated much scholarly interest. Labeled the "Sinic world in perspective," the "second case of industrial capitalism," the "Eastasia edge," or the "challenge of the post-Confucian states," this phenomenon raises intriguing questions about how typical East Asian institutions, still laden with Confucian values such as a paternalistic government, an educational system based on competitive examinations, an emphasis on loyalty and cooperation in the family, and local organizations that operate on the basis of consensus, have been adapted to the imperatives of modernization.

Some of the most creative and influential intellectuals in contemporary China have continued to think from Confucian roots. To be sure, articulate young intellectuals in the People's Republic today criticize their Confucian heritage as the embodiment of authoritarianism, bureaucratism, nepotism, conservatism, and male chauvinism, but the establishment of the Confucian Foundation dedicated to the preservation of Confucius's legacy, the publication of the journal *Confucian Studies,* and the concerted effort to rebuild Confucius's birthplace, Ch'ü-fu (Qufu), into a "holy land" clearly indicate that a revival of Confucian studies is under way. Indeed, some of the most seminal thinkers in China, Taiwan, Hong Kong, Singapore, and North America have persuasively articulated the relevance of Confucian humanism to China's contemporary modernization. The upsurge of interest in Confucian studies in South Korea, Taiwan, Hong Kong, and Singapore during the last four decades has generated a new dynamism in the Confucian tradition, and Confucian scholarship in Japan remains unrivaled. Confucian thinkers in the West, inspired by religious pluralism and liberal democratic ideals, have begun to explore the possibility of a "third epoch" of Confucian humanism. These trends signify that Confucianism's modern transformation in response to the challenge of the West is a continuation of both its classical formulation in the times of Confucius, Mencius, and Hsun Tzu, and its medieval elaboration in the thought of Chu Hsi and Wang Yang-ming. The new Confucian humanism, although rooted in the East, draws its nourishment from the West as well as from Asia.

Throughout East Asia the Confucian tradition, deeply rooted in over twenty-five hundred years of history, is being modernized and revitalized. The Confucian tradition remains a vital force that can touch our hearts, stimulate our minds, and enrich our lives, even in the late twentieth century.

SIX

□

Religious Traditions in Chinese Civilization: Buddhism and Taoism

T. H. Barrett

Anyone asked to write a short essay on Chinese religions must beware: to speak of Chinese religions is to speak of vast diversity over China's densely populated geographic space and many centuries of recorded history. The continuities and common factors of Chinese religions defy easy analysis. When one stumbles on one's first Chinese temple in Hong Kong or Taipei and finds its garish colors more reminiscent of Disneyland than the austere landscape paintings that typify Chinese culture in most Western eyes, what explanation will reconcile such dissimilar manifestations of Chinese spirituality? Perhaps the temple is a corruption of the ancient truths expressed in traditional landscape painting? Or perhaps the temple represents folk beliefs and landscape painting elite beliefs? Neither answer completely satisfies, and the honest answer is that we do not fully know.

Three thousand years ago when the king of the Shang dynasty consulted his departed ancestors by divination on the cause of his poor health, his response to his distress was basically the same that Marco Polo encountered among the Cathayans in southwest China in the thirteenth century: the first response to illness was to call in "magicians" to find out which spirit had caused the patient's affliction. When the first American anthropologist traveled to southwest China in the 1930s he too found a similar dependence on shamans in dealing with disease. Do these similarities represent a continuous tradition of religious healing? Or are they different ways of coping with the same problem? In the light of our current knowledge we cannot tell.

The full panorama of Chinese religious life dazzles our eyes in its variety. The only scholar to attempt a systematic survey of Chinese religious life labored for two decades to produce six substantial volumes, and he still died with his project only half completed.[1] It should also be noted that he worked before World War I, when the information that has since flooded in from anthropologists and historians of religion was not yet available. A host of religious phenomena, from astrology to zombiism, may be found in China, and one has only to experience the exuberant atmosphere of a Chinese festival to realize the richness and vitality of the ensemble of beliefs and practices that the student of Chinese religion must seek to comprehend.

Often, however, the student must be content to be an observer or to rely on other observers, whether Chinese or not. Much Chinese religion is in an important sense inarticulate. We only know of the Shang king's poor health because of the accidental discovery in this century of his divination records; neither he nor the later magicians or shamans took the important step of describing their religious practices in religious texts. There is much that may eventually be gleaned from the remarks of early Chinese writers about how such practices appeared, and present-day anthropologists are adding to our knowledge through their interviews and note taking. But only two major groups in China spoke and speak for themselves on religious matters: the Buddhists and the Taoists.

In the following pages I confine my remarks to Buddhism and Taoism not because they represent the full story of Chinese religion and not because they are necessarily the "best" Chinese religions but simply because their religious literature allows us to consider them on their own terms as spiritual traditions. Indeed, I would argue that it was largely their continued possession of religious writings that gave them coherence as traditions over space and time and that this textual legacy makes them uniquely approachable to researchers from outside the Chinese cultural world. How this situation has come about forms in itself the unifying thread in my own historical survey.

The reader should bear in mind that my concentration on the writings of Taoism and Buddhism is the most straightforward way I know to convey something of the dimensions of these two great currents in the broad ocean of Chinese religious life. As such, this chapter offers no more than a partial, personal view. Other views are readily available to the interested reader. The study of Chinese religion, along with Chinese studies in general, has made rapid strides over recent decades. The result has been a flood of publications on a wide variety of topics. Fortunately, we have now reached the stage where comprehensive introduc-

1. This was the classic work of J. J. M. De Groot, *The Religious System of China*, 6 vols. (Leiden: E. J. Brill, 1892–1910; Taipei: Literature House, 1964). An illuminating account of De Groot and his studies may be found in Arthur P. Wolf, ed., *Religion and Ritual in Chinese Society* (Stanford, Calif.: Stanford University Press, 1974), 19–41.

tions to Chinese religions are beginning to appear, but even the simplest of these runs to well over one hundred pages.[2]

Paradoxically, the upsurge of interest in Chinese religion has much more to do with changes in Western society than with any shift of attitudes in China. Even today there is no Chinese-language periodical devoted exclusively to the study of Chinese religion, although an English-language one has been in existence for a while in the United States. The lack of interest in religion in the Chinese-speaking world is not because most Chinese now live under an avowedly Marxist government that looks forward to the day when all religion will have become a thing of the past. As Jonathan Spence notes in Chapter 1 of this volume, the first Western observers to give extended thought to the nature of Chinese religiosity were the Jesuit and other missionaries who came to China from the late sixteenth century onward. These men remarked from the outset that most educated Chinese were tolerant enough of the missionaries' appearance on the religious scene, but this tolerance was ultimately because of an almost complete Chinese indifference to the spiritual issues that mattered so much to the standard-bearers of Western Christendom. One might think that these missionaries, coming as they did from a Europe riven with religious strife and themselves the products of long and concentrated religious training, may have overstated the secular nature of Chinese thought. But when the first Chinese started to write accounts of Europe, in the much less sectarian nineteenth century, it is quite obvious that some, at least, were profoundly shocked by the overt religiosity of Western society. No matter how advanced the West appeared in scientific or technological terms, Chinese intellectuals felt (and said) that their own tolerant agnosticism was something that Westerners needed to learn. In the Republican period, as Holmes Welch observed, a guide to Canton for Westerners enumerated its population as consisting of "14,000 Buddhists, 6,500 Christians, 2,500 Mohammedans, 1,500 Confucians, 1,000 Taoists, and 1,099,000 atheists—a figure of which Moscow itself could be proud."[3]

As one might suspect, such dubious statistics do not tell the full story. Catholic missionaries of the seventeenth century made converts who proved to be so devout that their zeal sometimes alarmed even those who

2. For an excellent introduction to popular Chinese religion, primarily in the modern era, see K. C. Yang, *Religion in Chinese Society* (Berkeley: University of California Press, 1961). Three valuable recent surveys, with bibliographies for further reading, are Christian Jochim, *Chinese Religions: A Cultural Perspective* (Englewood Cliffs, N.J.: Prentice-Hall, 1986); Daniel L. Overmyer, *Religions of China: The World as a Living System* (San Francisco: Harper & Row, 1986); and Laurence G. Thompson, *Chinese Religion: An Introduction*, 4th ed. (Belmont, Calif.: Wadsworth, 1988).

3. Holmes Welch, *The Buddhist Revival in China* (Cambridge: Harvard University Press, 1968), 210.

converted them. Protestant missionaries of the nineteenth century were at times staggered by the amounts of money Chinese spent on religious observances. In our own century when Chinese and Western social scientists started to examine objectively the practice of religion in China they certainly did not find that most Chinese were atheists.

What the social scientists found was that in China religion did not have the same high profile that it assumed in Western society. Rather, it was "diffuse," that is, so closely tied to the workings of the state, the local community, and the family that it lacked any independent representatives in Chinese society that were equivalent to the priests and ministers of Western Christianity. Although there were Buddhist monks and Taoist priests, they either remained isolated in their religious communities or else were called in by lay people to perform specific duties. Thus, an officiant at a Chinese funeral performed a technical function, but he did not resemble a Christian priest or minister in offering wisdom, guidance, and consolation. If any Chinese wished to seek spiritual counsel, there were ways and means of finding this, but the voices exhorting the people to live a holier life were scattered and less than strident.

These findings explain and corroborate the impressions of the first European missionaries that in their daily lives the Chinese of the seventeenth century appeared irreligious *by European standards.* However, almost a thousand years earlier the Nestorians from the Middle East, who were the first Christians to arrive in China, probably received different impressions. We know that they too were welcomed politely and extended complete religious toleration, but the borrowings from Buddhist and Taoist terminology in their writings show that they had entered a world of lively religious controversy. Far from being indifferent to religious matters, the Chinese rulers of that day held debates at court between representatives of the leading religions, and ordinary people flocked in vast assemblies to hear the sermons of popular preachers. Religious sentiments suffused art and literature and had done so for some time. For example, the colossal statues of Buddhas (described by Michael Sullivan in Chapter 11 of this volume), hewn from the mountain cliffs of north China, majestically demonstrate the power that religious faith then held. Although the most violent upheavals of the Cultural Revolution did not succeed in removing all these statues from the Chinese landscape, it is undeniable that the age of faith that created them has inexorably waned.

Despite the alleged changelessness of China, the diffuse state of Chinese religion over recent centuries represents only the latest stage in a long and complex historical process. When we move further back in Chinese history we may not find evidence of deeply held religious faith as dramatic as these gigantic Buddhas, but as David N. Keightley vividly illustrates (see Chapter 2 of this volume), archaeologists are providing us with signs of the power of the Chinese religious imagination from the very beginnings of their civilization. Keightley rightly emphasizes the importance of religious beliefs in Shang times, and the recent discovery of an elaborate religious painting on a Han funerary banner (ca. 168 B.C.) demonstrates a continuing Chinese fascination with religion over a thousand years after the end of Shang rule. What the Han painting means, however, is far from clear. For this period of history it is difficult to find written records to supplement the silent witness of religious artifacts. Despite the undeniable importance of religion in early China, not a single text of a purely religious nature has been preserved from Chinese classical antiquity. True, there are certain early Chinese works with strong religious overtones: the *I ching*, the *Tao-te ching* of Lao Tzu, and the book of *Chuang tzu* are the ones most familiar to Westerners. But these texts were valued by the elite carriers of China's cultural traditions not as straightforward sacred scriptures but for what they could teach about the workings of the universe, the ideal conduct of society, or even the imaginative use of language. Even in the sayings of Confucius himself we discern a certain reluctance to go into religious questions. Confucius's later follower Hsun Tzu (third century B.C.) articulates the argument that whatever the ostensible purpose of religious observances, their most valuable effect from the standpoint of Confucian thinking is simply that they increase social stability—an insight that has won him the respect of twentieth-century anthropologists.

Hsun Tzu's attitude promoted the diffuse manifestations of religion in society at the expense of others that might have had an unsettling effect on social institutions. The Confucian subordination of religion to the goal of social and political stability is important for understanding what happened during the Han dynasty, a period when the imperial government first achieved a stable form and when all the literature of preimperial China was collected and edited for posterity. The Han was an age of great religious diversity, but during this time the state came to support Confucian scholars, and Confucian scholars reciprocated by supporting the state. As a result, we only know about the religious diversity of this period through scattered references to religious experts, magicians offering to confer immortality on emperors, and so forth. These references were made by scholars who were not themselves concerned with publicizing or perpetuating such practices. All pre-Han and Han literature passed through the hands of men who either were influenced by Confucian attitudes or were Confucians themselves.

Thus, the Confucian canon formulated during the Han includes accounts of religious ritual, but only as norms of accepted social behavior in a broad sense. Even the surviving Han commentaries on earlier Confucian texts have little to add on the subject of religion. The commentaries that were affected by the exuberant religious temper of the age, which exalted Confucius to a sort of divinity, were themselves put out of circulation at a later stage. For material of a purely religious nature from the Han we are dependent on recent archaeology, which has unearthed, for example, a demonology remarkably similar to those included in popular almanacs today. This example is startling testimony to the continuity of popular religious tradition, but most Confucian scholars preferred to pass over this tradition in silence.[4]

Fortunately for the modern student of Chinese religion, the Confucian domination of written sources did not remain complete. Toward the end of the Han dynasty, during the second century of our own era, a much greater tension occurred between the literate elite and the government. The social order was gradually collapsing under internal and external pressures, and the misery of the common people was intensified by a succession of natural disasters, among which epidemics seem to have been particularly terrifying. At this time there seems to have been a widespread yearning for the appearance of a divine figure who would usher in a new and better age. Rather than looking to a sage like Confucius, whose ideas were now firmly identified with the imperial government, many nonelite adherents turned to the mysterious Lao Tzu, who was invested with a divine status, and in many circles the people awaited Lao Tzu's renewed revelation. Two great religious leaders, Chang Chüeh and Chang Tao-ling, were able to harness these feelings among the people and weld together powerful religious movements that challenged the authority of the dynasty. Both these men seem to have built up popular support not as religious writers or teachers but as healers who set up organizations of subordinates to supervise and administer their adherents, thus usurping the functions of government.

Chang Chüeh mobilized his followers, the Yellow Turbans, in A.D. 184 to rise in a massive revolt that effectively destroyed the political and military supremacy of the Han dynasty. Chang Chüeh's movement quickly collapsed, and he was killed within a year. By contrast, Chang Tao-ling, who styled himself the "Celestial Master," founded a small sect in Szechwan in the middle of the second century. This sect managed to survive under Tao-ling's grandson and to maintain itself as a virtually independent theocratic state for over three decades. Even after surrendering to

4. The reader should not be confused by the contrast between my characterization of Confucian indifference to, or suspicion of, religion and Tu Wei-ming's discussion (Chapter 5 in this volume) of Confucianism as an ethicoreligious worldview. The Confucians most admired by Professor Tu endowed the secular world with sacred importance and saw man as, among other things, a spiritual being. Nevertheless, in contrast with Taoists and Buddhists, most Confucians were far more secular in outlook, far more concerned with issues of social and political organization, and far less interested in details of an afterlife, the worship of spirits or deities, the quest for immortality or nirvana, and supernatural phenomena in general.

the warlord Ts'ao Ts'ao in A.D. 215, the followers of the "Celestial Masters" remained free to perpetuate their organization for religious, but not political, purposes.

Although this movement made some converts, it did not come to dominate intellectual circles. The classical heritage still remained the main object of study for most educated Chinese, even though the Han style of Confucian commentary yielded in importance to a more speculative approach based on a fresh look at a rather different group of ancient texts. On the basis of the *I ching,* the *Tao-te ching,* and (eventually) the *Chuang-tzu* the leading exegetes of the day constructed a new philosophy based on the primacy of *wu,* "nonbeing." This change dramatically reflected the negation of Han institutions by the new regime.

After a century of the propagation of "the way of the Celestial Masters" among the ruling group of north China, the subjugation of the area by non-Chinese precipitated a migration of the ruling Chin dynasty to the south. South China had until A.D. 280 been under the control of the independent kingdom of Wu, whose leading families had taken pride in maintaining the traditions of earlier times, unlike their northern opponents. The Chin refugees came to constitute the top layer of the aristocratic elite. The leading southern families possessed a wealth of knowledge concerning the pursuit of immortality but little political power, so they came to occupy the lower levels of the elite. Thus, in the *Pao-p'u-tzu* the southern writer Ko Hung (283–343) devotes half his space to moralizing over the decline in Confucian values and half to enthusiastic accounts of alchemy and other arcane matters; both topics are the product of his political failure to make any headway in his career at the new southern court.

After the establishment of the Way of the Celestial Masters in south China, aristocrats of a somewhat later generation than Ko Hung required some reassurance that their temporal lack of power was still outweighed by access to spiritual riches. Such reassurance was provided by a visionary named Yang Hsi, who by the year A.D. 370 had revealed a series of scriptures from the realm of Superior Purity, *Shang-ch'ing,* a realm loftier than any with which the Celestial Masters had communicated. These texts both renewed and reaffirmed the value of the alchemical and meditational practices of the southerners, and their success seems to have inspired a descendant of Ko Hung named Ko Ch'ao-fu to publish a further collection of revelations in A.D. 400. These scriptures, the *Ling-pao,* or "Sacred Jewel," canon, include elements such as ritual texts missing from the *Shang-ch'ing* scriptures (although present in the Way of the Celestial Masters) and, initially at least, they seem to have been a rival product.

Ko Ch'ao-fu's scriptures also make plain something already apparent occasionally in Yang Hsi's revelations: among the southern religious traditions incorporated into these new works was Buddhism. By the year A.D. 400 Buddhism had already had a long history in China, and its influence, although slight at first, grew during the course of the fourth century A.D. to the point where it is impossible to continue the story of Chinese religion without pausing to consider this Indian faith. Thus far I have traced the development of the religious tradition in China itself, first as a substitute for an imperial power that had grown weak and then as the religion of an elite. That this tradition should be called "China's higher religion" (as modern scholars sometimes refer to it) is quite justified: by the beginning of the fifth century it is possible to point to a large number of passages in surviving texts denouncing the excessive features of local religious cults, and the yearning for a new dispensation, apparent in the late Han, is associated with an urge to sweep away corrupt, vulgar religious practices. By the year A.D. 400 the "higher religion" tradition had evolved a variety of competing bodies of religious literature, and if it were to achieve any unified identity, some pattern of organization that could cope with its diversity was necessary. Buddhism provided an excellent model for such a task (see my later discussion of Taoism). It may reasonably be argued that Buddhism helped the indigenous Chinese religion achieve a sense of identity, but this debt was never acknowledged by the Chinese. On the contrary, under the collective title of the Taoists the adherents of China's higher religion stressed their connections with the ancient sage Lao Tzu and claimed that the foreign faith was simply a barbarized version of his teaching.

The Buddha was born in northern India almost two and a half millennia ago; the first reliable reports of Buddhism in China date to the first century of our era. Thus the Chinese were confronted from the start with a sophisticated religious system that had developed to some maturity in lands beyond their ken. All Buddhist believers, whatever their cultural background, turned then and turn now to the three great "jewels" of that tradition: the Buddha, the dharma (teachings), and the *sangha* (community of believers). A Buddha is an "enlightened one," a title that even the founder of the faith did not believe to be unique to himself (except in his own time). Later followers have allowed a multiplicity of Buddhas throughout space and time. All these beings are enlightened with respect to particular spiritual truths.

At the core of Buddhism are some very simple assertions: all existence entails suffering; suffering has a cause; the cause may be extinguished; and there is a path to this goal. Although Buddhism possesses no creed, these truths were widely accepted as being reducible to a few brief sentences. All things are subject to change; among all elements of existence there is nothing corresponding to an abiding, unitary, independent self; the fruitless desire for unjustifiably attributing permanent reality and experiences to this nonexistent self causes suffering; the extinction of such a desire leads to a tranquil realm known as nirvana, which is beyond the ceaseless process of reincarnation.

By the time the Buddha's doctrine, or dharma, reached China, such simple formulations contrasted starkly with the vast range of teachings that claimed in every case to represent the Buddha's (or a Buddha's) word. Some averred not only that there was no self but that all phenomena were equally devoid of real existence: all was *k'ung,* or empty. They claimed for themselves the name Mahayana, the Greater Vehicle (to salvation or nirvana), and criticized earlier Buddhists as adherents of Hinayana, the Lesser Vehicle, who were too concerned with the minute analysis of the elements that composed the notional (and illusory) self. Mahayanists also felt that to become an arhat, that is, to reach nirvana through following the Buddha's teaching, was a selfish goal compared to becoming a bodhisattva, a being of advanced spiritual standing who postpones his own enlightenment in order to help others along the path.

The full range of the dharma, or teachings, found written expression in a profusion of scriptures. Before the rise of the Mahayana various Buddhist groups transmitted a basic canon in three sections (the Tripitaka): the sutras (the discourses of the Buddha), the *vinaya* (monastic regulations) and the *abhidharma* (scholastic treatises). Mahayanist ideas were conveyed in new sutras attributed to the Buddha, and in time Mahayanist commentaries and treatises also appeared. Chinese translations of both Mahayana and Hinayana texts started in the middle of the second century A.D. Although there is no evidence that these translations had any immediate impact on the development of Chinese religion, the prominence of descriptions of meditation techniques among the texts translated suggests that they were produced for the benefit of Chinese who were already involved in the practice of meditation.

By the fourth century A.D. a much greater number of sutras were available in both north and south China, and the Chinese were beginning to realize the immensity of Buddhist literature. Even in elite circles the Chinese began to take seriously the ideas propounded in these translations. The Buddhist concept of *k'ung* seemed close enough to the notion of *wu,* nonbeing, to merit Chinese attention, and by the middle of the century Chinese Buddhist monks were taking part in abstruse philosophical discussions in the salons of south China. The non-Chinese rulers in the north were pleased to see the Indian religion flourish: it could bolster their prestige as religious patrons and help to unify otherwise diverse populations. The rulers were admittedly less interested in philosophy than in meditation, which both monks and monarchs believed could confer unusual powers, such as the ability to predict the outcome of battles.

The unpromising northern environment produced the first Chinese monk to grasp the full potential of Buddhism. Tao-an (312–385) encompassed the whole range of current Buddhist concerns, from an early training in meditation to a later interest in the more philosophical literature in vogue in the south. Realizing that the foreign religion by no means corresponded neatly to Chinese ideas, he stressed the importance of careful translation and undertook a catalogue of all the existing translated works he could find. This catalogue ran to over six hundred items—far more texts than in any early listing of Taoist literature. But Tao-an was painfully aware of the gaps in his knowledge of Buddhism and promoted further translation projects on a large scale. That he gave a high priority to more complete translations of the *vinaya* suggests that as well as striving for a better understanding of the dharma he was also concerned about improving the organization of the *sangha*.

The Buddhist community, or *sangha,* which principally denotes the monastic community, was a drastic innovation in Chinese religious life, and its health was essential to the maintenance and further propagation of the Buddhist faith. Prior to Tao-an's time Chinese Buddhist monks changed their names when they entered the clergy, taking the family names of their teachers; these "family names" in fact usually indicated the teacher's ethnic origins. In place of this diversity of nomenclature that suggested the affiliation of Chinese monks with various Indians, Iranians, Sogdians, and so forth, Tao-an ruled that all monks should take the family name of the Buddha Sakya, or Shih in Chinese. This conception of the Buddhist *sangha* as a single voluntary family translated the alien idea of a monastic order into terms that the Chinese could readily understand. Of course, that the Chinese could understand the concept did not mean that they readily approved of such a radically "un-Chinese" idea as a celibate clergy; even before Tao-an's time there is evidence of direct conflict over the status of the *sangha.* In India the severing of all secular ties to concentrate on the pursuit of a religious goal was a noble act; even a king would bow down to a monk. In China a recruit to a life of celibacy could be deemed guilty of cutting off the family line, the height of social irresponsibility. No Chinese ruler, moreover, was willing to surrender his prerogatives to any mere subject, however holy. Even at the height of Buddhist influence in China during the T'ang dynasty, imperial acceptance of the *sangha* was always grudging, and what favorable treatment the Buddhists received came to an abrupt halt in 842–845 when economic and religious motives combined to prompt the emperor to seize Buddhist property and return thousands of monks and nuns to lay life.

The *sangha* won a much longer-term, if always grudging, acceptance from Chinese society. Buddhist doctrine included some elements that were easy to reconcile with the Chinese emphasis on family life. The idea that one's future reincarnation was dependent on past individual karma may have been intrinsically strange to the Chinese, but by extending the scope of human possibilities for improvement over past and future lives, this doctrine allowed families to feel themselves more deeply involved in the fate of their departed members. There is ample evidence that Buddhists were already sensitive to this social dimension of their religion before they encountered the ancestor-worship of the Chinese. And the notion that religious merit acquired by an individual might be transferred to the benefit of others was an aspect of Mahayanist altruism that lent itself rather well to the practice of filial piety.

Of particular consequence for the establishment of the *sangha* was the belief that the donation of worldly wealth to the monastic community was an especially effective way of gaining merit. Individual members of the *sangha* led lives under the rule of the *vinaya,* which severely restricted all personal possessions, but monasteries as corporations were able to amass large capital sums that could be used not only on the collective buildings but also on acquiring landholdings to support more monks in their full-time endeavors. From Tao-an's time on, China's monasteries acquired economic power on a vast scale, enabling increasing numbers of monks and nuns to live off monastic endowments, translating, copying, and studying an ever-greater number of texts and propagating their religion throughout society. All this was different from the life of the Taoist priesthood, a largely hereditary profession dependent for support on clients who required specific expertise in dealing with the supernatural. Such a life was perhaps ultimately more secure in that it did not generate enough wealth to attract the attention of the state, but it did not allow for any great organizational development either. The Buddhist *sangha,* the vast family that embraced followers of different doctrinal schools, provided Taoists with an example of a type of unity that allowed for considerable diversity. The Buddhist practice of organizing all their sacred texts, Mahayana and Hinayana, into a single canon divided into various sections suggested a scheme whereby the various revelations of Taoism could also be grouped together into a single collection. Buddhist communities living off their endowments pointed to the advantages of securing similar patronage and especially the advantage of imperial patronage.

Thus, the career of the Taoist Lu Hsiu-ching (406–477) gives strong indications that the rich religious heritage of late-fourth-century south China was already being shaped into a coherent tradition that could stand as a rival to Buddhism. Although the emergence of a Taoist clergy modeled on the Buddhist *sangha* is as yet an obscure topic (the advent of a celibate Taoist clergy seems to date from the sixth century), Lu is said to have resided in an institution established by the emperor and to have grouped *Ling-pao* and *Shang-ch'ing* scriptures together with earlier occult southern texts into a single Taoist canon. That Lu also vigorously contested Buddhist doctrines shows that conflict between the two religions, doubtless spurred on by competition over patronage, was now much more the norm than mutual toleration, at least at the highest levels.

It should not be thought that the Taoists were unequal contestants in their competition with Buddhism. Against the established might of Buddhism, a religion that had already pervaded much of Asia, Taoism might seem a relative newcomer incapable of acquiring a similar institutional strength: from all periods of subsequent Chinese history the number of Buddhist monasteries compared with the number of Taoist abbeys always shows that the Buddhists predominated. But Taoist life had never centered on separate religious institutions, and the fact that Taoism was still developing during the Six Dynasties period (222–589) meant that it was flexible enough to absorb Buddhist ideas and incorporate them into fresh scriptural revelations. Thus, Taoism kept pace doctrinally with Buddhism whatever the weakness of its institutional base. By the T'ang period, for instance, Taoist texts enunciated the original Indian concept of *k'ung,* emptiness, as if Chinese (Taoist) divinities had always perceived reality in such terms.

Despite its borrowings from Buddhism, Taoism had very ancient roots in China, and it retained a distinctly Chinese outlook, particularly with regard to social and political questions over which Buddhism came into conflict with Chinese ways of thinking. To cite just one example, the Buddhist ideal of leaving family life to devote oneself entirely to a religious quest created a clergy with which the Taoist priesthood tended to be equated, but the Taoist priesthood was seldom as highly organized or as identifiable as the Buddhist clergy. The Taoist religious life was open to all (men and women alike) from childhood onward; once initiated into a rather loose system of arcane knowledge, one could "move up" through higher grades of knowledge and expertise, much like contemporary ladders of rank for learning martial arts such as judo. As a result, the dividing line between the Taoist clergy and the laity was, in T'ang times at least, determined somewhat arbitrarily by the state.

Taoism's "low profile," however, did not necessarily lessen state involvement in Taoism; its very "Chineseness" made state involvement easier. Because it offered the prospect of a religious synthesis that would make Buddhism unnecessary, Taoism appealed to autocratic rulers, particularly in north China. Persecutions of Buddhism in north China in 444–446 and 574–577 were largely the result of imperially sponsored moves to make Taoism the national religion. Taoism also helped inspire the great T'ang persecution of Buddhism in 842–845. The general T'ang policy was to avoid a head-on clash with Buddhism, but the T'ang emperors had always claimed descent from Lao Tzu, and they promoted the religion of their ancestor to such an extent that it became in some ways as closely tied to the T'ang state as Confucianism had been to the Han.

Surviving works from the T'ang dynasty—and even from a somewhat earlier date—show that Taoism was by this point a religious tradition of such breadth that its own adherents now required much more in the way of guidebooks to its doctrines and practices. These texts give an invaluable picture of how the Taoists themselves saw the various elements that constituted their religion, and one can deduce the major features of the religion in its mature state from these sources. Taoism approaches the unseen spiritual world beyond human society in two main ways. First, it deploys an array of rituals to summon help *in* from the "beyond" of the spirit world, either to help the individual or to help the community. Second, it advocates a complex mixture of techniques that the individual may practice in this world—alchemical, dietary, yogic, meditational, and so on—to pass to a better state of immortality *out* beyond ordinary human limitations. A glance at the orderly description of the rituals and techniques in these digests marks Taoism as the religion of the organizing elite, whose religious attitudes are also amply revealed in contemporary prose and poetry, rich in tales of wonder concerning the spirits and immortals and their dealings with this world. At times Taoist compendia may actually be misleading because some organize their materials by borrowing schemes evolved by scholastic Buddhism, even though Buddhism lacks the Chinese emphasis on the manipulation of elements in the physical world (whether through alchemy, yoga, or even sexual practices) that is so important as a means to Taoist goals.

Despite the T'ang preference for Taoism and the great persecution of 842–845, Buddhism remained an important force in Chinese culture. In the half millennium after Tao-an's pioneering work Chinese Buddhism interpenetrated Chinese society so deeply that any quick eradication was impossible. Throughout this period some of China's finest minds were engaged in the vast enterprise of understanding and appropriating for themselves the intellectual wealth of the Buddhist tradition. Tao-an's emphasis on the importance of translation proved most timely because in 401 the great translator Kumarajiva reached the northern capital of Ch'ang-an, and cooperated with Tao-an's disciples in the production of texts that fundamentally changed the character of Chinese Buddhism. He not only provided more polished translations of texts already known to the Chinese, such as the *Lotus Sutra* but also introduced hitherto unavailable texts of Buddhist philosophy to the Chinese, including those of such Indian Mahayanists as Nagarjuna. Kumarajiva allowed the Chinese for the first time to appreciate how the doctrine of emptiness was understood in India and put an end to the facile identification of Buddhist and native ideas that had prevailed earlier.

Thus, the fifth century was an important period in Buddhist circles in China for the dissemination of more accurate knowledge about Buddhism. This dissemination was complicated by the continued evolution of Buddhist thought in India, which was at first obscured from the Chinese. In the north, where interest in meditation was still strong, Buddhist scholars in the early sixth century noticed that some newly translated commentaries assigned the mind a role far greater than earlier Mahayanists had envisaged. Unfortunately, Paramartha, the translator who would have been capable of expounding on the full range of this new, more idealist thought (known as Yogacara in modern scholarship), arrived in south China in 548 in a period of political turmoil and was able to translate only a fraction of the Indian literature on this subject. The pilgrimage of the great Hsuan-tsang to India in 627 in search of further texts was largely motivated by his desire to sort out remaining problems; on his return to China in 645 he devoted himself to a series of translations that not only provided a complete (if somewhat partisan) account of the complexities of Yogacara thought but also raised the standards of accuracy in translation to yet higher levels.

Meanwhile, however, other pressures besides a thirst for academic knowledge had begun to mold Chinese Buddhism. Translations of an increasing number of difficult treatises had only been made possible because of the vast resources of manpower, time, and money available in Buddhist monasteries. Yet the economic success of the *sangha* threatened to cut it off from the realities of everyday Chinese life. The Taoists proved ever ready to supplant the Buddhists as a religious force, and the Confucians argued with increasing credibility that monks were parasites living idle lives at the expense of the peasantry. Among thoughtful Buddhists a sense of decline was reinforced by the translation of texts that emphasized the impermanence of all things, including the success of Buddhism itself.

By the sixth century Chinese Buddhists felt pressure to go beyond the scholastic elaboration of abstruse Indian doctrines and to discover in the here and now of their own troubled times a religious truth to live by. Men like Hui-ssu (515–577) laid the foundations of a truly Chinese Buddhism by relying on their own religious experience. In the light of his master's insights, Hui-ssu's disciple Chih-i (538–597), with the support of the Sui rulers of a reunited China, was able to unify the various competing schools of interpretation that had sprung up during the preceding several centuries. The lynchpin of Chih-i's system of thought was not, however, any academic treatise by a later Indian thinker but rather the *Lotus Sutra,* a vigorously Mahayanist depiction of the Buddha's preaching that had already achieved widespread popularity among ordinary believers.

Chih-i's synthesis, often called T'ien-t'ai Buddhism after the range of mountains where he made his home, was challenged as the result of two events. First, the fall of the Sui dynasty removed all imperial patronage from the T'ien-t'ai school. Second, the translations of Hsuan-tsang opened up new vistas of philosophical understanding for the Chinese. Fa-tsang (643–712) responded to this challenge by taking up the earlier work of men who had looked to the *Hua-yen Sutra* as their guiding light in the same way that the T'ien-t'ai Buddhists looked to the *Lotus Sutra.* Although the *Hua-yen Sutra* was a much larger work than the *Lotus Sutra,* it too enjoyed a degree of popularity. *The Hua-yen Sutra*'s emphasis on the role of the mind allowed for the elaboration of a system of philosophy on the same scale as that of the Yogacara literature. Just as much as Chih-i, Fa-tsang displayed a magisterial learning with regard to earlier Buddhist schools of interpretation. More important, at the heart of his thought lies a reconciliation of the Buddhist perception of reality with the strong Chinese faith in the interrelationship of all phenomena (a faith noted prominently in this volume by Nathan Sivin [see Chapter 7] and Michael Sullivan [see Chapter 11]).

The systems of Chih-i and Fa-tsang were further developed by other Buddhist thinkers in the eighth century, but thereafter it is not possible to point to any major innovations in Chinese Buddhist thought. This absence of innovation has been seen as a symptom of decline, but perhaps this assessment is unfair: the great effort of comprehension embodied in the Hua-yen and T'ien-t'ai systems had, after all, sorted out the vast mass of translated Buddhist literature—most of it claiming to represent the Buddha's very words—and graded it according to relative value; little else remained to be done. Both Chih-i and Fa-tsang chose a particular text already accepted as the basis for religious life in China as the fullest revelation of the Buddha's message, and other texts were interpreted as expedient, as lower levels of revelation for those of duller understanding. Religious practice could then proceed without the need for the academic virtuosity that a study of the whole Buddhist canon would require.

Popular Buddhism, of course, felt little need to resort to the whole canon in any case. One response to the sixth-century belief that the faith had fallen on evil times was to concentrate deliberately on the religious practices deemed most simple yet efficacious, disregarding all nonessential activity. Some T'ang monks devoted their learning to proving the scriptural justification for this kind of simplification. For example, some monks showed that calling on the name of Amitabha, Buddha of the Western Paradise, was all that was required to guarantee rebirth in his world, termed his Pure Land. Other monks appearing in T'ang sources (and earlier) offered hope of even more immediate benefits that derived from magical or ritual knowledge similar to that commanded by Taoist priests. This knowledge was not in fact a Chinese invention. A strain in Buddhism known as Tantrism had always acknowledged the importance of magical and ritual means to religious ends, and by the eighth century it had become developed enough to produce a literature that dominated translation activity for the remainder of Chinese history up to the twentieth century.

Yet for many this level of religious life was not enough: the goal of enlightenment, once described, could not simply be forgotten or deferred to better times. One mysterious figure, the monk Bodhidharma, held out the hope that all was not lost. We know that early in the sixth century a foreign meditation master of this name visited north China, but contemporary accounts reveal little of his activities. Later sources assert that he was none other than the last patriarch of Indian Buddhism, successor to a line of teachers stretching back to the Buddha himself and guardian of a religious truth that was a "separate transmission beyond scriptures, not dependent on the written word," but "passed from mind to mind."[5] Although a line of practitioners of meditation ("Ch'an" in Chinese, "Zen" in Japanese) claimed to perpetuate Bodhidharma's teachings in China, the revolutionary import of this type of Buddhism did not become clearly perceived until the eighth century.

During this period a number of small treatises attributed to Bodhidharma were in circulation, but because of sectarian squabbles among his spiritual heirs attention started to focus on a more recent figure: the Sixth Patriarch in China. This man, Hui-neng (638–713), reputedly an illiterate non-Chinese native of the far south, proved worthier to inherit the mantle of the patriarchs (at least according to the advocates of Hui-neng's line of succession) than a much more eminent meditation master whose disciples dominated the court. The famous *Platform Sutra* purported to represent a record of Hui-neng's preaching. Eventually, stories of the words and deeds of later masters who claimed their spiritual descent from Hui-neng began to appear and to be accorded a like degree of importance.

The Ch'an movement as it developed in the T'ang period explicitly subverted the whole scriptural basis of the Buddhist religion in China. The truth was no longer to be sought in obscure and alien phrases piled up in a welter of translated materials. The living truth was available in China in the person of masters who communicated directly with any seeker in the spoken language of the day. All that was needed to achieve enlightenment lay within. This perception was not novel to Chinese Buddhism, but it gained an especially vital relevance in the wake of the widespread destruction of monastery libraries and their contents in the persecution of 842–845 and more generally in the long series of rebellions that beset the latter half of the dynasty.

Taoism and Buddhism were both deeply affected by the collapse of the T'ang dynasty. The end of T'ang rule meant an end to both the au-

5. For an explanation of the origins of these phrases see Isshu Miura and Ruth Fuller Sasaki, *Zen Dust* (New York: Harcourt, Brace & World, 1966), 229–31.

tomatic imperial patronage of Taoism and the high prestige Taoist priests had enjoyed among the T'ang elite. In the social disintegration that accompanied the T'ang collapse religious institutions were difficult to maintain. This gave an advantage particularly to those Taoists and Ch'an Buddhists who believed that elaborate religious institutions and scriptural traditions were ultimately irrelevant to the pursuit of salvation (whether defined as immortality or enlightenment). Both Taoism and Ch'an Buddhism emphasized that the individual and the master-disciple relationship were far more important than elaborate institutions. Without rejecting the notion of a wider *sangha,* the Ch'an movement favored small self-supporting communities independent of wealthy patronage. Such a preference made economic sense in a period of chaotic warfare and the resulting destruction of the wealthy aristocratic clans that had dominated China since the late Han. Similarly, the new emphasis on the personal direct authority of the religious teacher (rather than on the written word) may be seen as a symptom of the collapse of old values in a new age of insecurity.

When the new order was finally consolidated under the Sung (in the tenth century), the environment that had brought both Chinese Buddhism and Taoism to maturity was gone for good. The destruction of the aristocracy meant that the Chinese state was now in the hands of bureaucrats recruited through an expanded system of civil service examinations. Although these examinations had become a permanent feature of government during the Sui and the T'ang dynasties, their function in earlier times had simply been to select a small number of potential high-level officials from a field of candidates who were generally very well connected, if not at the top of the social hierarchy. Membership in the new ruling class in Sung times, however, appears to have been based far less on hereditary social rank. Lacking the pride in genealogy that characterized their T'ang predecessors, the Sung elite tended to identify with a cultural tradition that dated back to an even earlier time, to the pre-Buddhist world of ancient China. Accordingly, the Sung examination curriculum stressed a commitment to Confucianism in a way that the T'ang had not. At the same time, Neo-Confucian theorists explicitly denounced the corrupting influences of Buddhism and Taoism, advocating a return to the secular roots (as they saw it) of Chinese civilization in high antiquity.

Although advocates of a hard-line religious policy had appeared as early as T'ang times, they did not win immediate acceptance. Far from it: several Sung emperors were so impressed with earlier precedents for imperial support of Taoism that they made intermittent attempts on their own to promote a Sung version of Taoist imperial ideology; also, eminent Ch'an masters did not lack for disciples among the highest circles in the land. Yet in general, from Sung times onward Buddhists and Taoists came under increasing pressure from the secular authorities to curb their influence in society. As the civil service examination system became more central to government recruitment, it promoted intolerant Confucian attitudes within the elite; the examination system also provided an avenue for advancement to real power for some who might otherwise have joined the clergy. Even more important, the government began to take deliberate steps to subvert the clerical establishment, corrupting the leadership by the sale of honors (the "purple robe" of imperial favor) and titles and lowering the standard of new clerical recruits through alternate moves to sell ordination certificates outright and to restrict ordinations severely.

No wonder few great creative thinkers appear in Buddhist circles after the Sung: the emphasis was now on the elaboration and conservation of established traditions, which were evident in the struggles during the Sung between T'ien-tai and Ch'an monks and in the seventeenth century between different Ch'an factions over the controversial doctrine of the patriarchal succession. Similar defensive and reactive measures, seen from the end of the Sung period onward, emerged in the considerable apologetic literature that sought to defend Buddhism against Neo-Confucian criticism.

The Taoist tradition, however, demonstrated its flexibility once again by absorbing new elements from the changed social order of the Sung period. Even during the late T'ang Taoist groups developed far from the centers of imperial patronage. One such example is a family in Kiangsi (claiming descent from Chang Tao-ling) that had attracted a considerable following by the early Sung. With the Sung court granting the Kiangsi family some recognition, as it did other new schools, the group "arrived" socially. Until the Ch'ing, members of the family behaved and were treated as full-fledged gentlemen. When the Sung lost north China to Jurchen invaders in the early twelfth century, Taoism still demonstrated continued vitality as religious movements burgeoned in the north amid the chaos and misery of the Chinese defeat.

Although some aspects of this northern religious ferment, such as an emphasis on healing, are reminiscent of developments in the late Han, the Ch'üan-chen school, which became the dominant Taoist movement in the north, shared a number of characteristics with Ch'an Buddhism. The Ch'üan-chen founder, Wang Ch'ung-yang (1112–1170), was said to have derived his teachings in part from the immortal Lu Tung-pin (popularly known as Patriarch Lu), who in many ways rivaled the Sixth Patriarch of the Ch'an school. Like the great Ch'an leader, Patriarch Lu was known through many stories that combined the commonplace and the mystical or supernatural in close association. Both patriarchs were authors of riddling verses, but, as a Taoist sage, Patriarch Lu possessed a distinct advantage over the Sixth Patriarch: he could speak from beyond the grave, adding fresh revelations generation after generation. Patriarch Lu normally communicated through the medium of automatic writing, using Chinese equivalents of the Western planchette, a popular religious practice of some antiquity that was well attested by Sung authors.

This intrusion of a "folk religious" element into the "higher religion" of Taoism was by no means unprecedented. Although Taoism from its earliest days had adopted the viewpoint and writing style (classical Chinese) of the elite, its interaction with the world of multifarious local cults had not always been marked with hostility. Some groups prominent in post-Sung Taoism, such as the Ching-ming tao from Kiangsi, seem to have grown out of highly localized indigenous groups that originally had not been connected with the Taoist tradition at all. Yet it is noteworthy that the Ching-ming tao achieved national prominence only after espousing values dear to the elite, such as filial piety and loyalty. Rather than seeing the religious history of the last millennium as one in which once-noble ideals are corrupted by vulgar superstition, it might make more sense to see it as a process in which the elite religion gradually diffused to a populace that formerly had been untouched by the beliefs of the educated classes.

It might also be argued that the most distinctive development during this period was not the diffusion or corruption of Buddhism or Taoism but the emergence of Buddhist and Taoist forms of popular religion that represented new traditions in their own right, independent of established Buddhism and Taoism and of purely local cults as well. From the Sung to the present, elite and popular traditions in Taoism have existed in close conjunction (at least in parts of China), even though they were often distinguished by a number of factors such as the use of the vernacular in popular ritual. Fully ordained Taoist priests operated in cooperation with more numerous, less-qualified practitioners, who served as their assistants or, alternatively, met the immediate religious needs of communities where priests were unavailable.

The greater number of Buddhist clergy did not prevent the emergence of popular forms of Buddhism, often led by charismatic laymen. Unlike Taoism, which had different levels of expertise, in theory one was either in the Buddhist clergy or not, even if in some areas Buddhist versions of the popular Taoist priesthood did exist. The Buddhist tendency to separate lay believers from the clergy was reinforced by government regulations that sought to confine monks to their monasteries. Thus, associations of lay Buddhists sometimes fell under the influence of religious leaders who were not controlled or supervised by anyone in the *sangha* proper. As a result, the millenarian, apocalyptic strain in Chinese religion, which had first emerged in the late Han, survived and prospered in an underground world of Buddhist folk sects, whose origins might often be traced to orthodox Buddhist groups but whose espousal of potentially subversive ideas led to their disavowal by the clergy and their persecution by the government.

The adherents of the White Lotus tradition were a prime target for suppression throughout the Yuan, Ming, and Ch'ing dynasties.[6] The White Lotus can apparently be traced back to a perfectly innocuous Buddhist association in the Sung, but an uprising in the mid fourteenth century by one of its later leaders, who prophesied the advent of the future Buddha Maitreya, proved to be the catalyst that destroyed the power of the Mongols in China and opened the way for Chinese rule once more. The Ming founder, Ming T'ai-tsu, rapidly dissociated himself and his dynasty from such sectarian fanatics as the White Lotus believers. Yet, when Ming T'ai-tsu's descendants began to lose control over the empire in the seventeenth century, the White Lotus tradition was still going strong and the disturbances that it had intermittently provoked escalated once more, even if not with such dramatic consequences.

The later White Lotus sects were not alone in offering an organized alternative to established Buddhism. In the second decade of the sixteenth century a lay Buddhist known to his later followers as Patriarch Lo initiated a revival movement that popularized Ch'an and Pure Land teachings in a number of vernacular texts. This movement remained on the fringes of orthodoxy for some time, and not all Buddhist monks felt obliged to repudiate it. However, by the end of the Ming dynasty some of Lo's later followers had absorbed the messianic ideas found in the White Lotus tradition, and orthodox Buddhists began to condemn his writings unequivocally. Even so, most adherents of the Lo religion remained relatively unthreatening to the social order. Their social welfare work among unemployed boatmen during the eighteenth century led the Ch'ing authorities to consider sparing them from the harsh repression that was the lot of most sectarians (whether they actually posed an active threat or not). In the end, however, even these social welfare activities were judged potentially dangerous, and the Lo followers were ordered to cease their operations.

The persistence of these groups, whose latter-day descendants still attract impressive numbers of adherents in such places as Taiwan, where membership is not concealed, would appear to be quite remarkable in view of the penalties usually inflicted on them. But the restrictions imposed on the Buddhist clergy, both by the government and by their own emphasis on their separateness from lay life, left a large gap in which

6. For a general study of organized popular Buddhist sects in the late imperial period, with special emphasis on the White Lotus traditions, see Daniel Overmyer, *Folk Buddhist Religion: Dissenting Sects in Late Traditional China* (Cambridge: Harvard University Press, 1976). A fine case study of one White Lotus–inspired rebellion is Susan Naquin, *Millenarian Rebellion in China: The Eight Trigrams Uprising of 1813* (New Haven: Yale University Press, 1976).

religious leaders closer to the people could operate. The lack of any institutional restraints on such men made this religious milieu highly volatile—a haunt of charlatans and fanatics as much as of men of spiritual integrity. Thus, the government was wise to keep a close eye on it.

Yet some elements made for stability and continuity even in these relatively heterodox groups. Sometimes leadership was hereditary and became a family business, which discouraged the rabble-rousing adventurer. Many groups, even in the nineteenth century, also transmitted scriptures going back to Ming times, such as the writings of Patriarch Lo mentioned earlier. These scriptures seem to have played a part in unifying the beliefs of different congregations that were widely separated in time and space. However, these scriptures should be seen in the much larger context of popular fiction and drama that were permeated with religious themes. Ch'üan-chen influences, for example, can be seen in early drama, and by the Ch'ing period there is at least one case in which a *pao-chüan* (precious scroll), as the sectarian texts were called, inspired a popular novel that in turn provided the basis for a further scripture. Similarly, a work like *Journey to the West,* although not produced for a mass audience, drew on folk religious themes also present in *pao-chüan* literature and publicized the popular cult of the Monkey King, if only indirectly through other works that capitalized on its success.[7] Thus, despite the government's suppression of overtly sectarian works, the values of popular religion came to be diffused over a wide area. Educated lay persons made some attempts, especially in the late Ming, to bring these values into line with those of the elite through the publication of *shan-shu* (morality books) for popular distribution. Such books purveyed the lowest common denominator of the ethical ideals of Buddhism, Taoism, and Confucianism, and the authors, after the fashion of that age, drew eclectically on all three traditions rather than promoting a particular orthodoxy. Although these morality books were not without their effect and although most folk legends only entered into print through the work of relatively educated writers, the vibrant world of popular culture could not be contained within even the most relaxed and syncretic bounds set by the elite. The great historian Ch'ien Ta-hsin (1728–1804) acknowledged this fact explicitly when he observed that

> in ancient times there were three teachings: Confucianism, Buddhism, and Taoism. Since the Ming dynasty there has been one more: popular novels [*hsiao-shuo*]. Novels and romances have never considered themselves to constitute a teaching, yet all classes of society are familiar with their contents; even women, children, and illiterates listen to them, which is as good

7. See Paul Ropp, Chapter 13 in this volume, for a brief discussion of the Buddhist influence on Chinese fiction and of the novel *Journey to the West.*

as reading. Thus, this teaching is even more widespread than Confucianism, Buddhism, and Taoism.[8]

Ch'ien's "fourth religion" has indeed left us a vast literature to study, but his point about the lack of self-awareness as a separate tradition is important: beyond texts associated with specifically Buddhist or Taoist forms of popular belief (such as the small collection of writings Patriarch Lo handed down in folk Buddhist sects or the manuscripts of Taoist priestly families), all the vernacular works we now possess have not been consciously selected for transmission to posterity; they only represent random selections from a mass of ephemeral publications, and their survival depended more on their literary than on their religious content. As a result, the study of Chinese religion through the rich tradition of vernacular literature is both tantalizing and frustrating—tantalizing for the sheer bulk of extant materials and frustrating for the immense difficulties involved in determining the precise relationship between this literature and actual Chinese religious beliefs and practices.

In contrast with popular vernacular fiction the survival of the canonical writings of Buddhism and Taoism has been the result of deliberate effort, often on a colossal scale. I have already noted the huge quantity of Buddhist works translated into Chinese and the stimulus that the example of the Buddhist Tripitaka provided for the formation of the Taoist canon, but we would know little of this formative period in the history of Chinese religion were it not for the successful preservation of hundreds of texts for well over a thousand years.

This preservation was achieved only with considerable expenditure of money and manpower. Occasionally, we find a single wealthy individual or family that underwrote the copying or printing of the Buddhist canon (it is unclear whether this was ever the case with the Taoist canon), but for the most part only the resources of the state or private subscription could keep these large bodies of literature in circulation. The involvement of the state in maintaining both Buddhist and Taoist canons, a practice already established in the seventh century, was not motivated by pure altruism, even though the religious merit acquired by publishing the scriptures was one factor alluded to at that time. The preparation of a carefully drawn up and catalogued canon provided the state with an ideal opportunity to scrutinize religious literature and to remove anything of subversive intent. Official cataloguers (albeit clerics) were responsible for detecting and condemning spurious Buddhist texts, and they kept a close check on all Buddhist literature composed in China, expunging some works once considered acceptable and including new

8. Ch'ien Ta-hsin, "Cheng-su," in *Ch'ien-yen t'ang wen-chi,* 17.14b, in the *Ssu-pu ts'ung-k'an* edition.

works only on a conservative basis. The success of this policy is evident today: despite the destruction of religious literature during the late T'ang and the Five Dynasties (from the late eighth to the tenth century), every single text out of the 1,076 deemed canonical in the mid eighth century survives, but many writings outside the canon have disappeared completely or have only been retrieved recently from Tun-huang or other such archaeological finds.[9]

This reluctance to grant canonical status to new Buddhist works may be traced through the early printed editions, the first of which was prepared under imperial auspices in 971–983. The chief victims of this policy seem to have been the Ch'an schools and their literature of Recorded Sayings (*yü-lu*) of the masters (although the invention of printing facilitated the preservation of many of these works outside the canon). At the end of the Ming the institution of the Continuation of the Canon, a supplement to printings of the canon by public subscription, made room for much more of this Ch'an literature and other works of commentary and exposition by later authors. This more liberal policy has also been continued by the Japanese editors responsible for twentieth-century versions of the canon. Admittedly, the Chinese state remained and remains less than enthusiastic about expanding the canon. For example, the Ch'ing Tripitaka did not include the Continuation of the Canon, and the current printing of the Buddhist canon, although designed to include all texts published in earlier canons, does not seem to envisage any further additions. But the total of over four thousand works that this project is scheduled to make available can only be accounted as generous; certainly no other Marxist state (and perhaps no modern secular state of any kind) has engaged in religious publication on such a scale.

Although the Taoist canon has also been reprinted, this was not such a massive undertaking because the transmission of the Taoist canon has followed a much more uncertain course. For one thing there were far fewer Taoist than Buddhist communities in which to store such a collection; in addition, Chinese (and Mongol) emperors perhaps felt wary about letting such a large repository of occult information become too readily accessible. The latter part of the thirteenth century was marked by fierce competition between Buddhists and Taoists to secure the patronage of the Mongol emperors. Such competition provoked Khubilai

9. In 1900 a walled-up cave containing thousands of documents dating from the fifth to the tenth century A.D. was discovered at Tun-huang in the far northwest of China. These texts have transformed our knowledge of the period. For a concise account of the discovery, see Arthur Waley, *Ballads and Stories from Tun-huang* (London: George Allen and Unwin, 1960), 236–42. For an assessment of their value to the historian, see D. C. Twitchett, "Chinese Social History from the Seventh to the Tenth Centuries," *Past and Present* 35 (December 1966): 28–53.

Khan to decree in 1281 that all Taoist texts and printing blocks, except for the *Tao-te ching*, should be burned.

This edict was relaxed by the next century, so the destruction was not total, but not long after the edict came the intense warfare sparked by the White Lotus rising against the Mongols, in which more works were lost. Apart from Taoism's lack of institutional strength, the Taoist readiness to discover truth afresh in the present (if need be through new revelations) may also have led to a neglect of scriptures that were no longer deemed of immediate practical value. As a result of these factors, the surviving Taoist canon today totals less than fifteen hundred works. Even so, through the photolithographic reproduction of surviving works from the Ming and Ch'ing dynasties and the addition of contemporary Taoist ritual texts to supplement the materials in the Taoist canon, the total amount of literature available in print is far in excess of anything available since Western studies of China began.

My account of the Buddhist and Taoist traditions is primarily concerned with explaining how and why these two great traditions may be studied in all their historical depth through written sources. To be sure, such sources have their limitations; even if we were able to retrieve all the Buddhist and Taoist texts that have disappeared over the centuries, there would still be many aspects of these religions—ranging from ineffable religious experiences to trivial gestures of etiquette observed in monastic life—that we would be powerless to understand because they were never written down. As most religious adherents instinctively feel and as the Ch'an masters of China so powerfully illustrate, religion is not something that can be confined to books.

But even the Ch'an masters allowed a certain value to the written word. The truth might be something as exalted and luminescent as the moon, but the written words might still have their use as a "finger pointing to the moon." There are, of course, more direct ways of approaching Chinese religion than reading books: witnessing the religious life of a Chinese community or even participating in Zen training or in martial arts exercises grounded in Taoist beliefs. However, most Chinese today would not claim these manifestations of religion as part of their traditional high culture, which they see as predominantly secular in its outlook (even though Zen, originally a Chinese product, is sometimes marketed as the very quintessence of Japanese civilization). If China did not possess a heritage of written records stretching far back in time—and we should remember that many cultures have preserved little or nothing in the way of written testimony to their history—it would be difficult, even making use of the artistic and archaeological evidence that remains of the material culture of China's past, to argue against the assertion, made often enough by some zealous defenders of the rational, humanistic image of Chinese civilization, that religion has never played more than a minor part in Chinese culture. Thanks to the preservation of the canonical writings of Buddhism and Taoism, our attention is directed not only toward the religious situation of China now but also toward the Chinese religious experience over many centuries.

Why insist on this point? Why burden the reader who is anxious to know how Chinese Buddhism and Taoism compare with Western religious traditions with so much history and bibliography? The reason for doing so is because it underlines the sad fact that little in the way of meaningful comparison has been undertaken because so little has been done by Westerners to master the accumulated legacy of Buddhist and Taoist literature. Some aspects of Chinese religion are obvious enough that a command of a wide range of sources is hardly necessary. It takes little specialist knowledge, for example, to appreciate that Chinese religion takes a distinctly positive attitude toward the human condition. Yet although we possess the means to explore the boundaries to this optimism, work has only just started on the many texts in the Buddhist and Taoist canons on such topics as the crucial phenomenon of repentance: the records of the dramatic rituals of penitence that were practiced at one time by both religions seem reminiscent of descriptions of Europe in the Middle Ages. Similarly, the generalization that the Chinese, unlike many other civilizations (including our own), never ascribed divine origins to their legal institutions makes an important observation on the humanistic tendency in Chinese thought. Yet there are traces of a legal code enforced by the way of the Celestial Masters, whose earliest leaders claimed divine authority, although no one has investigated this anomaly so far.

The whole question of the relationship between spiritual and temporal authority in China cries out for comparative treatment. Enough work has been done for us to know that the Chinese did not see this time-honored European division the way we do and that the struggles between kings and popes that mark our history could not have happened in China, where no religious leader could claim authority independent of the emperor. Yet there were struggles in China between religious believers and imperial autocrats, even desperate, fanatical struggles to the death. Although the visions of these sectarian insurgents at first sight seem to conform to Western images of the apocalypse, it is worth noting that in China no cataclysm is thought capable of bringing human history to a halt; even up to very recent times China's leaders have refused to believe that nuclear war could have such an effect. There are indications that such an assumption is evident in Chinese history, and religious sources, if we avail ourselves of them, should enable us to trace themes like this over nearly two thousand years, long enough for significant comparisons with Europe.

The span of documentation should also allow us to study long-term change comparatively. For instance, might not the waning support for both Buddhism and Taoism among the elite after the Sung be compared to the process of secularization in the West in more recent times? Or is such a suggestion fundamentally misleading? The more one studies Chinese Buddhism and Taoism, the more one suspects not only that they cannot easily be equated in their social roles with the Judeo-Christian tradition but also that they might not correspond to our own notions of religion at all. Although the Chinese have always distinguished natural and supernatural worlds in some fashion, they have not done so in the same ways as our Western ancestors. The distinction between religious and secular in China seems less clearcut—the relationship much more intimate—than in the West. In Chinese Buddhism enlightenment is not something far off; rather, enlightenment and unenlightenment are two sides of the same coin. "My supernatural powers and marvelous actions are seen in drawing water and carrying wood," runs the Ch'an adage. As for Taoism, some of its recommendations seem to us to belong with the practice of medicine rather than religion.

Both Chinese Buddhism and Taoism are generally much more interested in practice than belief. One can point to a Taoist "ten commandments" but not to any Taoist creed, and the same essentially holds true for Buddhism as well. Although "What do Chinese Buddhists and Taoists believe?" might seem a natural question to *us*, a concise answer would totally misrepresent both traditions and afford little reasonable basis for comparison. "What do Chinese Buddhists and Taoists do?" might be a more appropriate place to start, except that to focus on the present while ignoring the long historical processes that have shaped contemporary Chinese religion seems equally unlikely to clarify anything. "What happened?" may be only a preliminary question, but it must be asked and it can be answered. Today studies of such basic and hitherto neglected topics as the development of Taoist and Buddhist ritual are starting to appear; gradually, the true shape of Chinese religiosity will come into clearer focus. When it does, a future writer of an introduction to Chinese religion will probably be able to simplify matters to a few accepted generalizations in a way that is impossible at present. The current state of the field may be frustrating to the readers of this volume, but all I can do is conclude with the plea that they should not write off the study of Chinese religion as a baffling and uncertain area. Rather, because religion is the area of Chinese studies in which educated Chinese have contributed least to the exploration of their own tradition, this is the area in which we can expect the greatest advances from now on, and this is the area where non-Chinese are best placed to take part in them. China's heritage is in this case still mainly buried treasure—but we, too, can take part in the search.

SEVEN

□

Science and Medicine in Chinese History

Nathan Sivin

The historical discoveries of the last generation have left no basis for the old myths that the ancestry of modern science is exclusively European and that before modern times no other civilization was able to do science except under European influence. We have gradually come to understand that scientific traditions differing from the European tradition in fundamental respects—from techniques, to institutional settings, to views of nature and man's relation to it—existed in the Islamic world, India, and China, and in smaller civilizations as well. It has become clear that these traditions and the tradition of the Occident, far from being separate streams, have interacted more or less continuously from their beginnings until they were replaced by local versions of the modern science that they have all helped to form.

Central to this clearing of the air has been the study of China. There the record of technical endeavor has been fullest, most continuous, most accessible, and most exactly dated. That is only what one would expect of a state that was administered by a full-fledged bureaucracy two thousand years ago and a country where books were being routinely printed four hundred years before the Gutenberg Bible.

Understanding the technical traditions of other cultures is not just a matter for exotic tastes. To the contrary, this wider awareness has transformed our sense of Europe's development. Consider, for example, Francis Bacon's influential attempt, shortly after 1600, to explain that great efflorescence of human knowledge and activity that we now call the Renaissance:

This chapter is a revision of "Science in China's Past," in *Science in Contemporary China*, ed. Leo Orleans (Stanford: Stanford University Press, 1980), 1–29.

> Again, it is well to observe the force and virtue and consequences of discoveries, and these are to be seen nowhere more conspicuously than in those three which were unknown to the ancients, and of which the origin, though recent, is obscure and inglorious; namely, printing, gunpowder, and the magnet. For these three have changed the whole face and state of things throughout the world; the first in literature, the second in warfare, the third in navigation; whence have followed innumerable changes, insomuch that no empire, no sect, no star seems to have exerted greater power and influence in human affairs than these mechanical discoveries.[1]

Bacon's understanding was still conventional in 1920, although by then the attention of historians had largely shifted back from inventions to politics and religion ("empires" and "sects") if not to astrology ("stars").

Today the origins of Bacon's three inventions are a great deal less obscure. None of the three was in fact a European discovery. Printing I have already mentioned. Movable clay type was used to mold inscriptions in Chinese cast bronze vessels of the mid second millennium B.C. The earliest extant texts printed on paper from carved wood blocks originated in Korea by 751 and in Japan about 770 (nearly one thousand years after the Chinese invention of paper and four hundred years before its introduction to Europe).

Because printers needed thousands of different characters, labor was cheap, and books were published in a series of small printings, printing with movable type developed slowly and did not replace the older process until the twentieth century. We have an account of Chinese ceramic movable-type printing in the 1040s. The oldest such book that still exists (set in wood type) dates from the 1350s. It is not in Chinese but in the Tangut script of the northwest frontier. Metal type was in use still earlier. Printing with it was brought to a high state of perfection in Korea through a succession of royally subsidized experiments that culminated in the early fifteenth century.

As printing evolved across East Asia, its potentialities for changing "the face and state" of literature were by no means unexplored. By 1100, for instance, the Chinese government had authorized the printing of standard collections of texts in an attempt—often repeated but always with limited success—to control education. This was the case not only in the humanistic classics but also in such fields as mathematics and medicine.

As for gunpowder, formulas for flare mixtures appear in Chinese alchemical books of the ninth century A.D. or a little earlier. The propor-

1. Francis Bacon, *The New Organon and Related Writings*, Library of Liberal Arts, no. 97 (New York: Liberal Arts Press, 1960), 118. Joseph Needham, *The Grand Titration: Science and Society in East and West* (Toronto: University of Toronto Press, 1969), 62–76, has several interesting observations on this passage.

tions that make gunpowder explosive were known by 1050, and up-to-date commanders over the next two centuries had at their disposal increasingly destructive flamethrowing devices, bombs hurled by trebuchets, and rocket weapons. Between 1270 and 1320 metal-barreled cannon appeared on the Mongols' main battlefronts in Europe, the Islamic west, and China. Although it is not beyond doubt that the inventions that constitute the cannon were finally assembled in Cathay, the prehistory of the crucial propellant and of weapons that used it to fire projectiles was clearly Chinese.

Magnetic attraction was not a matter of recent knowledge in Bacon's time. It is clear that he was speaking of its use in the navigational compass, for the polarity and directive property of lodestone were known and applied to steering by Europeans late in the twelfth century. In China it is likely that a pivoted lodestone spoon was used for divination in the first century A.D. Well before 1100 the true compass—apparently developed earlier for geomantic siting—was being used in navigation, and the declination of the needle was known to steersmen as an effect, if not as a concept.

Bacon's statement about the springs of change in the West reminds us, then, that for many centuries Europe was on balance a beneficiary of technology transfers. Through the long centuries in which Europe gradually relearned the arts of civilization after the Roman Empire collapsed, China continued to build on its high culture. Many important inventions that apply the power of water or wind to machines are first found in Europe more than ten centuries later than in China. A few Chinese priorities of other types are an efficient harness for draft animals, the drawloom, deep borehole drilling, the segmental arch bridge, rigging that allowed ships to sail to windward, the axial rudder, porcelain, and cast iron.

A Chinese visiting one of the great cities of Europe in 1400 would still have found it backward. In Bacon's lifetime some Occidental cities could no longer be considered backward. By 1840 what appeared glorious about China to its more sophisticated visitors were mainly vestiges of the past.

Some of the reasons for the reversal in technological preeminence are internal to China: centuries of disastrous fiscal and other administrative policies, the remorseless pressure of increasing population, and a large measure of social stability and cultural homogeneity that left traditional values and forms practically unchallenged as the creativity behind them was sapped by intellectual orthodoxies. Other reasons for the reversal arose in Europe, above all a universal quantitative and logical approach to empirical knowledge and practice that gradually redefined nature, reshaped society, and remade human consciousness. In the final reckoning the predominance of Western science and technology cannot be explained by contributing factors entirely within Europe or outside it, for it was built on the intercourse of civilizations.

CHINESE AND WESTERN, TRADITIONAL AND MODERN

It is almost impossible to think about traditional Chinese science and technology without comparing them, explicitly or implicitly, with their present-day analogues. Otherwise it would be difficult even to identify what past activities are of technical interest. Nevertheless, the transforming influence of the scientific and industrial revolutions was so great that the earlier sciences of China and Europe resemble each other more than either resembles the modern variety. It is important, if one is to think clearly about science and technology as worldwide phenomena, to avoid confusing differences between China and the West with differences between traditional societies and societies that have become essentially modern.

Certain aspects of today's technical activity that may appear to be universal are in fact peculiarly European or peculiarly modern. We consider normal, for instance, a sequence of sciences derived from classical Greek schemes of knowledge but formed by the gradual spread in modern times of system and quantification, beginning with physics and moving through chemistry, the life sciences, and ultimately (or so Auguste Comte believed) through psychology, the yet-to-be-achieved exact science of the human mind. In Europe this scheme and its precursors did not, when they arose, describe established structures of knowledge but justified projects to bring them about by creating new institutions and habits of thought.

In China there was, for example, no biology. Observations and theoretical perspectives on the manifestations of life were scattered through a very different grouping of knowledge that I will sketch out below. Alchemists, East and West, set down a great deal of information about chemical processes. How much they learned from physicians and illiterate craftsmen we do not know. In any case the designation of Chinese alchemy as early chemistry ignores the fact that alchemical goals were not cognitive but spiritual. Most topics of modern physics had not been imagined before the demise of traditional Chinese science, and the more old-fashioned subjects—for example, heat, sound, and magnetism—were in China a matter of dispersed experiences and reflections rather than coherent disciplines.

Another practically universal modern assumption is that technology is applied science, that technological progress and economic benefit are the natural end of new scientific knowledge. Before the mid eighteenth century, emerging modern science did not affect technology in Europe. Craft traditions were developed by people who, even as literacy began to diffuse through society, had little access to science and little reason to use it.

The old certainty that the industrial revolution in Western Europe and the United States grew out of the direct application of modern science has come so seriously into question since the 1960s that we are prepared to see a much subtler influence operating since the eighteenth century. Coming out of the new Western mentality shaped by theoretical science, this influence led the educated to take an active interest in manufacturing and led artisans (along with everyone else) to begin reasoning impersonally and abstractly about facts, processes, commodities, and labor to an extent unprecedented in human history. The design of economic systems to exploit new scientific knowledge is, at least outside the chemical industry, mainly a twentieth-century phenomenon. Familiar though the direct linkage of science to technology may be to readers of this book, it would have appeared wildly exotic to all except a visionary few three hundred years ago in Europe or Asia.

Since China's industrial revolution began less than two generations ago, what we find previously—as in early Europe—are sciences and manufacturing techniques that had little to do with each other. The sciences reflected the concerns of the tiny literate elite, their cosmologies, and the managerial problems they encountered in their careers and recorded in their writings. Technology was on the whole a matter of craft traditions, passed down privately from father to son or from master to apprentice. It was on these mainly oral and manual traditions rather than on cumulative science, recorded in writing, that the technological preeminence of China was built.

What we know about the early industrial arts comes not from those who did the work but from scholars writing for fellow dilettantes or from officials writing for their peers who happened to be curious about the work of the lower orders. As the learned compiler of the great technological encyclopedia of 1637 put it, "While the best rice is cooking fragrantly in the palace kitchen, perchance one of the princes would wish to know what farming implements look like; or, while the officers of the Imperial Wardrobe are cutting suits of brocade, another of the princes might wonder about the techniques of silk weaving." Those were the circumstances in which a civil servant might actually feel a need for the book. "Let the ambitious scholar toss this book onto his desk and give it no further thought; it is a work that is in no way concerned with the art of advancement in offialdom."[2]

2. Sung Ying-hsing, *T'ien-kung K'ai-wu: Chinese Technology in the Seventeenth Century,* trans. E-tu Zen Sun and Shiou-chuan Sun (University Park: Pennsylvania State University Press, 1966), xiii–xiv (translation modified). Another translation of the technological encyclopedia worth consulting is Li Ch'iao-p'ing et al., trans., *Tien-kung-kai-wu: Exploitation of the Work of Nature,* Chinese Culture Series, no. 3 (Taipei: China Academy, 1980).

Thus in both China and Europe before modern times science and technology went their own ways. Natural philosophers learned from the techniques being practiced around them, at least to an extent that their practical curiosity dictated, but what they read in books counted for a great deal more. The achievements of artisans did not depend on the enhanced scientific understanding of their betters.

SCIENCE AND SCIENCES IN CHINA

In Europe since classical times the various sciences were part of a single structure that included all systematic rational knowledge. They were part of *scientia,* the part that has to do with nature. When in the early seventeenth century Francis Bacon (1561–1626) in England began inventing a physics to which experiment was the key to learning what was fact and what was not, and Galileo Galilei (1564–1642) in Italy imagined a universe full of physical motions that could be measured and computed, these two styles of science—the experimental and the mathematical—developed separately for a while. But they were still seen as parts of one endeavor.

In China there was no single structure of rational knowledge that incorporated all the sciences. Knowing was an activity in which the rational operations of the intellect were not sharply disconnected from what we would call intuition, imagination, illumination, ecstasy, aesthetic perception, ethical commitment, or sensuous experience. The various sciences, unlike those of Europe, were neither circumscribed by the philosophies of their time nor subordinated to theology (which did not exist in East Asia). The sciences developed a great deal more independently of each other than in the West. The practitioners of each science extended and revised the concepts and assumptions about physical reality with which that science began (the particular sciences emerged between the second century B.C. and the first century A.D.). Over the centuries they seldom responded directly to contemporary philosophic innovations. For example, Chu Hsi (1130–1200), perhaps the most influential moral philosopher of the last two thousand years, was intensely interested in astronomy and cosmology, but what he knew of these fields was grossly outmoded; astronomers returned the compliment by ignoring his frequently odd opinions about the sky. They were free to exert that autonomy because no institution enforced the authority of Chu Hsi over them. There is an obvious contrast with the educational institutions of Europe, from Plato's Academy and Aristotle's Lyceum to the medieval and early modern universities, in which the natural sciences were kept subordinate to philosophy.

Although in China the sciences were relatively autonomous provinces of knowledge, there were definite limits to what was expected of them.

Scientists were well aware of the growth of understanding and of the increasing ability to predict, but we do not find the conviction that in the fullness of time all phenomena would yield their ultimate secrets. The typical belief was rather that natural processes wove a pattern of constant relations too subtle and too multivariant to be understood completely by what we would call empirical investigation or mathematical analysis. Scientific explanation merely expressed, for finite and practical human purposes, partial and indirect views of that fabric. This point was made with great clarity by Shen Kua (1031–1095), a polymath who served as astronomer-royal and who made lasting contributions to practically every science.

> Those in the world who speak of the regularities underlying the phenomena, it seems, manage to apprehend their crude traces. But these regularities have their very subtle aspect, which those who rely on mathematical astronomy cannot know of. Still even these are nothing more than traces. As for the spiritual processes described in the *Book of Changes* that "when they are stimulated, penetrate every situation in the realm," mere traces have nothing to do with them. This spiritual state by which foreknowledge is attained can hardly be sought through traces, of which in any case only the cruder sort are attainable. What I have called the subtlest aspect of these traces, those who discuss the celestial bodies attempt to know by depending on mathematical astronomy; but astronomy is nothing more than the outcome of conjecture.[3]

This understanding did not diminish astronomy in Shen's eyes; he devoted his best energies to improving the calendar. His perspective, far removed from that of the modern scientist, would have been quite comprehensible to his contemporaries in eleventh-century Christendom, although he was applying it to a level of scientific knowledge much more sophisticated than theirs.

To sum up, the Chinese sciences were able to attain a high standard—at times the highest in the world—without the overarching structure of natural philosophy that subsumed science in Europe and without the naive claims to universal knowledge that modern positivists have sometimes attempted to read back into the Western tradition.

THE CHINESE SCIENCES: QUANTITATIVE

It will be clear by this point that a catalogue of priorities torn out of context can only give a distorted impression of what is worth knowing about

3. Hu Daojing, ed., *Meng-ch'i pi-t'an chiao-cheng* [Brush talks from Dream Brook], modern variorum ed., 2 vols. (ca. 1090; Peking: Chung-hua Shu-chü, 1960), item 123. For a more extensive discussion of Shen's attitude, see Nathan Sivin, s.v. "Shen Kua," in *Dictionary of Scientific Biography*. An earlier astronomical passage of similar purport is translated in Nathan Sivin, *Cosmos and Computation in Early Chinese Mathematical Astronomy* (Leiden: Brill, 1969), 61–62.

science in China. Regardless of how clearly certain features of early science may appear to anticipate today's knowledge, their contemporary meanings had little in common with those of modern science. In describing the sciences below, therefore, I pay as much attention to context as to accomplishment. The Chinese sciences will be portrayed, in other words, not as a succession of triumphs of objective knowledge abstracted from a morass of superstition but as one important thread firmly woven into the fabric of culture.

The sciences described will be those the Chinese defined by applying their concepts of order to various areas of experience—the sky for astronomy and astrology, the bodies of humans and animals for medicine, and so on. As I have already pointed out, this is a very different demarcation from that of modern science.

Mathematics

It is an old Western habit (which those mathematical pioneers, the ancient Mesopotamians, did not share) to think of mathematics as a quintessentially pure science dedicated to the fundamental exploration of number and extension, with practical applications a matter of little interest to the most esteemed sort of mathematician. In China mathematics was not the queen of the sciences but their servant.

Nearly one thousand Chinese mathematical treatises, beginning in the second century A.D. or a little earlier, survive from previous centuries. The great majority have to do with practical matters of the kinds officials, their clerks, and landowners (and increasingly, in the last ten centuries, merchants) would encounter: surveying, determining areas and volumes, calculating exchange rates and taxes payable in money and commodities, and figuring costs of transportation, materials, and labor. Techniques remained numerical and algebraic, with trigonometric approximations that made it possible from the eleventh century on to do much of the work of geometry with no more need to visualize figures in space than one would need today when solving simple problems on a calculator.

A severely logical and axiomatic corpus of proofs like that of Euclid never emerged to provide a unifying standard of rigor in the quantitative sciences. One cannot argue that national character ruled such rigor out, for we find the beginnings of a universal set of definitions, spanning science, language, ethics, and other fields, in the surviving writings of the abortive Mohist school (ca. 300 B.C.). That some Chinese were capable of constructing geometric proofs is clear from surviving examples beginning in the third century A.D., but this remained as minor a concern as numerical procedures were in Europe before algebra was introduced from the Orient beginning in the thirteenth century.

Chinese mathematics was instrumental from the start. At first, problems were set up with computing rods on a surface ruled off in squares

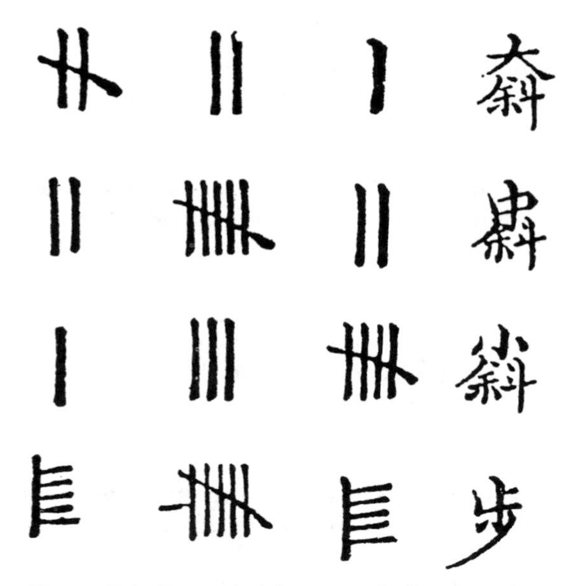

Figure 7.1. Example of matrix algebra notation from a textbook of 1303. The leftmost of these three simultaneous equations corresponds to $-2x + 2y + z = 15$. The equations are written from top to bottom, and a negative coefficient is indicated by a diagonal slash. Figures 7.1 through 7.5 are reproduced from Joseph Needham, *Science and Civilisation in China* (Cambridge, 1954–), by permission of Cambridge University Press.

like a checkerboard. As the rods were manipulated in appropriate squares, the counting board could represent a two-dimensional array of numbers (figure 7.1). The potentialities of this device were gradually exploited until by ca. 1300 it was being used to manipulate the coefficients of equations in several powers of up to four unknowns. By that time the counting board was being replaced by the abacus, an instrument roughly as speedy as but no more flexible than an early twentieth-century adding machine, and extremely well suited to the routine needs of the growing urban merchant class. Because the abacus could only represent a dozen or so digits in a linear array, it was useless for the most advanced algebra until it was supplemented by pen-and-paper notation. There were few important innovations at the highest level of mathematics from the mid fourteenth century until the seventeenth century, when the Jesuit missionaries prompted an efflorescence of interest in European geometry, true trigonometry, logarithms, and so on. This hiatus may have been part of the price paid for the convenience of the abacus.

The predominantly practical orientation of Chinese mathematics made it neither inferior nor superior to the Western tradition. Its lack of development at the abstract geometric level was balanced by its strength in numerical problem solving. Algebra reached Europe ready-made after it had emerged from a long process of convergent discovery and interaction in China, India, and the Islamic world. Many comparatively late European "discoveries," such as Pascal's triangle of coefficients (published in 1665, but known in the sixteenth century) and Horner's method for solving numerical higher equations (1819), were, we now know, named in ignorance of their Chinese origins (the former ca. 1100 or earlier, the latter ca. 1245).

There was a theoretical and speculative side of Chinese mathematics that modern historians have generally ignored, at some cost to our understanding of what the art meant to its practitioners. The senses of both words used for mathematics before modern times, *shu* and *suan,* include numerology. They refer as well to a variety of divination techniques that identify regularities—not necessarily quantitative—underlying the flux of natural phenomena.

Often, especially in the early centuries of mathematics, prognosticating the future and divining the hidden were thought to be among the powers of master computators. There is an obvious parallel with the complementarity of mathematical astronomy and astrology, which we find not only in China, India, and Islam, but in the West as late as the time of Kepler. The form of the relationship of course varied with the intellectual and social character of the two activities in each culture.

Mathematical Astronomy

According to the Chinese theory of monarchy, the ruling dynasty remained fit to rule because of the accord the emperor maintained with the cosmic order. This accord depended on his personal virtue and his correct performance of certain rituals. His special status in the order of nature enabled him to maintain a corresponding order in the political realm, for the state was a microcosm. If the emperor lacked virtue or was careless in his duties, disorderly phenomena would appear in the sky or elsewhere in nature as a warning of potential disaster in the political sphere.

This theory divided celestial phenomena into those that were regular and could be computed and those that were irregular and unpredictable and thus omens. Astronomers had two tasks. First, mathematical astronomy (*li*) was to incorporate as many phenomena as possible in a correct calendar—actually an ephemeris that included, in addition to days and lunar months, predictions of planetary phenomena and eclipses. Second, astrology (*t'ien-wen,* which in modern Chinese has come to mean astronomy) was to observe unpredictable phenomena and to interpret their political meaning. Thus, the emperor could be warned that all was not well in his realm, so that he could mend his ways and take appropriate administrative measures—or be reassured if the omen was favorable.

The calendar, issued in the emperor's name, became part of the ritual paraphernalia that demonstrated his dynasty's right to rule (a function not entirely different from that of economic indicators in a modern nation). Astrological observations could easily be manipulated and thus could be dangerous in the hands of someone trying to undermine the current dynasty (the analogy with economic indicators is again obvious). It was therefore a principle of state policy that the proper place to do astronomy was the imperial court. In certain periods it was illegal to do it elsewhere.

The most sophisticated accomplishments of Chinese mathematics are largely concentrated in astronomical and chronological reckoning. Astronomers' ability to use what amounts to higher-order equations, to deal with apparent rather than mean celestial motions, and to determine astronomical constants with great precision grew steadily until the ephemerides reached their zenith shortly before 1300. Although lunar eclipses could be predicted with considerable accuracy by 100 B.C., the lack of the spherical geometry or trigonometry needed to calculate accurately the intersection of the moon's shadow cone with the earth's sphere made solar eclipses an abiding problem. The tendency of the imperial court to look abroad for technicians who could deal with it was fateful for the development of astronomy within China, as we will see below. Beneath the steady evolution of computational astronomy over two thousand years in China lay a foundation not only of observational instruments but of data recording systems for centuries on end. Joseph Needham has summarized what is characteristically Chinese in this foundation:

1. The elaboration of large and complex observational and demonstrational instruments, from at least the second century B.C. to the great bronze armillaries of 1421 still on display at the Purple Mountain Observatory, Nanjing (figure 7.2).
2. The invention of the clock drive, and perhaps of the clock escapement itself, in a long series of great astronomical clocks culminating in the eleventh century. A water-driven mechanism rotated an armillary sighting tube for observation, a celestial globe, and a variety of time indicators (figure 7.3).
3. The maintenance of accurate, dated records of such phenomena as eclipses, novae, comets, and sunspots over a longer continuous period than in any other civilization.
4. Early star catalogues embodying quantitative positional data (the earliest possibly from the fourth century B.C., with extant observations from ca. 70 B.C.). No less important, although not as old

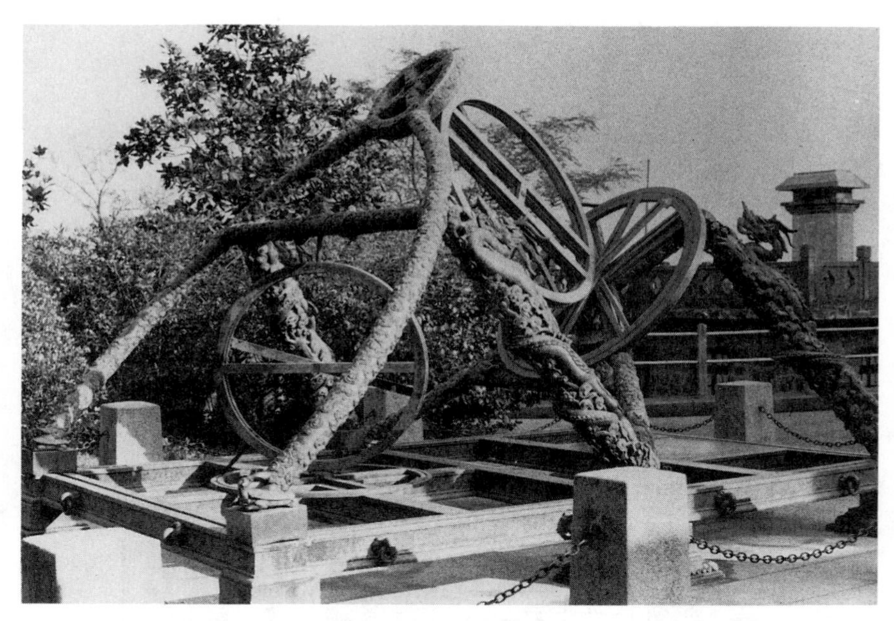

Figure 7.2. "Abridged armillary sphere" of 1421, now at the Purple Mountain Observatory, Nanjing.

as Mesopotamian cuneiform records, are a recently excavated second-century ephemeris and a table of planetary motions from 244 B.C. to 177 B.C.

5. A coordinate system mainly oriented on the equator and the equatorial pole, unlike the ecliptic system prevalent in Europe and Islam until it was replaced in the late sixteenth century with a system like that used in China.
6. Among several early Chinese conceptions of the universe, one in which it was boundless and in which the stars floated in empty space. Perhaps because of its audacity, the details of this cosmic scheme were lost early, and no influence on astronomical practice has been documented.[4]

Despite the limitations of pretelescopic observation, ancient astrological records have proved useful in many ways to modern astronomers. The orbital periods of such celestial bodies as Halley's comet and the frequency of sunspot cycles have been determined with confidence;

4. Based on Joseph Needham, *Science and Civilisation in China,* 7 vols. projected (Cambridge: Cambridge University Press, 1954–), 3:458; for a fuller discussion and references see Leo Goldberg and Lois Edwards, eds., *Astronomy in China: A Trip Report of the American Astronomy Delegation* (Washington, D.C.: National Academy of Sciences, 1979), chap. 2.

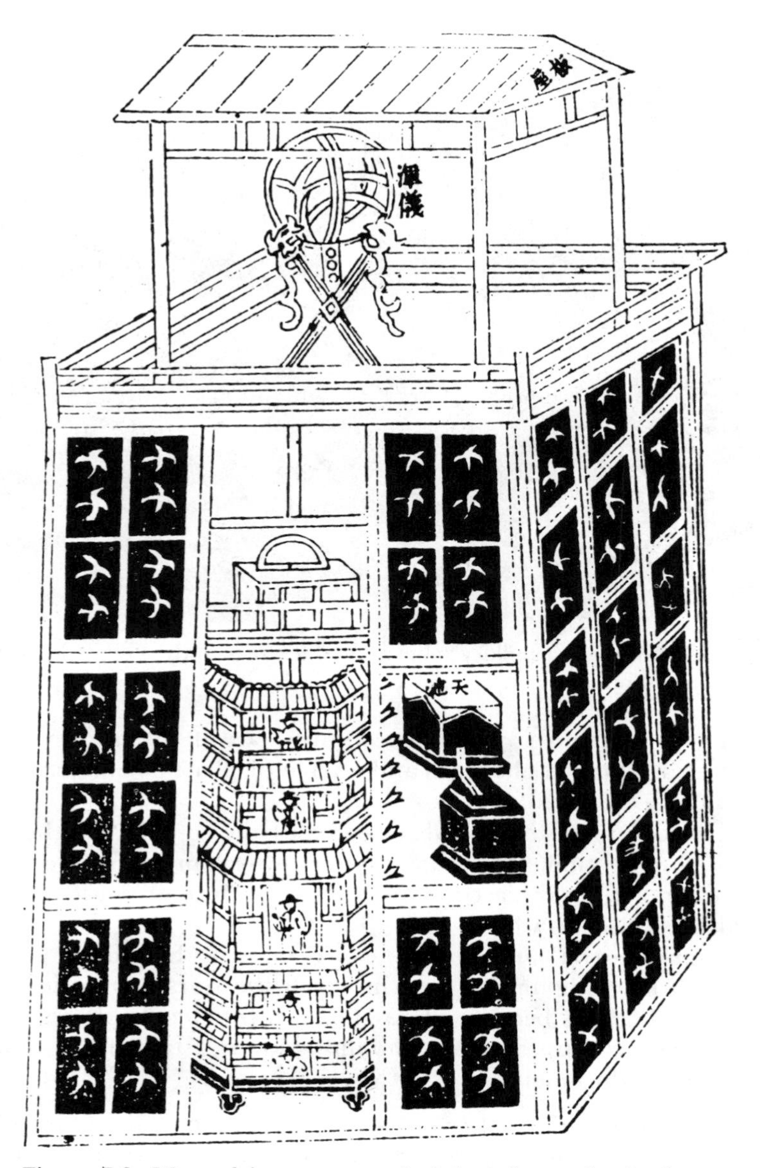

Figure 7.3. Water-driven astronomical clock from a book of ca. 1089.

detailed descriptions of supernova explosions that coincide with today's radio sources have been compiled.[5]

Chinese records have been most productive, supplemented primarily by those of Japan, Korea, and the Islamic world. European records have proved less useful for most of these purposes, since the churchmen and educated laymen who knew astronomy between the late Middle Ages and the seventeenth century generally accepted the Aristotelian dictum that there could be no change in the skies beyond the sphere of the moon. Comets and similar phenomena were considered events below the sphere of the moon (meteorological, more or less) and thus usually not worth noting.

A good part of the historical research under way in the People's Republic of China is devoted to exploring early records for information that bears on current scientific problems. Because of the wide scope of recorded astrological portents, the fruit of this labor has benefited other disciplines besides astronomy. For instance, over the past quarter century three major projects have resulted in detailed tables of earthquakes across the breadth of China and through its recorded history.[6]

Mathematical Harmonics

The third of the quantitative sciences studied the mathematical relations between sounds and the physical arrangements that produced them. The Pythagoreans in the sixth century B.C., it has often been said, motivated two and a half millennia of scientific exploration with their conviction that number and measure underlay the order perceptible in nature, even those aspects of it that appeared purely qualitative. The Pythagorean faith arose from the discovery that the main musical intervals produced by plucking strings of different lengths are related by simple ratios (a string half as long produces the octave, one two-thirds as long gives the fifth, and so on). Chinese harmonics was a similar blend of mathematics and numerology and was concerned with the dimensions of

5. For citations of Chinese research see Nathan Sivin, "Current Research on the History of Science in the People's Republic of China," *Chinese Science* 3 (1978): 39–58. David H. Clark and F. Richard Stephenson, *The Historical Supernovae* (Oxford: Pergamon Press, 1977), discuss ancient star explosions.

6. Chinese Academy of Sciences, Earthquake Working Committee, Historical Group, *Chung-kuo ti-chen tzu-liao nien-piao* [A chronology of materials on Chinese earthquakes], 2 vols. (Peking: Science Press, 1956); Chinese Academy of Sciences, Institute of Geophysics, *Chung-kuo ti-chen mu-lu* [A chronological list of Chinese earthquakes], 2 vols. (Peking: Institute of Geophysics, 1970; reprint, 1 vol., Washington, D.C.: Center for Chinese Research Materials, 1976); Hsieh Yü-shou and Ts'ai Mei-piao, eds., *Chung-kuo ti-chen li-shih tzu-liao hui-pien* [Collected materials on the history of Chinese earthquakes], 5 vols. (Peking: Science Press, 1983–). On the use of historical compilations in theoretical studies see J. Tuzo Wilson, "Mao's Almanac: 3,000 Years of Killer Earthquakes," *Saturday Review*, 19 Feb. 1972, 60–64.

resonant pipes. These pitch pipes provided the standards for ritual bells and stone chimes.

The approaches in East and West were by no means the same. Whereas the Pythagoreans proceeded by subdividing the octave, the Chinese multiplied the string lengths repeatedly by either 2/3 or 4/3 to generate a series (or "spiral") of fifths within the octave. The attempt to draw the most general significances of harmonics was equally ambitious at both ends of Eurasia. To give only one example, the Chinese adapted the pitch pipes as metrological standards of length, volume, and (indirectly) weight.

Harmonics in China is of interest not only for its use in connecting number and nature but for its application in musical performance, above all in the ceremonial music of the court. Music, like astronomy, was cultivated as an aspect of the imperial charisma.

In 1978 a set of sixty-five elaborate bronze chime bells with gold-inlaid inscriptions was unearthed in a tomb dated from the fifth century B.C. The bells produce tones over a range of five octaves; each bell produces two related tones when struck in two different places, a feat that involved remarkably sophisticated trial-and-error design by almost certainly illiterate craftsmen.[7]

THE CHINESE SCIENCES: QUALITATIVE

Most of the aspects of natural order studied in early science were not governed by number and measure. The patterns of function and dysfunction in the human body, for instance, could be accounted for only by qualitative theories. In the early West such theories incorporated a variety of explanatory entities, among them Empedocles' four elements and schemes of pneumata, exhalations, and humors. Such concepts labeled the aspects of a given thing or activity and thus divulged what it had in common with, and how it differed from, other things or activities that could be so analyzed.

By A.D. 200 at the latest, Chinese thinkers had elaborated two main ways to distinguish the phases of a process in time or a configuration in space. Temporal processes in nature were generally considered cyclical, and configurations were thought of as finite. One important theoretical entity was the complementary pair yin and yang, which when applied to processes stood for their taking and giving, abiding and transforming,

7. See Sinyan Shen, "Acoustics of Ancient Chinese Bells," *Scientific American* 256, no. 4 (April 1987): 104–10. For the theory of tuning to which these bells were adapted, see Cheng-Yih Chen (Ch'eng Chen-i), "The Generation of Chromatic Scales in the Chinese Bronze Set-Bells of the −5th Century," *Science and Technology in Chinese Civilization*, ed. Cheng-Yih Chen (Singapore: World Scientific, 1987), 155–97.

retracting and expanding, relaxing and stimulating aspects, and when applied to configurations stood for the ventral and dorsal, lower and upper, inner and outer aspects and analogous functions that could be thought of as feminine and masculine pairs. Yin and yang were without exception relational conceptions. As a modern textbook of traditional medicine puts it, "Considering the relation of chest and back, the chest is yin and the back yang; but when associating chest and abdomen, the chest, being above, is assigned to yang, and the abdomen, below, to yin." Similarly, yin and yang did not necessarily correspond to female and male; an old man may be yin when compared with a young man, and a young woman yang when compared with an old woman. Something is yin or yang only in reference to an ensemble of which it is a part.[8]

In addition to resolving any whole into its yin and yang aspects, one could understand it in terms of a similar system of five phases (*wu-hsing,* often mistranslated as "five elements" by false analogy with the Greek four elements). This understanding was not different from yin and yang but merely finer textured. In cycles of change the phases labeled "water" and "fire" stood for the most intensive aspects of yin and yang; "metal" and "wood" stood for the less intensive aspects; and "earth" stood for the aspect in which the opposed tendencies were balanced and in effect neutralized each other. The use of the five phases in the study of spatial relations was analogous. Most commonly four of the five stood for the cardinal points of the compass and the quarters of the sun's annual path corresponding to the four seasons, and earth stood for the central point on which others pivoted. Thus, for instance, in scientific discourse earth always implied balance and the neutral center; it did not refer to particles of earth as ultimate constituents.

Yin-yang and the five phases were not primarily technical concepts. Like the European notion of cause and effect, they belonged to everyday language and were likely to be used whenever anyone tried to explain structure and change. At the same time, like cause and effect they had more specialized meanings in learned discourse. As each of the qualitative sciences assumed its classical form, yin-yang and the five phases were given special definitions related to the subject matter of that field and were supplemented with other technical conceptions to provide a language adequate for theory. Because the sciences evolved independently, the exact meanings of common concepts tended to differ considerably from one discipline to another.

8. Kwangchou Armed Forces, Rear Support Units, Medical Administrative Organization, *Hsin-pien Chung i-hsueh kai-yao* [New essentials of Chinese medicine] (Peking: People's Hygiene Press, 1972), 2. This work is translated in Nathan Sivin, *Traditional Medicine in Contemporary China,* Science, Medicine, and Technology in East Asia, no. 2 (Ann Arbor: Center for Chinese Studies, 1988), 203.

Astrology

Mathematical astronomy has been described above as the science of celestial phenomena that can be predicted and thus need not be observed. Astrology, its complement, depended on data available only through contemplating the sky. It sought to discern the significance of unpredictable phenomena for current politics, interpreting observed data in part by precedent and in part by theoretical analysis.

In the standard histories published by successive dynasties we find records of a great variety of phenomena involving solar eclipses, sunspots, the stars and planets, and comets, as well as what would now be considered atmospheric phenomena and terrestrial prodigies. The character of the record and its contemporary use are perhaps best revealed by example. Here is the account of the great supernova of 1006 from the treatise on astrology in the official history of the Sung dynasty. It is one of several accounts in Chinese sources that, when pieced together, provide rich data on the supernova and allow its identification with a present-day radio source.

> On the fifteenth sexagenary day, fourth month, third year of the Luminous Virtue reign period [May 6, 1006], a Chou-po star appeared. It emerged in the south of the lunar lodge Base, 1° west of the constellation Mounted Guard [twenty-seven stars, mostly in Lupus]. Its form resembled that of the half-moon, and it had pointed rays. It glowed so brightly that objects could be distinguished by its light. It passed to the east of the constellation Treasury-and-Tower, and in the eighth month, following the rotation of the sky, "entered the turbid zone" [i.e., set with the sun and thus became invisible]. In the eleventh month it appeared once again in Base. Thereafter it was seen regularly heliacally rising in the east in the eleventh month and setting in the southwest in the eighth month.

Earlier in the same treatise the astrological characteristic of a Chou-po star, one of five canonical classes of auspicious stars, is noted in long-established language: "A Chou-po star is yellow in color and brilliant; the state in correspondence to which it appears will greatly prosper." The last phrase refers to a system of interpretation in which each part of the sky corresponds to an area of China. Where the manifestation appears indicates the part of the country affected. This instance corresponds roughly to modern Honan province.

Astrological interpretations are neither mumbo jumbo nor unsuccessful science. They are best understood, like modern economic indicators, as a technical framework for policy debates, resolved, as often as not, on other grounds. Faith in the validity of astrological categories, like confidence in extensively manipulated statistics today, persists despite their repeated failure to deliver accurate predictions.

In the biography of Chang Chih-po, an imperial commissioner in

1006, there is a fragment of the discussion that followed the appearance of a new star. We find Chang attempting to turn the attention of the court away from the auspiciousness of the omens and the details of interpretation toward the moral vigilance of the monarch, which Chang urged should not be relaxed at moments of good tiding:[9]

> When the Chou-po star appeared, the astronomer-royal reported it as an auspicious portent. The court officials prostrated themselves at the palace gates to offer congratulations. Chang expressed the view that the Ruler of Men ought to cultivate his virtue in response to the celestial phenomena, but that the appearances and disappearances of such stars had no particular significance [literally, "were not tied to anything"]. He proceeded to outline the essentials for mastering the Way [of correct government].

These essentials, we can be sure, supported the politics that Chang favored.

The inseparability of astrology from politics should not be taken to imply that the former was less pure a science than mathematical astronomy. Their institutional setting was the same, at least until classicists outside government circles in the seventeenth century took up the computation of ancient eclipses and other phenomena to understand early technical writings, correct the chronology of the Confucian scriptures, and test their authenticity. In early astronomy the great concentration of effort on solar eclipses, the relative neglect of such interesting topics as latitude theory and apparent planetary longitudes, and the use of gnomon-shadow observations for many centuries after armillary instruments had surpassed the gnomon in accuracy all represent the direct imprint on mathematical astronomy of court ritual patterns and the social norms behind them. The difference between astronomy and astrology was a contrast of emphasis on the quantitative as opposed to the qualitative and on objective motions as opposed to the correlation between celestial and political events.

Medicine

The data collected over the centuries about the body, health, and disorders were structured by the concepts of nature described earlier, form-

9. The three translations are from *Sung shih* (Standard history of the Sung period) (Peking: Chung-hua shu-chü, 1977), 56:1226, 52:1076, and 310:10,187. For additional sources and excellent discussions based on freer translations see Bernard R. Goldstein and Ho Peng Yoke, "The 1006 Supernova in Far Eastern Sources," *Astronomical Journal* 70 (1965): 748–53. For a worldwide study drawing on Goldstein and Ho, see Clark and Stephenson, *The Historical Supernovae*, 114–39. The lunar lodges were twenty-eight divisions of the sky along the equator that were used for recording locations of astronomical events. Base, one of these lodges, was centered about R.A. 14h 20m, and the brightest stars in Mounted Guard (mostly in the Western constellation Lupus) were between −35 and −40 degrees in declination. Treasury-and-Tower was a group of about ten stars in Centaurus.

ing a coherent body of theory used to diagnose and treat illness.[10] Classical medicine deserves the adjective "scientific" no less (but no more) than its counterparts in Western culture until recent times. It provided health care for a small portion of the Chinese populace. The majority of its patients and its more eminent practitioners belonged to the upper crust of society. Most of the afflicted among the Chinese population over the course of history had no access to the few fully qualified physicians. They depended on a great variety of less educated healers, ranging from herbalists to priests—a situation that would have been perfectly familiar in eighteenth-century France.[11]

What we call medicine incorporates and imposes order on experience related to every aspect of health, disease, and injury. One Chinese scheme of the major divisions of medicine included theoretical studies of health and disorder; therapeutics; the theory and practice of longevity techniques, including sexual hygiene; pharmacognosy; and veterinary medicine. Pharmacognosy, the study of vegetable, animal, and mineral substances used in therapy, brings together so much information on the sources and characteristics of thousands of drug ingredients that its literature was studied not only for therapeutic purposes, but also as compendia of natural history.[12] Prescriptions made up of both crude drugs and extracts were commonly used in combination with a great variety of other therapeutic means, including acupuncture and moxibustion, dietary regulation, calisthenics, breathing exercises, and massage.

In acupuncture needles were inserted into the flesh at certain points; in moxibustion cones of punk were burnt on the skin at those points. These stimuli affected what traditional physicians considered a circulation of vital fluid throughout the body (figure 7.4) and what clinical researchers today in China and abroad are more inclined to see as peripheral nerve endings and receptors. On the whole, acupuncture was classically considered a minor component of therapy, usually effective

10. The general level of Western publications on Chinese medicine is extremely low. The only penetrating analysis of classical medical concepts in any European language is Manfred Porkert, *The Theoretical Foundations of Chinese Medicine,* MIT East Asian Science Series, no. 3 (Cambridge, Mass.: MIT Press, 1974). For a Chinese outline of medical doctrine see Sivin, *Traditional Medicine in Contemporary China,* 201–427. The sections of *Science and Civilisation in China* on medicine are not yet in press. Several excellent essays by Needham in collaboration with Lu Gwei-djen have been gathered in *Clerks and Craftsmen in China and the West: Lectures and Addresses on the History of Science and Technology* (Cambridge: Cambridge University Press, 1970), in particular "Medicine and Chinese Culture," 263–93.

11. The only substantial study that looks beyond classical medicine to the diversity of health care in early times is Paul U. Unschuld, *Medicine in China: A History of Ideas* (Berkeley: University of California Press, 1985).

12. Paul U. Unschuld, *Medicine in China: A History of Pharmaceutics* (Berkeley: University of California Press, 1986), gives information about a large part of this literature.

only for certain disorders and when continued over a long period. In modern Chinese clinical practice it is of course impossible to evaluate acupuncture separately from the other Chinese and Western remedies with which the patient is treated.

Acupuncture has been promoted to the status of wonder cure by the American media in their restless quest for novelty. It has proved attractive out of proportion to the rest of traditional therapy. It is exotic to Americans, who were very late in learning about its long-standing popularity in East Asia. Few know about its use in Europe for roughly three hundred years or its vogue among physicians in early nineteenth-century America.[13] It is usually confused with acupuncture anesthesia (or analgesia), a new technique used in modern surgery since the late 1950s. In traditional surgery (limited to external medicine, amputation, and bonesetting), the only anesthetics we know to have been used were drugs—mainly alcohol, datura, and cannabis.

Classical Chinese medicine has often been represented as an empirical science based on the clinically sound use of effective natural drugs and other remedies. In this view, theories served primarily as mnemonic devices or as mystifications to confuse the untrained. Some modern physicians who have not troubled themselves to study classical medical doctrines dismiss them as futilities of the feudal past. Other authors have portrayed classical medicine as a remarkable corpus of theory—based on adaptations of the yin-yang and five-phases concepts—that succeeded in understanding the body as a many-leveled system and treated its ills holistically. They accordingly recommend it as a corrective to the impersonal, excessively lesion-centered and nihilistic tendencies of modern biomedical therapy. The mild and usually nonspecific remedies of traditional medicine are sometimes, but by no means always, expected to contribute to this reform. A closer acquaintance with the literature of classical medicine and with its practice in today's China suggests that these are partial pictures of a more complicated reality.

Before 1920 the strengths of medicine everywhere lay predominantly in the care of mild and chronic disorders. There was little physicians could do for most acute emergencies beyond strengthening the patient's defenses and preparing his family for the worst. With that emphasis on mild and chronic cases in mind, we are better able to judge the importance of gentle, gradual remedies, practices aimed at evaluating and improving the physical, mental, spiritual, and social circumstances of the patient, and theories used to relate symptoms to a multitude of therapeutic measures, both to design a flexible program of therapy and to

13. James H. Cassedy, "Early Uses of Acupuncture in the United States, with an Addendum (1826) by Franklin Bache, M.D.," *Bulletin of the New York Academy of Medicine,* 2d series, 50 (1974): 892–906.

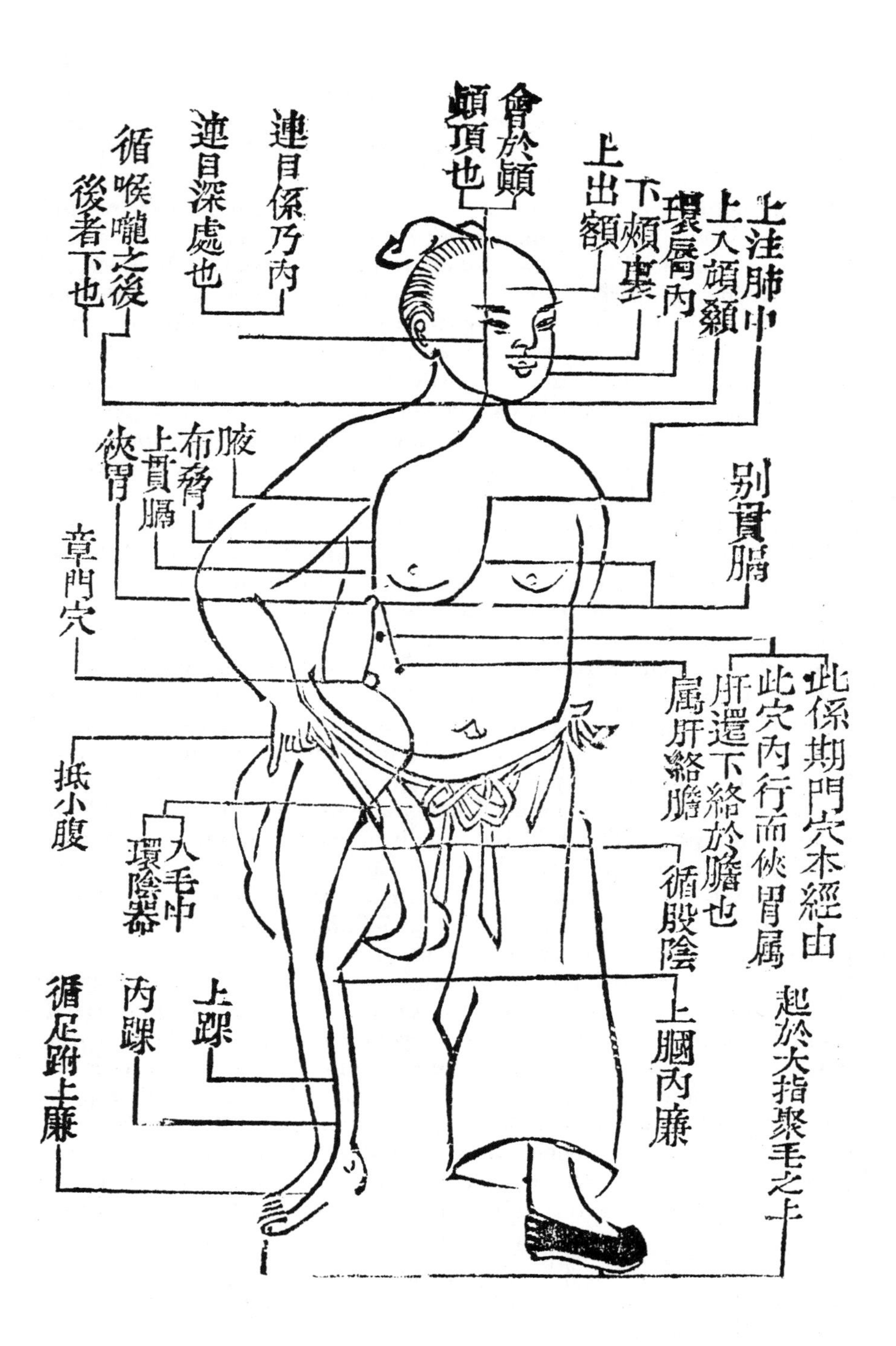
上注肺中
上入頏顙
環脣內
下頰裏
上出額
會於顛
顛頂也
連目係乃內
連目深處也
循喉嚨之後
後者下也
腋
布脅
上貫膈
挾胃
別貫膈
章門穴
此係期門穴本經由
此穴內行而挾胃屬
肝還下絡於膽也
屬肝絡膽
抵小腹
入毛中
環陰器
循股陰
上膕內廉
上踝
內踝
循足跗上廉
起於大指聚毛之上

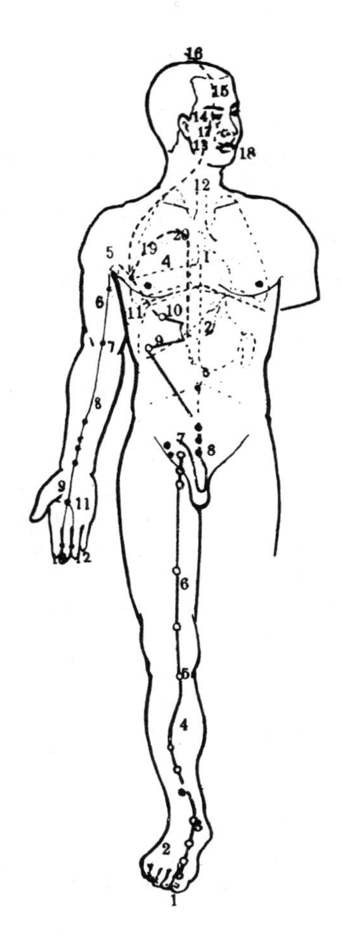

Figure 7.4. Similar diagrams of acupuncture loci from an eighteenth-century source and a textbook of 1960.

make those relations comprehensible to the patient. Theory also maximized control of acute disorders by emphasizing prevention and early treatment.

That Chinese medicine does not give a detailed and accurate picture of anatomy and physiology was not a handicap. The high state of anatomical knowledge in Europe by the time Andreas Vesalius died in 1564 was the glory of medicine as a branch of academic learning but had little application to medicine as the care of suffering people. It was not until the early nineteenth century that diseases in the living could be connected reliably with abnormalities seen when cadavers were dissected. Surgeons could exploit this knowledge fully only as disease came to be thought of in terms of localized lesions, as asepsis and anesthesia made local intervention safe, and as the organization of the medical profession imposed a single high standard of qualification. In the United States, for instance, the changes that made surgery safe and routine were not well under way until about 1920.

Unlike modern biomedicine, the traditional Chinese art could not draw on anything comparable to modern biology, chemistry, or physics. For that reason, its concepts look more like those prevalent in Europe four hundred years ago. They are not concerned with microorganisms or details of the body's organs and tissues. The strength of classical Chinese medical discourse lay rather in its sophisticated analysis of how functions were related on many levels, from the vital processes of the body to the emotions to the natural and social environment of the patient, always with therapy in mind. Chinese medicine is best evaluated in the light of this strength rather than according to criteria that could not have been applied anywhere until half a century ago.

Alchemy

Chinese alchemy used chemical techniques to prepare elixirs, which were perfected substances that brought about personal transcendence and eternal life. Elixirs could also be used for medical purposes and for transforming ordinary metals into gold. That is how an alchemist might have defined "external alchemy" (*wai-tan*); its analogue, "internal alchemy" (*nei-tan*), used the language of the laboratory to teach meditational (or sometimes sexual) disciplines in which the adept's body was visualized as the reaction vessel and furnace. In the first millennium the two alchemies were regularly practiced together, but after 1200 little activity in the external art was recorded.

The materials and apparatus of alchemy were on the whole the same as those of pharmacology, with some contributions from metallurgy and other practical chemical arts (figure 7.5). Certain developments, such as elaborate distilling vessels, appear so exclusively in alchemical literature that they may have originated there. The same may be said of gunpowder. What may be the earliest mention of flare mixture composition appears, oddly enough, in a list of external alchemists' misguided activities in a treatise on internal alchemy written not later than the end of the ninth century: "There was a case in which sulphur and realgar were mixed with saltpeter and honey, and burnt. Flames leapt up, burning the alchemist's hands and face and incinerating the building."[14]

The roughly one hundred remaining *wai-tan* books are probably the world's richest source for what was known about reactions and their products up to 1200. They reveal, in fact, that alchemy was not entirely

14. *Chen yuan miao tao yao-lueh* [Essentials of the mysterious Tao of the true origin], in *Cheng-t'ung tao tsang* [Collected Taoist works], 596:3a. On this book see Needham, *Science and Civilisation in China*, vol. 5, part 3, 78–79.

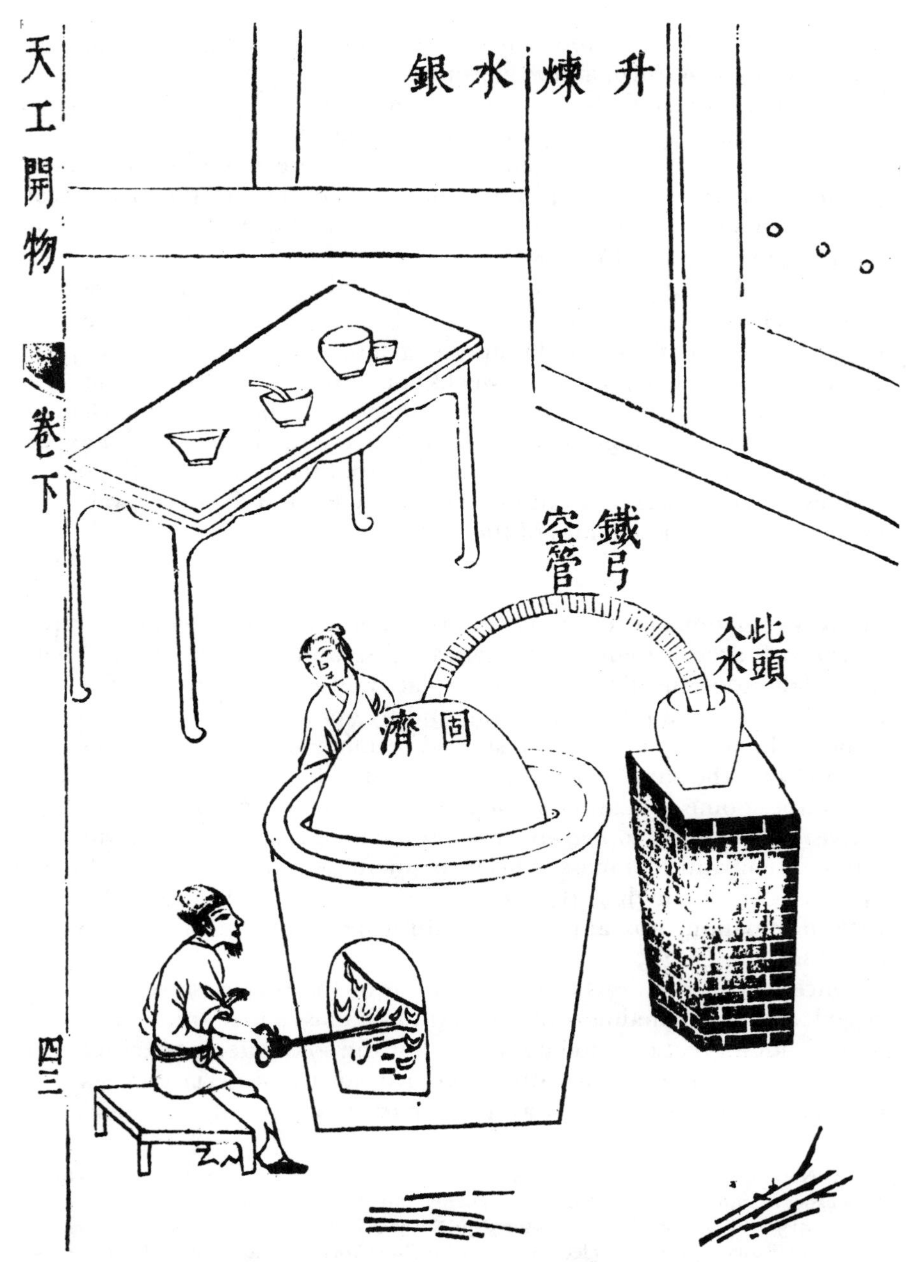

Figure 7.5. Commercial distillation of mercury, from the *Technological Encyclopedia of 1637*.

qualitative; some adepts took a lively interest in what weights of reagents would combine to form a new substance.[15]

Knowledge of chemical change was a means and a by-product, not the aim, of external alchemy. For some practitioners the goal was hardly distinguishable from that of medicine. Others were less interested in a product that would bring health or immortality than in the alchemical process, which they designed to serve as a model of the great cycles of nature, the rhythms of the tao.

No mortal could experience the cosmic cycles in their millennial sweep. These alchemists accelerated the scale of time, using theories based on yin-yang, the five phases, and numerology, to create, in a laboratory procedure that might require a few weeks to a year, an object of mystic contemplation. They believed, like the Pythagoreans before them, that to grasp the constant patterns that underlie the phenomenal chaos of experience is to be freed from the bonds of mortal finitude. As in the other Chinese sciences, the motivation that led to chemical discovery was connected to the deepest values of the seekers.

Siting

Masters of geomancy, or siting (to use the more informative term proposed by Steven J. Bennett), analyzed topographic features to find balanced land configurations in which to place houses and tombs.[16] Alchemy, as we have seen, used the yin-yang and five-phases concepts to understand and manipulate time as it shaped certain laboratory processes; siting adapted the same concepts to the study of space and form in the landscape. Some practitioners depended on their experience to judge the visual balance of topography, and some used readings taken with the famous geomantic compass. This instrument, which among its eighteen or more concentric dials (figure 7.6) incorporated indications of magnetic declination, was apparently a forerunner of the sailor's navigational instrument.

Once its contributions to the evolution of the compass are acknowledged, siting is sometimes shrugged off as a mass superstition. There is indeed not a great deal to be said for it if the sole criteria of evaluation are those of science today. But those are not the criteria that lead to understanding, since siting was not as narrowly focused as modern sci-

15. Nathan Sivin, in Needham, *Science and Civilisation in China,* vol. 5, part 4, 300–305. This essay is summarized in "Chinese Alchemy and the Manipulation of Time," *Isis* 67 (1976): 513–26, especially 521; reprinted in Nathan Sivin, ed., *Science and Technology in East Asia,* History of Science, Selections from Isis (New York: Science History Publications, 1977), 117.

16. Steven J. Bennett, "Patterns of the Sky and Earth: A Chinese Science of Applied Cosmology," *Chinese Science* 3 (1978): 1–26.

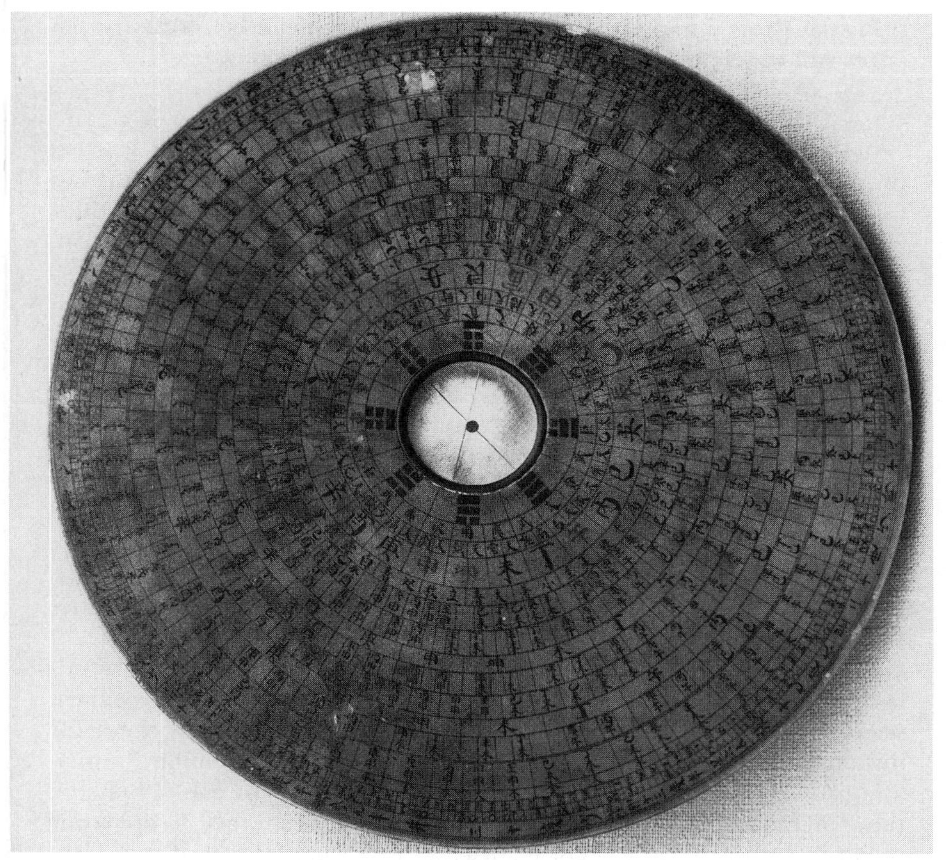

Figure 7.6. A nineteenth-century siting compass, from the author's collection. (Photo by Nathan Sivin)

ence. Siting nevertheless fits the broader definition of a premodern science, for certain schools of practice worked out a system of abstract and objective reasoning about the natural phenomena that concerned them.

Anthropologists have found siting worthy of study because of the way it was used (and is still being used) to resolve conflicts of status between practitioners' clients. Geographers and landscape architects have expressed interest in siting theory because it accomplished for centuries what modern theorists have been trying to do: provide a systematic framework for reasoning that will reliably yield beautiful sites. Because the balance that siting strove for was dynamic and complex, the benefits of the science are in large part aesthetic—not a matter of purely scientific interest, but of no small utility nevertheless. That may explain why siting has proved so durable. It and medicine are the only traditional sciences still widely practiced in Chinese communities today.[17]

Physical Studies

"Physical studies" is a grab bag of traditions that considered a great range of natural phenomena in the light of fundamental concepts. So far these traditions have been little studied, but a great deal in their literatures throws light on early knowledge of change and interaction, whether chemical, physical, or biological.

A few items from the section on trees in one of the most popular treatises suggest the wealth of information to be found there: "If peach is grafted onto persimmon, the fruit will be golden peaches. If peach is grafted onto Japanese apricot, the fruit will be meaty. If male and female gingko trees are planted together, the females will bear fruit. If pomegranate is grafted onto 'flowering cassia' [*Osmanthus fragrans Lour.*], the blossoms will always be red." Because we do not have records left by those who mastered grafting, it is from sources such as this one, as well as writings on materia medica, that the history of Chinese arboriculture must be reconstructed. An analogously broad range of documents must be studied by those who wish to understand many other ancient activities that required technical knowledge.

It would be misleading to leave the impression that the physical studies literature is a trove of information all of which is pertinent to modern science. The mixed character of the tenth-century book just cited, for instance, is obvious from two consecutive items in the section on "human affairs": "When a mother cries and her tears fall into the eye of her son, they will cause damage to its pupil and give rise to a cataract. In epidemic warm-factor disorders [a class of diseases involving fevers], if the clothing of the first person to fall ill is steamed in an earthenware steamer, the rest of the family will not catch the sickness."[18]

The abstract ideas in these extensive compilations also deserve to be investigated. In a study of how yin-yang and the five phases bear on alchemy, P. Y. Ho and Joseph Needham called the ancient application of these ideas "a hitherto unrecorded chapter in the prehistory of the conception of chemical affinity," by which they meant that it "seems to take its place in the linear ancestry of the idea that things can be arranged in

17. Siting is officially considered superstitious and is discouraged in the People's Republic, but it is still practiced. On siting in the New Territories of Hong Kong see Baruch Boxer, "Space, Change and Feng-shui in Tsuen Wan's Urbanization," *Journal of Asian and African Studies* 3 (1968): 226–40.

18. Tsan Ning, *Ke-wu ts'u-t'an* [Simple discourses on the investigation of phenomena] ed. Pai-pu ts'ung-shu chi-ch'eng (ca. 980), 1:4b and 2:16b. Compare the translation in Needham, *Science and Civilisation in China,* vol. 5, part 2, 149.

chemical classes the members of which are susceptible of chemically similar processes."[19]

The Transmission of Science between Civilizations

Things and ideas have flowed between China, Europe, and the other great civilizations regularly since the New Stone Age. Whether such characteristics of the earliest Chinese civilization as writing, the manufacture and use of the wheel, and bronze and iron metallurgy diffused into China from abroad or whether they were reinvented from scratch is still a matter for heated debate. These two hypotheses need not be considered mutually exclusive, for a mere rumor that something exists vastly simplifies making it. In any case the wheel and metalworking did not appear in China fully formed, as we would expect had they been imported.

Wrought iron, for instance, was being made in the mid seventh century B.C., perhaps six centuries later than the wrought iron of Anatolia. Cast-iron objects from the sixth century B.C. have been excavated. Cast iron could not be produced at will in the West for another seventeen centuries. Steel was produced at first from wrought iron, but the industrial processes for making it from cast iron were perfected in the second century B.C. This feat was possible because all the necessary elements were available: efficient furnaces derived from ceramic kilns, reciprocating bellows to provide an air blast, good refractory clays, and phosphorus-rich ores or fluxes to lower the melting point of iron.[20]

Science was part of the flow between East and West from early times. The Greek medical doctrine of the four elements reached China via India by about A.D. 500. Physicians from Byzantium or Syria, possibly Christians, are said to have cured a Chinese emperor in the mid seventh century. Jesuit missionaries in China published a treatise on Western physiology and an anatomical atlas in the mid seventeenth century, but the two books were very little circulated and received practically no attention. The first European book on Chinese medicine was published in 1682, the first on acupuncture in 1683. Alchemical elixirs of Western origin are noted in seventh-century China, and there is some evidence that Chinese alchemical gold was traded or sold abroad. But the greatest foreign scientific influence on China in early centuries, as in the seven-

19. Ping-Yü Ho and Joseph Needham, "Theories of Categories in Early Mediaeval Chinese Alchemy," *Journal of the Warburg and Courtauld Institutes* 22 (1959): 173–210, especially 201; a revised version appears in Needham, *Science and Civilisation in China,* vol. 5, part 4, 322.

20. For a summary of recent research see Tsun Ko [K'o Chün], "The Development of Metal Technology in Ancient China," in *Science and Technology in Chinese Civilization,* ed. Cheng-Yih Chen (Singapore: World Scientific, 1987), 225–43.

teenth-century heyday of Jesuit missionary activity, was exerted in astronomy. A fuller discussion of that field is in order.

Before the middle of the seventh century A.D., after Buddhism had become rooted in China, Indian astronomers worked in the Chinese capital. Their techniques were partly derived from Greek astronomy. They were more reliable for predicting solar eclipses than those current in China. The political significance of solar eclipses led the Chinese court from the turn of the eighth century to depend on resident foreign astronomers. When the Mongols brought China under their rule in the second half of the thirteenth century, their astronomical officials were Islamic, from Persia and Central Asia. Their computational procedures were more accurate than those of their Indian predecessors. Muslims were still performing the same services for the court when Jesuits began competing with them three hundred and fifty years later.

The Jesuit missionaries in China in the early seventeenth century were there not to propagate astronomical science but to convert the empire from the top down to Roman Catholicism. The only established access to the top was in the Astronomical Bureau, which had provided court positions to foreigners for nearly one thousand years. By 1645 the Europeans had gained operational control of the bureau after submitting to the throne a series of treatises that set out in Chinese the mathematical and cosmological foundations of European astronomy and winning several dramatic eclipse prediction contests. They maintained their status in the astronomical civil service past the middle of the eighteenth century.

The church's injunction against teaching the Copernican doctrines of the central sun and the planetary earth in 1616 and the condemnation of Galileo in 1633 made it impossible for the missionaries to disseminate the state of the art as it developed over the next century or so or to explain fully what the accomplishments of Copernicus, Kepler, and Newton had been. As the new astronomy evolved, discussions of it in Chinese by Jesuit writers before 1760 were thus full of gaps and contradictions, which were never explained. What is often considered the great watershed in European scientific consciousness was not revealed in China until late in the nineteenth century, long after it had become commonplace in the West. Nor were the Jesuit writings sufficiently technical and detailed to permit the Chinese to advance world knowledge. Nevertheless, they stimulated a high pitch of astronomical activity.

The geometric and trigonometric approaches and the cosmological framework of the Jesuit writings in Chinese, obsolete though they became as the seventeenth century wore on, precipitated what can only be called a scientific revolution. The best Chinese astronomers of the time (who mainly worked outside the imperial court) adopted new concepts, tools, and methods. They changed their convictions about what constituted an astronomical problem and what significance astronomy could have for the ultimate understanding of nature and even of human society.[21]

This metamorphosis of astronomy did not lead to the fundamental changes in thought and society that are naively supposed to be the inevitable outcomes of a scientific revolution. Conceptual revolutions, like political revolutions, occur at the margins of societies. The astronomers who responded to the Jesuit writings were members of the educated elite who above all felt the responsibility for strengthening and perpetuating traditional ideas. They were, in other words, at the center of their society. It is scarcely surprising that they used what they learned from the West to rediscover and carry to new heights the astronomical techniques of their greatest Chinese predecessors.

Only after the Opium Wars of the early 1840s could the Chinese receive a systematic education in the exact sciences as then taught in Europe. This time the educators were not individual priests dependent on the toleration of their hosts. They were mostly Protestant missionaries exempt from Chinese laws, their right to operate missions and schools guaranteed by imposed treaties and enforced by gunboats. They were no longer appealing, as the Jesuits had done, to an elite intent on adapting new techniques to traditional ends. The Protestant missionaries educated mostly the poor and people of modest means. Even their richer converts came to them because changes in the civil service gave their children little chance of conventional success in the old society.

Late-nineteenth-century Chinese astronomers trained in Western institutions had no reason even to be curious about what their compatriots in earlier times had done. By 1880 Protestant missionaries, generally working with Chinese, had translated from European languages a number of basic textbooks in astronomy, mathematics, and physics and made them generally available at low prices. Their schools, libraries, bookshops, and other institutions were founded to instigate change, not to preserve Chinese civilization.

As the threat of dismemberment by the colonial powers became more imminent, the Chinese government was belatedly persuaded to begin educating modern scientists. In 1866 a department of mathematics and astronomy was added to the T'ung-wen-kuan in Peking, which had previously been a college for interpreters. In 1867 a translation department was added to the Shanghai Arsenal, which had been established two

21. John B. Henderson, *The Development and Decline of Chinese Cosmology* (New York: Columbia University Press, 1984); Benjamin Elman, *From Philosophy to Philology: Intellectual and Social Aspects of Change in Late Imperial China,* Harvard East Asian Monographs, no. 110 (Cambridge, Mass.: Council on East Asian Studies, Harvard University, 1984); Nathan Sivin, "Copernicus in China," *Studia Copernicana* (Warsaw) 6 (1973): 63–122.

years earlier. There Chinese foreign employees of the imperial government systematically undertook the translation and publication of modern works in science, engineering, medicine, law, and so forth. These and the less systematic technical publications of the missionaries were widely distributed and eagerly studied by amateur groups that maintained the tradition begun by the Jesuit writings. The new translations often played a part in the education of statesmen and reformers, for whom they provided a window on the world. The future lay, however, not with those who saw modern technology as a tool to breathe new life into an empire and a traditional culture, but with those at the margin of the old society, educated in modern schools and given employment in imported institutions.

From about 1900 onward, Chinese astronomers began to emerge who were fully prepared to benefit from advanced training abroad. They were educated in missionary institutions as well as in government universities as these appeared. When ten foreign powers extracted heavy indemnities from China after the Boxer Uprising in 1900, the United States used income from its share to support students during their technical training abroad. Scientists trained in the United States, Europe, and Japan, as well as those educated in China, created the first large-scale system of research institutions and an educational system to train scientists. A few of these institutions were founded by foreigners in the image of their own, but—to redirect the words of a leading historian of China—"on all sides of this gleam of Western light, China was being torn apart by forces so powerful that they made the Westerners' efforts poignantly irrelevant."[22]

Since 1949 China has by fits and starts invented policies toward education and science that reflect its own priorities rather than the expectations of other nations.

THE HISTORY OF SCIENCE IN CONTEMPORARY CHINA

In China today it is normal for scientific journals to publish historical studies, for research centers, observatories, and other organizations to house research groups for ancient science and technology, and for modern scientists to be knowledgeable about their country's scientific heritage.[23] This situation contrasts so greatly with that of most other countries that it calls for an explanation.

I have already noted that early astronomical and earthquake records

22. Jonathan Spence, *To Change China: Western Advisors in China, 1620–1960* (Boston: Little, Brown, 1969), 172.

23. Recent astronomical publications and research are summarized in Sivin, "Current Research."

are a valuable resource for current scientific research. But this is only one motivation for the awareness of history. Other reasons are related to China's place in the world. For millennia the Chinese considered their land the one true center of civilization. Over the past century China has had to make an entirely new place for itself as only one member of a large family of nations. For most of the last one hundred years it has been dependent on and has been looked down on by foreigners for that reason. The present government is resolved to make China independent within limits set by the imperatives of survival and is trying to enlist the energies of every citizen.

China's recent policies for technological development have been unique in many respects. They have made unique demands for adaptation on the part of the whole scientific sector of society, which until a couple of decades ago was considered quintessentially Western. Science and engineering were what one learned from foreigners in order to safeguard oneself against them. This view has gradually been changed over the past twenty years by popularizing the history of Chinese science. Children's books, postage stamps, museum exhibits, and school lessons have all carried the message that science is not European but a world enterprise and that over most of history China was one of the great contributors to that enterprise.

It is not difficult to find this point explicitly stated. Consider the afterword to a book for teenagers on every aspect of technical history, published just after the Cultural Revolution: "The achievements of China's ancient science and technology prove that the Chinese people have the ability needed to occupy their rightful place among the world's peoples. These achievements will also encourage our faith and strengthen our resolve, so that in the shortest possible time we may catch up to and surpass the world's most advanced levels of development. China has yet greater contributions to make to humanity."[24] Scientists and medical researchers experience this consciousness as a close linkage between scientific work and political activity.

Enhanced consciousness of Chinese scientific history is not entirely an internal matter. The importance and fascination of the Chinese scientific tradition have long been known in Europe, Japan, and the United States. Scholars in many countries have contributed to understanding it as well

24. Chinese Academy of Sciences, Institute for the History of Natural Sciences, ed., *Chung-kuo ku-tai k'e-hsueh ch'eng-chiu* [Achievements of ancient Chinese science and technology] (Peking: Chung-kuo Ch'ing-nien Ch'u-pan-she, 1978), 706. Written for teenage readers, this comprehensive work contains contributions by China's best-known historians of science and technology. The sentences translated in the present essay do not appear in the English version, *Ancient China's Technology and Science* (Peking: Foreign Languages Press, 1983).

as to making the work of many great Chinese historians of science accessible in other languages.[25]

Educated people all over the world are now prepared to respond to new revelations about Chinese scientific traditions—whether they be new applications for the ancient art of acupuncture or the unique archaeological finds that have been appearing without interruption since the 1950s. The heightened interest has meant a small but perceptible rise in the world's esteem for China. More to the point, it has meant that scientists all over the world are increasingly involved in the give and take that help Chinese scientists to be fully involved in the international scientific community.

25. Historical scholarship, mainly since 1980, is summarized in Nathan Sivin, "Science and Medicine in Imperial China—The State of the Field," *Journal of Asian Studies* 47, no. 1 (1988): 41–90.

EIGHT

□

Women, Marriage, and the Family in Chinese History

Patricia Ebrey

Much has been written about women and the family in traditional China. Early Western observers were naturally struck by the features of the Chinese family that stood in contrast to their own practices, features such as ancestor worship, legally recognized concubinage, large families with several married brothers living together, and lineages that brought together hundreds of kinsmen. Women's situations distressed most Western writers. Nineteenth- and early-twentieth-century observers described in detail the plight of girls who might be killed at birth by parents who did not need another daughter, who could be sold at five or six as indentured servants, whose feet were bound so small that they could hardly walk, who when a little older had to marry whomever their fathers ordered them to marry, who had to submit to frequently tyrannical mothers-in-law after marriage, who might not be allowed to remarry after their husbands' deaths, who had few legal rights to property, and who could be divorced easily and denied custody of their children.[1] "The condition of the Chinese woman is most pitiable," one missionary observed. "Suffering, privation, contempt, all kinds of misery and degradation, seize on her in the cradle and accompany her pitilessly to the tomb."[2]

As noted elsewhere in this volume—the Introduction and Chapters 3, 7, 9, 10, and 13—scholars today have largely overcome the habit of viewing premodern China from the perspective of the modern West. Many features of the traditional Chinese family are now recognized to have

1. See, for instance, Arthur H. Smith, *Village Life in China* (1899; reprint, New York: Little, Brown, 1970), 196–237, and Justus Doolittle, *Social Life of the Chinese* (New York: Harper, 1895), 1:98–112, 2:197–213.

2. M. Huc, *The Chinese Empire* (London: Longman, Brown, Green, and Longmans, 1855), 1:248.

been much more common in world history than corresponding European practices, especially modern European ones. A well-studied example is age at marriage. Through most of Chinese history both women and men married relatively young, women soon after puberty and men not much later. In Western Europe, by contrast, in the eighteenth and nineteenth centuries both men and women were commonly waiting well into their twenties to marry, men often until their late twenties. This difference in age at marriage affects many aspects of family structure. Where women marry early they generally have more children, and the population grows more rapidly. Where men marry in their teens they usually stay in their parents' home, and their wives are under the authority of their mothers. Such arrangements make it easier for the senior generation to set the tone in child-rearing practices, religious and economic activities, and so on, which adds to social conservatism. Large extended families are easier to achieve when generations are short and new members (mostly brides) socialized at young ages. These differences between the Chinese and Western families in the eighteenth and nineteenth centuries are all real and important, but it is now well established that the Western European case is the unusual one, not the Chinese.[3]

If one turns to Eastern, Southern, or Western Europe before the seventeenth century, other contrasts between Europe and China dissolve. Examples of similarities include extensive ties to patrilineal kinsmen (that is, kinsmen with the same surname, linked through males alone), arranged marriages, marriages involving significant financial transactions, and strong patriarchal authority over women and children. If we turn back to the Roman era we discover even more similarities to the Chinese case, such as an emphasis on succession to the family altar and concubinage.[4]

Bringing up these historical changes in the Western family, however, reinforces another common perception of differences between China and the West: social forms changed in the West, often dramatically, whereas they seem to have remained nearly constant in China over several millennia.

Since the early 1960s changes in the Western family have been studied in increasing detail and sophistication. After the Fall of Rome Europe

3. J. Hajnal, "European Marriage Patterns in Perspective," in *Population in History*, ed. D. V. Glass and D. E. O. Eversley (Chicago: Aldine, 1965). In the West late marriage for men was practiced even in the fourteenth and fifteenth centuries in Italy. See David Herlihy, *Medieval Households* (Cambridge: Harvard University Press, 1985), 107–11. Recent research suggests that Japan stood somewhere between China and Western Europe. See Arthur P. Wolf and Susan B. Hanley, eds., *Family and Population in East Asian History* (Stanford: Stanford University Press, 1985), esp. the introduction.

4. On the Roman family see Numa Denis Fustel de Coulanges, *The Ancient City: A Study of the Religion, Laws, and Institutions of Greece and Rome* (1864; reprint, Baltimore: Johns Hopkins University Press, 1980), 32–108.

developed a family and marriage system quite unlike anything else in Eurasia. Whereas the Romans had allowed concubinage, adoption of heirs, and marriage of cousins, all with an eye to continuing a family line and preserving its property, the Catholic church outlawed all these practices. After several centuries of struggle the church was remarkably successful in forging a new system of family and marriage. Scholars studying changes in Western family practices have stressed the conflict between Roman and barbarian customs, the Christian celebration of celibacy, social mobility and status consciousness among elites, and so on. They have shown that the Protestant Reformation had major consequences on the emotional relations among family members, as did industrialization and the modern state.[5]

By contrast, study of the history of the Chinese family is only just beginning. Most textbooks on Chinese history discuss the family, if at all, in an introductory section as part of the background. If they mention change in the family before the twentieth century, it is a decline in the status of women in the late T'ang or the Sung (discussed later). Scholarly analyses of the family in the Chinese past have also been relatively unconcerned with change, concentrating on either general principles or particular institutions in specific periods but not changes from one period to another.[6] As described in most studies, the Chinese family had little reason to change because it was nearly perfectly constructed of reinforcing strands: ethics, property law, marriage practices, concepts

5. See, for instance, Diane Owen Hughes, "From Brideprice to Dowry in Mediterranean Europe," *Journal of Family History* 3, no. 3 (1978): 262–96; Jack Goody, *The Development of the Family and Marriage in Europe* (Cambridge: Cambridge University Press, 1983); Herlihy, *Medieval Households;* Georges Duby, *The Knight the Lady and the Priest: The Making of Modern Marriage in Medieval France* (New York: Pantheon, 1983); Christiane Klapisch-Zuber, *Women, Family, and Ritual in Renaissance Italy* (Chicago: University of Chicago Press, 1985); Lawrence Stone, *The Family, Sex and Marriage in England, 1500–1800* (New York: Harper & Row, 1977); and Louise A. Tilly, "Demographic History Faces the Family: Europe since 1500," *Trends in History* 3 (1985): 45–68.

6. Studies of change, of course, are not possible until scholars have undertaken detailed studies of both particular periods and general principles. Many useful studies of these types in English are cited elsewhere in this chapter. Other studies include the various chapters in David C. Buxbaum, ed., *Chinese Family Law and Social Change in Historical and Comparative Perspective* (Seattle: University of Washington Press, 1978), especially the chapters by Jack L. Dull, Tai Yen-hui, and Shūzō Shiga; several chapters in Kwang-ching Liu, ed., *Orthodoxy in Late Imperial China* (Berkeley: University of California Press, forthcoming), especially the chapters by Charlotte Furth and Jonathan Ocko; the various chapters in Richard W. Guisso and Stanley Johannesen, eds., *Women in China* (Youngstown, N.Y.: Philo Press, 1981); Ann Waltner's articles, including "The Loyalty of Adopted Sons in Ming and Early Qing China," *Modern China* 10 (1984): 441–59 and "The Moral Status of the Child in Late Imperial China: Childhood in Ritual and in Law," *Social Research* 54 (1986): 667–87; and some of my own studies, such as *Family and Property in Sung China: Yüan Ts'ai's Precepts for Social Life* (Princeton: Princeton University Press, 1984) and "Concubines in Sung China," *Journal of Family History* 11, no. 1 (1986): 1–24.

of descent and gender differentiation, even criminal law all served to strengthen fixed principles of family behavior. Moreover, when change has been noticed, it has been interpreted as the result of changes in ideas much more than changes in the economy, the state, or even popular religion. For example, the cult of widow chastity is traced to the Sung philosopher who asserted that losing one's virtue was worse than starving to death, and lineages are traced to the scholar who set up a charitable estate for his kinsmen. Should not the strength of the state, the commercialization of the economy, the character of elites, and shifts in popular piety have had effects on Chinese family life of the sort that they did in the West? A major goal of this chapter is to show that they did. I only give a sketchy overview of how the early Chinese family system was linked to the social, political, and economic systems of the Chou through Han periods. The key changes that occurred from T'ang times on and their links to other historical changes are examined in more detail because I have concentrated my own research on this middle period.

The early development of the Chinese family may be traced using three sets of ideas and practices: those concerned with descent (patrilineality), with ethics (filial piety), and with authority and property (patriarchy).

PATRILINEALITY

Patrilineality, one of the fundamental principles of the Chinese family system, is a bundle of intertwined practices. The most crucial in the Chinese case were the use of patrilineal surnames, the worship of recent patrilineal ancestors, the belief in the need for a male heir to continue the sacrifices, and the organization of kinsmen on the basis of common patrilineal descent. In the classical period these practices gradually gained hold among aristocrats.

For much of this century scholars have argued that the earliest cultures in north China were matrilineal (that is, they traced descent through mothers). Whether or not this inference is accurate, by Shang times patrilineal descent was clearly established, at least for the ruling house and related lines. As David N. Keightley emphasizes in Chapter 2 of this volume, in highest antiquity ancestor worship was the preserve of the royal family, and ancestral rites were a political resource—royal ancestors were considered extremely powerful deities. Kings conducted elaborate ancestral sacrifices, constructed huge tombs to keep their ancestors strong and happy, and communicated with their ancestors through divination. In the Chou period rules for elaborate differentiation in ancestral rites according to political rank were codified. Commoners were not to make sacrifices of meat, but they could offer vegetables to deceased fathers once each season.

This ancestral cult was intimately tied to the kinship organization of aristocrats. The Chou royal lineage and the descent groups of the feudal lords and patricians always had a main line of successive heirs, each of whom was the first son of the wife. The main line had claim to both political and ritual leadership of the descent group, which was formed of those with a common ancestor. Its current head inherited the fief or office and presided over the ancestral rites. He was to look after the needs of all members of the descent group but in a graduated manner; he looked over the closest lines first. The obligation to continue ancestral rites also led to the obligation to secure male heirs. Late in the classical period Mencius declared that the worst of unfilial acts was a failure to have descendants (*Mencius* 4A.26).

By the late classical period an agnosticism about ancestors as spirits who responded to offerings was gaining hold among the highly educated.[7] At the same time, however, ancestral rites were apparently spreading beyond the elite. By the Han dynasty ancestor worship and elaborate funerals and burials were widely practiced among the upper class and were also of some importance among common farmers. People of modest means often risked their health to perform extended or exaggerated mourning for parents, sleeping in huts with inadequate clothing and skimpy food. By late Han times large tombs were built by all those who could afford them, and mortuary art suggests very strong popular beliefs in ghosts and the ability of descendants to ease their parents' afterlife. Even relatively low members of the elite sometimes built stone ancestral temples near their parents' graves to be able to make offerings to them. Some of these actions were for "show," but the strength of the religious attitudes should not be missed.

Perhaps as important as the spread of ancestral rites was the spread of patrilineal surnames. In the classical era commoners often did not have family names, and even the family names of aristocrats were highly confusing. In Chou times *hsing* defined the set of people one should not marry, and *shih* were used as family names in referring to people. In other words, nobles not only had a "clan name" (*hsing*) based on common descent from a distant, perhaps mythical, ancestor but also had a local "family name" (*shih*) that did not always indicate kinship connection. The real beginning of the modern system of patrilineal surnames seems to be a product of the unification of the country by the Ch'in dynasty and its successful efforts to register the entire population. There-

7. Hsun Tzu is most notable in this regard. He wrote that "sacrificial rites originate in the emotions of remembrance and longing for the dead." For gentlemen who understand this purpose, "they are a part of the way of man; to the common people they are something pertaining to spirits." See Burton Watson, trans., *Basic Writings of Mo Tzu, Hsun Tzu, and Han Fei Tzu* (New York: Columbia University Press, 1967), 109–10.

after, the hodgepodge of names by which people had been called all came to be classed as "surnames" (now uniformly called *hsing*) to be passed down to patrilineal descendants. These surnames came to be considered a sign of kinship connection, making it easy for everyone to identify with a patrilineal descent line and see themselves as part of a "continuum of descent." The spread of surnames thus greatly facilitated the spread of patrilineal ideology.

FILIAL PIETY

I use filial piety to evoke the set of ethical ideas, generally associated with Confucianism, that came to provide an explicit ideology of the proper basis for family life. At the most general level these ethics called for everyone to act according to his or her station, and these stations were determined largely by seniority and gender. These kinship ethics were well suited to maintaining the system of kinship of the Chou aristocrats. Juniors were to comply with the wishes and needs of their seniors; solidarity with patrilineal kin was to be graduated according to degree of closeness. Because the first son would have a social fate different from that of a younger son, the rank order of brothers was much stressed; younger brothers were instructed to practice deference to their seniors from childhood. Although the primary line was singled out from all others, the distinctions between fathers and paternal uncles and between sons and fraternal nephews were blurred. The ethical relationship between uncles and nephews was supposed to be very close to that between fathers and sons.

Confucius is particularly associated with the concept of filial piety. The *Analects* contains the statement that the basis of human goodness (*jen*) is filial piety and brotherly deference (*Analects* 1.2). In Confucius's conception of a society regulated by ritual, people occupying a great variety of statuses and roles deal with each other in the ways appropriate to their station; by doing so, they continually maintain and create the social system without the use of force. The family is the primary arena in which this process of creation would take place; therefore, the social and political importance of correct behavior within the family is enhanced. For instance, Confucius said, "When gentlemen are generous to their own kin the people will be incited to human goodness. When the elderly are not neglected, the people will not be fickle" (*Analects* 8.1).

In the age of the philosophers following Confucius, when many established principles were challenged, the desirability of filial piety and the deference of juniors was assumed by all, even opponents of Confucianism like Mo Tzu and Han Fei Tzu. Han Fei Tzu devoted a full chapter to it (chapter 51 in Han Fei Tzu) and saw its cultivation as useful to the state because it leads to loyalty. Confucius's followers went further, however, than other schools of thought: they promoted carefully defined ethical relations to a wider range of relatives. Elaborately graded mourning obligations were specified in the *Book of Rites* for patrilineal relatives descended from a common great-great-grandfather and for the closest matrilateral and affinal kin (relatives through mothers and wives). These mourning rules conform well to the descent groups of Chou patricians because of their distinctions of seniority both of generation and within a generation among brothers and their weak sense of separation into households. The *Book of Rites* also fully articulates the distinctions between men and women in household affairs and ritual, stressing over and over their hierarchical but complementary roles. For instance, one chapter explains the symbolism of marriage rituals as showing the differences between men and women. The man goes in person to fetch his bride, showing that men take the initiative. "This is the same principle by which Heaven takes precedence over earth and rulers over their subjects."[8] In the chapter titled Domestic Regulations the segregation of men and women is called for even in the home: "Except at sacrifices or funerals, they do not hand vessels to one another. If they must pass something, they use a tray, or if none is available, they should both sit down and put the object on the ground."[9]

The Han period witnessed unprecedented celebrations of filial piety, establishing an enduring strand in Chinese family ethics. Filial piety came to be considered a political virtue, tied to loyalty to the emperor, and extreme manifestations of filial piety were declared to be an adequate basis for recruitment to government office. Han views of parent-child relations were more one-sided and authoritarian than classical Confucian ones, which may reflect not only political needs but also the new patriarchal family structure discussed later.[10] The text of the *Classic of Filial Piety*, which espoused the Han view of filial piety, came to be a common primer; it was used to inculcate generations of students with the ideas that caution, restraint, and obedience will allow one to avoid disgrace to parents and to maintain the livelihood necessary to support them.

The filiality of daughters and daughters-in-law was not described in the *Classic of Filial Piety*, but two other influential works made up for this omission: Liu Hsiang's *Biographies of Great Women* and Pan Chao's *Admonitions for Women*.[11] As yin-yang cosmology came to be developed during the Warring States period and the Han, it was also used to elaborate fam-

8. Cf. James Legge, trans., *Li chi: Book of Rites* (Sacred Books of the East 1885; reprint, New York: University Books, 1967) 1:440–41.

9. Legge, *Li chi*, 1:454–55.

10. Dau-lin Hsü, "The Myth of the 'Five Human Relations' of Confucius," *Monumenta Serica* 29 (1970–1971): 27–37.

11. See Albert Richard O'Hara, *The Position of Woman in Early China* (Taipei: Mei Ya, 1971), and Nancy Lee Swann, *Pan Chao: Foremost Woman Scholar of China* (New York: Century, 1932).

ily ethics, especially with regard to the differences between males and females. Echoing this sort of thinking, Pan Chao wrote: "*Yin* and *yang* have divergent natures; male and female have different conduct. *Yang* has moral power through toughness; *yin* is useful through gentleness. A man is valued for his strength; a woman excels through gentleness. Therefore there is a common saying, 'If a boy at birth resembles a wolf, one only fears he will be puny. If a girl at birth resembles a mouse, one only fears she will be a tiger.'"[12]

Conceptualizing the differences between men and women in terms of yin and yang stresses that these differences are part of the natural order of the universe, not part of the social institutions artificially created by men. Moreover, the natural basis of these distinctions is not limited to the differences in men's and women's bodies. Chinese writers did not argue for women's subordination based on women's child-bearing capacity or men's larger bodies and stronger muscles. They started instead with the fundamental polarity of yin and yang, which explained all sorts of other natural phenomena such as the alternation of day and night, the changes of the seasons, and the progress of diseases. In yin-yang theory the two forces complement each other but not in strictly equal ways. Most writers, especially those who can be labeled Confucian, tacitly accepted that yang is superior to yin, that action and initiation are more valued than endurance and completion.[13] Virtually all who used yin-yang ideas to discuss male-female differentiation used them to explain that the proper social role of men was to lead and of women to follow.

PATRIARCHY

The authority of family heads, relations among siblings, ties to close relatives, and even age at marriage are all shaped by the way family property is controlled and distributed. The structure of authority and control of property in the Chinese family is aptly described by the word "patriarchy." The key features of this system, as it developed historically in China, were (1) a conception of property, especially land, as family rather than individual property, (2) the idea that this property belongs to the men of the family and must be divided equally among brothers whenever divided, (3) the legal authority of fathers over women and children, which includes the father's right to arrange the marriage of his children, to sell his children, and to dispose of their labor, and (4) the notion that women are morally and intellectually less capable than men and therefore are to be under male control.

12. Swann, *Pan Chao,* 85.

13. For the Taoist exception to this generalization see Roger T. Ames, "Taoism and the Androgynous Ideal," in *Women in China,* ed. Richard W. Guisso and Stanley Johannesen (Youngstown, N.Y.: Philo Press, 1981), pp. 21–45.

Chinese patriarchy, in this sense, was not a product of the classical period, but of the early imperial state. In theory at least, during the classical period neither descent groups nor families had much family property at their disposal. Patricians had fiefs or offices with attached lands that commonly passed to heirs (normally only one), but these privileges were not supposed to be private property or to be sold or divided. Rather they were political responsibilities undertaken by family lines with the concurrence of their lords. Thus, among patricians the family as a unit of production and consumption was not clearly demarcated: the key political and economic unit was not the coresident household but the wider descent group focused on the main line.

During the Warring States period the small family (*chia*) as a unit of consumption and production under the authority of a family head gradually became more prevalent. By the early Han it was universal. In the Han the government promoted the status of family heads by granting them titles, recognizing their legal authority over their wives, children, and other juniors, and making them responsible for the fiscal obligations of the family. The state also promoted the small family by economic and political policies that strengthened the independence of smallholders. Even tenants, who were probably still very numerous, were more like smallholders than Chou serfs and tenants, with greater prospect of improving their financial situation through diligent savings or migration to undeveloped areas.

In the classical era offices and fiefs could only be transmitted to one son. Land in the Han, however, could be divided, and the equal division of family property among all sons became the established custom, apparently among all strata of society. The custom of partible inheritance had great consequences for the subsequent history of the Chinese family. It fundamentally undermined the primacy of the main line, leaving eldest sons with little more than extra ritual responsibilities. The origins of this custom are obscure, but it did not derive from classical texts or the doctrines of Confucians. Perhaps the practice of equal division of land started among peasants in areas where land was relatively abundant, which appear to be the areas where the easy buying and selling of land was first established (that is, the state of Ch'in). There is also evidence to suggest that the government promoted equal division as a means of curbing the growth of landed magnates, who might otherwise challenge its rule.

Social, economic, and geographic mobility were high in the early Han. Peasants could buy land, fall into debt, migrate, and so on. As a consequence, it became common to think that whether a family declined or prospered depended on hard work and managerial success. Neither a lord nor a village nor a kin group could guarantee a family's economic survival, but neither would any of these entities prevent its advance.

These attitudes toward the long-term rewards of cooperation and hard work for a family's future came to form the core of what has sometimes been called Chinese "familism."

The development of Chinese patriarchy in the Han period was just as important in the evolution of the Chinese family as the formulation of ethics, ancestral rites, and patrilineality in antiquity. The Han family system was the product of an imperial government, mobile society, and agrarian economy. From Han times on there was always a major conflict built into the family system. Elements of classical origin—ancestor worship and an ethics that fostered seniority and took no account of property relations—were at odds with the system of distributing property by which all brothers were equal, and each father had much more authority over his own sons than over his nephews.

The centuries after the Han saw a reversal of many Han developments. Small proprietorship was already in decline in the late Han, and during the next four centuries it probably reached its lowest levels during the entire imperial period. Moreover, the relatively weak governments of this period did not respond to these economic changes in ways that favored a "smallholder mentality." Generally, they paid less attention to family heads as a basis for governing and allowed local officials more autonomy in how they collected taxes and recruited labor. At the end of the fifth century a radically new land policy was promulgated in the north that distributed smallholdings to all those able to work them but prohibited the recipients from passing on the croplands they received to their children. This "equal-field system," which lasted into the eighth century, gave family heads more freedom from control by masters but limited their control over their progeny. Thus, during much of this period farmers found it difficult to build up their property and "advance their family"; either they found themselves in a state of serflike dependency on the owner of a manor or they made use of land temporarily allotted them by the state.

The laws of the T'ang, the first set to survive in large quantity, show that even if the equal-field system acted to limit patriarchal control over adult sons, the government was not intentionally trying to weaken family heads. In the code family heads had full authority to arrange their children's marriages, which could be at relatively young ages (thirteen *sui* for girls and fifteen for boys). So long as a man and his wife lived with his parents, the younger couple was subject to the older one. Nor could they leave or divide the property without the consent of the parents. Should violence occur in the family, the junior was held responsible or judged more severely.[14]

14. On the family in Chinese law see Ch'ü T'ung-tsu, *Law and Society in Traditional China* (Paris: Mouton, 1961).

MARRIAGE INSTITUTIONS

The development of marriage institutions in China was closely tied to the development of patrilineality, filial piety, and patriarchy. Key features of the marriage system in China included exogamy rules based on a strong concept of patrilineality (one did not marry patrilineal kin, a rule that was eventually extended to include all those of the same surname), and monogamy (a man could have only one wife, although concubines were not limited in number).

Much of the classical ideology of monogamy seems related to the strong sense of social hierarchy of that age. Marriage alliances were a major part of aristocratic politics, and the high legal and ritual status of the wife undoubtedly had much to do with the rank of her family. Wives had an important role in all ancestral rites, and no man was ritually complete without a wife. In the classics concubines were of several sorts, depending on the political status of the husband. Kings had a whole series of consorts of graded ranks, the most high-ranking of which could be younger sisters or nieces of the queen.[15] After the decline of the classical aristocratic system the basic principles of this marriage system survived. The law codes of the imperial period enforced monogamy and provided a variety of punishments for bigamy and for promoting a concubine to the status of wife.

Through the T'ang dynasty China had a system of marriage finance in which the man's family made gifts to the family of the bride, which the bride's family normally used to prepare a dowry for her.[16] By the Sung period (960–1279) the balance in marriage finance had shifted so that the wife's family had large net outlays for dowries, especially in the upper class where dowries often included land. This shift can be seen in changes in the kinds of complaints people made about mercenary marriages. In the T'ang people complained of the snobbishness of those who would only marry out their daughters if they were presented with lavish betrothal gifts. For instance, in 632 Emperor T'ai-tsung complained that the aristocratic families of the northeast were arrogant in their assumption of superior birth. He charged that "every time they marry out a daughter to another family they demand a large betrothal gift, taking quantity to be the important thing. They discuss numbers and settle an

15. Classical ideology as expressed in the ritual classics assumes only one wife for any given man. In actuality, however, rulers of states in the Chou period not infrequently had more than one wife simultaneously. See Melvin Thatcher, "Marriages of the Ruling Elite of the Spring and Autumn Period," in *Marriage and Inequality in Chinese Society,* ed. Rubie S. Watson and Patricia Buckley Ebrey (Berkeley: University of California Press, forthcoming).

16. The following discussion is based on Patricia Buckley Ebrey, "Shifts in Marriage Finance, Sixth to Thirteenth Centuries," in *Marriage and Inequality in Chinese Society,* ed. Watson and Ebrey.

agreement, just like merchants in the market."[17] In the Sung, by contrast, writers complained of young men who paid more attention to the size of a potential bride's dowry than to who she or her parents were. Chu Yü (ca. 1075–ca. 1119) complained that families with daughters might have to come up with over a thousand strings of cash if they wanted a recent recipient of the *chin-shih* degree as a son-in-law.[18] As this shift in marriage finance took hold, people began to draw up detailed lists of dowries before concluding marriages. Moreover, the legal code was revised to protect a daughter's rights to a dowry if her father died before she was married. The cost of dowry even came to be recognized as a major problem among ordinary people. Some officials went so far as to set limits on the size of dowries to ease people's burdens and discourage female infanticide. For instance, Sun Chüeh (1028–1090), prefect of Foochou, issued an order that dowries not exceed one hundred strings of cash.[19]

By the mid eleventh century there clearly was a dowry crisis in the upper class. Ts'ai Hsiang (1012–1067), while prefect in the 1050s, posted a notice protesting that in choosing brides, people thought only of the dowry. Once the dowry was delivered to the groom's home, "they inspect the dowry cases, in the morning searching through one, in the evening another. The husband cruelly keeps making more and more demands on his wife. If he is not satisfied, it can spoil their love or even lead to divorce. This custom has persisted for so long that people accept it as normal."[20] Ssu-ma Kuang (1019–1086) reported that because disappointed parents-in-law often maltreated their daughters-in-law, parents had to put together lavish dowries out of fear for their daughters' safety.[21]

In Europe dowered marriages developed out of bilateral inheritance, that is, inheritance by both sons and daughters, but this was not the case in China. In no period of traditional China did daughters inherit like sons when the family property was divided, usually after the death of the parents. Except for orphans and daughters without brothers who could be residual heirs, girls received property from their natal families only at marriage in the form of their dowry. Thus, in the Sung when the cost of the dowry became substantial and exceeded the value of the betrothal gifts received, families began for the first time regularly transmitting a significant portion of their wealth through their daughters and thus outside the boundaries of their patrilineal descendants.

What brought about this Chinese shift in marriage finance? In mod-

17. Wu Ching, *Chen-kuan cheng-yao* (Shanghai: Ku-chin Ch'u-pan-she ed.), 7:226.
18. *P'ing-chou k'o-t'an* (Ts'ung-shu Chi-ch'eng ed.), 1:16.
19. T'o T'o et al., *Sung shih* (Peking: Chung-hua Shu-chü, 1977), 344:10927.
20. Lü Tsu-ch'ien, ed., *Sung wen-chien* (Kuo-hsueh Chi-pen ed.), 108:1439.
21. Ssu-ma Kuang, *Ssu-ma shih shu-i* (Ts'ung-shu Chi-ch'eng ed.), 3:33.

ern China dowry has generally been more lavish among the rich than the poor and so has been attributed to the status-consciousness of the wife-giving family who, to quote Freedman, "do not wish to demean themselves before the other family."[22] Linking dowry with status differentiation, however, provides no insight into the historical shift toward large dowries in China because T'ang society, if anything, was more concerned with status and prestige than the Sung elite. The T'ang case shows that the size of betrothal gifts could just as well serve as symbols of high status as direct dowry.

The shift toward large dowries demonstrates, I believe, the ties of the family to larger social, economic, and political structures. The T'ang–Sung period was one of major social and economic change. In the mid T'ang the government largely gave up attempting to control the private ownership of land or its transfer from one generation to the next. The use of money also began to rapidly increase, the government issuing twenty times as much money per year in the mid eleventh century as it had in the T'ang. With these economic changes, people at all social levels had new opportunities to use property (money, land, or the goods that could be bought with money) to prepare dowries.

But why did they want to supply daughters with dowries? A major answer seems to be a change in the nature of the elite. Betrothal gifts in the T'ang were linked to marital exclusivity and the preservation of an aristocracy of old families. It was not that these old families willingly gave their daughters to whomever came up with the most money. Rather they were so reluctant to marry with anyone but their own kind that outsiders had to go to extraordinary lengths if they wished to penetrate the aristocratic circle.

The Northern Sung (960–1126) elite was different. The leading families were rarely descendants of the leading T'ang families, and pedigree by itself was less of an asset. The growing bureaucracy offered more opportunities for members of local elite families through the expanded examination system. The notion of an educated class of families whose members occasionally held office gained general recognition, displacing the T'ang notion of a superelite of families whose members nearly all held office.[23] With these changes the culture of the elite in Sung times became, if anything, more competitive. The basic rules of civil service recruitment were repeatedly changed; there was a persistent tendency for those with good connections to devise ways to favor people of their

22. Maurice Freedman, "Rites and Duties, or Chinese Marriage," in his *The Study of Chinese Society*, ed. G. William Skinner (Stanford: Stanford University Press, 1979), 258.

23. See John W. Chaffee, *The Thorny Gates of Learning: A Social History of Examinations* (Cambridge: Cambridge University Press, 1985), and Robert P. Hymes, *Statesmen and Gentlemen: The Elite of Fu-Chou, Chiang-Hsi, in Northern and Southern Sung* (Cambridge: Cambridge University Press, 1986).

own sort (through "protection" privileges, "sponsorship," "facilitated" or "avoidance" examinations, and so on).

Large dowries came to be more widely used because officials and aspirants to office, lacking the built-in networks of the T'ang aristocrats, needed to make connections to facilitate promotions, to gain allies in factional disputes, and so on. The dislocations of the tenth century seem to have resulted in many men finding themselves cut off from both patrilineal and affinal kin. In such cases it was easier to build up networks of affinal kin through marriages with families long settled in a place than to wait the four or five generations needed for the family to grow into a sizable patrilineal descent group. Offering large dowries made a good "bribe" because dowries involved transfer of property from one line to another. Moreover, ties through marriage were stronger when they involved dowry, for both families had lingering claims to seeing to its proper use.[24]

The custom of channeling wealth through dowries probably spread to lower levels through a trickle-down effect as people regularly attempted to raise their own status by copying the mores of those a step above them, a process greatly facilitated by the commercialization of the economy and the relative fluidity of social status in the period. In time, through market forces, it apparently became difficult to arrange any respectable marriage without a dowry.

ANCESTRAL RITES, DESCENT GROUPS, AND FUNERALS

Chinese ideas of the patrilineal descent line go back to the classical period, but their full elaboration in all levels of society occurred much later. This development was a by-product of new forms of social organization that brought about higher levels of interaction between the educated and ordinary people from Sung times on.

A major arena for such interaction was family or life-cycle rituals, that is, weddings, funerals, and ancestral sacrifices. After the end of the classical period, these rites developed separately on three levels: government authorities stressed differentiation according to political status, with separate forms of the rites for the emperor, nobles, officials, and commoners; the educated elite, or at least leading intellectuals, tended to rationalize the ceremonies, for instance, treating sacrifices as a way to commemorate rather than worship the dead; and ordinary people, from real religious impulses and belief in ghosts, tended to add to their rites, for instance, performing sacrifices on more occasions and to more ancestors.

24. See Patricia Ebrey, "Women in the Kinship System of the Southern Song Upper Class," in *Women in China,* ed. Richard W. Guisso and Stanley Johannesen (Youngstown, N.Y.: Philo, 1981), 113–28.

As noted by T. H. Barrett in Chapter 6 of this volume, Buddhism spread quickly after the collapse of the Han dynasty. Buddhism was a serious threat to traditional family rituals because it articulated distinctly antifamily values: freeing oneself from social entanglements and "leaving the family" to become a monk. To the extent that Buddhist and Taoist deities became the focus of popular piety, ancestors probably came to seem somewhat less important or powerful. Buddhist monks also came to play a large role in family rituals, conducting both funerals and ancestral rites for people as Buddhist ceremonies.

Not until the Sung period did educated men and government officials begin to concern themselves much with the family and religious practices of commoners. Educated men who sought to renew the Confucian program were confronted with a great variety of practices that were at odds with the classics. These practices included the negotiation of dowries (discussed earlier), a very active ancestral cult centered on graves, the cremation of the dead, the use of portraits as representatives of the dead in ancestral rites, Buddhist priests chanting sutras at funerals, bodies left in temples while descendants waited to find a geomantically favorable burial ground, marriages in which husbands lived with their wives' families, the adoption of strangers, and so on. These uncanonical or non-Confucian practices were perceived as dangerous above all because they threatened morality, especially family morality. Classical Confucianism posited that the performance of correct rites morally transformed people. Incorrect rituals were thus seen as morally corrupting.

What were scholars to do about the customs of the common people? In some cases they worked hard to justify or accommodate innovations, channeling them into acceptable forms. In other cases they tried to have uncanonical practices outlawed or otherwise discouraged by the government. They also compiled new guides to the performance of rites that made many compromises between classical and modern practices, and they made great efforts to have these books circulated and propagated.[25] The courses that the scholars took had considerable influence on the development of family and kinship practices. Two customs can serve as examples: the cult of the grave and cremation.

In Sung times graves had become a major focus of ancestor worship as actually practiced.[26] People thought of their ancestors as residing at their graves. They made both reports and offerings to their ancestors

25. See Patricia Ebrey, "Education through Ritual: Efforts to Formulate Family Rituals in the Sung Period," in *Neo-Confucian Education: The Formative Stage,* ed. John W. Chaffee and Wm. Theodore de Bary (Berkeley: University of California Press, 1989).

26. The following discussion is based on Patricia Buckley Ebrey, "Early Stages in the Development of Descent Groups," in *Kinship Organization in Late Imperial China, 1000–1940,* ed. Patricia Buckley Ebrey and James L. Watson (Berkeley: University of California Press, 1986).

there. Even literati went to great efforts to find old graves, to preserve graves from encroachment by outsiders, to organize rites to be held there, to erect shrines for these purposes, to assure the continuance of these rites by endowing them with land, and so on.

The cult of the grave seems to have been closely tied to the first appearance of modern descent groups in the Sung period. One of the first signs that sets of patrilineal relatives were getting together was their visiting of the graves of common ancestors at the Spring Festival. In the T'ang it seems only recent graves were visited. But by the end of the eleventh century, in certain regions at least, grave rites focused on "first ancestors" were bringing together hundreds of relatives whose common ancestors had lived centuries earlier. This joint activity was performed in a context that stressed descent ties and seems to have greatly strengthened recognition of boundaries around local sets of patrilineal relatives. Identity was not based just on sharing the same surname and coming from the same county but depended on joining in at the rites at the same grave.

Scholars of the Sung realized that there was no canonical basis for rites at graves. In fact, in the classics commoners are not supposed to sacrifice to their ancestors at all, nor even to make offerings to ancestors further back than their grandparents. Even those with the right to make sacrifices, moreover, were not supposed to do it at graves, but at tablets in altars in their homes.[27] Yet the custom of visiting graves and making sacrifices there received imperial approval in the great T'ang guide to rites, the *K'ai-yuan li,* on the grounds that this was the only place commoners could perform ancestral rites. Accommodation went much further in the Sung when the philosopher Ch'eng I (1033–1107) argued that rites at graves were an expression of filial piety and that commoners should be able to worship as many generations of ancestors as officials. This position was reiterated by Chu Hsi (1130–1200), the most important intellectual figure of the period, who included these revisions in his highly influential guide to the performance of family rites.

With the acceptance of these ritual practices it became possible for educated men to take greater roles in local descent groups. When a local group of agnates produced literate men, which often happened by the thirteenth century, these men would try to give the group the prestige associated with classical terms and ideas and reinterpreted the group in terms of the ideology of the classical descent group. They wrote genealogies for it, commemorated it in inscriptions, and encouraged the erec-

27. Chinese believed that people had two souls, a more earthly one that stayed with the body and a more spiritual one that separated from the body and "went everywhere." People were supposed to make offerings to the spiritual soul, first concentrating it in a tablet, not the earthly soul in the grave.

tion of an ancestral hall. As these descent groups became more common, they entered the general political repertoire. Members of the elite might consciously set out to organize their kinsmen as a way to strengthen their local base. Thus the accommodation of grave rites allowed the educated to shape and channel social and cultural phenomena occurring among commoners and often even to control it.[28] This process was a dynamic one: changes in religion and local social organization led to intellectual changes; these changes in turn influenced elite behavior and thus transformed the local organization.

The growth and development of descent groups in Ming and Ch'ing times is gradually coming to be better understood. Lineages did not develop at the same time or in the same ways or in every place. In Hui-chou, Anhwei province, lineages, many led by merchants, were prominent in the mid Ming. Throughout the lower Yangtze region the seventeenth century seems to have been a time of great growth for lineages. These lineages were usually led by literati, often degree-holders. Lineage growth was connected to the intellectual concerns of the literati and to the economic growth and commercialization of that period. In Kwangtung and Fukien lineages were becoming increasingly dominant in the Ch'ing period, but in contrast to the lower Yangtze, these lineages were often composed entirely of commoners. In these areas peasants often had to organize lineages to protect themselves from other organized lineages.[29]

Thus, grave rites are a case where accommodation on the part of the

28. See Robert P. Hymes, "Marriage, Descent Groups, and the Localist Strategy in Sung and Yuan Fu-chou," in *Kinship Organization in Late Imperial China, 1000–1940,* ed. Patricia Buckley Ebrey and James L. Watson (Berkeley: University of California Press, 1986).

29. Major historical studies include Hilary J. Beattie, *Land and Lineage in China: A Study of T'ung-ch'eng County, Anhwei, in the Ming and Ch'ing Dynasties* (Cambridge: Cambridge University Press); Jerry Dennerline, "The New Hua Charitable Estate and Local Level Leadership in Wuxi County at the End of the Qing," in *Select Papers from the Center for Far Eastern Studies* (University of Chicago), 4 (1979–1980): 19–70; idem, "Marriage, Adoption, and Charity in the Development of Lineages in Wu-hsi from Sung to Ch'ing," in *Kinship Organization in Late Imperial China, 1000–1940,* ed. Patricia Buckley Ebrey and James L. Watson (Berkeley: University of California Press, 1986); Keith Hazelton, "Patrilines and the Development of Localized Lineages: The Wu of Hsiu-ning City, Hui-chou, to 1528," in *Kinship Organization in Late Imperial China, 1000–1940,* ed. Patricia Buckley Ebrey and James L. Watson (Berkeley: University of California Press, 1986); Rubie S. Watson, "The Creation of a Chinese Lineage: The Teng of Ha Tsueh, 1669–1751," *Modern Asian Studies* 16 (1982): 69–100; David Faure, *The Structure of Chinese Rural Society: Lineage and Village in the Eastern New Territories, Hong Kong* (Hong Kong: Oxford University Press, 1986); Timothy Brook, "Funerary Ritual and the Building of Lineages in Late Imperial China," *Harvard Journal of Asiatic Studies* (1989). Anthropological studies of lineages in recent time (or some vaguely defined "traditional" time) are even more plentiful. The classic works are Maurice Freedman, *Lineage Organization in Southeastern China* (London: Athlone Press, 1958) and idem, *Chinese Lineage and Society: Fukien and Kwangtung* (London: Athlone Press, 1966).

intellectuals and the state facilitated elite leadership of local kinship groups. Cremation provides a contrasting example of the ways in which family religious practices were shaped by the efforts of the state and intellectuals.[30] Cremation gained popularity during the tenth century and flourished through the fourteenth century. Cremation was about as far from earlier death-related rituals as possible. In China, rather than disposing of the dead in ways that would bring about the quick disappearance of the bodily remains, those who could afford it had always used methods believed to delay decay. They not only used very thick inner and outer wooden coffins, but they also built tomb chambers of stone or brick and took other measures they thought would preserve the body, such as placing jade objects in the coffins or even, in the famous Han example, dressing the body in jade.

Cremation had come to China with Buddhism. It had been the standard burial method in India, and Buddhist monks practiced it in China. Cremation made perfect sense in terms of Buddhist notions of transmigration. One was to be reborn into another body: there was no need for the old body to be preserved or its decay delayed. In China cremation often was managed by Buddhist establishments; some crematoria were run by Buddhist temples, and temples provided storage for the ashes that remained after the cremation or pools where the ashes could be scattered.

The evidence for the spread of cremation in Sung times is conclusive from both textual and archaeological sources. In 962 the practice was outlawed but by no means suppressed. In 1158 an official wrote in a memorial that, "Today the people have the custom of 'transformation by fire.' While their parents are alive they worry only that they cannot provide everything their parents need, but when their parents die they roast them and throw them away. . . . The worst offenders burn them and toss the remains in water. . . . Nowadays the cruelty of cremation increases every day."[31] In 1261 another official described a crematory outside Soochow: "There is a temple called 'Aid for All' one *li* [about one-third mile] to the southwest of the city. For a long time this temple has had about ten ovens for cremating people that it operates to make a profit. All the ignorant people of the city are attracted to it. As soon as their parents die, they cart them off and consign them to the flames. The ashes that are not consumed are collected and thrown in a deep pool."[32]

Neo-Confucians like Ssu-ma Kuang, Ch'eng Hao (1032–1085), and Chu Hsi were aghast at the practice of cremation and criticized it se-

30. The following discussion is based on Patricia Ebrey, "Cremation in Sung China" *American Historical Review,* forthcoming 1990.

31. T'o, *Sung shih* 125:2918–19.

32. Huang Chen, *Huang-shih jih-ch'ao* (Ssu-k'u Ch'üan-shu ed.), 70:14b.

verely as barbaric and a mutilation of parents' bodies. Their reactions seem to have encouraged officials to seek ways to eradicate cremation. Local officials often tried to help the poor, who they believed turned to cremation because they could not afford burial sites. Han Ch'i (1008–1075) set aside land for burial for the poor so that they would have no need for cremation. A few years later the government ordered every county to set up such charitable graveyards, to be run by temples, issuing detailed regulations on the records the monks should keep on the location of each grave and the offerings they made there. Some of these charitable graveyards have recently been excavated by archaeologists.

The problem of the poor selecting cremation because of its economy could also be attacked at the private level. Descent groups were especially important in this process, as they often subsidized the burials of their poorest members or even established group burial grounds for all their members. Through public and private efforts of this sort as well as stricter laws and more thorough propaganda, cremation slowly lost its popularity during the Ming and Ch'ing periods. In recent centuries funerals and burials came to play heightened roles as arenas for family and kinship activities.[33]

The inclusion of the cult of the grave into acceptable Confucian ritual forms and the gradual suppression of cremation are just two examples of the ways elite and popular culture interacted and modified each other in the creation of Chinese family and kinship structures. This process required intellectual compromises, legal readjustments, political incentives, new forms of social organization, the codification and dissemination of new ideas of orthodoxy, and so on. The result of this gradual process, which lasted through the Ming and into the Ch'ing, was a much more thorough penetration of orthodox patrilineal ideology throughout society at large. For instance, the belief in the need for a patrilineal heir, to be secured by adoption if necessary, does not seem to have been particularly strong among ordinary people until this process was well underway. In a similar way knowledge of the complex Chinese mourning grades and exogamy rules (for instance, the rule against marriage to a mother's grandniece) seems to have depended on the spread of written texts and the spread of local forums—such as descent groups—which brought knowledge of these texts to the illiterate.

Just as there was a certain tension between the patrilineal principles of the classical era and the property law of the early imperial period, there was also tension between the dowered marriages and more thorough penetration of patrilineal principles. Dowered marriages tended to strengthen the cognatic principles in Chinese kinship, that is, to increase

33. See Evelyn S. Rawski and James L. Watson, eds., *Death Rituals in Late Imperial and Modern China* (Berkeley: University of California Press, 1988).

the importance of relatives through mothers and wives. Narrowing the gap between elite and popular performance of ancestral rites and funerals, to the contrary, promoted the idea of the primacy of ties to patrilineal relatives, near and distant.

These two conflicting tendencies interacted over time. Some Sung Neo-Confucians perceived that the shift toward dowry was a threat to China's traditional patrilineal family system; this perception was one motivation for their call for a revival of the ancient descent line system. Descent line rhetoric and the growth of descent groups can also be given some credit for curbing the trend toward dowry. Where descent groups existed, they reduced the incentives for dowry among ordinary people by providing them with an adequate set of social connections. In recent times dowry seems to have been more common among ordinary people in areas without strong lineages. In areas where there were strong lineages the rich, but not ordinary poor farmers, gave dowries.

FOOTBINDING AND WIDOW CHASTITY

Textbook surveys of Chinese history often note a decline in the status of women that is usually dated to the T'ang–Sung transition or to the Sung period.[34] The two signs of this decline most frequently mentioned are the pressure on widows not to remarry and the practice of binding young girls' feet to prevent them from growing more than a few inches long.

In looking for explanations of the spread of these practices, so misogynist to modern Western eyes, should we be looking to the T'ang, the Sung, the Yuan, the Ming, or the Ch'ing periods? The key question is not when such practices first appeared, as any number of ideas can appear without becoming historically important, but when they became firmly established.

Footbinding began its spread in the Sung, first among dancers and courtesans. Nevertheless, in the large body of Sung poems and songs scholars have found only a few lines that refer to bound feet. The poet Hsü Chi (1028–1103) referred to a woman as "knowing about arranging the four limbs [for burial], but not about binding her two feet." Su Shih (1036–1101) wrote a song that described in some detail the bound feet of a dancer; it reveals that he found tiny feet an object of wonder and wanted to hold them in his hand to get a better look. The first surviving inquiry into the origins of footbinding was written in the early twelfth

34. See Edwin O. Reischauer and John K. Fairbank, *East Asia: The Great Tradition* (Boston: Houghton Mifflin, 1958), 224–25. See also Charles O. Hucker, *China's Imperial Past* (Stanford: Stanford University Press, 1975), 175–76, and Dun J. Li, *The Ageless Chinese: A History,* 2d ed. (New York: Scribners, 1971), 364.

century by a scholar who referred to bound feet as both small and "bowed" and associated with the lotus.[35]

From the late twelfth century on, casual references to footbinding become gradually more common. The earliest protest against footbinding that I have found is by Ch'e Jo-shui from the late Sung: "I do not know when the practice of wives binding their feet began. Little children not yet four or five *sui,* who have done nothing wrong are nevertheless made to suffer unlimited pain to bind [their feet] small. I do not know what use this is."[36] A thirteenth century tomb of the young wife of an imperial clansman contained several sets of shoes for bound feet, and the woman's feet were in fact bound with a strip of cloth.[37]

Such is the evidence for assessing the spread of footbinding in Sung times. Through the eleventh century the evidence is extremely thin, and it is plausible that the practice was most common among dancers or courtesans. Literati were familiar with this world, and they recognized bound feet without necessarily having wives or mothers with bound feet. A late-fourteenth-century writer quoted a twelfth-century discussion of the relatively recent origins of footbinding and then quoted another source, otherwise unknown, that said a dancer in the palace of the ruler of the Later T'ang (923–935) bound her feet to make them small and curved like new moons. He concluded that people began to imitate her, and that although the practice was still rare through the eleventh century, it spread through imitation so that in his day people were ashamed not to practice it.[38]

Can anything be inferred from these limited references concerning the reasons for the spread of footbinding? Howard Levy argues that erotic attraction was basic to the appeal of bound feet. In his discussion of the origins of footbinding, however, Levy connects it to intellectual currents in the Sung dynasty, especially the emphasis on womanly docility and chastity. He repeats a story that Chu Hsi, while prefect of Changchou in southern Fukien, encouraged footbinding as a way to promote chastity by making it more difficult for women to move about (because women with bound feet had to use canes to walk). This story is almost surely spurious as far as the reference to Chu Hsi goes.[39] But does it contain a deeper truth? Did footbinding spread because of increased con-

35. *Chieh hsiao chi* (Ssu-k'u Ch'üan-shu ed.), 14:7a; Howard S. Levy, *Chinese Footbinding: The History of a Curious Erotic Custom* (New York: Bell, 1967), 47; and Chang Pang-chi, *Mo-chuang man-lu* (Ts'ung-shu Chi-ch'eng ed.), 8:89.

36. Ch'e Jo-shui, *Chiao-ch'i chi* (Pai-pu Ts'ung-shu ed.), 1:22a.

37. Fu-chien sheng Po-wu kuan, *Fu-chou Nan-Sung Huang Sheng mu* (Peking: Wen-wu Ch'u-pan-she, 1982), 8.

38. T'ao Tsung-i, *Cho-keng lu* (Ts'ung-shu Chi-ch'eng ed.) 10:158.

39. Levy, *Chinese Footbinding,* 44. Levy cites a Chinese secondary source that in turn cites another Chinese source that I have been unable to identify in any bibliography.

cern about controlling women and, in particular, limiting their mobility? Is there a socioeconomic explanation for the attraction of delicate women? Are there historical reasons why this attraction would have become more potent in Sung and Yuan times? Does it have anything to do with remarriage?

Discouraging young childless widows from remarrying and, especially, encouraging their suicides can be considered as misogynist as footbinding, but the history of its spread is different. The idea of widow chastity was not new in Sung times. The *Book of Rites* says, "Faithfulness is the basis of serving others and is the virtue of a wife. When her husband dies a woman does not remarry; to the end of her life she does not change."[40] The Han dynasty *Biographies of Great Women* contained several accounts of women whose primary accomplishment was their determined resistance to remarriage. These women generally cited maxims about wifely fidelity, such as "Even if there is a sagely mate, she does not go a second time," "The moral duty of a wife lies in not changing once she has gone [in marriage]," or "The moral duty of a wife lies in not having two husbands."[41] Many of these women ended up sacrificing their lives rather than accepting disgrace. Pan Chao wrote, "According to ritual, husbands have a duty to marry again, but there is no text that authorizes a woman to remarry."[42] The biographies of great women in the histories of the Later Han (25–220) and the Wei (220–265) include cases of chaste widows, including some who mutilated themselves rather than remarry or who died of grief at their husband's death. One scholar suggests that in the sixth century Chinese historians took a special interest in cases of chaste widows because of the threat of Hsien-pi cultural domination: widow chastity was a distinctly Chinese virtue, and promoting it helped create barriers between Chinese and Hsien-pi culture.[43]

Two texts for women's education composed in the T'ang dynasty taught that widows should be faithful. The last item in the *Analects for Girls* is titled Preserving Chastity (*Shou chieh*): "When husband and wife 'join the hair,' the moral principles involved are as weighty as a thousand gold pieces. Should it happen that misfortune occurs and [your husband] dies first, for three years you will wear heavy mourning. You must keep your commitment and make your heart firm. Attend to protecting the family, managing the estate, and preparing the tomb, then train and educate the descendants to preserve the reputation of the deceased."[44]

40. See Legge, *Li chi,* 1:439.

41. See O'Hara, *Position of Women,* 122, 123, 139.

42. See Swann, *Pan Chao,* 87.

43. Jennifer Holmgren, "Widow Chastity in the Northern Dynasties: The Lieh-nü Biographies in the *Wei-shu,*" *Papers on Far Eastern History* 23 (1981): 165–86, esp. 185–86. The Hsien-pi were proto-Mongol tribes who, along with several other non-Chinese groups threatened and overtook parts of north China in the fourth, fifth, and sixth centuries.

44. *Ku-chin t'u-shu ch'i-ch'eng* (Chung-hua Shu-chü, 1934 ed.), *ts'e* 395:10a.

The *Classic of Filial Piety for Girls* noted the correspondence of husband and wife to yin and yang and the need for both: "The wife is earth; the husband is Heaven. Neither can be dispensed with." But then it went on to draw a distinction between them: "Husbands perform a hundred activities; wives focus on a single commitment. Men have the duty to remarry; for women there is no text authorizing 'a second dip.'"[45]

Given these precedents, it is not surprising that widow chastity was widely recognized as an ideal in Sung society. The government rewarded women who were widowed young and who remained unmarried for lengthy periods with honorary banners and sometimes grants of grain as a way of "improving customs," on the same principle that it rewarded exemplary filial piety demonstrated through maintaining an undivided household for five or more generations, undergoing unusual mourning austerities, or slicing off a piece of one's thigh to prepare medicine for an ailing parent.[46] Many Sung writers reveal an admiration for the virtues of widows who did not remarry. Lou Yueh (1137–1213), for instance, wrote that the widow of one of his cousins went beyond the model of Kung Chiang in the *Biographies of Great Women*. Although Kung Chiang resisted her parents' pressure to remarry, she was not known for any other qualities. Lou's kinswoman, née Chiang, however, had been left a widow at twenty-six with five children, ranging in age from two weeks to six *sui*. Her own mother tried to get her to remarry, and her parents-in-law did not discourage her, but she refused, on the grounds that otherwise the orphans' fate could not be assured. She then devoted herself to managing the family, which grew large and prosperous under her direction.[47]

Even among relatively ordinary people the notion that there was something wrong in widows remarrying seems to have had power quite independent of Ch'eng I's or Chu Hsi's teachings. The force of this idea can be seen from ghost stories in which a dead husband warns his wife against remarrying. In one such case the dead husband, alarmed that his wife was having too good a time during the mourning period, told her through a shaman, "You may not remarry. If you do I will kill you."[48]

Moralists, of course, also extolled widow chastity. Ssu-ma Kuang wrote, "'Wife' means an equal match. Once she is matched with him, she does not change for the rest of her life. Therefore loyal subjects do not serve two masters, and chaste women do not serve two husbands."[49] Most famous, of course, is the comment made by Ch'eng I in response to a ques-

45. *Ku-chin t'u-shu chi-ch'eng, ts'e* 395:11a.

46. Hsu Sung et al., *Sung hui-yao chi-pen* (reprint, Taiwan: Shih-chien shu-chü, 1964), *li* 6:1a–15a.

47. *Kung-k'uei chi* (Ts'ung-shu Chi-ch'eng ed.), 105:1486–89.

48. *I-chien chih, ping* 4, 482.

49. *Chia fan* (Taipei: Chung-kuo Tzu-hsueh Ming-chu Chi-ch'eng ed.), 8:2b.

tion about whether a poor widow with no one to depend on could remarry: "The problem is that people in recent times are afraid of freezing or starving to death; therefore, they say such things. But starving to death is a small matter; losing chastity is an extremely great matter." Chu Hsi included this passage in his *Reflections on Things at Hand,* adding to its fame.[50]

Despite wide agreement that it was better not to remarry, remarriage seems to have been remarkably common in the Sung.[51] My reading of the evidence is that throughout the Sung period widow chastity belonged to the realm of virtue, not that of decency. Everyone agreed that households that did not divide for five or more generations deserved admiration and emulation, yet few could attain this standard and they were not publicly ridiculed, much less shunned, for this failure. Widows who remarried and men who arranged for their daughters, nieces, or daughters-in-law to remarry were looked on in a similar way. As several scholars have shown, recorded cases of chaste widows and especially widow suicides did not begin their dramatic rise until mid Ming times.[52]

To summarize, footbinding seems to have steadily spread during Sung times, and explanations for it should be sought in Sung circumstances, but widow chastity had very little specific connection to the Sung, the idea predating the Sung and the exaggerated emphasis on it developing much later. The spread of footbinding may well have had something to do with larger shifts in Chinese construction of gender (that is, their ways of thinking about what makes people male or female). The act of binding girls' feet and of preferring girls with small feet for brides and courtesans were powerful statements about femininity. As such they should be seen in the context of the cultural construction of masculinity to which they contrasted. It has long been noted that the Sung marked a general shift in Chinese cultural orientation, in particular, the shift toward accentuating those strands of Chinese culture that most contrasted with the cultures of China's northern rivals: the Turks, Khitans, Jurchens, and Mongols. These cultural shifts were manifested at a wide range of levels, from increased use of sedan chairs and the love

50. *Erh Ch'eng chi* (Peking: Chung-hua Shu-chü, 1981), *i-shu* 22b, 301; Wing-tsit Chan, trans., *Reflections on Things at Hand: The Neo-Confucian Anthology compiled by Chu Hsi and Lü Tsu-ch'ien* (New York: Columbia University Press, 1967), 177.

51. Ebrey, "Women in the Kinship System of the Southern Song Upper Class." See also Chu Jui-hsi, *Sung-tai she-hui yen-chiu* (Taipei: Hung-wen, 1986), 132–39.

52. Susan Mann, "Women in the Kinship, Class, and Community Structures of Qing Dynasty China," *Journal of Asian Studies* 46, no. 1 (1987): 37–56; Andrew C. K. Hsien and Jonathan D. Spence, "Suicide and the Family in Pre-Modern Chinese Society," in *Normal and Abnormal Behavior in Chinese Culture,* ed. A. Kleinman and T.-Y. Lin (Dordrecht, Holland: Reidel, 1980).

of antiques and delicate porcelains to the decline in the popularity of hunting among the official elite and the elaboration of the model literatus, who could be refined, bookish, contemplative, or artistic but need not be strong, quick, or dominating.

New notions of masculinity invited and required new notions of femininity. If the ideal man among the upper class was relatively subdued and refined, he might seem too effeminate unless women came to be even more delicate, reticent, and stationary. Moreover, the Chinese had long believed that they practiced stricter male-female segregation than the steppe peoples to their north. This segregation may in general have been increasing in the Sung as another means of ethnic differentiation. Footbinding was not only uniquely Chinese, but it made it all the more likely that Chinese women would stay at home.

The cult of widow chastity came later and seems to owe less to the need to accentuate Chinese distinguishing features. Jennifer Holmgren argues that one of the sources for the pressure on widows not to remarry was a change in property law enacted under the Mongols, particularly the law that widows could not take their dowries with them if they remarried. This change, she demonstrates, was motivated in part by problems created by outlawing the Mongol practice of the levirate (which had a widow marry her husband's younger brother). The levirate kept the dowry in the husband's family, and the new law achieved the same end by direct legislation.[53] This law did not prevent parents-in-law from forcing their widowed daughter-in-law to remarry, and in fact provided the financial incentive of the dowry.[54] The moral stricture against remarriage and especially the emphasis on remaining in the husband's home can thus be interpreted as a pro-woman policy because it protected widows from being forced to give up their property and their children.

The cultic dimensions of widow chastity reached much greater proportions in late Ming and Ch'ing times and, as a consequence, are best related to changes more specific to those periods, such as the increased commercialization of the economy and increased competition in the examination system.[55]

53. J. Holmgren, "Observations on Marriage and Inheritance Practices in Early Mongol and Yüan Society: With Particular Reference to the Levirate," *Journal of Asian History* 20 (1986): 127–92.

54. See Ann Waltner, "Widows and Remarriage in Ming and Early Qing China," in *Women in China,* ed. Richard W. Guisso and Stanley Johannesen (Youngstown, N.Y.: Philo Press, 1981), 129–46.

55. See Paul S. Ropp, "The Status of Women in Mid-Qing China: Evidence from Letters, Laws and Literature" (Paper presented at the annual meeting of the American Historical Association, Washington, D.C. 1987); Mark Elvin, "Female Virtue and the State in China," *Past and Present* 104 (1984): 111–52; and Mann, "Women in the Kinship, Class, and Community Structures of Qing Dynasty China."

CONCLUSION

The goal of this chapter has been to put the history of the family in China in comparative perspective not by comparing separate characteristics but by making possible a comparison of the stages and processes of change. By way of conclusion let me try to draw some of these comparisons.

First, there is no historical rupture in family or marriage practices in China comparable to those associated with Christianity in the West. Buddhism, for all its great cultural importance in China, never undermined ancestor worship or the associated belief in a spiritual and material link from ancestors to descendants over many generations. Belief in Buddhist hells, karma, and rebirth did not eliminate offerings to ancestors presumably already reborn elsewhere. By contrast, of course, conversion to Christianity carried with it the rejection of family cults and a variety of family practices, such as concubinage and cousin marriage.

Changes of the order associated in the West with the Protestant Reformation, the rise of the modern state, and industrialization did, however, occur in China. Among these I would include the spread of patrilineal surnames, the introduction of partible inheritance, the development and spread of modern-style descent groups, the shift toward substantial dowries, the increased practice of adoption, the decline in widow remarriage, and probably many others as yet unstudied.

One large question posed by the comparison of Chinese and Western family history is the role of economic change. Families are always to some extent economic units and are unlikely to remain unaltered by major economic changes. It is well recognized that capitalism and socialism in the twentieth century have each led to fundamental changes in Chinese family organization, patterns of authority, marriage decisions, and so on.[56] Did any earlier changes have comparable effects? The establishment of the basic agrarian regime of small proprietorships was certainly tied to the development of Chinese patriarchy. Commercialization of the economy in the late T'ang and the Sung seems to have been important in establishing dowries as a major part of marriage finance in China. The next major increase in commercialization in the late Ming and early Ch'ing probably had much to do with the great proliferation of lineages in this period and perhaps with the social changes that led to the cult of widow chastity.

In this brief overview I have not made economic change the only force behind changes in Chinese family practices.[57] I also refer to changes

56. See Kay Ann Johnson, *Women, the Family and Peasant Revolution in China* (Chicago: University of Chicago Press, 1983).

57. For a much more rigorously economic interpretation of the history of women in China see Hill Gates, "The Commoditization of Chinese Women," *Signs: Journal of Women in Culture and Society* 14.4 (Summer 1989): 799–832.

in the state, popular religion, the political situation of the elite, cultural identity with regard to alien others, and the impact of alien rule. Comparable factors have been shown to have been important at different times in the history of the Western family, and the history of the family in China seems to be just as complex.

An intriguing historical contrast between China and the West is the relatively high level of standardization of family practices in China across regions, classes, and dialect groups. Throughout the country descent reckoning was patrilineal, offerings were made to recent ancestors, family property was divided among brothers, marriages among patrilineal kin were disapproved, essentially all women married, late marriages were rare, adoption was common, young married couples started their lives together in the home of senior relatives if feasible, and so on. In the West, by contrast, there was much greater variation in inheritance practices, naming practices, the proportion of people marrying, and the incidence of couples starting marriages in their own homes. Standardization in the West was generally limited to matters over which the church had asserted authority. The chief agent fostering standardization of family practices in China was not an organized church but the state. The integrating powers of the state are seen repeatedly through Chinese history but through different mechanisms in different periods. Ancestral rites were strongly rooted in the ancient cult of royal ancestors. Patrilineal surnames probably became universal because of the need of the imperial government to register the entire population. The patriarchal household was strengthened by the Ch'in and Han governments' desires to curb feudal forces and deal directly with family heads. Patriarchal principles were regularly reinforced by the law codes the government issued. Moreover, the bureaucratic technique of appointing natives of distant areas as magistrates tended to undermine distinct regional traditions of inheritance practices or other family legal matters. The state exerted tremendous influence on the education of the elite, especially from Sung times on, through the examination system. This education led the elites of the diverse regions to imitate common models of family behavior and to share an interest in reforming the family practices of commoners that the state deemed deviant. The state even played a major role in Ming and Ch'ing times in rewarding and celebrating the virtues of chaste widowhood.

NINE

Chinese Economic History in Comparative Perspective

Albert Feuerwerker

Much ink has been spilled and many pages filled with explanations of economic "backwardness" or "underdevelopment" or "late development" in the non-European world. Even as late as the sixteenth century, China's economy produced for its population a standard of living in no way inferior to that of any other nation in Europe or Asia. Western students of China have asked with some frequency why late imperial China did not therefore "industrialize" or "modernize" as Europe did from the eighteenth century onward and Japan proceeded to do in the late nineteenth and early twentieth centuries. Scholars in the People's Republic of China phrase the equivalent question in terms of a failed or delayed transition from "feudalism" to "capitalism" along the Marxist path of historical progress.

If that were my topic here, I would argue that underdevelopment, in fact, is an overdetermined condition; it was the "norm" of world history until very recent times. Even today, development is more the exception than the rule. Proponents of economic, cultural, political, social, and other causes of underdevelopment have each found overwhelming evidence for their favored explanations. In fact, any one of these factors is sufficiently important to prevent a premodern economy from developing into a modern one. Other factors are simply overkill. Of course I do not mean that there was no economic growth before industrialization of the modern variety. The necessary distinction is between growth of total production and growth of production per capita, which I call respectively "premodern economic growth" and "modern economic growth." Underdevelopment may include the possibilities of growth, stagnation, or decline, but always within the constraints of premodern economic growth and without any sustained change in per capita production. We know a great deal about the enormous obstacles to moving from the framework of premodern growth to that of modern growth. Despite a century of study and research economic historians are much less certain about how the process of modern economic growth got started in England and Holland in the seventeenth and eighteenth centuries. And we are least of all informed about the history and dynamics of premodern economies per se, apart from the question of their not being transformed into modern economies.

From the "invention" of settled agriculture ten thousand or more years ago until the advent of the classical empires in Europe and the Near East or the beginning of the imperial era in China, there are convincing indications in the historical record both that the total population grew in each of these regions and that over the long run per capita production and consumption also increased. In other words, "real" economic growth (in the form of small increases in per capita production) occurred also in the ancient world. It is possible, even in a premodern economy, for the production of food, housing, tools, and so on, to grow for a time at a more rapid rate than the rate of population increase. But there is still a great difference between modest growth "for a time" and sustained per capita growth "over the long run."

More frequently than not over these millennia, characterized as they were by sometimes violent regional or local fluctuations in population size and total production, the decades and centuries saw only meager, temporary, or localized increases in per capita production. The growth that did occur was mainly in the absolute size of the population and in total production. This growth in production proceeded at a snail's pace and resulted in little or no improvement of living standards. Indeed, I would suggest that Europe at the peak of the Roman Empire and China at the height of the Han dynasty (roughly two thousand years ago, at the time of Christ) had both reached a plateau of sorts with respect to the possibility of sustained increases in per capita production using the best technology then available. In the case of Europe the best economic performance of the Roman Empire was (with some local and short-term exceptions) probably not bettered until the eighteenth century. In China a burst of technological and organizational creativity occurred in the Sung dynasty (960–1279) and fostered both absolute and per capita growth in production, which broke through the earlier plateau. Not all specialists agree, but I believe that the best economic performance of the Sung as measured by per capita production was probably not surpassed in China before the twentieth century.

Despite the economic growth of China in the Sung period I believe we are justified in characterizing most of the economic change that occurred in both China and the West from Han and Roman times until the nineteenth century as premodern economic growth. Implicit in this term is the notion of growth in total population and total production, but little change in per capita production and consumption. Modern economic growth, by contrast, implies economic changes of the kind that occurred in Europe in the eighteenth century and after. Based on the continuous advance of science and technology, modern economic growth brought with it the possibility of sustained growth in per capita production and, as a consequence, the possibility, even if not the certainty, of sustained improvements in standards of living.

Within this general framework I attempt to paint, with very broad strokes, a comparative picture of Chinese and European (mostly Western European) economic growth over roughly the past thousand years. In particular, I examine trends and developments in demography, technology, social, political and economic institutions, and international economic relations at the two ends of the Eurasian land mass. Statistical series for important economic variables—in contrast to occasional numbers and frequent qualitative indicators—are generally not available for China before the twentieth century (the late nineteenth century for foreign trade figures). Relatively better European data, that is, compared to the Chinese data just discussed, begin to be available in the eighteenth century. The seeming exceptions to the absence of statistical series for imperial China before the twentieth century are population figures of various kinds, episodic surveys of cultivated acreage, and partial reports of government income and expenditure. Of course none of these series are "modern" statistics. They can sometimes be used after considerable "interpretation" of why and how they were collected to suggest important economic trends. The econometric manipulation of these statistics, however, produces few reliable results before very recent times.[1]

If one plots the population data (weak as they are before the nineteenth century) for Western Europe, primarily, and China over the past thousand years, the results are similar; the distinctive curves of growth for each are composed of a succession of logistic curves (figure 9.1). China's population reached perhaps 60 million by the Han dynasty (206 B.C.–A.D. 220) and did not exceed that total in the millennium before the Northern Sung dynasty (960–1126), when it grew sharply to 100

1. Kang Chao, *Man and Land in Chinese History: An Economic Analysis* (Stanford: Stanford University Press, 1986), is a stimulating guide to the traditional population and acreage data and also provides a good example of some of the perils awaiting those who would use them.

Figure 9.1. Comparative demographic history of China and continental Europe. The European estimates are from Colin McEvedy and Richard Jones, *Atlas of World Population History* (New York: Penguin Books, 1978), 18. I am indebted to Professor James Lee of the California Institute of Technology for the Chinese population estimates.

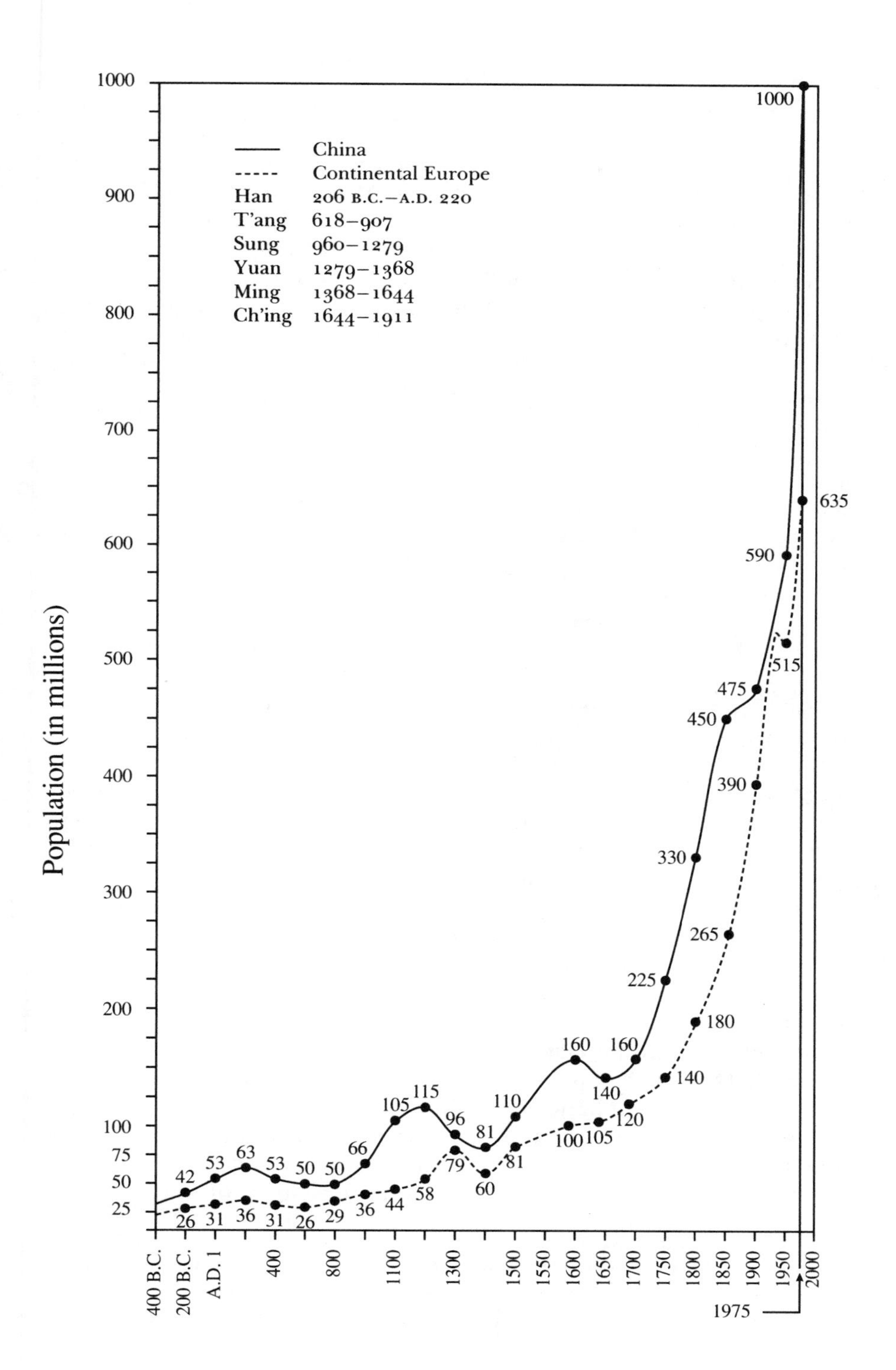

China
Continental Europe
Han 206 B.C.–A.D. 220
T'ang 618–907
Sung 960–1279
Yuan 1279–1368
Ming 1368–1644
Ch'ing 1644–1911
Population (in millions)
1000
900
800
700
600
500
400
300
200
100
75
50
25
42
53
63
53
50
50
66
105
115
96
81
110
160
140
160
225
330
450
475
590
1000
26
31
36
31
26
29
36
44
58
79
60
81
100
105
120
140
180
265
390
515
635
400 B.C.
200 B.C.
A.D. 1
400
800
1100
1300
1500
1550
1600
1650
1700
1750
1800
1850
1900
1950
2000
1975

million. It then increased more slowly to 120 million in the Southern Sung (1127–1279). This first period of growth was reversed by a spectacular decline in population from 120 million to 60–80 million in the Yuan, or Mongol, dynasty (1279–1368). A second cycle began with recuperation and slow growth during the Ming dynasty (1368–1644): China's population reached at least 150 million in the sixteenth century. The second cycle ended with a crisis in the seventeenth century that was attributable to civil war and the Manchu conquest, whose demographic effects were negative but difficult to measure with any certainty. However, the seventeenth-century crisis was short-lived. Population growth resumed and accelerated in the late seventeenth century. A third cycle, spanning the eighteenth and early nineteenth centuries, saw an increase from 150–200 million in 1700 to 430 million in 1840. This rapid burst of growth was halted or reversed by a series of great rebellions in the mid nineteenth century. Finally—this time with no cyclic downturn yet evident or likely—population growth resumed at the beginning of the twentieth century. China's population, which was about 400 million in 1900, reached 500 million in 1937 and then very rapidly increased from 540 million in 1949 to 1,030 million at present.[2]

Leaving aside the most recent demographic phase in China, the three Chinese cycles of growth and decline are matched by similar, but not identical, logistic curves in Western Europe: three periods of growth are punctuated by two periods of decline or stagnation in Europe. From A.D. 1000 to 1347 Europe's population increased, perhaps doubling in size. Some historians believe that this period of growth ended even before the onset of the black death in 1347. Widespread epidemic disease was only one striking aspect of the overall "Malthusian" response to "overpopulation"—the pressure of people on inadequate land, resources, and technology—that the expansion phase had brought about.

Western Europe's population may have fallen by as much as a quarter or a third before it began growing again in the late fifteenth or the sixteenth century (the timing differed considerably in different parts of Europe). By the second half of the sixteenth century population was once again pressing on land and resources. The "crisis of the seventeenth century" saw population decline or stagnation in Germany (most dramatically), France, Spain, Portugal, and Italy, that is, in central and southern Europe. But in northwest Europe—England, the Netherlands, and Scandinavia—there was no catastrophic decline. In northwest Europe the rapid growth of the sixteenth century continued into the mid seventeenth century before giving way to a century of very modest

2. I rely heavily on David Griggs, *Population Growth and Agrarian Change: An Historical Perspective* (Cambridge: Cambridge University Press, 1980) for my discussion of European demographic history. Although my text refers usually to Western Europe, excluding the less densely inhabited eastern areas, population estimates for the west alone over the two millennia shown in Figure 9.1 are not always available.

population increase between 1650 and 1750. A third phase of growth in Western Europe began in the mid eighteenth century, at first at rates not much higher than those experienced in the sixteenth century, but then (in most countries) proceeding much more rapidly from the mid nineteenth century onward. Most important, this third phase of European population increase has been continuous to the present: the population of Western Europe in 1970 (462 million) was more than five times what it had been in 1700 (86 million).

Comparing China's and the West's economic histories can also be a response to several questions about the relationship between economics and population. What is the connection between demographic changes and economic growth and decline? What justification is there for assuming that an increasing population is a direct or indirect indicator of economic growth (as is commonly done)? If economists frequently reason in terms of cycles, demographers, strictly speaking, do not. A population either grows or remains in equilibrium. There are few if any historical examples, at least at the level of a country or a sizable region, of populations in which mortality (the death rate) has remained for long in excess of fertility (the birth rate). In other words, human populations *normally* increase, and the mere fact that a population is increasing does not call for an explanation. But a population increase provides an opportunity (and challenge) to specify how the society responded to that increase and how that response in turn affected population trends.

No population can grow to any significant degree or for any length of time without the total production of the economy increasing in some proportionate measure. Thus, premodern growth necessarily includes increases of both people and productive activity. The growth of population in China in the Sung dynasty was coupled with a Sung "commercial revolution," and the demographic expansion of the Ming was associated with a "second commercial revolution." And clearly the eighteenth century was a time of economic expansion as well as a time of rapid population increase in China. Furthermore, there are good reasons to believe that economic growth also occurred in China in the twentieth century prior to 1937 (even though this version is not the prevalent view), when population grew from 400 million to 500 million.

In Western Europe population growth occurred simultaneously with the revival of commerce and cities in the twelfth and thirteenth centuries. The second phase of demographic increase in Europe was accompanied by the sixteenth-century "price revolution." In the views of many scholars population growth either caused or was a consequence of "protoindustrialization" in eighteenth-century Europe.[3]

3. For example, see Peter Kriedte, Hans Medick, Jurgen Schlumbohm, *Industrialization before Industrialization: Rural Industry in the Genesis of Capitalism* (Cambridge: Cambridge University Press; Paris: Editions de la Maison des Sciences de l'Homme, 1981).

I now look more closely at the economic and demographic responses to population changes that underlay the most important features of premodern economic growth. As Ester Boserup has shown, population growth can induce its own production response in the form of successive modifications in available technology.[4] For example, changes from shifting cultivation to settled dry cultivation, then to irrigated agriculture, and finally to irrigated multiple cropping, make possible the support of an enlarged population. This outlook underlies Dwight Perkins's magisterial study of Chinese agriculture from 1368 to 1968.[5]

In addition to changes in technology (including land use and agriculture), the "Neo-Malthusian" demographic analysis of optimum populations, based in part on the later, more sophisticated editions of Thomas Malthus's famous *Essay,* is also important for understanding the economic and demographic responses to population changes. Neo-Malthusian optimization focuses on what the "best" population is for a country; the answer is usually the population that maximizes production per capita. This approach is at times applied statically to show that average per capita production declines with population growth in the absence of improved technology or increased resources. But the historical experience of some populations, including those of China and Western Europe, suggests that population growth itself may stimulate (or *seem* to stimulate) a variety of responses that either put off or slow down a fall in per capita production. These options are broadly either technological (thus confirming Boserup's analysis in some degree) or demographic (illustrating the Neo-Malthusian view of optimum populations). I now consider Western Europe and China in each of their three cycles of growth in order to discover which responses they took.

In Europe between 1000 and 1300 there were limited technological possibilities for increasing crop yields. Leguminous crops that might help maintain soil fertility occupied only a small proportion of the arable land. The supply of manure, critical to yields, diminished per capita over time as grazing land was plowed up to produce food crops for the expanding population. The replacement of the ox by the horse allowed more frequent cultivation of the seedbed, but few changes occurred in farm implements once the plow had supplanted the hoe. Most of the increase in grains came from expanding the cultivated acreage, including reductions of fallow by shifting from the two-field system (leaving half of one's land idle each growing season) to the three-field system (leaving only one-third idle). But by 1250 little good land was left, and the prob-

4. See Ester Boserup, *Population and Technological Change: A Study of Long-Term Trends* (Chicago: University of Chicago Press, 1981).

5. Dwight Perkins, *Agricultural Development in China, 1368–1968* (Chicago: Aldine, 1969).

lem of maintaining the fertility of the land under cultivation remained a pressing one.

We have little evidence of a European demographic response to overpopulation in the form of Neo-Malthusian fertility adjustments. Overseas migration was not yet a possibility, and rural-urban migration occurred only to a limited extent. Apart from rising mortality, internal migrations of European populations that founded new villages and hamlets were the major demographic response to population pressure in this first cycle.

I would argue that the first Chinese cycle of population growth beyond the plateau of 60 million, achieved at the beginning of the imperial era, was in large part the consequence of a shift from millet to wheat as the dominant crop in north China (which was the core of the Chinese empire before the Sung dynasty). Once the population growth phase began, the principle technological response (we may also say "production response") in Sung China was the spread of wet rice cultivation, especially in newly developed lands south of the Yangtze river. Amano Motonosuke's remarkable history of Chinese agricultural technology makes it clear that what we typically think of as *Chinese* agriculture was basically elaborated in the Sung period (960–1279).[6] The basic foundations for land utilization, cropping patterns, tools, use of human and animal manures, water control and irrigation techniques were laid in Sung China and would predominate for the next ten centuries (with minor improvements but no major changes in the Ming and Ch'ing periods).

As in Europe, there is no evidence of changes in fertility as the population grew. It is not certain to what degree the increased mortality in the Mongol century (1279–1368) was a direct result of the brutal wars that accompanied the fall of the Sung dynasty or the indirect result of a Malthusian crisis of overpopulation. The Chinese demographic response included more rural-urban migration than in Europe; urbanization in Sung China (and continuing into the Mongol era) was probably the highest anywhere in the medieval world. But, again as in Europe, the major demographic response was internal rural-rural migration, which resulted in the populating of vast areas of China south of the Yangtze river.

The population of most of Western Europe went through a second cycle of growth followed by stagnation, not decline, between 1450 and 1650. The pressure of population on land and resources produced clear symptoms of rural poverty in late-sixteenth-century England and Germany and seventeenth-century France. Even by 1600, however, no fundamental advances beyond medieval agriculture had been made, and

6. Amano Motonosuke, *Chūgoku nōgyōshi kenkyū* [Studies in the history of Chinese agriculture] (Tokyo: Ochanomizu, 1962).

there was no substantial increase in crop yields to support a larger population. With little or no new land to open or reclaim, the agricultural production response to overpopulation was limited to the increased average yields that resulted from the gradual spread of known techniques. However, the rapid growth of rural industry throughout Western Europe in the sixteenth century provided some employment for the landless and, most important, supplementary income to smaller peasant households.

Compared with the fourteenth century, this second cycle was characterized by a much wider range of demographic options. In the late sixteenth and early seventeenth century two new West European patterns emerged: late marriage and a high rate of celibacy compared to that in both China and previous centuries in Europe. These patterns were at least in part a response to falling living standards. The lower marriage rate that resulted from them naturally reduced marital fertility and lowered the rate of population increase—until the nineteenth century when a sharper drop in mortality more than canceled this effect. Migrations overseas, for the first time in large numbers, and rural-urban migrations into a growing number of great cities where population was apparently "consumed" as death rates exceeded birth rates probably also helped reduce rural population pressure. Thus, even in the absence of any significant technological advances in agriculture, European standards of living in the downphase of the second cycle never fell to the low point of the fourteenth century.

The second Chinese cycle—let us call it the Ming cycle—like its counterpart in Western Europe, was characterized by a phase of population growth followed by a downphase of stagnation rather than a sustained decline in numbers. By the end of the seventeenth century or the early eighteenth century at the latest, population growth had once again resumed. I treat the third, or Ch'ing, cycle together with the second because the seventeenth-century crisis that accompanied the Ming collapse and Manchu conquest only interrupted rather than fundamentally changed the direction and nature of the premodern economic growth that China experienced from the fifteenth to the mid nineteenth century. In the latter part of the Ch'ing cycle overpopulation was once again certainly a cause of the mid-nineteenth-century rebellions, which produced both absolute population losses, at least in the Yangtze valley provinces, and a subsequent decline in the rate of growth. Only by the turn of the century had total population returned to the level of 1850.

If the large "movements" in our once-over-lightly examination of both Europe and China were analyzed in more detail, we would notice that the demographic-economic cycles were experienced differently from region to region and, especially, from locality to locality. For example, the rate of population growth in China's lower Yangtze valley, which roughly consists of the highly commercialized provinces of

Kiangsu and Chekiang, over most of the millennium under view here was as much as twice that of the other regions of China taken together. The upper Yangtze region—present day Szechwan province—suffered particularly severe population losses at the end of the Sung and Ming cycles. But this region and the south and southwest in general grew more rapidly in the third cycle, which began in the eighteenth century, than did the middle Yangtze or north China regions. And in the mid nineteenth century the demographic losses were greatest in the lower and middle Yangtze regions.

The responses to overpopulation in the Ming and Ch'ing cycles that took the form of population movements, although not yet studied in detail, are reasonably clear. The migration of "overseas Chinese" (*hua-ch'iao*) to Southeast Asia from the coastal provinces of China was probably only important locally as a "safety valve" for population pressure, but nonetheless it may have been proportionately as important as the migration of colonists from Spain, England, and France to the Americas. It is unlikely that any significant urbanization beyond Sung levels occurred in the Ming cycle; nevertheless, the total size of the population living in cities increased in proportion to absolute population growth, and the number of urban centers clearly grew. A significant number of additional market towns was established in the seventeenth and eighteenth centuries, but again it is not evident that there was any increase in the proportion of urban residents. Thus, rural-rural migration—from the more densely settled regional cores to the less densely populated regions or to the peripheries of the same region—was the principal response to demographic pressure. In the Ming cycle China south of the Yangtze river was filled out, in particular the southwestern provinces of Yunnan and Kweichou; the upper Yangtze provinces were repopulated; and the population grew in the peripheries of the middle and lower Yangtze regions and in Lingnan (southeast China, mainly Kwangtung). These were the same areas that experienced major migrations during the Ch'ing cycle, which also saw the beginnings of a substantial flow of population into Manchuria in the northeast.

The matter has not yet been adequately studied, but I find no evidence of a systemwide change in marriage and fertility rates during the Ming or Ch'ing cycles comparable to the striking differences that resulted from the patterns of late marriage and widespread celibacy that emerged in early modern Europe. Nor does it appear that the sort of internal changes in family structure and psychology that are attributed to proto-industry in early modern Europe occurred in China, even though this kind of internal self-regulation of population levels also seems to have occurred in Tokugawa Japan (1600–1868), where decisions within the household about the age of marriage and by the village community about new household formation successfully curtailed population growth in the eighteenth century. How such limitations on population growth were induced in Japan remains unclear, but it seems highly significant that such self-regulation of population growth occurred in the two areas of the world that have industrialized most rapidly, namely Western Europe and Japan. In another context it might be useful to pursue the hypothesis that the absence of such population control in late imperial China was a major determinant of the divergent modern economic histories of China and Japan.

Although changes in grain yields in the first two European cycles were only modest ones if they occurred at all, the production response in China to the Ming and Ch'ing cycles of population growth was much more striking and also of greater impact than the demographic responses I noted. China's population increased by a factor of four or five between the fourteenth and nineteenth centuries, and the area of cultivated land more than doubled. The qualitative evidence, although it shows temporal and regional fluctuations, suggests that over these five centuries average standards of living as measured by grain consumption per capita were relatively constant. Dwight Perkins suggests that the remarkable feat of feeding this greatly expanding population was achieved by a combination in roughly equal proportions of increased arable land and a rise in the national average yield of grain per unit of land.[7] Both these factors were critically linked to the growth of the population itself because each required highly labor-intensive inputs.

To be sure, there was some horticultural innovation over this long era but no fundamental advances beyond the agricultural technology and its accompanying engineering components that had been elaborated in the Sung period. Average grain yields were sharply increased by the widespread diffusion of the best practices already known: improved seeds, more productive cropping patterns (including double cropping), and increased investments in "traditional" capital in the form of implements, water control, and fertilization. Although important in some regions, such as the Han river highlands, the importation in the sixteenth century of corn and potatoes from America supplemented the indigenous process of seed improvement to only a small degree. In Ming and Ch'ing China, as in early modern Europe, rural handicrafts also provided significant employment and income for many peasant households. But this aspect of the production response to overpopulation, although superficially similar in Western Europe and China, in fact encompassed premodern industrial institutions that differed in critical ways. In particular, I would argue that the absence in China until very late of "putting-out" in the cotton textile industry made the role of that largest rural handicraft quite different from its European counterpart. More-

7. Perkins, *Agricultural Development in China, 1368–1968.*

over, the limited appearance of "handicraft factories" in China was not the herald of a new mode of production (in the Marxist sense used by many Chinese historians).[8]

After comparing the Sung, Ming, and Ch'ing demographic-economic cycles in China with the medieval and early modern cycles in Western Europe, I conclude that before the seventeenth century (and possibly the eighteenth century) the European production, or technological, response was much less far-reaching and significant than the comparable Chinese response. The progression from millet to wheat in north China and then to rice in the South and ultimately to double-cropping (of wheat and rice or multiple rice crops)—and the elaboration of the tools and the cultivation and water control techniques that accompanied this progression—produced a much greater possibility for premodern growth in the Chinese economy than the horse collar, improvements in the plow, and the shift from a two-field to a three-field system did in medieval and early modern Europe.

By the eleventh century the Western European economy had certainly left the (probably exaggerated) shadows of the Dark Ages. Yet in the half millennium or more from this starting point until the "age of absolute monarchy," no comparison of agricultural productivity, industrial skill, commercial complexity, urban wealth, or standard of living (not to mention bureaucratic sophistication and cultural achievement) would place Europe on a par with the Chinese empire. It was apparent to most European observers, the most famous one being Marco Polo, that China was "ahead" of Europe in every one of these areas. But success in this first half millennium may have "spoiled" the possibility of further successes from the eighteenth century onward.

Let me restate this admittedly broad comparison between Western Europe from the Fall of Rome to the seventeenth century and China from the Han dynasty to the mid Ch'ing: premodern economic growth interacting with demographic changes in China over this millennium and a half produced overall, in the long run, on average, a perceptibly

8. In the "putting-out" (*Verlagen*) organization of manufacturing, a merchant investor commonly advanced raw materials, and sometimes also production machinery such as looms, to rural or semirural households who in turn delivered products made to his specifications to the merchant at a previously stipulated price. *Verlagen* implies a greater degree of involvement in production by the merchant-capitalist, in order to achieve the quality control required by a more distant market, than was the case in the artisanal *Kaufsystem* under which a peasant producer sold his cloth, for example, to a local merchant or broker who did not directly participate in the production process. Putting-out merchants in Eu rope were later among the investors in early factory industry. Many scholars in the People's Republic of China have acclaimed the establishment of "handicraft factories" (*kung-ch'ang shou-kung-yeh,* i.e., Karl Marx's "manufactories") by putting-out merchants—for which the Chinese evidence is scanty at best—as marking the appearance of "sprouts of capitalism" in Ming and Ch'ing China.

higher level of material culture than that enjoyed by most of Europe before 1700. There were two foundations for this achievement: first, the productive technology (mainly agricultural because that was the principal industry, but including other economic sectors as well) that was elaborated in Sung China and adopted over the next thousand years; second, the social, political, and economic institutions (also perfected in the Sung period, even though originating much earlier) that facilitated or "lubricated" China's extraordinary premodern economic growth. Lack of space and the logical structure of this chapter, not a belief in technological determinism, limit me to only a brief reference to the second of these foundations.

In contrasting China with Europe what is most striking is that the potentialities of the Sung traditional technology and institutions in China were not exhausted until the nineteenth and twentieth centuries. These institutions, even when in decline, could feed, clothe, house, govern, edify, and amuse China's large and rapidly growing population. In contrast, agricultural and other technology in late medieval and early modern Western Europe does not seem to have advanced much beyond the best performance of the Roman Empire. The European absence of production institutions equivalent to those of Sung China was one reason why Europe's demographic response to overpopulation in the second cycle, namely, reducing population growth through the patterns of late marriage and frequent celibacy, was so much more important than its production response.[9] One possible interpretation of this major demographic change is that it was an attempt to defend against the erosion of European living standards that was attributable to the exhaustion of available technology. But in China no such demographic response occurred, and it seems reasonable to conclude that one reason that it did not was because there were no comparable, or perceptible, economic incentives to do so.

If late medieval and early modern Europe responded demographically more than technologically to the recurrent crises of overpopulation, significant changes in both the technology and the organization of Western European agriculture (still the major "industry") began to appear from the seventeenth century onward. The production potentialities of these changes, which first appeared in the Low Countries, were not fully realized for more than two centuries. This process of realization included the geographic extension of cultivated land, technological "deepening," and major social reorganization. Although the new

9. I say this in full awareness of the perils of teleological reasoning. I am simply noting the coincidence of two factors—Europe's reduction of population growth and its lack of a Sung-style production response—and am not claiming that either is the "ultimate cause" of the other.

agricultural techniques were first developed in the Low Countries, their impact in this area was limited because of the great pressure of the population on the land. The new mixed farming and crop rotation practices were first effectively employed in the light soil areas of southern England, where they resulted in increased production not only per unit of land but also per worker. From England the improved agriculture spread gradually over the Western European mainland. Paralleling this diffusion, but occurring mainly in the nineteenth century and later, we can note the systematic application of chemical and biological science to horticultural problems as well as the increased mechanization of the principal agricultural processes.

The social changes that accompanied these economic developments were enormous. In England hundreds of "enclosure acts" ended the old village system of common lands and served to concentrate land in the hands of the large landowners, who let it out to the most efficient farmers. This development and the introduction of crop rotations marked the end of the necessity to maintain fallow land. The enclosures also increased agricultural efficiency by reducing the size of the peasant labor force while raising production. On the European continent serfdom came to an end as absolute monarchs in search of increased revenues sought to raise agricultural output by reducing the feudal privileges of the nobles, who obstructed productivity, and by increasing the incentives for peasant producers to make greater productive efforts.

An agricultural revolution is probably not a necessary and distinct phase of economic development prior to modern industrialization. But concurrent agricultural transformation seems to have been essential in order to release manpower for industry, feed the growing cities, and supply raw materials for manufacture. It is highly significant, for example, socially, politically, and economically that from the eighteenth century on there were never again famines in France such as those that had punctuated the previous millennium. Although the full realization of the new agricultural technology required centuries, its consequences were already evident when eighteenth-century Europe confronted the Chinese empire of the Ch'ing.

The onset of fundamental change in Western Europe was not matched in China, which remained largely in the mold that had been set in the Sung dynasty and refined in succeeding dynasties. A new era of change in Europe was facilitated by the demographic responses I noted because they guaranteed that the early gains in per capita production would not be immediately swallowed up in support of a rapidly increasing population. Only in the last half of the nineteenth century—when the base had already been secured, so to speak, for modern economic growth—did the growth rate of Western Europe's population jump over that of the sixteenth century.

Stagnation or "homeostasis" in China, however, was in part the product of a demographic and institutional stability—even rigidity—that blocked further technological and economic development. The possibilities of the traditional technology were not exhausted before the twentieth century in China, and therefore there were fewer incentives for the internal self-regulation of population growth in the Ch'ing dynasty than was the case in early modern Europe or Tokugawa Japan.

One of the sad ironies of modern Chinese history is that when the necessity and, at last, the possibility of developing and adapting the new European production technologies arrived, it occurred simultaneously with the advent of a fourth Chinese demographic cycle—one in which the rate of population increase reached or exceeded for a time 2 percent per annum. This pattern is typical in what we call the developing countries and is the consequence of a large fall in mortality without any significant decline in fertility. The difficulties of achieving sustained modern economic growth in the People's Republic of China since 1949 in the face of such overwhelming population pressure is self-evident.

I have compared the production and demographic responses to conditions of overpopulation in premodern China and premodern Western Europe over a millennium and more and have suggested an agenda for further comparative inquiry that might link our study of both ends of the Eurasian land mass more closely. Before concluding, I would like to consider two further matters, namely, social and political institutions, and the international environment. Both premodern and modern economic growth in Europe and China were of course shaped by their differences in these two areas as well as in the two I have discussed at length. In the space remaining, I can only say a few words about each of these very large topics.

Although the third European demographic-economic cycle was one of modern economic growth, the comparable Chinese cycle definitely was not. The institutional structures of traditional Chinese society—its political, legal, kinship, and educational formations, among others—had not obstructed and perhaps had even facilitated premodern economic growth from the Sung dynasty to the eighteenth century. Chinese performance during this period was at least as successful as in contemporary Europe. Certainly the acceleration of traditional growth in the seventeenth and eighteenth centuries argues against the received view in China today that late imperial "feudal autocracy" was the major obstacle to economic performance and that it prevented China from following the Marxist path to capitalism and beyond. But Chinese political institutions—let us use the state as our example in this brief exposition—unlike those of early modern Europe, seem to have contributed little if anything toward modern economic growth.

I would argue that a situation in which there are several competing polities (such as the state-building monarchies of early modern Europe) is much more conducive than a unified empire (as in Ming and Ch'ing China) to the development and implementation of the critical abstractions and institutions of law and property of the kind that facilitated Europe's modern economic growth. Furthermore, the relative material scarcity of early modern Western Europe accentuated the intensity of the international and domestic competition for survival and expansion. China in the sixteenth century was, overall, richer than Europe, but the competitive drive of the emerging European nation-states was missing in China. Mercantilist competition among several regional political actors, as occurred in Europe, was not a genuine alternative for China's imperial power monopoly. This discussion suggests a link between the technological and demographic concerns I have emphasized in this chapter and the parallel matter of institutional innovation designed to deal with the omnipresent problem of "transaction costs" (in Douglass North's language).[10]

For all its bureaucratic sophistication the Chinese empire never undertook several basic policies that would have aided economic development. It never developed a funded national debt that untied wealth from the land, it never promulgated comprehensive codes of business law nor created judicial institutions that were devoted to maintaining property rights, and it never developed insurance schemes that could have been used to reduce commercial risk. Before the nineteenth century there was little need—that is, no credible domestic or foreign challenge—for the Ch'ing emperors and the bureaucratic elite that served them to follow the path of the Houses of Stuart, Bourbon, and Habsburg and their administrators, who built the modern European nation-states and favored economic enterprise in exchange for the financial resources to pursue their competitive struggles. The Chinese rulers already possessed "all under Heaven," and they could not be aware of how parochial that conceit would soon become. By the nineteenth century Ch'ing decline and China's unprecedented population growth, its ignorance of the West, and the simultaneous European assault on Ch'ing sovereignty all helped insure Chinese frustration and "failure" to develop the infrastructures necessary for modern economic growth, even when the pressing need for such infrastructures became painfully clear.

The protection of property, the reduction of risk, and the facilitation of capital mobility are all important concerns, but they do not address the critical question of how new technical and organizational knowledge

10. Douglass C. North, *Structure and Change in Economic History* (New York: Norton, 1981).

(without which modern economic growth cannot occur) was itself discovered and applied in the seventeenth, eighteenth, and nineteenth centuries in Europe. The production of knowledge is dependent in large part on the "knowledge institutions" of a society. In a more comprehensive discussion these and other institutional realms would require our attention. Why, for example, does the remarkable technological, institutional, and ideological creativity of Sung China appear to have exhausted itself and not to have been renewed before the twentieth century?

Before modern times, then, we can "award" technological and institutional leadership to China and demographic flexibility to Western Europe. In the early modern world scientific and technological discovery advanced in Europe but not in China. Institutional innovation swept over Europe, but China offered the sacred "virtue" of its emperor to all who came from afar and sought to be civilized.

The international context also favored Western Europe while it moved from premodern to modern economic growth. In this context, the economic effects of Western imperialism have generally been grossly exaggerated, by both the critics and the defenders of the capitalist West. Neither the profits of empire for the imperialist powers nor the economic damage (as opposed to political and cultural harm) to the colonized were the most critical matters. What is important, I suggest, is that Europe had centuries for its transformation—which occurred from roughly 1600 to 1900—but that such a leisurely pace was not politically or psychologically acceptable (and perhaps not economically feasible either because of the "critical minimum effort" now needed to start economic growth) for the Chinese, who were now awakened to the shrill tones of modern Chinese nationalism. Europe, by exploiting the "phantom acreage" of the New World and its markets as well as those of Africa and Asia, made the outside world a participant in the beginning of its modern economic growth. For China, Europe before the nineteenth century was mainly a curiosity and the source of substantial local trading profits. Afterward, Europe (and America and Japan) brought China political loss—abridgment of sovereignty and cultural denigration. These losses were serious forms of damage in a zero-sum game, where for every "winner" there must also be a "loser." But the economic shock of foreign trade, investment, and technology transfer—and the special privileges foreign businesses enjoyed in China that were protected by political concessions—was simultaneously an opportunity. In principle, unlike the political realm of unequal treaties and extraterritoriality (whereby Westerners in China were subject only to Western law), the economic realm was an arena where there could be more than one winner.

In the last decades of the twentieth century China is importing Western technology and making its own growing contributions to its economic development. Although the policy is undoubtedly harsh and sometimes brutal at local levels, China has undertaken a major effort to limit its population expansion and has achieved considerable success, at least in urban areas. Institutional innovations in the areas of law, contracts, property rights, and so forth (which would have been unthinkable in the days of Chairman Mao) are proceeding apace. Foreign trade turnover continues to grow, and China's links to the world are being continually enlarged in every realm. If, as I have implied, these are the critical variables for the achievement of modern economic growth, that long-delayed transition is now beginning to be realized in China.

TEN

□

Modern Chinese Social History in Comparative Perspective

William T. Rowe

The day has long passed when scholars of China were able to view that society's history up until the late nineteenth century as essentially stagnant, in contrast to a West which for at least the past half millennium was relentlessly progressive. The absence of overseas expansion and basic technological innovation need not be taken for the absence of social change or even for the absence of change in a direction that we are pleased to call "modern." In recent years a number of Western scholars, following in their own heretical fashion the lead of Chinese and Japanese Marxists, have come to see the history of China both before and after the nineteenth-century European impact as following a course of social development that had surprising similarities to parts of Europe in the same period. Given the eventual outcomes, however, the precise forms this development took in China and the West were obviously different. In this chapter, based on a mixture of recent and not-so-recent scholarship, I advance some hypotheses about what changed and what did not change in the past five hundred years of Chinese history; I also offer some thoughts about how this process of change is comparable to the Western experience and how it is unique.

A number of caveats are in order at the outset. First, although Chinese social history exhibited very great regional and even local variations, variations at least as great as those within Western Europe, these will be largely ignored in the dramatically simplified scenario that follows. Second, let no one assume that the developments described were exhaustive of the range of social change in the period under consideration. In particular, I hope that as a historian whose own research has focused largely on urban China I shall be forgiven for concentrating here on developments in cities. Although urban developments immediately affected only a minority of the Chinese people, I believe that they represented the vanguard of change and had a broad indirect impact throughout society as a whole.

I begin by noting some preconditions and attempting to suggest why the sixteenth century constitutes a useful point of departure for surveying the emergence of modern Chinese society. Through the end of the nineteenth century and the beginning of the twentieth, the stable factors in China were largely cultural and political and the destabilizing forces socioeconomic. Chief among the constants were the imperial state and the Confucian ideology of minimalist government on which it was based. One cannot help but be struck by the parallel between the late Chinese Empire and the Holy Roman Empire as assessed by Mack Walker:

> The Constitutional strength of the Holy Roman Empire is easy to mistake for weakness. . . . It was built not on internally developed force but on a remarkable mechanism for the restraint and limitation of force; its stability came from the perpetual frustration of disruptive energy and aggressive power. The principle permeated the Empire. . . . It was applied by the emperor himself, and against him; by the component states [for China, read: local interests and bureaucratic factions], and against them.[1]

Beyond this political "restraint," other enduring characteristics of late imperial China included the following: an ethos that stressed harmony, social order, continuity, and community service, all promoted by the state via that unparalleled vehicle of elite indoctrination, the civil service examination system; a fairly successful state monopolization of the approved channels of upward mobility; an emphasis on merit and a customary law of partible inheritance, which made downward mobility over generations an ever-present possibility for the elite; and an orthodoxy that to a greater or lesser extent viewed commerce with suspicion and disdain. Perhaps paradoxically, the late imperial Chinese economy was marked by the existence of comparatively strong property rights and, based on these rights, an agrarian system emphasizing free alienation of land, household-scale proprietorship, and an elaborate and flexible system of mortgaging and leasing.

A major process of socioeconomic transformation, however, began in the mid sixteenth century and continued to unfold despite recession, rebellion, invasion, and dynastic change through the mid eighteenth century. The two major causes of this process seem to have been population growth (discussed in detail by Albert Feuerwerker in Chapter 9 of this volume) and increased foreign trade. Increased population

1. Mack Walker, *German Home Towns: Community, State, and General Estate, 1648–1871* (Ithaca: Cornell University Press, 1971), 11–12.

density and a significant percentage increase in the nonagrarian population were supported by the spreading cultivation of early-ripening rice, which encouraged double-cropping, and by the adoption of New World crops, such as maize and sweet potatoes. Vast imports of New World and Japanese silver fueled a quantum leap in the level of domestic commerce, including, apparently for the first time, routinized long-distance exchange of low-value-per-bulk staples under private auspices. The increasing quantity of available specie and grain for purchase on the market also induced the state to begin the protracted process of transforming the land tax, its fiscal base, from collections in kind to collections in cash, which in turn inclined many landlords to demand rent in cash and stimulated the production of cash crops by the cultivator. A process of regional specialization in export commodities began in the late Ming, leading to effective interregional commercial integration by the mid Ch'ing. Finally, upland areas in central China and peripheral areas such as Taiwan underwent a rapid process of opening and development in the early 1700s and by the latter decades of that century had begun to exhaust their capacity to easily absorb new arrivals. The closure of these frontiers and the net outflow of specie begun by the opium trade conveniently mark the end of this two-hundred-year cycle of development.

We might begin to survey the range of social changes set in motion by this early modern commercial revolution with a look at settlement patterns. One of the most dramatic developments was the rise of the *chen,* or nonadministrative commercial town. Traditionally, cities in China were regularly dispersed, walled seats of bureaucratic administration. There were of course exceptions, such as the enormous *chen* of Ching-te in Kiangsi, center of the national pottery industry, and Hankow, hub of interregional domestic commerce situated at the confluence of China's two longest navigable rivers, the Yangtze and the Han. Founded in the fifteenth century, Hankow hosted a population of perhaps a million persons by the end of the eighteenth century.

But whereas Ching-te and Hankow were unusually large, they were simply the most visible examples of a more widespread pattern of emerging *chen* of greatly varying sizes and economic specializations. In the increasingly commercialized "six prefectures" of the Yangtze delta, centering on Hangchow and Soochow, scores of important towns evolved out of the rural "grass markets" (*ts'ao-shih*) of the middle ages to link rural producers of cotton and silk with urban consumers and the interregional trade.[2] Distributed in a dendritic hierarchy at key points along the lat-

2. These paragraphs draw on the recent spurt of scholarship in China on lower Yangtze *chen,* especially Ch'en Hsueh-wen, "Ming-Ch'ing shih-ch'i Chiang-nan te i-ke ch'uan-yeh shih-chen" [A specialized market town in Ming-Ch'ing Kiangnan], *Chung-kuo she-hui ching-*

ticework of natural and man-made waterways running through the delta area, these *chen* by early Ch'ing times lay within a day's round-trip travel of every villager in the region. Prior to the sixteenth century most *chen* constituted no more than a single line of shops paralleling the riverbank; they were places where peasants exchanged raw produce for daily necessities such as salt and vegetable oil. With increasing commercialization, however, the more centrally located *chen* began to develop more complex T- or X-shaped street plans, subdivide into specialized neighborhoods (sometimes segregated by internal gates), and attain populations in the tens of thousands.

Some *chen* also became functionally complex. They included not only brokers and buyers for interregional traders in raw cotton, silk, mulberry, and silkworm cocoons but also silk and cotton textile dealers who were involved in processing raw materials and marketing their own distinctive finished products. Processing was sometimes accomplished through putting-out to rural cottage industry (the combination of population and fiscal pressure in the late Ming had dramatically increased the importance of sideline spinning and weaving to the budget of Yangtze delta peasant households). In these arrangements the dealer was essentially a capitalist middleman, directly employing only a staff of shopclerks and stockboys. A minority of dealers, however, also set up their own handicraft workshops (*tso-fang*) using wage labor in the *chen* themselves. In these cases the dealers became direct employers in a capitalist production process. In either case the relationship between the *chen* and the countryside was transformed and intensified; rural producers now looked to the town not only for marketing their agricultural surpluses but also for subsidiary employment and, by the mid Ch'ing, as the chief source of staple foodstuffs.

The social composition of these growing commercial towns was unprecedented in Chinese history. Although some of the larger *chen* came to host submagistrates and serve as centers of subcounty administration, for the most part the economic hierarchy of central places remained distinct from the administrative hierarchy. Thus, the sociocultural influence of the bureaucrats and their civil and military entourages remained negligible. Similarly, although the urbanization of landlords in this region of highly concentrated landownership proceeded apace, probably the majority of these gentrified rentiers ignored the *chen* and headed instead for the more refined atmosphere of the county seats. Therefore, although the *chen* spawned a lively cultural life of their own, it was less

---

chi shih yen-chiu 1985.1:54–61, and Wang Chia-fan, "Ming-Ch'ing Chiang-nan shih-chen chieh-kou chi li-shih chia-chih ch'u-t'iao" [A preliminary investigation of the structure and historical significance of market towns in Ming and Ch'ing Kiangnan], *Hua-tung shih-fan ta-hsueh hsueh-pao* 1984.1:74–83.

the culture of the literati than that of the folk tradition, based on the market teahouse and the wineshop and rich in tales of fantasy, romance, and martial exploits. The elite of these towns were merchants, often of great wealth and broad connections. The bulk of the population was made up of semiskilled artisans, shopclerks, stockboys, and unskilled laborers involved in loading and unloading boats and carrying goods between piers, marketplaces, and warehouses.

Although the development of the *chen* occurred earliest and most dramatically in the silk-cotton region of the Yangtze delta, it was by no means restricted to that area. In another region noted for its export of handicraft textiles, the dozen or so counties surrounding the Yangtze-Han confluence in Hupeh, the famous eighteenth-century historian Chang Hsueh-ch'eng recorded the existence of scores of nonadministrative market towns.[3] Even omitting the gargantuan Hankow, the largest among these had populations comparable to their lower Yangtze counterparts, that is, in the tens of thousands.

Paralleling the rise of the *chen* throughout the empire was the great expansion of suburban areas. Extramural trading quarters had begun to spring up outside the gates of major administrative cities at least as early as the tenth and eleventh centuries. These quarters hosted merchants who sought to take advantage of officially maintained transport routes while avoiding excessive control by bureaucrats within the walls. These suburbs continued to grow in the late Ming and thereafter; they were attached not only to walled administrative cities but also to the larger *chen* themselves, and households in these neighborhoods became increasingly involved in cottage industry. Thus, although the spatial distribution of protoindustrial activity in China is a topic in which a great deal of research needs to be done, it seems likely that the great intensification of handicraft production in the sixteenth through the eighteenth centuries was as much a suburban as either an urban or rural development.

The notion of a distinctive "protoindustrial" era, initially developed to characterize changes occurring in rural household structures in early modern Europe, has recently found favor among Western historians studying changes in cities and urban-rural relations during the centuries preceding the steam revolution.[4] In Europe this period was marked by a tremendous overall growth in the level of handicraft production that was directed to distant markets. This growth was heavily concentrated in certain regions, and in these regions the rural self-sufficient "natural economy" disappeared altogether. These regions were also recipients of

3. Chang Hsueh-ch'eng, *Chang-shih i-shu* [Surviving works of Chang Hsueh-ch'eng], 24:23.

4. Jan de Vries, *European Urbanization, 1500–1800* (Cambridge: Harvard University Press, 1984); and Paul M. Hohenberg and Lynn Hollen Lees, *The Making of Urban Europe, 1000–1950* (Cambridge: Harvard University Press, 1985), part 2.

considerable immigration, much but by no means all of which took the form of urbanization in the regions' central cities. These cities played the key role in exporting the manufactures of these regions and in coordinating the overall production process, even while production activities themselves were dispersed among urban, suburban, and rural dwellers. In essence, the favored regions as a whole were becoming semi-urbanized.

A similar process operated in China between the sixteenth century and the introduction of mechanized factory industry at the end of the nineteenth century. If, as historians in the People's Republic have argued, one social consequence of the early modern commercial revolution was the emergence of a distinctive "urban ethos" (*shih-min ssu-hsiang*) at odds with the pastoral values of Confucian orthodoxy, the high velocity of turnover of the urban population very quickly led to the dispersion of these new values throughout the overall society, at least within such highly developed regions as the Yangtze delta, the Yangtze-Han confluence, and pockets along the southeast coast. At the same time, these areas also experienced a process of social dislocation, clearly reflected in the popular literature of the period. For example, one late Ming novel (summarized by Judith A. Berling) describes the perceptions of anomie on the part of several traditional-minded elites in a lower Yangtze *chen:*

> They view with alarm the disorderly elements of society (young bullies, riffraff, runaway servants, religious charlatans). . . . The old (village-based) patterns of relationship are breaking down, and new ones have not yet emerged to fit the urbanized world. . . . Suspicion of people's motives in this competitive urban setting leads to a breakdown of traditional networks of mutual support and generosity. . . . There seems to be no effective mechanism for mediating . . . disputes. . . . Theoretically, a system of elders and mutual security teams (*pao-chia*) should handle it, but it is not functioning. . . . The relative impersonality and scale of town life contribute to the breakdown of human relationships.[5]

Lying behind this social dislocation was an important transformation in styles of labor relations and work organization. In its own fashion China's workforce underwent a process of proletarianization (that is, becoming more legally free, geographically mobile, and dependent for its livelihood on the sale of its labor for cash wages), which was not that dissimilar from the experience of workers in Western Europe. Before the seventeenth century a significant portion of China's labor force lived in

5. Judith A. Berling, "Religion and Popular Culture: The Management of Moral Capital in *The Romance of the Three Teachings,*" in *Popular Culture in Late Imperial China,* ed. David Johnson, Andrew J. Nathan, and Evelyn S. Rawski (Berkeley: University of California Press, 1985), 195, 204–5.

an unfree status, although it is not clear how large this portion was—almost certainly it was a minority. In agriculture, in addition to small-scale owner-cultivators (the Ming had come to power in the late fourteenth century on a platform of land to the tiller) and freely contracted tenants, there were also large agrarian manors (*chuang*) operated in part by hereditary bondservants (*nu-p'u*) who held cultivation rights over their plots but not the personal freedom to leave their lord. The Ming code of 1397 specifically restricted the right to command bondservants to the imperial family and members of the examination gentry, but through various subterfuges, such as the "adoption" of bondservants by landlords, bondservants were in fact possessed by many rich commoner landlords as well. In handicrafts, large numbers of skilled artisans were held in impressed service by the state, to man such enterprises as the imperial pottery kilns at Ching-te and the imperial silkworks at Soochow and Nanking. Also, in local areas such as Hui-chou in Anhwei province, customary law sanctioned such practices as holding a relatively small number of domestic servants as household slaves.

In the early seventeenth century various processes began to contribute to what ultimately became a nearly complete emancipation. First, the final decades of the Ming saw many small-scale uprisings of agricultural bondservants and of urban impressed artisans, especially in the commercially developed lower Yangtze region, as well as the much larger rebellions of Li Tzu-ch'eng and Chang Hsien-chung, which devastated large swaths of the empire and disrupted institutions of personal dependency everywhere in their path. The policies of the early Ch'ing only intensified this process. In a concentrated effort to resettle those areas of southwestern and south-central China that had been significantly depopulated by the rebellions, the Manchus offered such incentives as free seeds and tax holidays to pioneers who would reclaim fallow land, thus setting in motion a massive migration and establishing a precedent for rural geographic mobility. The early Ch'ing sponsorship of private copper mining in the southwest, reversing the late-Ming prohibitions of this activity (based largely on fears of concentrated numbers of free laborers), launched what has been called China's eighteenth-century "gold rush" and spawned a new labor force that was not only free and mobile but permanently withdrawn from settled agriculture. A further stimulus to geographic mobility came in the Yung-cheng reign (1723–1735) when lands formerly officially reserved to minority tribes were opened to Han Chinese immigrants.

Imperial legislation in the early and mid Ch'ing consistently worked in favor of free wage labor, which policy-makers clearly saw as a necessary component of economic recovery and growth. As early as 1645, the new Manchu rulers abolished the castelike hereditary artisan registration system (*chai-chi*), which had been carried over from the early Ming, and merged these groups into the general status category of free commoners (*min*). In the late 1720s the Yung-cheng emperor issued a series of edicts emancipating members of a variety of "mean occupations" (*chien-min*) from servile status, including the hereditary servants (*shih-p'u*) of southeastern Anhwei, the "fallen people" (*to-min*) of Shao-hsing prefecture, Chekiang province, and certain categories of Chinese slaves within the Manchu banner forces (*ch'i-nu*). In the middle decades of the Ch'ien-lung reign (1736–1795) the court issued a succession of revised "hired labor laws" (*ku-kung-fa*). Although not prohibiting servile labor altogether, this sweeping legislation limited it to situations where a specific dependency clause had been written into the contract. In the vast majority of cases, including those where no formal contract existed, laborers would enjoy a great many rights, including the right to address their employer as a status equal, the right to refuse to perform personal or other services not spelled out at the time of hiring, and the right to leave at the termination of the agreed-on period of employment, when the terms of employment—such as the hours or the nature of the work—had been violated, or when wages fell into default. The imperial administration probably did not actively intrude into society on a regular basis to enforce these regulations, but researchers have produced considerable documentation to show that, when hearing criminal cases, state authorities consistently invoked these labor laws in arriving at verdicts.[6]

The relaxation of personal dependency relations and the encouragement of geographic mobility also contributed to a situation where a growing percentage of the workforce engaged primarily in nonagricultural pursuits. No one has yet produced conclusive evidence of any broad pattern of concentration of landownership over the Ch'ing period, but the average size of the family farm must have fallen rather dramatically. Moreover, at some point the rising productivity that had been made possible by the expansion of cultivated land and the intensification of land use was overtaken by the rate of population growth. Many scholars now accept the working estimate of Ping-ti Ho that this point came around the year 1800, though of course there was wide regional variation.[7] One result of this process was what Philip C. C. Huang, studying north China, terms "partial proletarianization": peasant households continued to maintain nonprofitable and inefficient family farms while achieving subsistence by selling their surplus labor to more successful farmers or to rural industrial operations, such as oil presses and pa-

6. For example Wu Liang-k'ai, "Ch'ing-tai Ch'ien-lung shih-ch'i nung-yeh ching-chi kuan-hsi te yen-pien ho fa-chan" [The development of agrarian economic relations in the Ch'ing Ch'ien-lung reign], *Ch'ing-shih lun-tsung* 1 (1979): 5–36.

7. Ping-ti Ho, *Studies on the Population of China, 1368–1953* (Cambridge: Harvard University Press, 1959).

per mills.[8] In the more commercialized areas of greater economic opportunity, however, a growing number of persons left the countryside altogether.

Increased population pressure was probably felt earliest in southeast and central China, where in the mid nineteenth century the lid blew off in the form of the cataclysmic Taiping Rebellion. In addition to providing a sudden check on population growth (directly or indirectly the rebellion is usually estimated to have caused about thirty million deaths), the Taiping wars also caused massive dislocations in rural areas in the form of refugees and, more important, conscription into military organizations of all types. The vast majority of the persons displaced from the countryside in these years were never reintegrated into their native villages after the restoration of peace. Looking only at the government-controlled Hsiang and Huai armies (not the rebel armies or the vast proliferation of local forces), Saeki Tomi shows how the ambitious schemes to resettle the demobilized troops went awry in the 1860s, releasing hundreds of thousands of highly mobile and systematically unsocialized adult males into the society at large.[9] Apparently, most ended up in large- or middle-sized cities, contributing to the phenomenal growth of the urban population in the second half of the nineteenth century. Many became bandits (whole units of former anti-Taiping campaigners remained together after demobilization to plunder when and where they could); others became members of secret societies and sectarian movements. Eventually, all of these formed the basis of early twentieth-century warlord armies.

One of the most striking things about the increasingly proletarianized labor force during the Ch'ing was its geographic mobility. Scholars in the People's Republic such as Liu Yung-ch'eng have recently begun to document the existence, as early as the eighteenth century, of labor markets of regional scope in which prospective employers could find short-term wage-laborers for work either in or out of agriculture.[10] Large numbers of semiskilled workers regularly traveled great distances from home, lured by work in the manufacturing and construction sectors. For example, in the 1880s Wu-ch'ang county (Hupeh province) routinely sent many of its native sons to work as stonemasons in adjacent Ta-yeh county, as carpenters making tea chests in more-distant P'u-ch'i, as tan-

8. Philip C. C. Huang, *The Peasant Economy and Social Change in North China* (Stanford: Stanford University Press, 1985).

9. Saeki Tomi, "Shindai Tōseichō ni okeru kyōyū no teppai mondai" [The problem of demobilized braves in the Ch'ing T'ung-chih reign] in *Chūgokushi kenkyū,* by Saeki Tomi (Kyoto, 1971), 2:392–405.

10. Liu Yung-ch'eng, "Lun Ch'ing-tai ch'ien-ch'i nung-yeh ku-yung lao-tung te hsing-chih" [On hired labor in agriculture in the early Ch'ing], *Ch'ing-shih yen-chiu chi* 1 (1980): 91–112.

ners in Chiang-hsia, as bamboo workers in Ch'i-shui, and as blacksmiths in Hsing-kuo and T'ai-hu (An-hui province).[11]

But by far the majority of those permanently released from agriculture probably found work in the expanding transport sector, as boatmen, interlocal carters and animal-drivers, and intralocal porters, longshoremen, nightsoil- and water-carriers, sedan-chair bearers, and, beginning around the turn of the twentieth century, rickshaw pullers. These occupations were the antecedents of the ubiquitous industrial-era "coolie." In my own research I have found, for example, that nineteenth-century boatmen on the nine-hundred-mile long Han River hailed from half a dozen different provinces. They signed on at various ports along the way for specific hauls of cargo and were released at the destination to seek further work at that point. Of course these activities were only possible because of the dramatic intensification of domestic interregional and foreign trade that marked China's early modern era.

I now turn to the other half of the equation. If a free, mobile labor force was appearing over the course of the late imperial era, were the forms of business structure and work organization accommodating themselves to this fact? In Western history the scenario is often portrayed roughly as follows. Prior to the transition to capitalism—a transition that occurred, depending on the locale, one or more generations *before* the advent of mechanized industry—the household production system predominated. The head of household was a master artisan who marketed his own wares, typically by producing them to custom order. The master might employ journeymen and usually had one or more apprentices, all of whom lived in the master's household as pseudofamily members. At some point, however, merchants, who were often unusually successful masters themselves, began to take control of the system. They raised capital, commissioned ready-made goods for a wider market, either reducing master artisans to the status of subcontractors or establishing handicraft workshops of their own, intensified the division of labor, destroyed the apprentice system and the household economy and replaced it with the large-scale hiring of wage labor. One of the chief consequences of this process was the solidification of a class structure based on relationships of production.[12]

If the legal and organizational preconditions for this kind of transition were not as fully developed in China as in the West, neither were

11. *Wu-ch'ang hsien-chih* [Gazetteer of Wu-ch'ang county] (1885), 3:14.

12. This process is treated, for example, in E. P. Thompson, *The Making of the English Working Class* (New York: Vintage, 1966); William H. Sewell, Jr., *Work and Revolution in France: The Language of Labor from the Old Regime to 1848* (Cambridge: Cambridge University Press, 1980); and Alan Dawley, *Class and Community: The Industrial Revolution in Lynn* (Cambridge: Harvard University Press, 1976).

they completely absent. A law of contracts that might have allowed sophisticated economic arrangements on the scale required for mercantile capitalism was never codified, but a wide range of contractual arrangements was in actual use in commercial dealings and enforceable in local courts. By the late Ming partnerships had become very sophisticated: the numerous gradients between managing and silent partners each bore specified limits of financial liability that tended to be respected in legal proceedings. Although that great Western capitalist breakthrough, double-entry bookkeeping, apparently had not been achieved, accounting techniques adequate to measure such items as profit margins, assets, and liabilities were in general use. The banking institutions that had developed by the late eighteenth century offered a sophisticated range of credit instruments, and the joint-stock company, with its capacity for growth-oriented refinancing, had appeared even earlier. The technology of mobilizing and managing capital had also reached an impressively high level.[13] Moreover, China developed systems of agency, brokering, and factoring arguably much more refined than those of the early modern West. They gave China the unique ability to develop a powerful and efficient commercial capitalism without the large-scale individual firms that had been necessary in Europe.

Utilizing such techniques, a number of changes in the organization of production took place. Most celebrated was the introduction of merchant-owned handicraft workshops (*tso-fang*). Chinese scholars have located the emergence of these workshops as early as the late sixteenth century in highly developed lower Yangtze cities in such trades as cotton and silk weaving, dyeing, papermaking, and chandlery,[14] although they represented only a minor trend at this time. Some Western scholarship suggests that handicraft workshops in cotton weaving became pervasive—in the lower Yangtze and in other traditional textile production areas such as Hunan and Hupeh—only in the late nineteenth and early twentieth centuries. By this era the workshops existed in a symbiotic relationship with new mechanized industry, with yarn for handicraft workshops drawn from spinning factories both in China and overseas.[15] As in Europe, from their first appearance handicraft workshops met stiff re-

13. See Imahori Seiji, "Shindai ni okeru goka no kindaika no hasu" [The modernization of business partnerships in the Ch'ing period], *Tōyōshi kenkyū* 17, no. 1 (1956): 1–49; Teng T'o, "Ts'ung Wan-li tao Ch'ien-lung" [From Wan-li to Ch'ien-lung], in *Lun Chung-huo li-shih chi ke wen-t'i* [On several problems in Chinese history], by Teng T'o (Peking: San-lien Shu-tien, 1979), 189–239.

14. A pioneering study of this subject is Fu I-ling, *Ming-Ch'ing shih-tai shang-jen chi shang-yeh tzu-pen* [Merchants and commercial capital during the Ming and Ch'ing eras] (Peking: Jen-min ch'u-pan-she, 1956).

15. Albert Feuerwerker, "Handicraft and Manufactured Cotton Textiles in China, 1871–1910," *Journal of Economic History* 30, no. 2 (June 1970): 338–78.

sistance from the craft guilds, which represented master artisans and which sought to preserve the traditional household production unit by tightening controls over the apprentice system.[16]

Through the end of the nineteenth century the guilds enjoyed considerable success in forestalling the rise of the handicraft workshop, but they were notably less successful in preventing the emergence of a more pervasive form of large-scale work organization: the labor gang and the contract labor system. This system involved groups of ten, twenty, or more workmen, usually drawn from the same native area and practicing the same occupation, who lived and worked together and hired out to employers as a unit for a specified period of time. One member of the group was the gang headman (*fu-t'ou, pao-t'ou*), who often had actually recruited and assembled its members and served as their agent in negotiating employment. Sometimes a further intermediary appeared in the process in the person of a labor broker (*fu-hang*), who set up shop in an urban area, brought the gang headman together with prospective employers, guaranteed the good faith of both parties, and took a percentage of the wages paid. Where costly tools were involved these might be the property of the broker, and in a Chinese equivalent of the abominated "truck system" of eighteenth-century England either the broker or the gang headman might house and feed the workmen during their term of employment, paying them essentially in kind. This system appeared by the second half of the seventeenth century or perhaps earlier and soon became the dominant form of labor organization in the transport sector. More important in terms of its impingement on the artisan household economy, it was widely adopted in the construction trades and in certain manufacturing activities such as cloth calendering.[17]

It is obvious from the rapidity with which factory industry (both foreign- and Chinese-capitalized) took hold in the early twentieth century that a large, free, and competent labor force was available to be tapped for employment in this sector. I have suggested in broad terms how this labor force came into being. I believe that the immediate basis for China's new industrial proletariat was not, as is often assumed to have been the case in Europe, "debased" artisans who had found transitional employment in handicraft workshops, but rather the rootless, free-floating labor pool available in the labor gang system, especially in

16. See Imahori Seiji, "Shindai no jutei seido" [The apprenticeship system in the Ch'ing period], in *Chūgoku kindaishi kenkyū josetsu* [Studies in modern Chinese history], by Imahori Seiji (Tokyo: Keisō shobō, 1968), 133–52, and P'eng Tse-i, "Shih-chi hou-ch'i Chung-kuo ch'eng-shih shou-kung-yeh shang-yeh hang-hui te ch'ung-chien ho tso-yung" [The reestablishment and functions of Chinese urban handicraft and merchant guilds in the late nineteenth century], *Li-shih yen-chiu* 1 (1965): 71–102.

17. Yokoyama Suguru, *Chūgoku kindaika no keizai kozo* [The economic structure of China's modernization] (Tokyo: Aki shobō, 1972).

the huge transport sector that served the large and ever-growing domestic circulation economy.

Were similar processes at work in the agricultural sector? If the family firm showed surprising powers of survival in urban commerce and handicrafts in the face of daunting challenges, even more did the family farm continue to dominate in the countryside. Historians in the People's Republic are fond of pointing to the emergence in the late Ming and middle Ch'ing of "managerial landlordism," plantation-style agriculture using hired labor to grow commercial crops on the scale of up to about a hundred acres, but it is clear that these arrangements were limited to a few relatively developed areas and were unusual even there. I earlier noted a secular trend toward the sale of surplus labor by peasant households, but the individual household clearly remained the predominant managerial unit, and those fortunate enough to accumulate surplus land continued through the mid twentieth century to rent it out in parcels the size of family farms or even smaller.

It was in rental arrangements, however, that something approximating "capitalism" did creep into Chinese agriculture. In the most productive and market-oriented agrarian regions, notably Soochow prefecture in Kiangsu, the attractions of city life and the rural class warfare of the late Ming and Taiping rebellions combined to produce a high degree of urbanized absentee landlordism. In the post-Taiping years a system of rent collection agencies (*tzu-chan*) emerged that served as intermediaries between tenants and city-based investors in rural land. Investors and tenants did not know each other's names; investors bought and sold rural plots and agents managed their portfolios much like stockbrokers.[18] Absentee landlordism involved the high development of one feature often identified with capitalist production: the clear separation of ownership and management. But the resulting capitalism was of a peculiarly sterile sort, hardly conducive to the entrepreneurial spirit or the mobilization of funds for capital improvement.

In the cities the combination of trends already described led to a new style of social organization and a new intensity of collective action for social purposes. One of the most dramatic new forms of social organization were the guilds formed by the new urban elite. These guilds were *not* relatively conservative artisan guilds, but rather guilds of long-distance wholesale merchants (as in Europe the goals and outlooks of these two organizationally similar institutions could be very different). When guild-centered elite activism brought together leading merchants of various local origins and the trades that operated in a given locality to form um-

18. Yuji Muramatsu, "A Documentary Study of Chinese Landlordism in Late Ch'ing and Early Republican Kiangnan," *Bulletin of the School of Oriental and African Studies* 29 (1966): 566–99.

brella organizations (which Japanese historians, following historians of German cities, call "guild-merchants"), an alternative power structure to that of the imperial bureaucracy was the potential result.

For example, in the nonadministrative commercial town of Hung-chiang, located along the major trade route between central and south-west China, a municipal federation of ten sojourner-merchant guilds (*shih-kuan*), including groups from Kiangnan, Kiangsi, and Kweichow, over the second half of the nineteenth century gradually acquired a wide range of quasi-governmental powers. In 1866 it established a municipal militia to defend the city against rebel attacks and secret society disorders. During a flood-induced subsistence crisis in 1878 it set up a charitable granary. The same year it purchased several American-made fire engines and founded a municipal fire department. The federation also established an orphanage in 1879, a smallpox vaccination clinic in 1883, a municipal cemetery in 1884, and a municipal police force in 1885, managed by a committee of leading merchants to which two members of each guild were appointed. Significantly, this piecemeal incursion of merchants into the domain of the state was accomplished with local bureaucratic acquiescence and usually ex post facto official sanction.[19]

A similar alliance of the major merchant guilds emerged in the Manchurian treaty port of Newchwang (Ying-k'ou) in the 1880s. The group collected taxes on shops and commercial transactions, imposed tolls on local bridges, managed the local money market, oversaw the flow of grain, undertook the maintenance of local streets, the municipal water supply, and drainage and sewage facilities, and sponsored a wide range of public welfare and relief agencies. For convenience in carrying out their tasks the merchant-managers divided the city into their own administrative subdistricts, and occupied, in the words of the local Maritime Customs superintendent, "a position somewhat similar to the municipal councillors" in a Western city.[20]

To be sure, this particular elite response to the new problems of increasing complexity in urban society did not occur in all cities, but something comparable seems to have happened in quite a number of them. The cities where it took place were not necessarily the largest (although in several of China's biggest cities—Shanghai, Hankow, Canton—comparable developments can be observed). The pattern seems to have been particularly pronounced in cities on the margins of Chinese civilization, for example Pao-t'ou (Inner Mongolia), Tainan (Taiwan), and Newchwang, but it was clearly not unique to places on the cultural frontier. Some of the most dramatic examples occurred in *chen* like Hung-chiang

19. Niida Noboru, "Shindai Konan no girudo-machanto" [A guild merchant in Ch'ing Hunan], *Tōyōshi kenkyū* 21, no. 3 (December 1962): 315–36.

20. Inspectorate General of Customs, "Newchwang," in *Decennial Reports, 1882–91* (Shanghai: Inspectorate General of Customs, 1892), 34–37.

and Hankow, which had no position in the administrative hierarchy, but again this was not a necessary precondition. What seems common to all cities where this sort of development took place was a pronounced orientation toward trade (particularly trade of an interregional sort) rather than administration, and social domination by the merchants in control of that trade, who were usually extralocal in origin and as a group rather diverse.

One key factor that promoted merchant self-government was the inadequacy or temporary withdrawal of an effective regular bureaucratic administration. Hence, merchant self-government was more prevalent not only in *chen* and at the cultural frontiers but also in times of sudden military or political crisis. One of its most celebrated early appearances, for example, came in Chungking, the commercial metropolis of the upper Yangtze valley, when during an attack by Taiping forces in the 1860s a loose federation of sojourner merchant guilds known as the Eight Provinces (*Pa-sheng*) temporarily assumed a wide range of quasi-governmental powers.[21] Similar temporary actions in the name of "preserving stability" (*pao-an*) by chambers of commerce and merchant militia corps were widespread throughout China at the moment of the Ch'ing collapse in 1911–1912.

A second type of urban elite response to new social problems, the corporate-style philanthropic association, was, on the surface at least, less threatening to the imperial bureaucracy's monopoly of political authority. These associations were also more broadly based; although they were found in greater numbers in the more commercially developed cities, they were not merely a function of merchant guilds. They began in the sixteenth century, stagnated somewhat during the heyday of bureaucratic effectiveness during the eighteenth century, then started to proliferate again in the nineteenth. These associations varied widely in their inspiration and their specific aims, but their organizational styles were recognizably similar. They included Buddhist societies for the ceremonial release of captive birds and animals (*fang-sheng-hui*), Confucian organizations for the collection and ritual burning of waste paper bearing written characters (*hsi-tzu-hui*), and more secular associations such as those that sponsored lifeboats (*chiu-sheng-hui*), operated urban fire brigades (*shui-hui, paó-huo-hui*), or financed community granaries (*she-ts'ang*). Most ubiquitous and most comprehensive in the range of services provided was an institution known in the late Ming as the "united benevolent association" (*t'ung-shan-hui*) and in the nineteenth century as the "benevolent hall" (*shan-t'ang*).

Most of these institutions had antecedents as far back as the eleventh century, during the Southern Sung, and were championed in the writ-

21. Tou Chi-liang, *T'ung-hsiang tsu-chih chih yen-chiu* [A study of local origin associations] (Chungking: Ch'eng-chung shu-chü, 1946).

ings of neo-Confucian social thinkers of that era such as Chu Hsi. These antecedents raise a thorny question regarding the degree of continuity in Chinese social organization over this period of nearly a millennium: Is it possible that we consistently overstate the degree of innovation in the period following the sixteenth century? Certainly, there was rapid socioeconomic change in this era (as I hope I have demonstrated), but is it not possible that the changes we observe in the repertoire of collective action constituted little more than a renaissance, a revival? Or do the vigorously private, urban-commercial worlds of the Southern Sung, the late Ming, and the late Ch'ing perhaps represent Chinese society operating on its "normal" track, and the despotic command economies of the Yuan and early Ming and the exceptionally able bureaucratic management of the high Ch'ing no more than short-term deviations? In my view there is increasing evidence to justify this perspective. However, the revivals of societal activism in both the late Ming and the late Ch'ing clearly offered important innovations of their own. The general trend was one of extrabureaucratic initiative, ever more unambiguous and unembarrassed merchant sponsorship, and, probably most important, a more articulated pattern of corporate-collective management and finance. In China, as in the West, this last shift almost certainly drew its inspiration from similar contemporary innovations in the structure of commercial and industrial enterprises.[22]

In Hankow, the subject of my own research, the late-Ch'ing phase of this process began with the private founding of two benevolent halls in the 1820s and 1830s. They undertook to provide specialized services (the operation of harbor lifeboats and public burial) on a municipality-wide scale and were financed by rents on urban endowment land. By the last decades of the century some thirty halls existed, each corporately managed on the scale of an urban neighborhood but linked into a citywide system and financed by a combination of endowments, neighborhood subscriptions, and irregular property taxes. The halls provided an expanding range of services including the distribution of food and winter clothing to indigents, medical care, burial, and neighborhood firefighting. The halls did not themselves sponsor public security forces, but at least in the winter months local officials formally coordinated their activities with those of the increasingly high-profile, merchant-sponsored municipal militia.

A further refinement of this trend was the founding in 1889 of a single municipal benevolent hall in the Shantung treaty port of Chefoo.

22. This point is stressed in the European context in David Owen, *English Philanthropy, 1660–1960* (Cambridge: Harvard University Press, 1964), 3, 13. On the Chinese experience see especially Fuma Susumu, "Zenkai to zentō no shuppatsu" [The origins of *shan-hui* and *shan-t'ang*], in *Min-Shin jidai no seiji to shakai* [Government and society in the Ming-Ch'ing period], ed. Ono Kazuko (Kyoto: Kyōto daigaku jinbun kagaku kenkyūjo, 1983), 189–232.

The cost of construction of the *shan-t'ang*'s magnificent premises was met by citywide public subscription; its annual operating costs of more than seven thousand taels was also largely offset by subscribers, but with the assistance of a specially imposed local opium tax and a surcharge on Domestic Customs collections at the port. The Chefoo Benevolent Hall was internally divided into sixteen departments whose functions spanned the gamut of usual *shan-t'ang* activities—the distribution of rice gruel, the burial of unclaimed corpses, the operation of harbor lifeboats, smallpox vaccinations, waste-paper collection, and the operation of an anti-opium clinic. It also functioned as a consumer credit society, offering interest-free loans of up to five thousand copper cash to persons recovering from illness in order to enable them to return to the workforce; the loan was to be repaid in daily installments of ten cash for each thousand cash borrowed.[23]

A very evident rise in the level of elite-sponsored philanthropy occurred from the Sung to the late Ch'ing. These activities were in part the result of the growth in the urban poor, persons for whom no communal group such as the lineage or native village any longer served to provide a natural safety net. Again based on a late Ming novel, Berling summarizes the perceptions of the new urban elites: "In the city charity is difficult, for the poor keep coming. Unlike the small village where the lines of responsibility can be drawn in terms of a hierarchy of relationships and obligations, in town there is a vast sea of 'the poor.'"[24]

The shift over this period for the sponsorship of public services and public welfare from the state to local elites was quite obviously related to the enfeeblement of the imperial bureaucracy, both on a secular and a cyclical basis. Mary B. Rankin has convincingly portrayed this process in its late Ch'ing phase as the expansion of a "public" (*kung*) sector that was extrabureaucratic, community-centered, and firmly under the stewardship of the local elite.[25] By the close of the nineteenth century, however, the government was anxious to reenter the arena of expanding social services and not merely sanction and coordinate societal self-help. On the one hand, the government increasingly tended to draw on the state's resources—most evidently commercial revenues, such as those derived from the imperial Maritime Customs, which continued to thrive in the midst of general government impoverishment—to underwrite part of the costs of new philanthropic endeavors. On the other hand, the state started to governmentalize such revenues as local shop taxes, initially imposed by neighborhood associations and benevolent halls, and the local bureaucratic administration started to assume responsibility for

23. Inspectorate General of Customs, "Chefoo," in *Decennial Reports 1882–91*, 60.

24. Berling, "Religion and Popular Culture," 205.

25. Mary B. Rankin, *Elite Activism and Political Transformation in China* (Stanford: Stanford University Press, 1986).

carrying out the social functions underwritten by these revenues. These developments were one path to the belated creation of a European-style modern state in nineteenth- and twentieth-century China.

The sorts of changes just described were accompanied by others in the nature and the role of elites and in the relationship between elites and the state. To a considerable extent China's experience in this regard also parallels that of Europe. Writing of England, E. A. Wrigley notes: "In the provinces in the later seventeenth and early eighteenth centuries there were increasingly large numbers of men of position who stood outside the traditional landed system. These were the group whom Everitt has recently termed the 'pseudo-gentry.' They formed 'that class of leisured and predominantly urban families who, by their manner of life, were commonly regarded as gentry, though they were not supported by a landed estate.'"[26] A similar urbanization of the gentry started to occur in China during the late Ming. It was most prominent in the lower Yangtze and was encouraged by both the "pull" of commercial opportunity and the "push" of agrarian rebellion. A pronounced expansion of the number of elites in professional managerial roles, for example, as "gentry-directors" (*shen-tung*) of water control and other public works projects, also occurred around this time. The process accelerated in the late nineteenth century when nongovernmental elites assumed military leadership to combat the Taiping rebellion and subsequently were important in postrebellion "reconstruction" (*shan-hou*). As the government relaxed the prohibitions that prevented degree-holders from entering trade, and sales of gentry degrees to merchants ballooned, gentry and merchant roles merged into the so-called "gentry-merchant" (*shen-shang*) class, an urbanized and increasingly reformist elite that became the forerunner of China's twentieth-century bourgeoisie.

An even more dramatic transformation began in the last decade of the nineteenth century and the first decade of the twentieth. Sparked in large part by a perceived threat to China's national survival, large numbers of agrarian elites in the more developed regions of China, members of long-established landed families which for generations had resisted direct involvement in urban commerce, finally relocated to cities and began to retool themselves as industrialists or other modern-sector professionals; they joined the urban gentry-merchants and compradores and left the countryside to its own devices. The abolition in 1905 of the civil service examination system, the traditional vehicle of elite legitimation, came as a shock to many conservative aspirant scholars, but for probably a larger number the act was anticlimactic. In many ways the

26. E. A. Wrigley, "A Simple Model of London's Importance in Changing English Society and Economy, 1650–1750," *Past and Present* 37 (July 1967): 54.

most striking social phenomenon of the early twentieth century was the rapid transformation of the traditional gentry into powerful new professional elites: factory managers, bankers, lawyers, doctors, engineers, scientists, educators, journalists, and—not least—military officers. Beginning with the late Ch'ing and especially under the fragmented and transient authority structure of the warlord era (ca. 1916–1927), these new elites within small- and larger-scale urban places organized themselves into officially sanctioned professional associations (*fa-t'uan*), contended for quasi-governmental regulatory powers over sectors of the economy (that is, the newly governmentalized "public sphere"), and experimented with local coalitions such as "All-Interests Federations" (*ko-chieh lien-ho-hui*) in order to exert their control over local society.[27]

It would be inaccurate to portray late Ch'ing and republican China as a period characterized by the unbroken downward and outward shift of power. A more appropriate reading, in fact, might see in the period beginning with the early twentieth-century Ch'ing reforms and continuing through the early republic, the Nationalist era, and the first fifteen years of the People's Republic, a progressive growth of a larger, more pervasive, and more powerful state than China had seen at any time in its long history. Although the history of political centralization proceeded unevenly (experiencing a dramatic setback in the interlude between the ascendancies of Yuan Shih-k'ai and Chiang K'ai-shek), the growth of the "governmental sphere" (*kuan*), in the sense of bureaucratic command over resources, personnel, and range of functions undertaken, was nearly unbroken and continuous. The climax of these two parallel processes—the expanding power both of societal elites and of the state—may have come (as some scholars have recently suggested) in a kind of state "corporatism" under the Nationalists, in which a modern revolutionary party with totalitarian claims to authority sought to legitimate, coordinate, and in some cases create organized elite interest groups in service of party and national goals.[28]

According to Charles Tilly the major changes in European society between about A.D. 1500 and the early twentieth century were largely the consequences of two key developments: the rise of capitalism and of the modern national state.[29] Assuming Tilly to be correct—and he is by no means without his critics—with what justification may we borrow these Western categories to describe processes of social change in China? On

27. R. Keith Schoppa, *Chinese Elites and Political Change: Zhejiang Province in the Early Twentieth Century* (Cambridge: Harvard University Press, 1982).

28. See especially Joseph Fewsmith, *Party, State, and Local Elites in Republican China* (Honolulu: University of Hawaii Press, 1985).

29. Charles Tilly, "Retrieving European Lives," in *Reliving the Past: The Worlds of Social History*, ed. Olivier Zunz (Chapel Hill: University of North Carolina Press, 1985), 11–52.

the one hand, imposing models derived from one culture on another runs the risk of blinding the analyst to important factors in the target culture that are not of relevance to the borrowed model. On the other hand, as Susanne Rudolph has argued, "the virtue of imposing external categories into the indigenous account is precisely that they raise questions that the indigenous accounts would like to let sleep."[30] Whereas an ideal comparative history would proceed by first deriving developmental models independently of the cultures compared and only then asking where the different cultures coincide and differ, the present state of research does not appear to allow this. In this chapter, then, I have settled for the more practical course of trying to suggest how modern Europe's two "grand processes"—the rise of capitalism and of the state—may be useful in interpreting modern Chinese social history.

Capitalism may be defined in at least three alternative ways, as (1) a system that mobilizes financial resources and applies them to profit-making ventures, (2) an organization of production relations that relies on the use of free, hired labor on a scale considerably expanded beyond the household level, and (3) a Marxist "social formation" that comes into being when the capitalism of the first and second definitions becomes so pervasive in an economy that it dictates social and political relations beyond the confines of the marketplace and workplace. The capitalism of the first definition existed in China as early as the Sung period, if not long before, and the capitalism of the third definition (if indeed one is inclined to accept that definition as meaningful) has probably never pertained in China at any time. It is then the rise of capitalism of the second definition, the increasing pervasiveness of capitalist production relations, that has characterized social change in China in the early modern and modern periods.

State-making may be seen as both the bureaucratization of personnel and posts and the increasing penetration of society by the formal state organization, whose budget and personnel grow as a function of overall product and population. The development of political bureaucratization in China, of course, largely antedated that in Europe and served as a model for the latter. But the dramatic expansion of the state apparatus along European lines was new to China in the twentieth century.

Thus, if capitalism and state-making were key factors in modern China's social history, as they were in the West, the sequence of these two processes in the Chinese and the European cases were very different. In Europe the rise of capitalism and the modern state were very nearly syn-

30. Susanne Hoeber Rudolph, "Presidential Address: State Formation in Asia: Prolegomenon to a Comparative Study," *Journal of Asian Studies* 46, no. 4 (November 1987): 736. For a forceful articulation of the opposing view see Gary G. Hamilton, "Why No Capitalism in China? Negative Questions in Historical, Comparative Research," in *Max Weber in Asian Studies*, ed. Andreas E. Buss (Leiden: Brill, 1985), 65–89.

chronic, whereas in China the expansion of the state lagged by perhaps as much as three centuries behind the appearance of capitalism. Why? Immanuel Wallerstein and his followers offer one possible explanation, which highlights the role of cross-cultural interaction. In their view the emergence of a capitalist world-system after the sixteenth century both precipitated the development of central states in the metropolitan West and impeded such developments in peripheral areas such as China, with the aim of preventing these countries from escaping a subordinate position in global relations of production.[31]

The evidence presented here suggests that the world-system approach is not so much wrong as it is insufficient. Despite the unquestionable importance of Western expansion in shaping China's developmental experience, the overall direction of social change in the two civilizations was more closely parallel than it was inverse.[32] The origins of Chinese capitalism were domestic rather than imported. Similarly, the lateness of the rise of the modern state in China also owed more to indigenous than to exogenous forces. Prior to the twentieth century the small-government predispositions of Confucian ideology combined with the integrative power of Chinese cultural values to make a large state both undesirable and unnecessary. Even more important was the absence of a system of relatively coequal political antagonists, as was present in that crucible of state-building, seventeenth-century Europe. Finally, of course, there was the tremendous diseconomy of scale: a culturally and physiographically discrete unit, the Chinese Empire was nevertheless simply too large to support a pervasive state apparatus under the burden of the overhead costs imposed by premodern technology. Whatever the reason, the divergences between Chinese and Western social histories since 1500 are not due to the fact that the progressive West discovered capitalism and the modern state and China did not, but rather to the fact that the two civilizations developed these institutions in somewhat different fashions, conditioned by the distinctiveness of their two respective cultures.

31. Immanuel Wallerstein, *The Modern World-System: Capitalist Agriculture and the Origins of the European World-Economy in the Sixteenth Century* (New York: Academic Press, 1976); and Frances V. Moulder, *Japan, China, and the Modern World Economy: Toward a Reinterpretation of East Asian Development, ca. 1600 to ca. 1918* (Cambridge: Cambridge University Press, 1977).

32. A stimulating article supporting this view, which came to my attention after effective completion of this chapter, is Joseph Fletcher, "Integrative History: Parallels and Interconnections in the Early Modern Period, 1500–1800," *Journal of Turkish Studies* 9. 1 (1985): 37–57. In the Chinese case I would extend the temporal parameters of the "early modern" period perhaps a century beyond those chosen by Fletcher, up to the widespread introduction of factory industry around 1900.

ELEVEN

□

Chinese Art and Its Impact on the West

Michael Sullivan

Unlike philosophy, history, or economics, art can be understood even when we do not understand it intellectually, for the enjoyment of art—that is, our aesthetic response to it—is itself a form of understanding, as mysterious as it is complete. Art does not need a translator, for it is "read" in the original. Aesthetic response is a response primarily to form; it has little to do, in the first encounter, with the purpose of the work of art, its subject matter, content, or history. But it is good to know these things about a work of art, not only because they enrich our appreciation of it but also because they enable us to see in the work clues to the understanding of a civilization and ways of comparing one culture with another. Certainly Chinese art is inseparable from the civilization of which it is an expression. What I have to say about it should be far more intelligible in the light cast by the other chapters in this volume.

I would like to set down very briefly some of the essential features of Chinese art and to consider how we in the West have become aware of it, how we have responded to it, and, more briefly still, what effect our confrontation with it has had on our own art. Answering these questions is of course an impossibly large task for a single chapter, so I will have to imitate the impressionist, painting my picture with very broad strokes and in the process making some sweeping generalizations.

One might summarize the aesthetic ideals expressed in Chinese art in three words: order, harmony, vitality. The Chinese value order as the source of social well-being. Order implies authority, the acceptance of constraints on the individual for the good of society as a whole. One has only to compare Chinese painting, even of the twentieth century, with its Western counterpart to realize how constrained Chinese artists were, and often still are, within certain formal and technical conventions. They accept these constraints, as they accept the social constraints imposed on them, for the good of society and for the good of art itself; for they feel that there is a point at which the freedom of the individual must give way before the harmony and cohesion of the society of which they are members.

Authority, so long as it is manifest in good government, must be accepted. Authority is embodied in the emperor. Did the Chinese emperor ever say what Louis XIV said to his court painters, "I entrust to you the most sacred thing on earth—my fame"? If he did not, it was because his sanctity was taken for granted. Portraits of the Chinese emperor (figure 11.1) are both likenesses of the man himself and symbolic representations of his imperial role. Such paintings belong at what we might call the Confucian end of the spectrum of Chinese thought and belief, embracing the concept of the emperor, the imperial system, the civil service, and the binding force of political order and social ethics. This concept of order is also expressed, on a tremendous scale, in the aerial photograph of the Forbidden City, which was, and with its "forecourt" T'ien-an-men Square still is, seen as the symbolic heart of the state, from which power radiates and toward which all eyes are turned (figure 11.2). The Forbidden City with its attendant places of sacrifice was the stage on which the drama of loyalty and obedience, awe and reverence, was acted out in ritual and ceremony.

Yet the concept of order does not belong only in the Confucian sphere of belief and action. For the location, orientation, and layout of the palaces and imperial altars were governed by principles distilled from the natural order in geomancy, or siting (*feng-shui,* discussed by Nathan Sivin in Chapter 7 of this volume), a pseudoscience concerned with natural forces and influences, which belongs to what we may call the Taoist end of the spectrum. The principles of geomancy have to do with the relationship not between man and man but between man and nature. The calendar, the imperial sacrifices, the cult of the sacred mountains, the placing of temples and tombs, palaces and mansions, are ordained to conform not to man's order but to nature's order.

If we examine a ritual bronze vessel of the Shang or early Chou dynasty, we discover these two concepts of order interacting in a wonderful formal harmony. A wine vessel of the type called *yü* (figure 11.3) is the very embodiment of royal or clan power as expressed in ritual—grand, noble, earthbound. If we look more closely, we find that it is covered with motifs real and imaginary taken from the natural world: dragons, snakes, tigers, birds, elephants, and that mysterious composite creature

---

Figure 11.1. Anonymous. Portrait of the K'ang-hsi emperor (r. 1662–1722). Colors on silk. 161.6 × 77.5 cm. Ch'ing dynasty. The Metropolitan Museum of Art, Rogers Fund, 1942. (42.141.2)

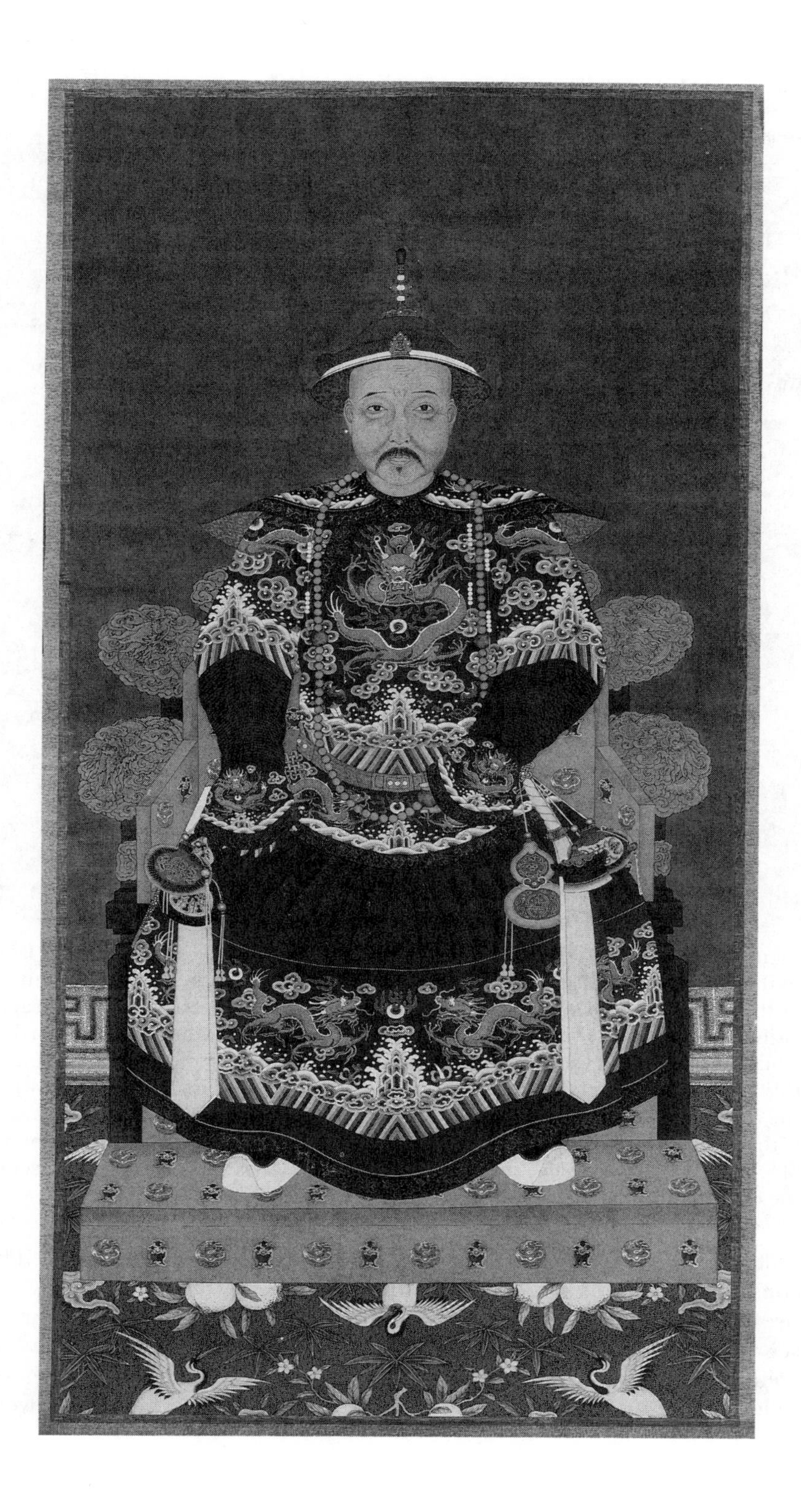

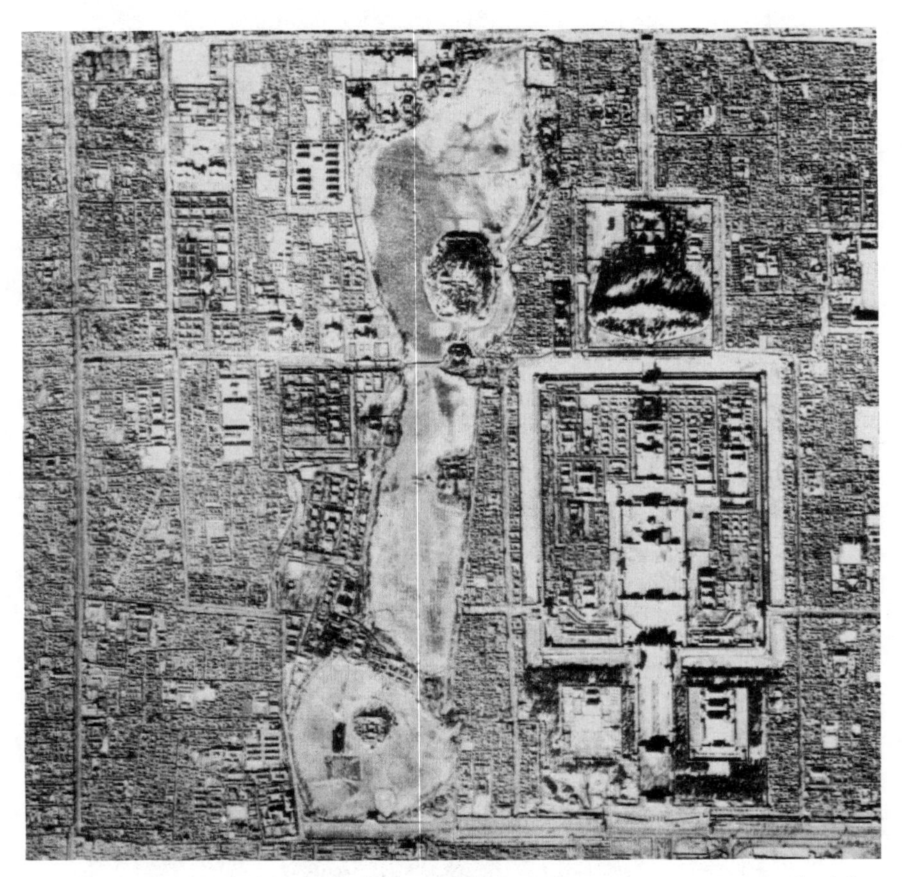

Figure 11.2. Aerial view of the heart of Peking. Down the center runs the lake of the New Summer Palace, Wan-shou-shan; to the right is the moated rectangle of the Purple Forbidden City, with the three halls of state, San Ta Tien, clearly visible on the north-south axis. Prospect Hill lies in the rectangle to the north, while to the south is the main gate of the Forbidden City, T'ien-an-men. Since this photograph was taken, in about 1945, the city walls have been torn down, the area to the south of T'ien-an-men has been cleared to make a huge square, with the Great Hall of the People on the west side, and new streets and apartment blocks have taken the place of many of the narrow lanes and courtyard houses of the old Peking.

called the *t'ao-t'ieh,* which dominates the lower half of the vessel. The consensus of opinion on the meaning of the *t'ao-t'ieh* is that it was a protective spirit of a benevolent nature. If we look still more closely, we see that these zoomorphs are set against a pattern of endless coils and volutes that have no symbolic meaning, although they were formerly called the "thunder pattern" by Chinese antiquarians because they were

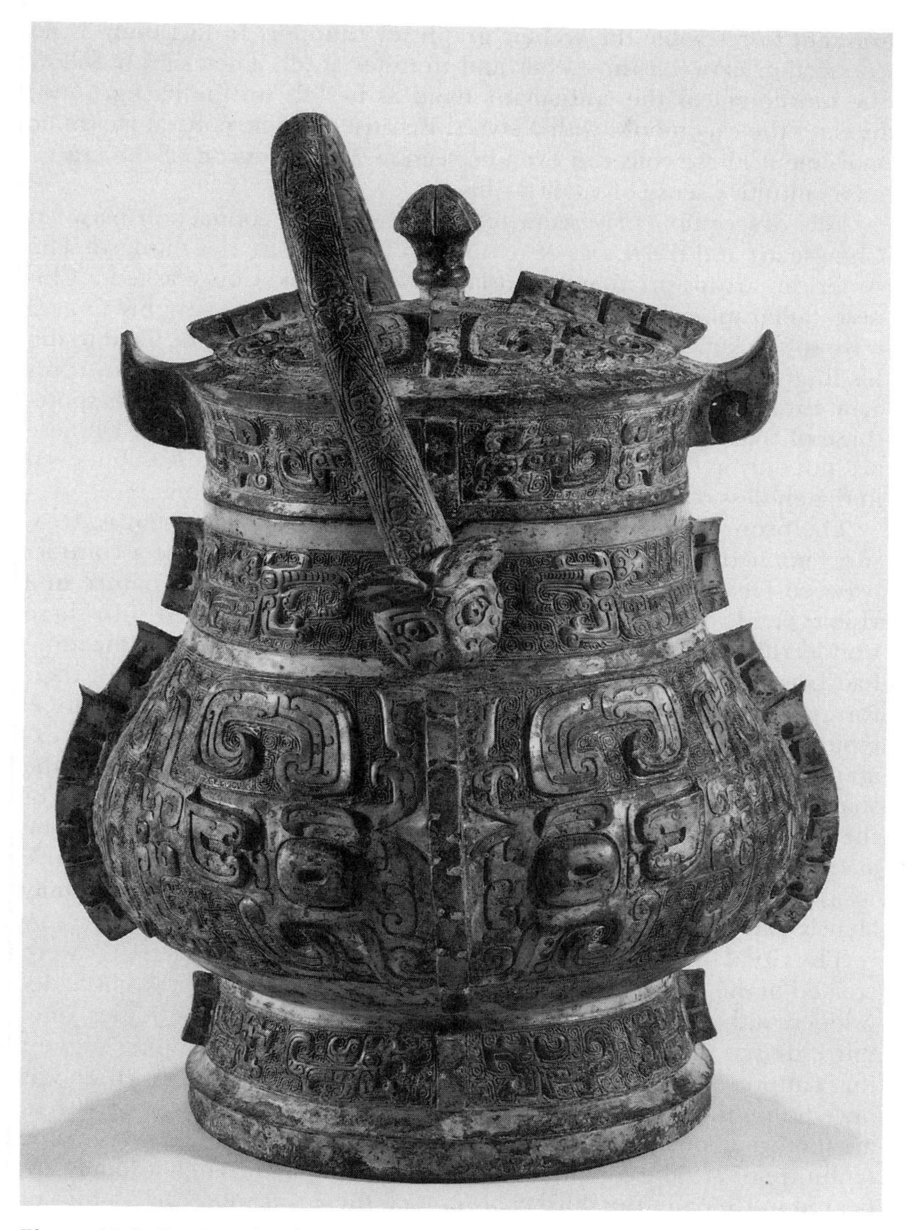

Figure 11.3. Bronze ritual vessel of the type *yü*. 36.1 × 26.9 cm. Shang dynasty, late An-yang. Courtesy of the Freer Gallery of Art, Smithsonian Institution, Washington, D.C. (40.11)

thought to resemble the archaic graph for thunder. In fact there is no connection between these coils and thunder at all. They simply follow the movement of the craftsman's hand as he fills up the background, incising the clay mould with a stylus. Because of their natural rhythmic movement, these coils can even be seen as an expression of the craftsman's intuitive sense of vitality—his *ch'i.*

This description may seem to be pressing the connection between Chinese art and the forces of nature too far, but I do not think so. The American art historian and translator William Acker once asked a Chinese calligrapher, who wrote with very large brushes, why his fingers were so blackened with ink. The calligrapher replied that he liked to dig his fingers into the brush, so that he could feel the *ch'i* flow down his arm, through the brush, and onto the paper. I think that there is something of that *ch'i,* which is one of the fundamental concerns of Chinese art, not only in the lively forms of the creatures on the bronzes, but even in the endless coils of the thunder pattern that sets them off.

The bronzes on the royal ancestral altar were *ling-pao,* that is, treasures imbued with religious power. They were the witness of a contract between Heaven and the ruler, uniting Heaven, man, and nature in a visible bond. So powerful were the associations compacted into these wonderful vessels that long after their original purpose and meaning had been diffused and diluted (although not entirely forgotten), their forms continued to inspire the potter and worker in metal and jade. A typical Lung-ch'üan celadon tripod vessel of the Sung dynasty, for example, is both an ornamental object and, in effect, a reminder of the shape, if not of the original function, of the ritual bronze *ting* tripod of the Shang and Chou, although what was once a cooking pot used in the ancestral rites has become a vessel in which to stand incense sticks (figure 11.4). For a Chinese to have such objects on his desk or on the family altar is to have a reminder of the roots of his culture.

The ritual bronzes are a three-dimensional art form. When they were created in the Shang and Chou periods, sculpture as a craft was little developed, although very recent discoveries of clay figures of deities, one-third life size, in a Neolithic site of about 3,500 B.C. in Liaoning suggest that sculpture of some kind has a more ancient history in China than was once thought. But so far as is now known, there is nothing in pre-Ch'in art (before about 250–240 B.C.) comparable to the monumental stone sculpture of ancient Egypt, Mesopotamia, or Greece. When it finally appeared in China in the third century B.C., there was more than a hint of foreign influence and inspiration. It seems to be no coincidence that stone sculpture began to develop in China at about the same time that the Chinese were making their first sustained contacts with western Asia.

At the time when the First Emperor, Ch'in Shih-huang-ti, was destroying the last of the feudal states, he commissioned the casting of

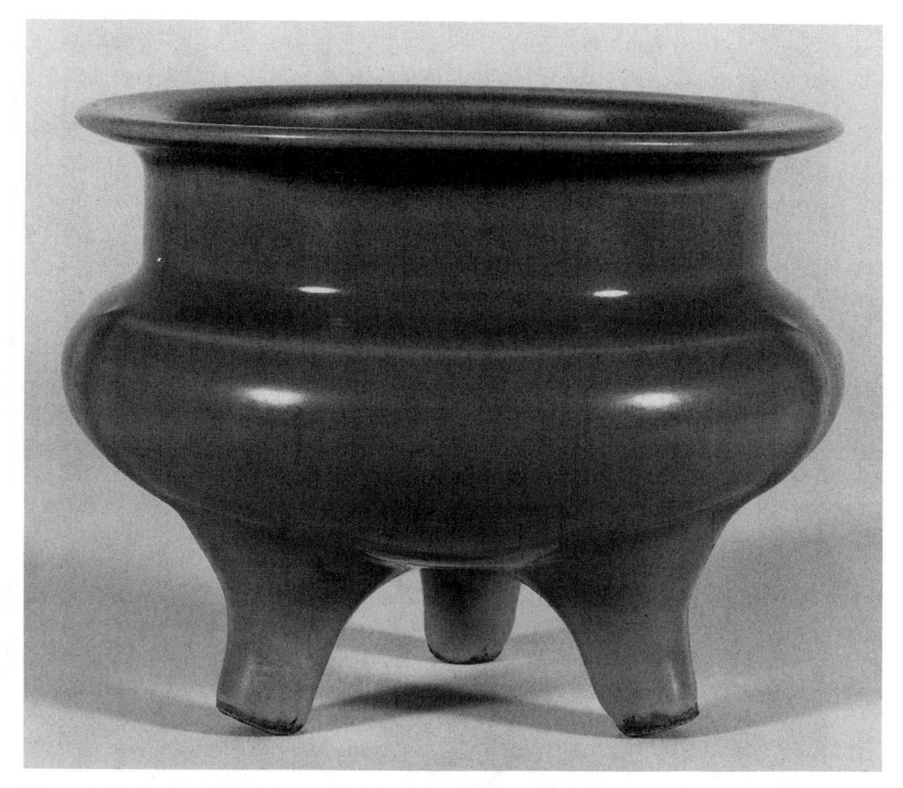

Figure 11.4. Incense burner in the form of a *ting* tripod. Lung-ch'üan celadon ware. 13.4 × 18 cm. Sung dynasty. Arthur M. Sackler Museum, Harvard University, Cambridge, Massachusetts. Collection of Robert M. Ferris IV. (LTL 21.1980)

twelve enormous bronze figures of what the historian Ssu-ma Ch'ien simply calls "men." Where did the idea of making such gigantic figures come from? Ch'in Shih-huang-ti was as creative as he was destructive. Perhaps he conceived of the idea himself, but it is not impossible that he had heard reports of the colossal sculpture of ancient Iran and Syria, and even perhaps of the Colossus of Rhodes.

Chinese stone sculpture is essentially a linear rather than a plastic art, its beauty being of movement rather than of mass. This quality is splendidly shown in the stone chimaeras and winged lions that flank the approaches to the imperial tombs of the period between the Han and the T'ang. Many observers have noted the resemblance between the flatness and linearity of the Buddhist figures and reliefs of the late Northern Wei dynasty (early sixth century; figure 11.5) and that of Romanesque sculpture. Both periods were "ages of faith," and this ethereal quality in the

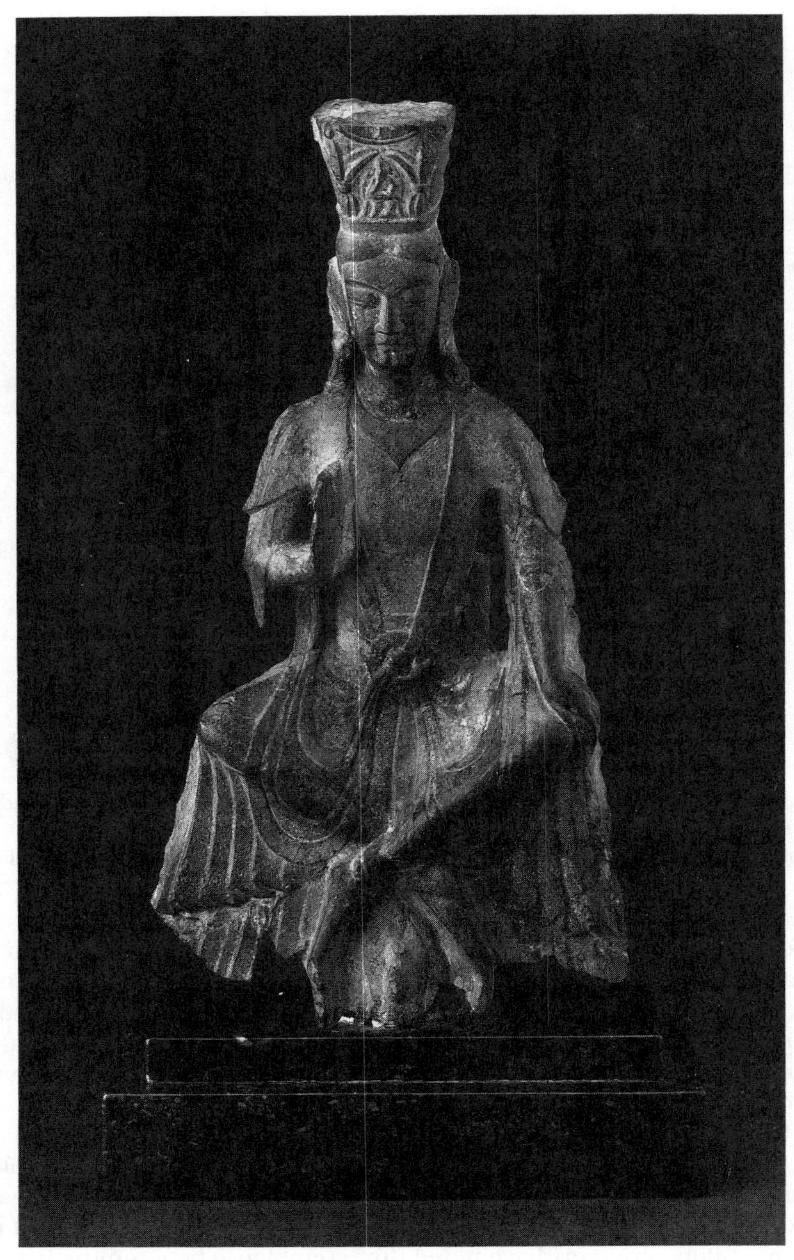

Figure 11.5. Maitreya Buddha. Gray limestone. From Pin-yang cave, Lung-men. Ht. 44.8 cm. Early sixth century. The Minneapolis Institute of Arts. The William Hood Dunwoody Fund. (45.3)

sculpture at Lung-men, for example, has been seen as an expression of intense spirituality. In fact, however, the flat, linear, insubstantial quality of Northern Wei Buddhist sculpture derives not from religious fervor but from the style of secular figure painting that had been practiced by Ku K'ai-chih (ca. 366–406) and his contemporaries in Nanking almost a century earlier. When in the Sui and T'ang dynasties Chinese Buddhist sculpture "filled out" and became massive and plastic, as in the cave shrines at T'ien-lung-shan, that was in part because it was coming under the influence of Indian art; but even in these sensuously modeled figures the Indian mass is swept over with lines of drapery that suggest the brush of the Chinese painter rather than the chisel of the stone carver (figure 11.6). In the final fusion of the Indian and the Chinese formal ideals, it is the Chinese that triumphs, particularly in the temple sculpture of later dynasties modeled in clay, which responds so easily to the movement of the craftsman's hand in the creation of flowing drapery, scarves, and ribbons.

We can feel the sense of life expressed in movement and line just as clearly in the potter's art. If we compare a Greek amphora with a Chinese vessel of, for instance, the T'ang dynasty, we find in the former a perfection and symmetry of form that is completely realized, and therefore somewhat static (figures 11.7 and 11.8). The T'ang bottle, by comparison, is full of flaws, the glaze uneven. But there is life in it. Take a T'ang pot in your hands. Not only do you find its contour and mass, its swelling curve and uplifted shoulder, and the natural flow of the glaze over the body satisfying to the eye, but you can follow with your fingertips the movement of the potter's hands as he put his fingers to the clay to bring it to life. In painted Tz'u-chou wares of the Sung dynasty we find these qualities still further enhanced by the painter's brush, moving freely over the surface, adding another dimension of vitality (figure 11.9). When in later dynasties the porcelain body became no more than a dead white surface on which the decorator painted his birds and flowers, as if on a sheet of paper, much of the life was drained out of the vessel, however beautiful the painting on its surface might be.

The same free movement of the craftsman's hand holding a brush governed lacquer decoration as far back as the Han dynasty, and probably even earlier, and on a Han bronze vessel the motifs inlaid in gold and silver echo the scrolls and volutes of lacquer painting. On a bronze shaft of the Han dynasty (figure 11.10), the decoration inlaid in gold, silver, and semiprecious stones creates semiabstract forms of great beauty—wavelike movements that, simply with the addition of grasses and trees, birds, leaping tigers, or bounding deer, could be "read" as clouds, hills, or waves. This lively, rhythmic formal language was adapted also by the designers of the backs of bronze mirrors. It was borrowed also for the motifs on Han woven stuffs and embroidered textiles, such as have been

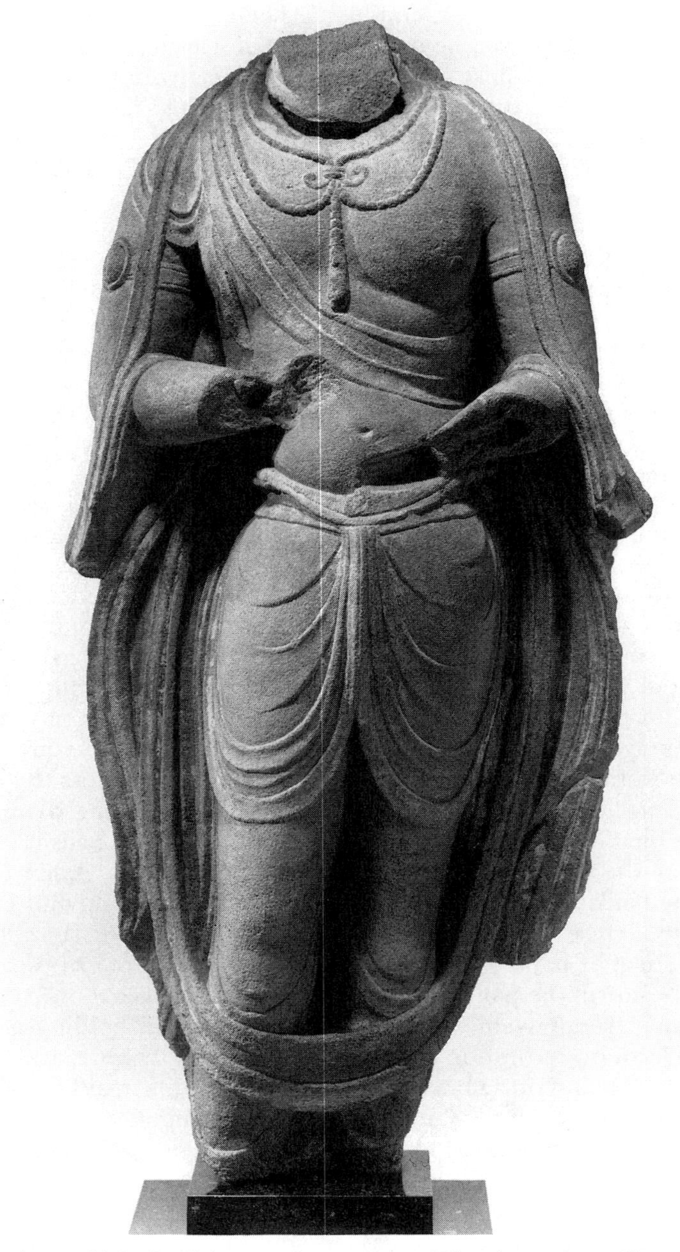

Figure 11.6. Bodhisattva. Stone. From T'ien-lung-shan, Shansi. T'ang dynasty. Rietberg Museum, Zurich. Eduard von der Heydt collection. Photo by Wettstein and Kauf.

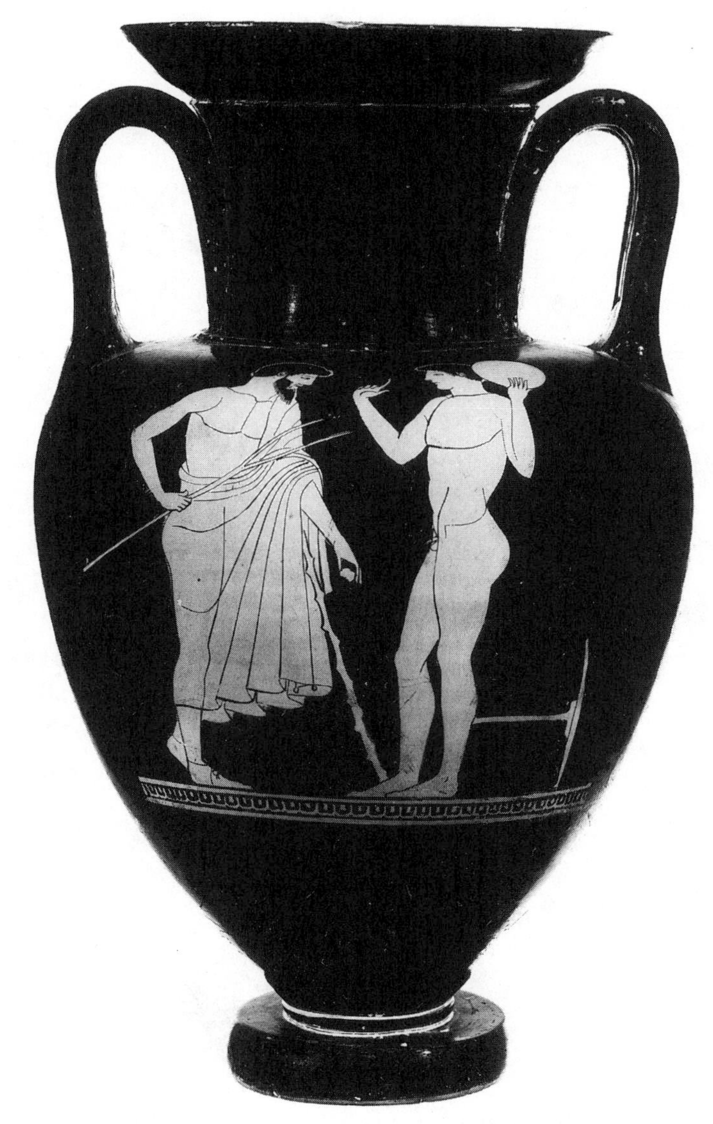

Figure 11.7. Amphora. Greek. c. 480 B.C. Ashmolean Museum, Oxford. (1891.689 [v.273])

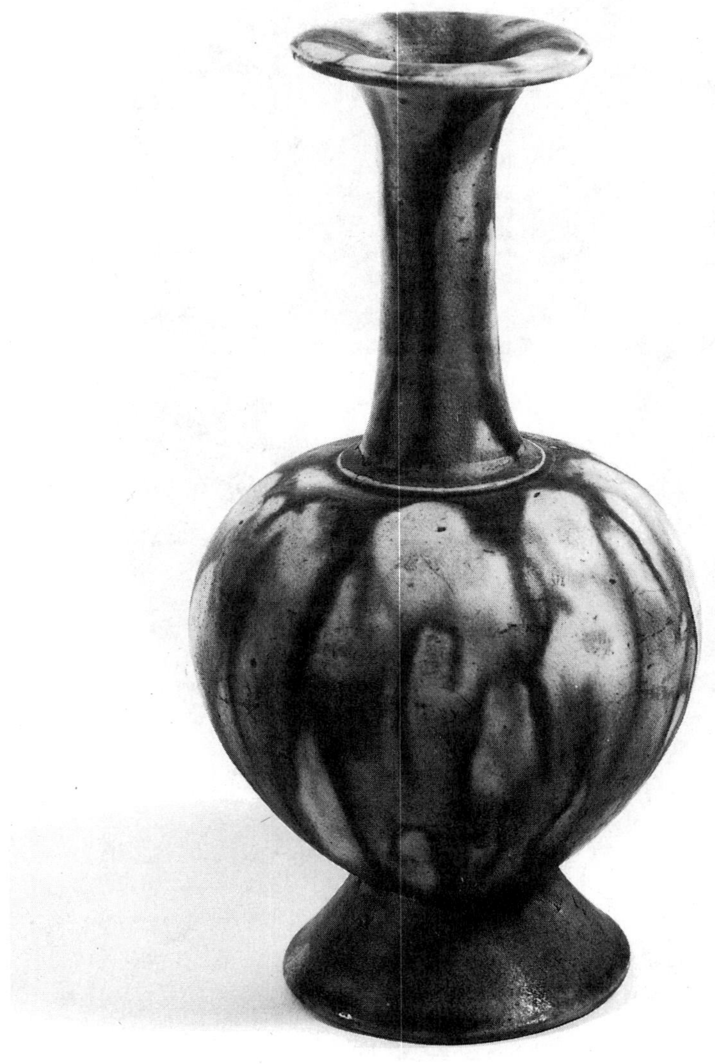

Figure 11.8. Bottle. Lead-glazed earthenware. North China. T'ang dynasty. Ashmolean Museum, Oxford. (1956.1079)

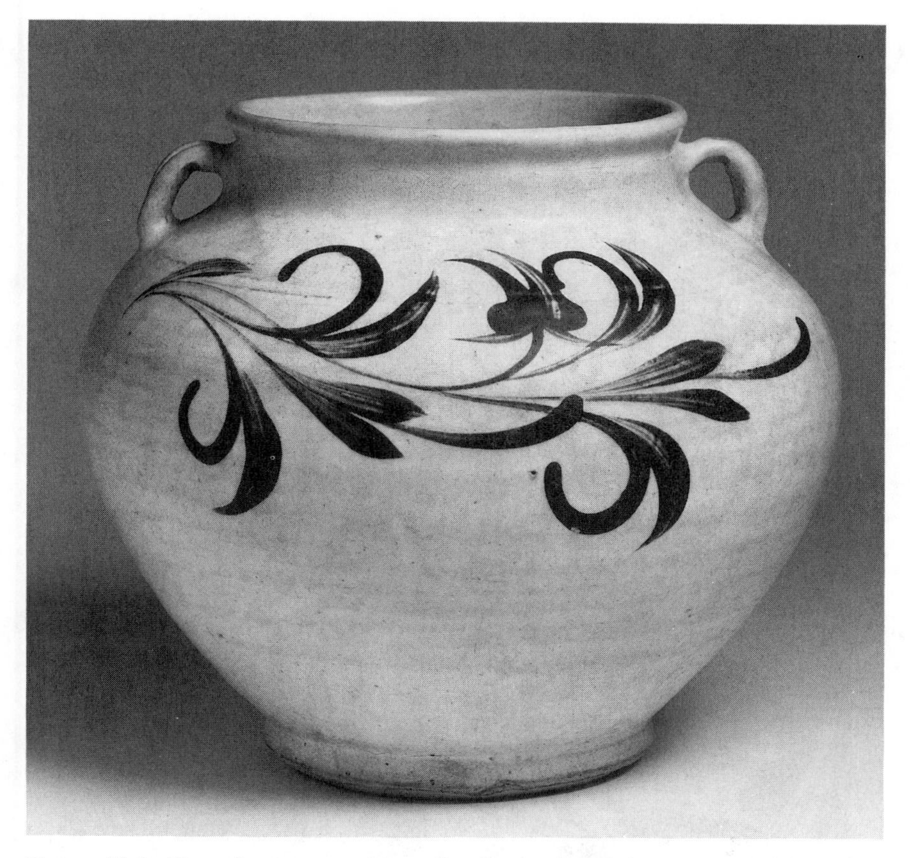

Figure 11.9. Vase. Stoneware with underglaze painted decoration. Tz'u-chou ware. North China. 20.3 × 21.6 cm. Sung dynasty. Asian Art Museum of San Francisco. The Avery Brundage Collection. (B60 Pl+)

found in the desert sands of Lou-lan and Noin-Ula and in the water-logged tombs of Ma-wang-tui outside Changsha.

It was out of this formal language based on the rhythmic movement of the craftsman's hand that the essential beauty of Chinese painting was born. But if the formal language of Chinese painting derives at least in part from crafts such as lacquer decoration that have little to do with representational art, the *meaning* of that language is to be sought elsewhere, in the realm of metaphysics, philosophy, and poetry.

In the brief space of this chapter I can do no more than hint at the richness of the legacy of Chinese painting. Let me just say that its stylistic and technical range is far greater than the Westerner generally imagines. To the untutored Western observer, all Chinese paintings look much the same, partly perhaps because they are all painted with brush

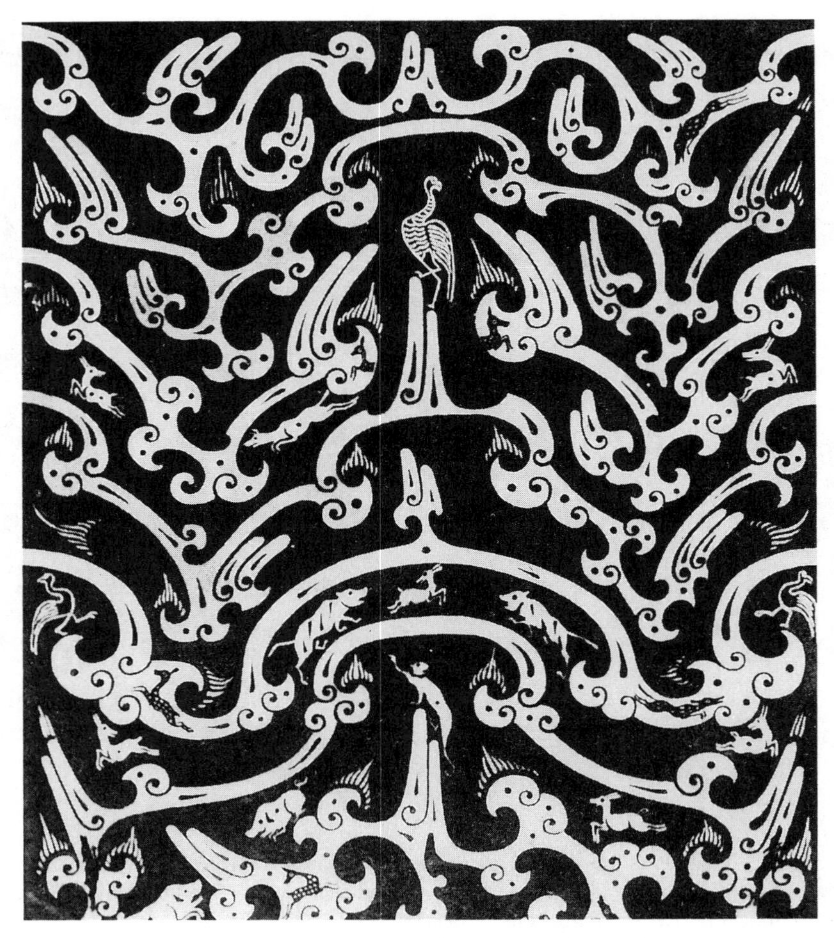

Figure 11.10. Detail of decoration on bronze tubular fitting. Bronze inlaid with silver. Han dynasty. Eisei-Bunko Foundation, Tokyo.

and ink on silk or paper; the range of media in Western pictorial art is far greater. But as we scan across the spectrum from right to left, as it were, that is, from the orthodox, conservative, didactic "Confucian" figure painting of masters such as Li Lung-mien (ca. 1040–1106) at one end to the free, uninhibited gestures with the brush of such eccentric "Taoists" as Chu Ta (1625–1705?) at the other, we find a wider range of technique and expression within the one medium than we would find in any period in Western art before the late nineteenth century. It must be said, however, that although the range of formal expression in traditional Chinese painting is wide, the range of subject matter is much more restricted than that of Western painting. There are many subjects depicted by the Western artist—warfare, violence in its many forms, death, cityscapes, the dark side of life, the nude, to name a few—that would (with very rare exceptions) be unthinkable as subjects for the Chinese artist's brush. To depict such things was not what art was for.

Court painting and the art of the professionals who took their techniques and standards from the court artists tended naturally to be craftsmanlike, meticulous, impersonal, striving for a degree of realism (figure 11.11). This tradition is one in which the personality of the artist is often so little revealed as to be barely distinguishable. This is as true of the work of a court painter of the T'ang dynasty, such as Chang Hsuan, as it is of the anonymous court painter of the Kang-hsi emperor's portrait (see figure 11.1). Landscape painters in this courtly and professional tradition, striving for visual accuracy, welcomed—or at least tentatively experimented with—some European techniques when in the seventeenth century they began to encounter them for the first time. The scholars, for the most part, ignored Western art. Realism, they felt, was a matter for craftsmen painters, not for gentlemen.

When we move away from the court and from the workshops of the professional artists into the milieu of the literati, we are moving into another world altogether, a world in which any hint of professionalism is to be avoided, or cunningly disguised by a playful archaism or a pretence of clumsiness, a world in which it is the touch of the artist's brush, like the touch of the pianist, that is the vehicle for meaning, because the theme itself—landscape, bamboo, birds and flowers—is purely conventional, even hackneyed. In these works not everything is said. To the scholar-poet, painting for other scholar-poets, a mere hint is enough. To say more than is absolutely necessary is to risk the charge of vulgarity, than which, in the eyes of the Chinese literatus, there is no greater sin.

This suggestiveness in the painting of the literati, combined with a certain whimsical awkwardness, can be seen in a famous album of Huang-shan by the great seventeenth-century Individualist Shih-t'ao. He says in his inscription that he is merely playing with the brush. Yet Shih-t'ao would regard incompetence in poetry or calligraphy as something quite inexcusable. His vocation is letters; his painting—ostensibly at least—merely his pastime as an amateur.

When the scholar paints a landscape, he seldom depicts a real place; if he does, it is often barely recognizable. Rather he is, as Su Tung-p'o said, merely "borrowing" the forms of mountains, rocks, and trees as a vehicle for the expression of feelings and ideas. The paradox is that the feelings depicted are about nature itself. But they are generalized. And while avoiding an accurate representation (something he leaves to the professionals), he must make his landscapes enjoyable *as* landscapes; they must draw us into nature and make us one with it. They are not simply

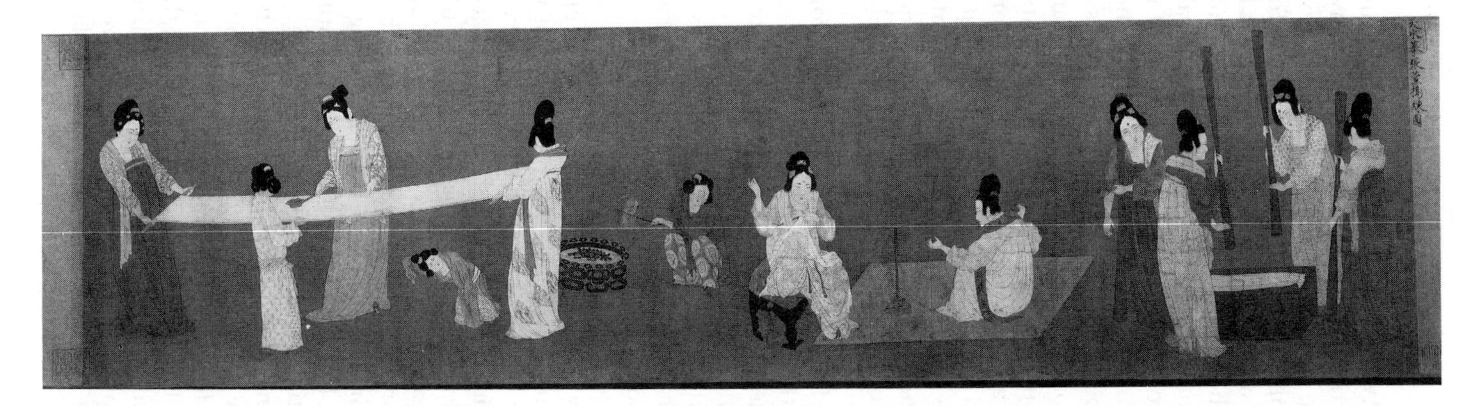

Figure 11.11. Attributed to Sung Hui-tsung (r. 1101–1125). Copy after Chang Hsuan (T'ang dynasty), *Court Ladies Preparing Newly Woven Silk.* Handscroll. Ink, color, and gold on silk. 37 × 145.3 cm. Chinese and Japanese Special Fund. Courtesy, Museum of Fine Arts, Boston. (12.886)

expressive gestures with the brush and no more. Representation and expression, it might be said, are in a state of creative conflict.

The scholars' painting has yet one further dimension, for sometimes its main purpose was not so much to represent nature or to express feeling as to act as a vehicle for social intercourse. This dimension is beautifully exemplified in many paintings by the Ming and Ch'ing literati, which are testimonies to friendship, witness to shared values, and recollections of time spent together enjoying wine, poetry, conversation, and nature itself. The landscape themes are often conventional; it is the inscriptions that reveal what very human documents these paintings are. This uniquely Chinese quality is beautifully illustrated by a painting by Wen Chia (figure 11.12), which was included in the exhibition *The Literati Vision: Sixteenth Century Wu School Painting and Calligraphy* organized by Tita Hyland and held at the Memphis Brooks Museum of Art in conjunction with the symposium on Chinese civilization at Memphis State University, where this and several other chapters in this volume were first presented.

The Chinese scholar-painter, as a philosopher, seeks to distill the essence of nature and to see beyond the visible forms to the reality that lies behind them. Yet even the most abstract landscapes, such as some of those by the seventeenth-century eccentric Chu Ta (Pa-ta Shan-jen [1625–1705?]), are distillations of the "landscape experience." The same can be said about the oil paintings by the twentieth-century master Zao Wou-ki (Chao Wu-chi; figure 11.13), now living in Paris. When I first met this artist, I told him that to me his "abstract expressionist" paintings looked like landscapes. At that time the French critics were condemning him for not painting "pure" abstractions. But he was delighted by my comment, remarking, "Of course they're landscapes!"

The contemporary painter Wu Kuan-chung, working in Peking, has often said that, like a kite-string, a slender bond connects the artist with the visible world of nature and that it matters not how tight the string is stretched, so long as it is not snapped. But, we may ask, why should it not be snapped? Why not create, like Mondrian, pure abstractions with no apparent referents in nature? The Chinese answer to this question is bound up with their belief that completely nonfigurative art is "neutral" and incomplete. It has been said that the cultural authorities in Mao's China banned abstraction as "bourgeois formalism." That concern was a factor at the time, needless to say. But the hostility to pure abstraction in China is older and deeper than Maoist ideology. Abstraction is acceptable in decorative art; indeed it is the basis of it. But to the Chinese painting is not just the creation of forms, however beautiful. It is something much more. When I asked the painter Huang Yung-yü what he thought of the abstract works he had seen in New York's Whitney Museum, he said, "*Mei-yu i-ssu*"—"They have no meaning." In other words, they are

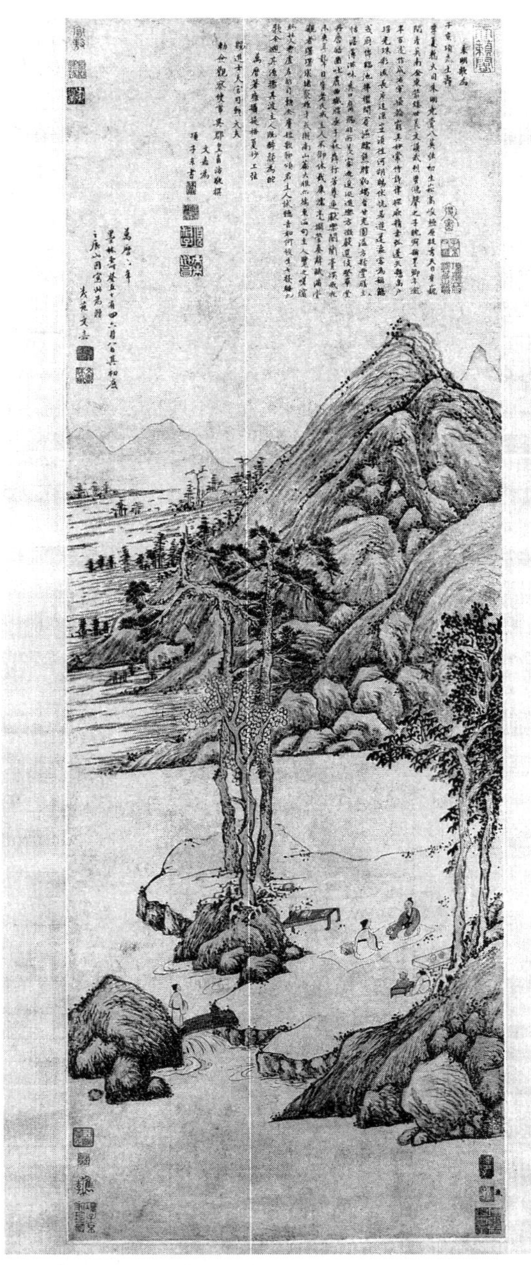

Figure 11.12. Wen Chia (1501–1583). Landscape dedicated to the collector and patron Hsiang Yuan-pien (1525–1590). Hanging scroll. Ink and color on paper. 117.5 × 40.0 cm. 1578. The Metropolitan Museum of Art, Edward Elliott Family Collection, Purchase, the Dillon Fund Gift, 1981. (1981.285.9)

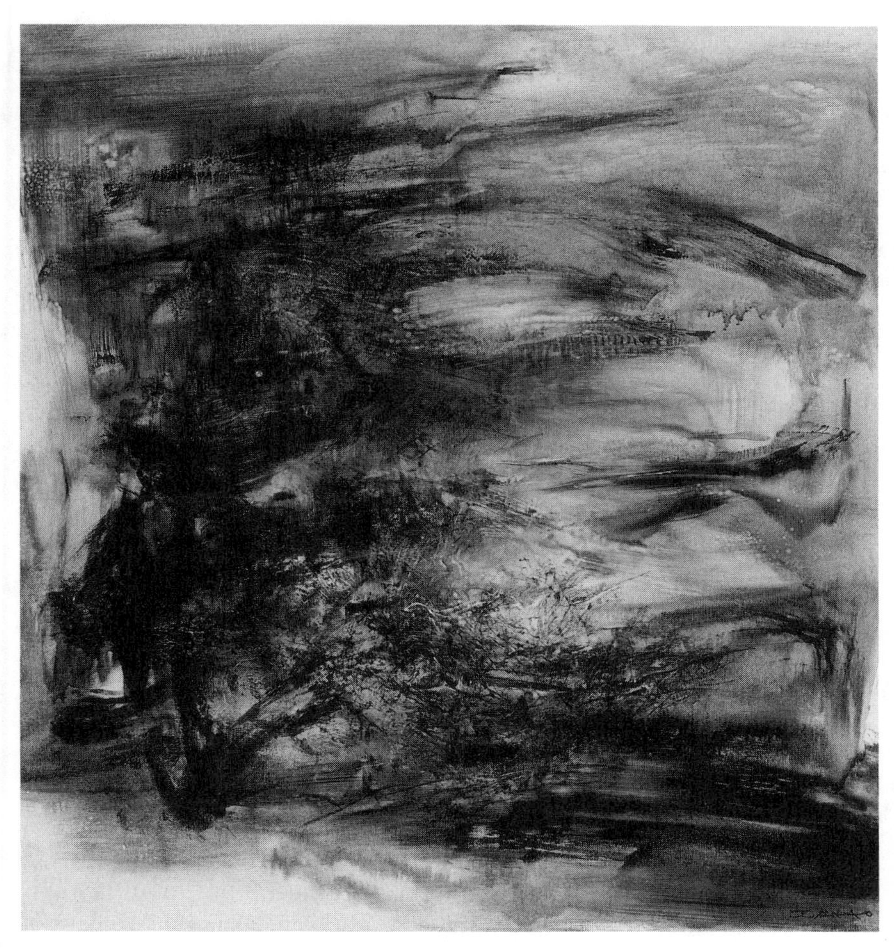

Figure 11.13. Zao Wou-ki [Chao Wu-chi, 1921–]. Abstract landscape. Oils. 162 × 150 cm. H. H. Arnason Collection, New York. (24-5.65)

only form. And to Huang Yung-yü, who like all Chinese artists takes a holistic view of the unity of art with all other aspects of knowledge and experience, form is not enough. As Tu Wei-ming has noted, in China all modalities of being in the universe are considered interconnected.[1] Nevertheless, the time may well be approaching in China when pure abstraction is recognized, by some artists at least, as it is in the West, as a subtler and more sophisticated approach to reality than pictorial realism.

1. Tu Wei-ming, "The Continuity of Being: Chinese Visions of Nature," in his *Confucian Thought: Selfhood as Creative Transformation* (Albany: State University of New York Press, 1985), 43.

What of calligraphy, we might ask. Is not calligraphy an art of pure form? Not at all, say the Chinese. For however beautiful the writing, it is "abstract art" only to those who cannot read it! The content of the passage cannot but be an essential element in the beauty of the whole. It need not be inspiring or profound, although such virtues enhance the writing's value. On the other hand, no example of Chinese calligraphy of which the content is vulgar or unedifying, however well-written, could be considered by the Chinese as good or beautiful. In this connection it is perhaps worth noting that when a Chinese admires a work of art, he does not say that it is "very beautiful" (*hen mei*). Rather, he says that it is "very good" (*hen hao*).

Before leaving the subject of painting, I should mention that long before the idea of four-dimensional art was discovered in the West, the Chinese had made it their natural mode of pictorial expression. By four-dimensional I mean an art that combines the three dimensions of space with that of time. In the long handscroll *Ch'ing-ming shang-ho t'u* (Going upriver at Ch'ing-ming festival time; figure 11.14), a famous example of early twelfth-century realism, a panorama unfolds that would take perhaps several hours to cover if one were actually walking along the riverbank into the Northern Sung capital. Here is a perfect parallel to Nathan Sivin's discussion of Shen Kua (see Chapter 7) and an illustration of the Northern Sung scientific attitude to the real world, which was not again to be reflected in Chinese painting until China felt the impact of Western art in the twentieth century. The decay of realism from the Yuan dynasty onward was due in large part to the fact that aesthetic aims were no longer set by the court but by the literati, whose artistic ideals were quite different.

One key to this achievement of the Chinese painter was a sense of space that was not discovered in the West until the twentieth century when Naum Gabo declared in the *Realist Manifesto* (1920), "We cannot measure space by objects; we can only measure space by space." Space is not confined in the Chinese painting within the frame, for it has no frame. Furthermore, the painting is itself a picture of space, in which there may be rocks, mountains, trees, people, fishes, or simply air or water. When Pa-ta Shan-jen paints a fish on the blank paper of an album leaf (figure 11.15), we know that the fish is swimming in the water and that we will still be looking at the water when, with a flick of his tail, the fish has darted out of sight. In Pa-ta's picture space is just *there,* whether it is occupied by objects or not. It can just as well be occupied by a poem.

I have tried to suggest some of the essential ideals and qualities of Chinese art in a very sketchy way. Until the sixteenth century the art of China was virtually unknown in the West, except for a small company of dragons and phoenixes who had wandered across Asia to settle on the cathedral vestments of medieval Italy, notably on the embroidered copes

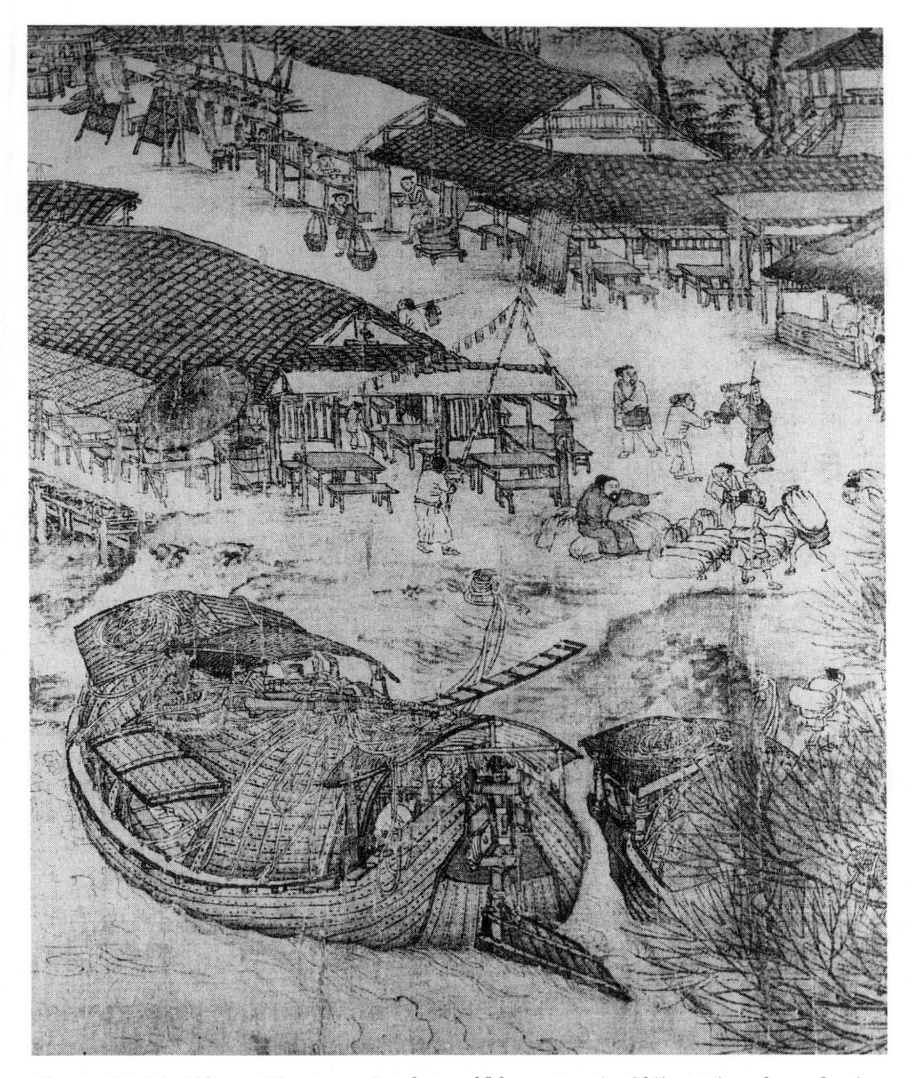

Figure 11.14. Chang Tse-tuan (early twelfth century). *Ch'ing-ming shang-ho t'u* (Going upriver at Ch'ing-ming festival time). Detail of a handscroll. Ink and slight color on silk. Sung dynasty. Palace Museum, Peking.

made at Lucca. Textiles were one of China's finest gifts to the West. Yet to the Italian weavers and embroiderers, who perhaps had read Marco Polo, Cathay must have seemed unbelievably remote and unreal. Gradually, we have become more familiar with the forms and styles of Chinese art. How did we get this knowledge? How much have we learned and understood? And how much has this learning enriched our own culture?

Here I would like to make a distinction between art and craft. The

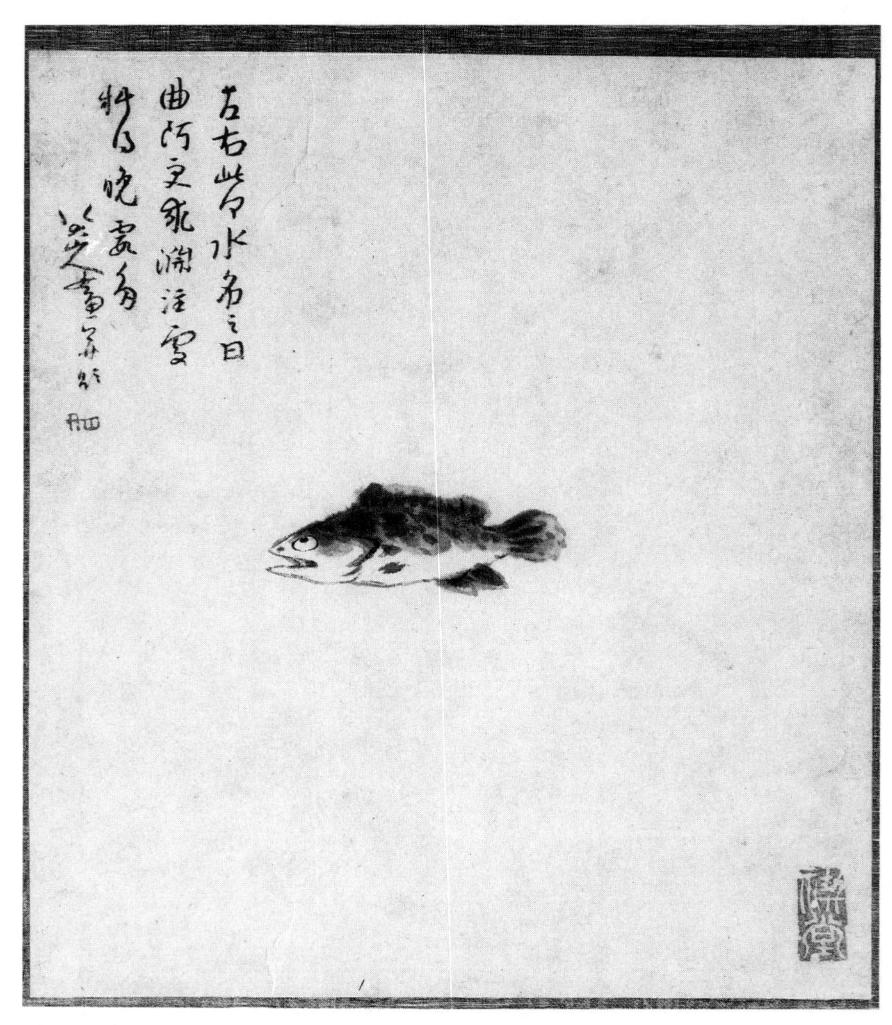

Figure 11.15. Chu Ta [Pa-ta Shan-jen, 1625–1705?]. Fish. Album leaf. Ink on paper. Ch'ing dynasty. Sumitomo Collection, Oiso, Japan.

distinction is important, for Chinese crafts have been enjoyed ever since the West began to import them. In the seventeenth century fortunes were made and lost over cargoes of blue and white porcelain. A well-known story tells of a German prince who traded a squadron of dragoons for a pair of Chinese vases. Chinese screens could be found in many of the great houses of Europe. But the appreciation of Chinese art at the higher levels did not come until the present century. In 1858 a note on a forthcoming exhibition of Chinese art at the Egyptian Hall, Piccadilly, declared, "So far as we are yet informed, everything about China seems to be quaint and strange and madly comical." So it is not surprising that fourteen years later a writer in the *Gazette des beaux arts* could confidently state, "We are now as well informed about Chinese art as we can hope to be." As late as 1935 the critic Roger Fry was writing that ordinary English art lovers "may feel happy in the presence of trifling bibelots, the 'chinoiseries' of later periods, which have been acclimatized to our drawing rooms, but the great art, and above all, the religious art, will repel them by its strangeness." I think Fry put it rather too strongly. The English were not repelled by Chinese religious art, as many were by the too explicitly physical religious art of India. Rather, Chinese painting was too subtle, too unemphatic, too elusive, the ideals it conveyed too intellectual or too philosophical, to appeal to a public attuned to the realism, strong colors, and solid compositions of Michelangelo, Poussin, or Delacroix, in which space exists not for itself but to surround or locate solid objects and color is an essential element in the design.

With such aims of art in mind, seventeenth- and eighteenth-century Europe thought that Chinese pictorial art was charming, certainly, but incompetent, even ridiculously so. The great Jesuit missionary Matteo Ricci (1552–1610) wrote, "In the making of statuary and cast images, they have acquired none of the skill of Europeans, while they know nothing of art or painting in oil, or of the use of perspective in their pictures, with the result that their productions are lacking in any vitality."[2] The Portuguese writer Alvarez de Semedo, in his *History of That Great and Renowned Monarchy of China* (1641; English translation, 1655), wrote: "In *Painting* they have more curiositie, than perfection. They know not how to make use either of *Oyles* or of *Shadowing* in this Art. . . . But at present there are some of them, who have been taught by us, that use *Oyles,* and are come to make perfect pictures." The idea that Chinese painting must be inferior because it did not use oils, Western perspective, or chiaroscuro was to persist into the twentieth century.

But there was one art in China that struck a deep response in the European mind in the eighteenth century, that touched our sensibilities and had a profound influence on taste. This was the art of the Chinese garden. Although he never visited China, Sir William Temple in his *Upon Heroick Virtue* (1683) described the Chinese garden, using a term that was probably a corruption of a Persian word, *sharawadji* or *sharadj,* aptly defined by the German scholar Gustav Ecke as "an apparent disorder which is actually rhythm in disguise." Nowhere can one better see and enjoy this "rhythm in disguise" today than in the gardens of Soochow.

A vague awareness of the aesthetic principles behind the Chinese garden was strengthened when the Jesuit missionary Matteo Ripa arrived in

2. Quoted in Michael Sullivan, *The Meeting of Eastern and Western Art,* rev. ed. (Berkeley: University of California Press, 1989), 43.

London in 1724 and showed his pictures of the gardens of the imperial summer palaces at Chengte (Jehol) to Lord Burlington and William Kent. As later the Japanese print was to stimulate the birth of impressionism, so now did the Chinese garden, so far as it was known and understood—or misunderstood—stimulate in England, then elsewhere in Europe, a reaction against the formal, geometrical gardens of Italy and France, and it helped to bring to birth the natural garden that was so much more in accordance with English taste. No matter that by some the Chinese garden was absurdly misrepresented. Sir William Chambers, who had actually visited Canton briefly in 1742–1743 and should have known better, distinguished several categories of Chinese garden, one of which was the "terrible." His descriptions, in fact, were inspired more by the violently romantic landscape visions of Salvator Rosa than by anything he had seen in China. Chambers was ridiculed in his own day; but he could not have painted such a picture of the Chinese garden if England had not itself been on the threshold of the romantic revolution. The most perfect realization in Europe of this new Anglo-Chinese concept of the garden was attained at Stourhead (1741); and the beautiful drawing of Stourhead by the Swedish architect F. M. Piper could easily be mistaken for the plan of a Soochow garden (figure 11.16).

By the end of the eighteenth century the Chinese influence on English and European sensibilities had done its work and left the stage; there was no place for Chinese taste in the cool, austere world of neoclassicism. As the nineteenth century progressed, China and Chinese culture rapidly lost their power to charm. The Opium wars, the influence of the missionaries, and the decline of the Manchus all gave the impression of a cruel, inscrutable people, of a corrupt civilization in decay. From 1868 onward it was Japan, flatteringly remolding itself in the West's image, that was admired. One could, like Whistler and Oscar Wilde, enthuse over Chinese blue and white, but Chinese culture was not taken seriously. As late as 1906 the director of the Metropolitan Museum in New York could remark of the attempt to distinguish between Chinese and Japanese art, "It is all nonsense." Well into the twentieth century it was the collectors of Chinese porcelain, men like J. P. Morgan and George Eumorfopoulos, who seemed to represent what was left of the old admiration for Chinese culture. But their approach was that of the connoisseur who admires the work of art simply for itself, for its sensuous qualities, and knows or cares little for the ideas that lie behind it or the civilization that produced it.

Interest in Chinese art might have remained at this level had it not been that China began to emerge from her feudal slumbers and that the West discovered Chinese poetry and literature. Through the work of such scholars as Arthur Waley a window was opened on Chinese thought and feeling to which Westerners could respond because of its humanity and because the world that Waley and other gifted translators revealed

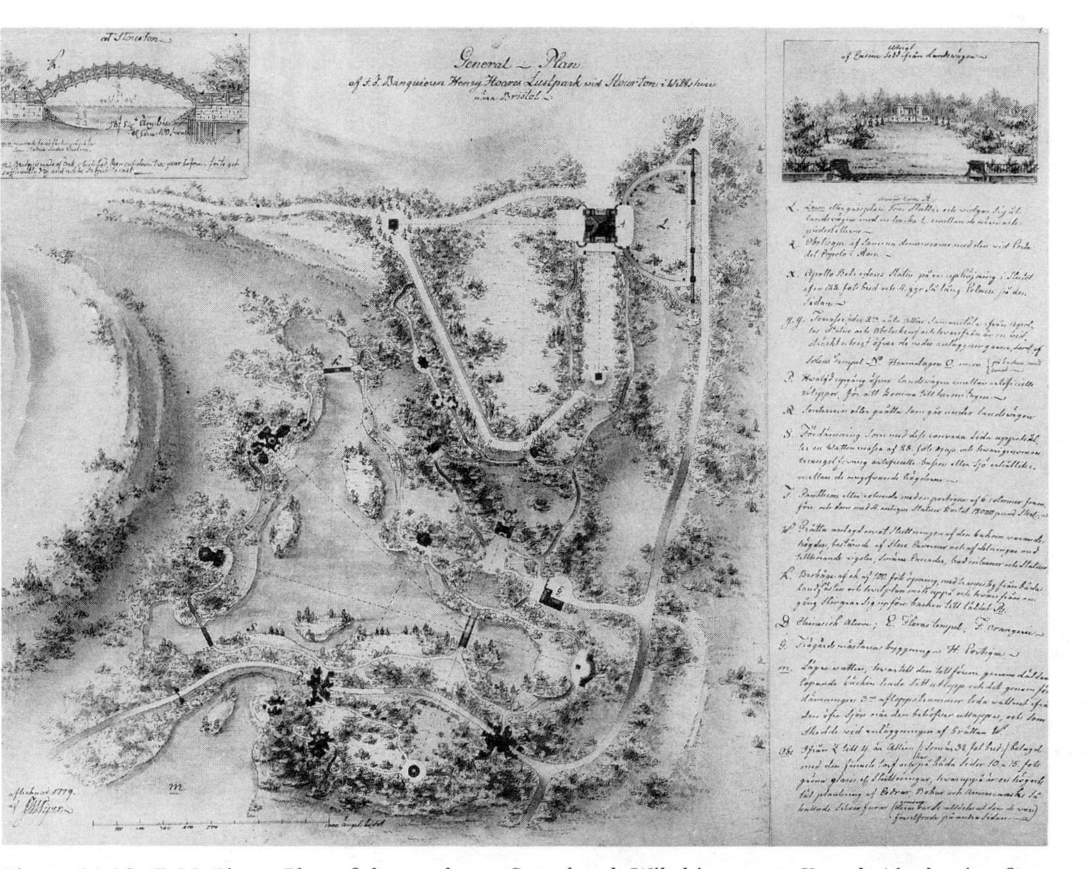

Figure 11.16. F. M. Piper. Plan of the garden at Stourhead, Wiltshire. 1741. Kungl. Akademien för de fria konsterna, Stockholm.

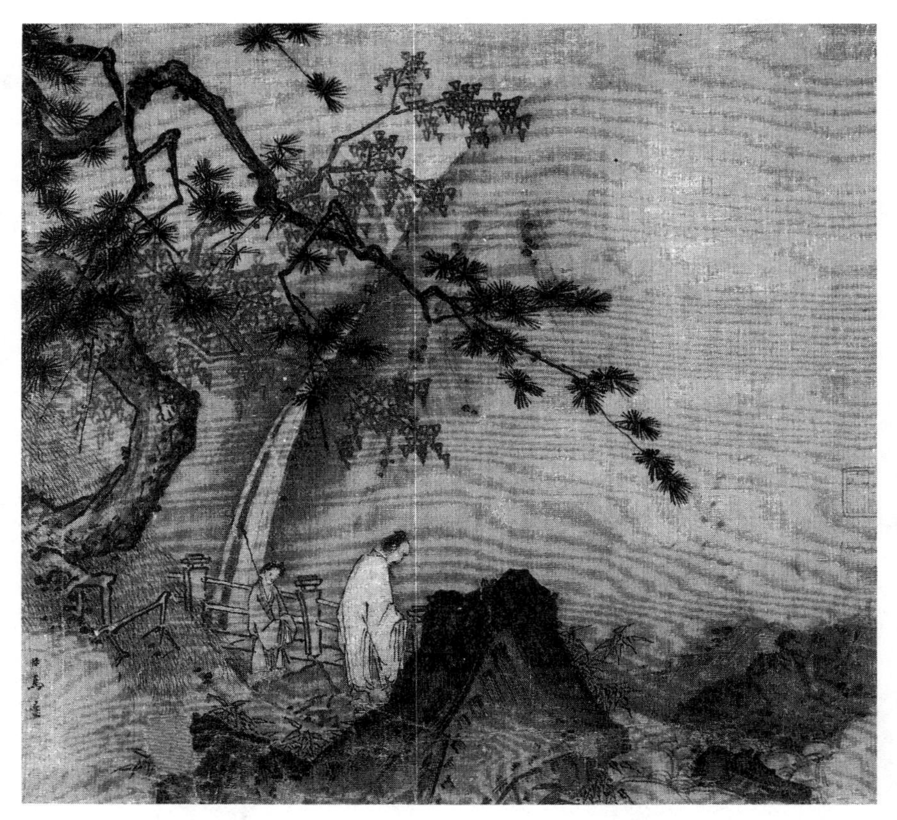

Figure 11.17. Ma Yuan (active ca. 1180–1230). Scholar by a Waterfall. Album painting. Ink and light color on silk. 24.9 × 25.9 cm. Southern Sung dynasty. The Metropolitan Museum of Art, Gift of the Dillon Fund, 1973. (1973.120.9)

was so different from that presented by the newspapers and the movies. By reading in translation the thoughts of Chinese poets and thinkers, the West came at last to the beginning of an understanding of Chinese painting.

The language of Chinese painting is rich and varied. Some traditions are more accessible than others. Some schools are easy to appreciate, for instance, the landscape painting of the Southern Sung academicians such as Ma Yuan (Figure 11.17) and Hsia Kuei in which the romantic, vaguely melancholic mood is so explicitly expressed in the style and the sentiments are often as conventional as those of Elizabethan love lyrics or the landscape poetry of Thomas Gray or William Collins. Also, our eyes and minds are now tuned by abstract expressionism to respond easily, if superficially, to certain kinds of Ch'an (Zen) painting, such as the extraordinary landscape visions of the Southern Sung master Ying Yü-chien (figure 11.18).

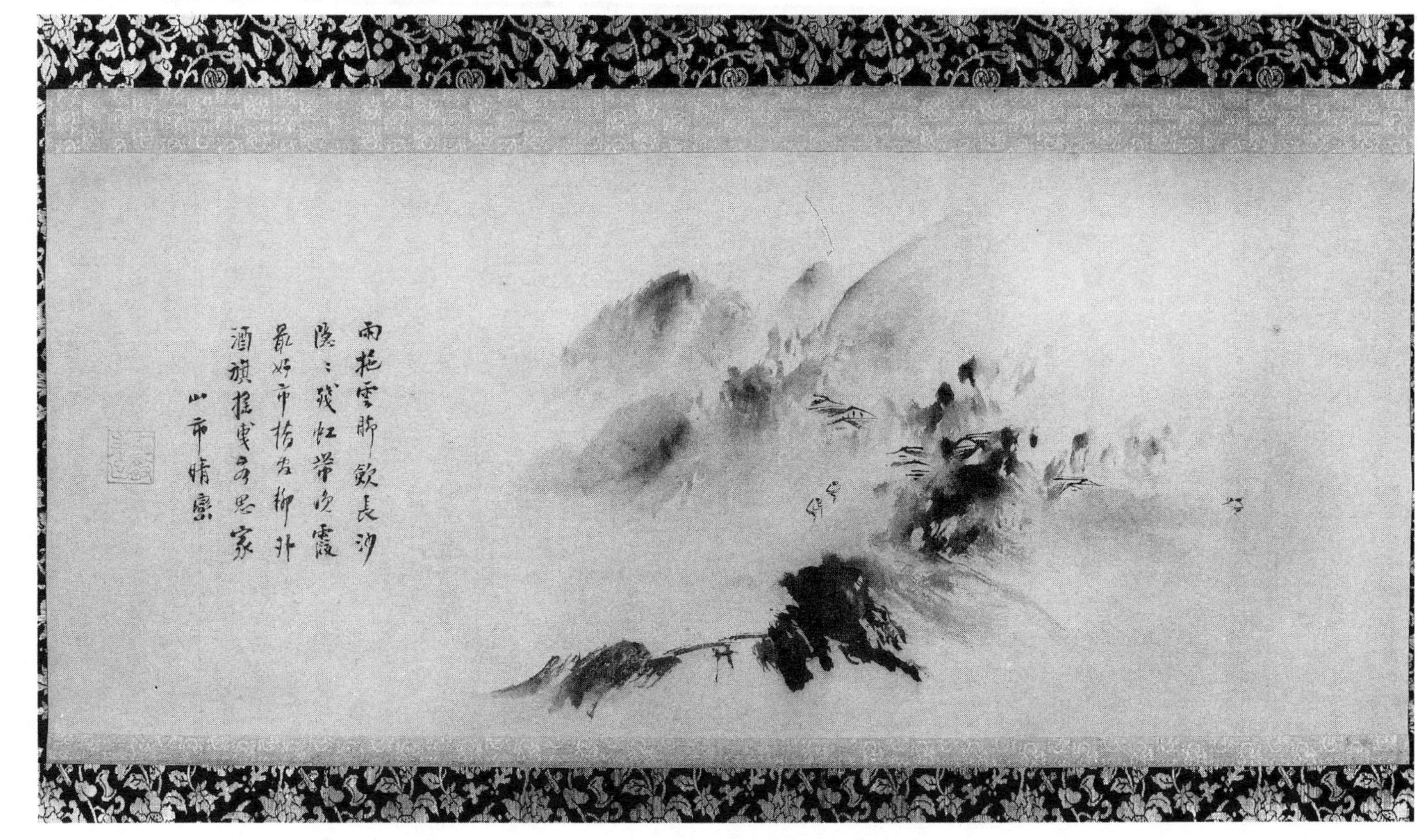

Figure 11.18. Attributed to Ying Yü-chien. Landscape. One of the Eight Views of Hsiao and Hsiang. Handscroll. Ink on paper. 30.3 × 83.3 cm. Southern Sung dynasty. Idemitsu Museum of Arts, Tokyo.

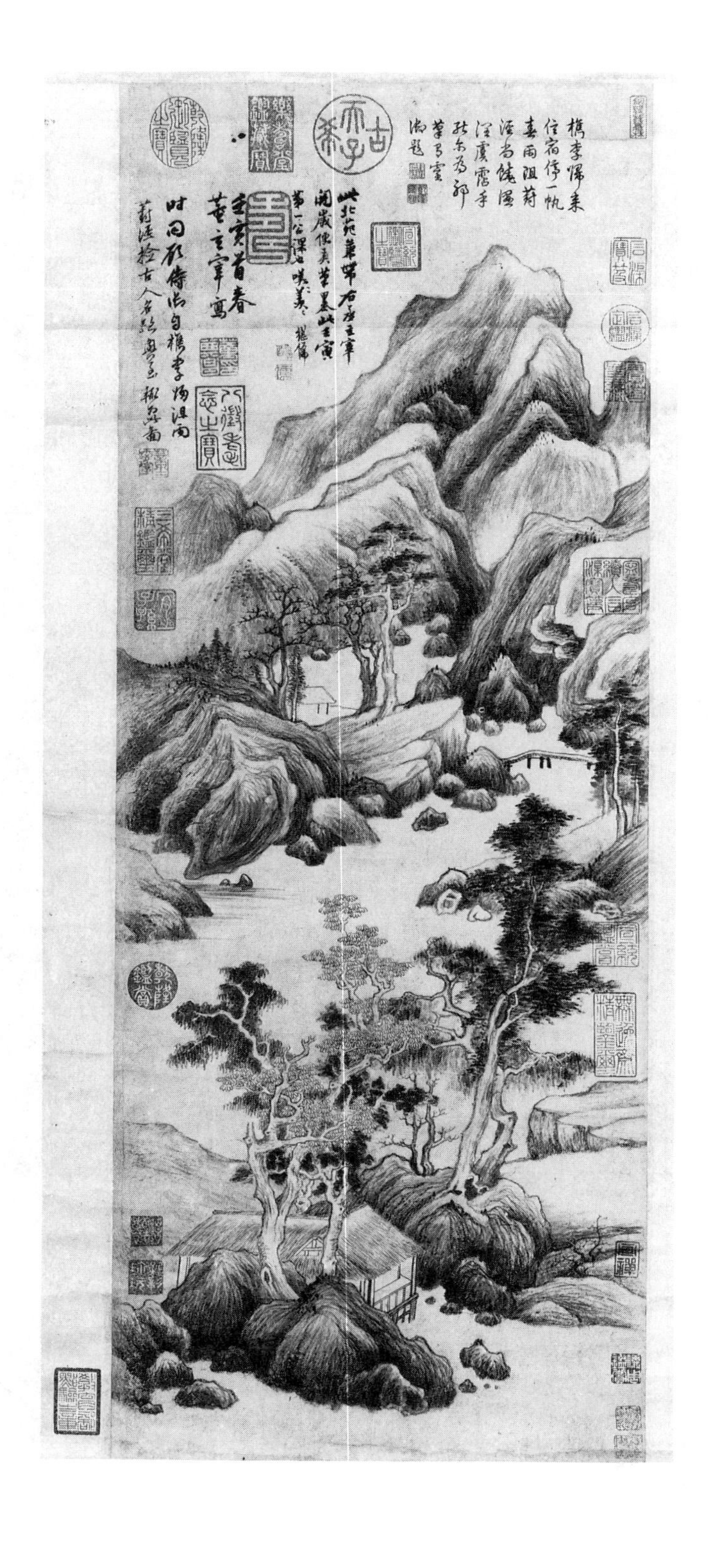

If, by contrast, we find scholarly landscape painting difficult—particularly that of a high-powered intellectual such as Tung Ch'i-ch'ang (figure 11.19)—that is because the rejection of realism and the abstraction from natural forms are carried to a point where specific meaning in a picture, whether it refers to a particular place or occasion or to the style of an earlier master, is apparent only to someone steeped in this language and able to catch the stylistic allusions and read the inscription. We can echo Tu Wei-ming here in speaking of the Chinese scholar responding to the symbolic resources of his own culture.[3] When we become conversant with these symbolic resources we intensify our understanding of Chinese scholarly painting many times over. But the average Westerner has no key to these mysteries. We hear of Western artists being inspired by the formal qualities of Chinese calligraphy or by expressionistic Ch'an painting. But I have never heard of a Western artist who claimed to be influenced by Tung Ch'i-ch'ang.

Yet doors to the higher reaches of Chinese painting are opening every day. A growing interest in Oriental philosophy and the translating of the scriptures of Buddhism and Taoism (whose riches are described by T. H. Barrett in Chapter 6 of this volume) are helping to make the West aware of the Chinese view of the universe and the natural order and Chinese concepts of energy, space, and time. We are discovering that these concepts have much more in common with the world as revealed by modern physics and psychology than they have with that of traditional Western cosmology and religion. We may grasp this congruence of Chinese tradition and modern Western concepts by looking at an extraordinary album painting by Shih-t'ao of about 1700, showing a man sitting in his little hut among the mountains (figure 11.20). Not only is this technically and stylistically a very original work; it is also psychologically a profoundly exciting one because the figure (the painter himself?) seems to be enveloped in the mountain, like a spider in the middle of its web, while at the same time the network of quivering lines that surrounds him seems in some strange way to be an emanation of his own consciousness.

The world that the modern physicist describes as "real" is not just what is tangible and visible to the eye. It is, rather, of infinite minuteness and infinite extent. Matter, we now know, is in a constant state of flux

3. Tu Wei-ming, "Confucian Humanism in a Modern Perspective," lecture given at Memphis State University, October 12, 1984, for the symposium "China's Gifts to the World."

Figure 11.19. Tung Ch'i-ch'ang (1555–1636). Landscape. Hanging scroll. Ink on paper. 1612. National Palace Museum, Taipei, Taiwan, Republic of China.

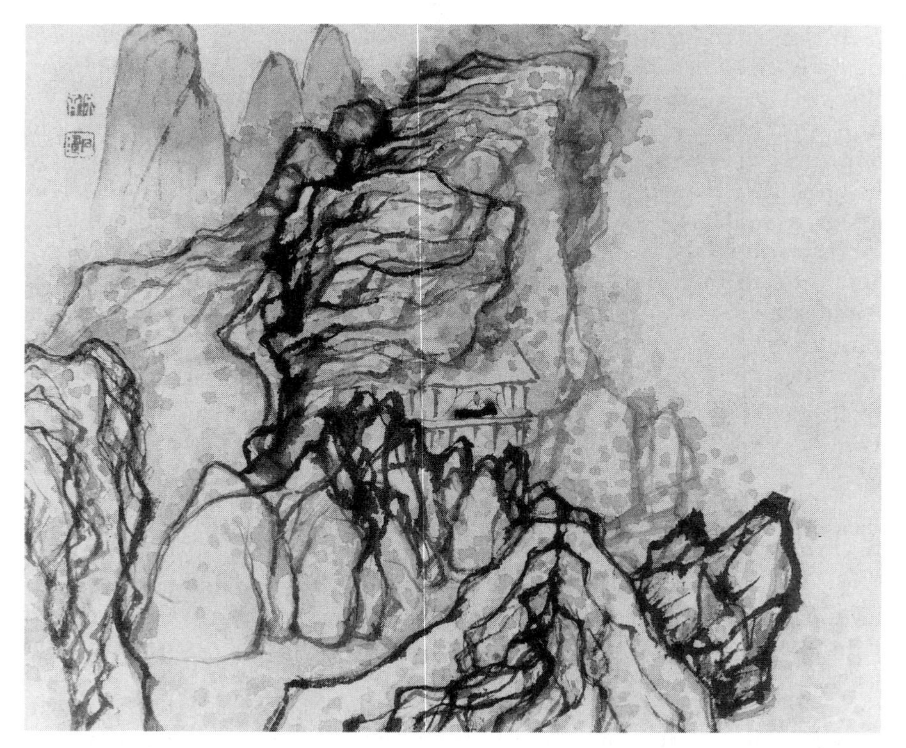

Figure 11.20. Shih-t'ao [Tao-chi, 1642–ca. 1707]. Man in a hut beneath a mountain. Album leaf. Ink and color on paper. Ch'ing dynasty. Collection of C. C. Wang, New York.

and what appears real—the evidence of the senses—is only transient or, as the Buddhists say, *māyā,* illusion. At this level of awareness there can at last be a meeting of minds between East and West. Now at last it has become possible for us to understand what the Chinese artist is saying; witness the response to the great postwar exhibitions of Chinese art and recent writings on Chinese painting, particularly in America, which have reached a level of expert knowledge and understanding unthinkable thirty years ago.

Does this new understanding point to an influence of China on modern Western art comparable to the tremendous influence of the West on contemporary Chinese art? I think not. Although many thinking people in the West are interested in Chinese culture, and some admire it, they see no useful reason to emulate it. We may feel the cold blast of East Asian economic pressure and sell our Chevrolet to buy a Nissan, but we still feel free to accept or reject East Asian cultural and artistic forms and values as we see fit. By contrast, it is precisely in this sense that East Asia has not been free.

A small number of modern Western artists, such as Mark Tobey, Henri Michaux, and Morris Graves, have acknowledged their debt to Chinese art, particularly to calligraphy. But listen to Mark Tobey:

> Artistically speaking, I have had several lives. Some critics have accused me of being an Orientalist, and using Oriental models, but this is not so. For I knew when in Japan and China, as I struggled with their *sumi* ink and brush, in an attempt to understand their calligraphy, that I would never be anything but the Occidental that I am. But it was there that I got what I call the calligraphic impulse to carry my work into some new dimensions. With this method I found I could paint the frenetic rhythms of the modern city, the interweaving of lights and streams of people who are entangled in the meshes of this net.[4]

It was because he wanted to paint the neon lights of Shanghai that Tobey developed his "white writing." Other Western artists have acknowledged the Oriental influence in their work, for example, Sam Francis, who spends half his time in Tokyo. Franz Kline, however, whose work looks so "calligraphic," denies any such influence, and Jackson Pollock, whose marvelous description of his own act of painting accords so perfectly with that of the T'ang dynasty action painters, never, so far as I know, mentioned the Orient as a source of inspiration in his art. In any case, so rapid has been the internationalization of art in recent years that whether or not a particular Western painter is stimulated by the Orient or whether a Chinese artist such as Zao Wou-ki is influenced by Abstract Expressionism is rapidly ceasing to have much historical significance.

As today the East absorbs, masters, exploits, and now advances Western science, technology, and art, so too the West develops, through science, a view of nature that is not so very different from that which, millennia ago, the great civilizations of Asia arrived at through intuition and reflection. Books with titles such as *The Tao of Physics, Zen and the Art of Motorcycle Maintenance,* and *The Dancing Wu Li Masters* are popular signposts on this journey that the East and the West seem to be taking together, as year by year their paths converge. I do not envisage a synthesis, for a synthesis implies something final, static. Rather, what I do envisage is a dynamic interaction of Eastern and Western cultures that will always be different from each other, particularly in their attitudes to society and the individual. But as we draw closer together, through such gatherings as the symposium that prompted the chapters in this book, we can see the walls that once separated us crumbling about our feet.

4. Quoted in Wieland Schmied, *Mark Tobey* (London: Thames and Hudson, 1966), 11.

TWELVE

□

Poetry in the Chinese Tradition

Stephen Owen

Despite the claims of poets and lovers of poetry, it is a simple fact that lyric poetry has never played a direct or forceful role in Western civilization. Other forms of literature have played a large, if usually unacknowledged role: dreams of Homer drove Alexander the Great to conquests, and Nero played at being the divine tragedian both in the empire and on the stage. In more recent times motion pictures embody desires and values, and this art form shapes timid imitations in our daily lives. But unlike the narrative and dramatic forms, lyric poetry has always been a peculiar and singular occupation, uneasily honored by a few and largely ignored by most. However, in Chinese civilization poetry has been and remains an important part of the way in which the Chinese have understood themselves and their past. The differences in the role of poetry in the two civilizations is largely a consequence of different conceptions of what poetry is and what is achieved through it.

The Western concept of literature developed out of ancient epic and drama: narrating and acting out stories. The most popular forms of literature today—novels and motion pictures—have grown out of that tradition. The best Western lyric poetry has remained close to epic and drama and has shared their values of creation and making (the etymological meaning of "poetry" is "making"). Poetry tells tales, recounts or recreates visions, and speaks of the self through masks, as in a play. Such poems are the work of poets, who see themselves and are seen by others as a breed apart: writing poems is simply not a part of the average person's everyday life. Perhaps many people write poems in youth and

All translations in this chapter are my own. The T'ang poems appear in slightly different versions in my book, *The Great Age of Chinese Poetry: The High T'ang* (New Haven: Yale University Press, 1981).

have dreams of being a poet, but the public acclaim that accompanies that dream is given to few; and denied such acclaim, the impulse to write poetry usually withers.

The Chinese lyric was conceived very differently and occupied a very different place in Chinese society. It was a companionable art, for private and social use; and though one might dream of achieving fame for one's poetry, the rarity of such fame in no way undermined the pleasure or value in the act of writing. The lyric poem is defined as *yen chih,* "to articulate what is in the mind intensely." Put simply, the Chinese lyric at its best was conceived as the highest form of speaking to someone else, an activity appropriate to all human beings on certain occasions and in certain states of mind.

The desire for such a general human poetry has not been entirely absent in the Western tradition, but powerful illusions about the specialness of the poetic vocation made this desire questionable. The poet William Wordsworth once gave a definition of poetry that seemed to approach the Chinese definition: he said that poetry was "a man speaking to men." This famous definition was a special moment in the history of Western poetry; Wordsworth tried to articulate the impulse toward a lyric poetry that would be truly different from the novel or drama. But the history of Western literature led him to phrase his definition in the wrong way, and that misphrasing made it impossible to escape the archaic Western concept of literature. When he said "a man speaking to *men,*" he saw lyric poetry as addressing a collective plural, as in epic and drama. Whoever speaks to everyone speaks to no one in particular.

The Chinese understood the lyric as speaking not to humanity as a whole but to *someone* else, some person or group the poet knew or even someone of another age and place, someone the poet would like to know. This someone would be a person the poet hoped would come to know *him* through the poem. The Chinese had a rich vocabulary for writing about poetry, but within that rich vocabulary there is no term quite like the Western word "audience," the collective plural of Wordsworth's "a man speaking to men." The term that Chinese writers on poetry used instead for a good reader was *chih-yin,* "the one who knows the tone," and that term goes back to an old story in the Taoist text *Lieh-tzu:*

> Po-ya was a master in playing the lute, and Chung-tzu-ch'i was a master in listening. When Po-ya played his lute, his mind might be fixed on climbing a high mountain; then Chung-tzu-ch'i would say, "Wonderful! Uprearing and towering like Mount T'ai." Then Po-ya's thoughts might turn to the flowing water, and Chung-tzu-ch'i would say, "Wonderful! Rolling on in floods like the Yangtze and Yellow Rivers." And whatever was in Po-ya's mind, Chung-tzu-ch'i knew it.
>
> Once Po-ya wandered by the dark northern slope of Mount T'ai and suddenly came on a terrible storm. He stopped beneath a cliff, his heart

full of melancholy. Then he took his lute and played it, first a melody of the downpour, then the tones of the mountain itself crashing down. And every melody he played, Chung-tzu-ch'i followed his excitement to the fullest. Then Po-ya put down his lute and said with a sigh, "Wonderful is *your* ability to listen. The images you see in *your* mind are just like those in my own. How could I conceal any sound from you?" (*Lieh-tzu*)

The *chih-yin,* the "one who knows the tone," is the good reader of poetry, and the phrase has a rich resonance; it is also a particular kind of friend, a person whose sympathetic nature and willing familiarity make that person able to see through the music (or the words of a poem) to the other person and his or her state of mind. In the course of its long history, a poem might discover a million *chih-yin,* but these *chih-yin* never make an "audience." Every time the poem meets a good reader like Chung-tzu-ch'i the relation is private, personal, and unique. This definition is not at all an unreasonable model for literature; it is, after all, the way we relate to other people in our lives, whereas finding a willing audience is as rare as being a poet.

In contrast to Wordsworth's "man speaking to men," the Chinese lyric is someone speaking to someone else. The motives in such speaking may be grand or petty: to complain about a social abuse, to explain one's position in a political crisis, to state one's most cherished values, to give an account of visiting a mountain, to talk about depression, or even just to tell what the poet did that day. This speaking may have much "meaning" in the Western literary sense or it may have little. But if you become the good reader and friend of the poet, you are interested in the poem because you care about the person, and the poem's complexity is the complexity of a human being.

The relation formed in the poetic act does not need to be confined to people in the present. The Confucian philosopher Mencius once spoke of the impulse to form friendships with others: a person looks for friends on an ever wider scope until finally that person is compelled to go beyond the present and read the works of the ancients. Mencius called this "going beyond to make friends." In hope of such a relation a person might write poems with his eyes on the future.

In a basic way Chinese poetry becomes a way to create community, both speaking to others in the present and creating a living community across time. To a reader in the nineteenth or twentieth century, the eighth-century poet Tu Fu can be as real a person as anyone in the everyday world. Poetry is seen as a means to know others and to make oneself known to others. This function helps to explain some of the uses of poetry in the Chinese tradition that are often surprising to Western readers. For example, writing poetry was used in the civil service examination to qualify a person for holding public office. This example would be a bizarre use of poetry in the Western sense of the term, but if the poem reveals "what kind of person" the writer is, then it can become an important way to judge someone's suitability for office.

To understand the powerful role of poetry in Chinese civilization it is necessary to look to the beginnings of poetry. These origins, out of which the kind of poetry I have been describing took shape over a span of many centuries, can be traced to the history of one of the Confucian Classics, the *Shih ching*, or *Book of Songs*. The *Book of Songs* is a collection of over three hundred songs composed between about 1000 B.C. and 600 B.C., when the collection reached its present form. These songs represent every aspect of life in the Chou dynasty: ritual hymns to the Chou ancestors, ballads about the founding of the Chou dynasty and its wars of expansion, moral poems, marriage poems, banquet songs, and folk poems.

To the reader familiar with early Western poetry and the archaic religious writings of Near Eastern civilization, the most striking characteristic of these Chinese songs is the absence of terror. There is reverence for the spirits and much human unhappiness, but there is little of the terror at the arbitrary actions of an incomprehensible deity or the terror at the same fearsome forces at work in human beings. Greek myths of origin often begin with a rape or murder. But in the first stanza of the song "Birth of the People" Chiang Yuan founds the house of Chou as an act of her own will, controlling the god through ritual:

The one who first gave birth to the people
Was the Lady Chiang Yuan.
How did she give birth to the people?
By the rites she made and the sacrifices,
To be no longer childless
She walked on the toeprint of the god,
Then became fertile, then increased,
Was made pregnant, was soon delivered,
Gave birth and nurtured,
And this was Hou Chi.

As so often occurs in stories about divine infants in folktales everywhere, Hou Chi, Prince Millet, the founder of the House of Chou, is exposed to the elements. But unlike similar stories in other civilizations, "Birth of the People" shows little interest in why the exposure occurs. The infant Hercules strangled serpents that Hera sent to kill him; but Hou Chi, exposed in the wilderness, is protected and fostered by nature's creatures. Even so, the exposure and the protection scarcely matter, occupying only one stanza of the song. Most of the song is devoted to a loving enumeration of the kinds of grains that grew from Hou Chi's planting and to a celebration of the phases of the agrarian cycle. The song ends by bringing the ancient cycle and its rites up to the present.

Tell us about the sacrifice—
The grain is pounded, the grain is baled,
The grain is winnowed and trampled.
We wash it until it is thoroughly soaked,
Steam it until it is all steamed through.
Then we consider, then we plan,
On a southernwood fire we sacrifice fat,
And take a ram for the rite of the road-god.
Then we roast it, then broil it,
To initiate the succeeding year.

It fills the platters
The platters and the tubs.
And when the fragrance begins to rise,
The god on high takes it with pleasure,
For the scent is good indeed.
Hou Chi founded these rites,
And the people have in no way failed in them,
From then all the way until now.

This immense confidence in the stability of the rites and of the relations between gods and humans is not likely to lead to tragedy or to curses that follow from generation to generation. It does, however, lead to a different sense of beauty, one based not on mystery but on the balance and order of the relationship between humans and the natural or spirit world.

In the centuries that followed the completion of the *Book of Songs* Chou civilization crumbled, and its feudatories became the Warring States. Although society endured terrible suffering in this period, those evils seemed to be the result of human error—terrible enough but possible to correct and not based in any transcendent mystery of the universe and its deity.

Much of the *Book of Songs* consists of what seem to be folk songs that contain motifs common to folk poetry everywhere.

There is a dead doe in the wilds,
All wrapped in white rushes.
There is a girl whose thoughts are of spring,
A gentleman led her astray.

There are bushes in the forest,
A dead deer in the wilds,
All bound around with white rushes,
There is a girl white as marble.

"Slowly now, and gently—
Don't touch my apron,
Don't make the dogs bark!"

The comparison of lost virginity and the death of an animal can be found in folk poetry the world over. However, the closing changes the common song of seduction. The girl speaks up in protest, but her admonition is directed to her worries about waking the dogs and, through their barking, waking her family.

The *Book of Songs* was the beginning of Chinese poetry, and it was a beginning in lyric rather than in epic and drama. In its maturity Chinese poetry owes much to these origins but less to the *Book of Songs* itself than to the long and complicated history of the use and interpretation of its ancient songs. Through that history of interpretation the *Book of Songs* became the archetype for all poetry. During the period after the anthology took its final form, learning the *Book of Songs* by heart became an essential part of the education for anyone who wanted to take part in the life of the feudal courts, and the ability to quote these songs appropriately was considered necessary for polite discourse. In the *Analects* Confucius admonished, "If you don't know the *Book of Songs,* you will have no way to speak well." Envoys sent from one court to another and philosophers frequently quoted the *Book of Songs* in their speeches, both to prove points and to *hsing,* that is, to "stir" the listeners to sympathy with their point of view.

Before the Ch'in dynasty the *Book of Songs* had already acquired great authority, and because it was one of the central texts of Confucian learning the *Book of Songs* was ordered burned by the first Ch'in emperor, who wanted to destroy traditional values and replace them with his own utilitarian statism. But with the founding of the Han dynasty, the *Book of Songs* was reconstructed from memory and was reinterpreted to satisfy the interests of Han scholars. More than any other moment in the tradition, the Han reinterpretation of the *Book of Songs* established the importance of poetry in Chinese civilization.

According to the Han scholars one could find the moral history of the Chou dynasty in the *Book of Songs;* it was a kind of "interior history." The history embodied in the *Book of Songs* did not tell of historical events, but rather gave the reader a real sense of what it was like then, as seen through the responses of the individual authors of the poems. By reading the poems of the *Book of Songs* the later reader was supposed to be able to see the world through the mind and eyes of people of an earlier era. Poetry was not a craft or an art, but rather an involuntary expression of strong feeling bound up with the particular moment in history and society when it was produced.

This Han interpretation was codified in the Great Preface to the *Book of Songs,* which became the orthodox definition of poetry for the rest of the history of traditional China:

> The poem is that to which what is intensely on one's mind goes. In the mind it is the intensity of intent; coming out in language it is a poem.
>
> Emotions are stirred within and take on form in words. If words alone are inadequate, we speak it out in sighs. If sighing is inadequate, we sing it.

If singing it is inadequate, unconsciously our hands sway to it and our feet dance it out.

The emotions emerge in sounds; when those sounds have patterning, they are called "tones." The tones of a well-managed age are at rest and happy: its government is balanced. The tones of an age of turmoil are bitter and full of anger: its government is perverse. The tones of a ruined state are filled with lament and brooding: its people are in difficulty.

Although the Han interpretation is a general statement open to a wide latitude of interpretation, it provides guidelines that shaped the development of future poetry. First, poetry is conceived not as an activity practiced by poets but as a general human activity, something that "happens to" people when they experience feelings of a certain intensity. It differs from ordinary language not absolutely but by degree. Poetry comes forth naturally; it cannot be helped. And the good reader can see in such poetry both the state of mind of the writer and the circumstances of the world in which that writer found himself.

The Confucian scholars, whose interpretive traditions lay behind the formation of the Great Preface, were primarily interested in moral history, the ways in which the moral climate of a particular age would manifest itself in writing. Thus, a poem like "There is a dead doe in the wilds," quoted earlier, would be taken to show the decline of courtship and marriage customs that accompanied the political decline of the Chou. Although the particular interpretation made by these early Confucian commentators may now seem somewhat farfetched, the principle behind such interpretation remains valid and is, in fact, the principle that sustains much Marxist and historicist interpretation in the West: the social and political conditions of an age cannot but appear in poetry.

Confucian interest in moral history helped to shape one strain in the Chinese poetic tradition, namely, where poets write with the purpose of exposing social abuses. By making the evils of such abuses emotionally vivid through their poetry, these poets hope to encourage the ruling powers to correct them. The T'ang poet Po Chü-i (772–846) has several series of such poems, which have perhaps been more often praised in this tradition than read. The following song, "The Old Charcoal Seller," is directed against the practice in which the emperor's agents requisitioned any goods for use in the palace, setting their own prices.

An old charcoal seller
Who cut the wood and burned it to charcoal
  in the South Mountains,
From the smoke his face has turned the color of ash,
The locks of his hair are graying,
  his fingers all black.
When he sells his charcoal, what does he use
  his money for?—

Clothes for his body, food for his belly.
Though the clothes he now wears are terribly thin,
He worries about the charcoal's price
  and wants the weather cold.
Last night outside the city a foot of snow fell,
And at dawn his charcoal cart
  crunched through the icy ruts.
His ox was worn out, the man was hungry,
  and the sun was already high,
When he stopped the cart in the slush
  outside of the market's south gate.
Two riders come prancing toward him,
  he wonders who they are—
A palace eunuch officer
  with his white-robed servant boy;
In his hand he holds an edict
  which he reads to the man out loud,
Then turns the carriage and shouts at the ox,
  dragging it northward to the palace.
In that carriage the charcoal was more than a
  thousand pounds,
But the palace official who drives it away
  doesn't care at all.
A half a bolt of red gauze, a yard of fine silk
Have been tied upon the ox's head,
  payment for his charcoal.

The imperial government used silk as a medium of exchange, but the price set by the palace eunuch would only buy the old man five or ten pounds of rice, hardly enough to see him through the winter.

The impulse to discover social circumstances behind a poem occurs not only in poems like "The Old Charcoal Seller" but also in pieces that permit such interpretation less directly. The following piece is from a collection of poems called the "Nineteen Old Poems," probably from the early second century A.D. A social interpretation would see in it a sense of despair owing to the decline in Eastern Han society rather than a sense of despair about the universal human situation.

Those who have gone seem more remote each day,
The newly come each day seem more like kin.
I go out the gates, gaze straight ahead,
And see only the mounds of tombs.
Ancient graves have been plowed into fields,
Their cypress and pines cut down for fuel.
Sad winds roar through white willows
Their moaning brings grief too much to bear.
I long to return to my village home,
But about to go, no road takes me there.

The Great Preface may have encouraged such political and social interpretation, but its implications were much broader than political poetry. If poetry revealed a human state of mind, it not only implicated the political and social circumstances in which the person found himself but also revealed the nature of the person.

Perhaps the first poet to make full use of poetry as a means to articulate the apolitical dimensions of personality was T'ao Ch'ien (365–427). In T'ao Ch'ien's age, as in most of Chinese civilization, an educated man found full justification only in service to the state and society. However, there were many intellectuals who sought fulfillment in other, private goals, and the poetry and prose of such individuals is more widely read today than the writings of men who chose the regular course of state service. The fact that these individualists wrote more voluminously and persuasively cannot be taken as a sign that the age was dominated by individualism; rather, the decision to reject state service created a greater need for the poet to offer self-explanation and self-justification.

T'ao Ch'ien held office briefly, then made the radical decision to give up his post and return to his farm to spend the rest of his life as a farmer. Considering the dangerous political circumstances of the age in which he lived, this may have been a wise decision, but it was not an easy one. He used his poetry as a means to justify his choice, both to himself and others. T'ao's poetry became a kind of poetic autobiography and as such was an important stage in the development of the concept of poetry as a means to make the self known. In the following poem, the first in a series of five entitled "Returning to My Gardens and Fields," T'ao gives the essential narrative of alienation followed by return to his true nature.

Since youth I felt no sympathy for common things,
By nature I loved the mountains and hills.
But I made a mistake, fell into the world's net,
And once gone, remained there thirty years.
The caged bird yearns for its former forest,
Fish in a pond long for their native deeps.
I cleared wasteland by the edge of the southern wilds,
And to keep my simplicity went back to my gardens and fields.
A square plot, ten acres or so,
A thatched cottage of eight or nine rooms.
Elm and willow shade the rear eaves,
Peach trees and plums form rows before my hall.
Faint in the distance are villages
From which coils of smoke wind upward;
Dogs bark deep in the lanes,
Cocks crow from the tips of the mulberry.
No dust and dirt mix in my yard,
My empty chambers give ample peace.
Long I have been caught in a cage,
And now again I return to the nature of things.

Such life choices do not inherently require writing in poetry. Poetry is the means that gives such choices value, that makes them "public" (even though T'ao Ch'ien would claim that both the choices and poems were private). By writing again and again about his choice to retire to his farm, T'ao Ch'ien creates for himself a myth of the "natural life," which he sets against the more commonly accepted values of state service.

The poetry of the T'ang dynasty set the model for poetry in traditional China for the next thousand years. The great poets of the eighth and ninth centuries remained the most powerful figures for later ages, reminders of how successful poetry could be in embodying a human personality. In the latter part of the seventh century the Empress Wu introduced the composition of poetry into the civil service examination, which served as a means to recruit government officials from outside the aristocratic circles that surrounded the court. At about the same time the composition of poetry became a pervasive practice among the educated. Previously, poetry had been the practice of the few, of courtiers and eccentrics like T'ao Ch'ien. But beginning in the eighth century Chinese poetry began to realize its ancient promise that it be a means for anyone to "speak what was on the mind intensely."

In the T'ang, poetry was often more an activity than a literary "thing"; it was something an educated person was called on to do in certain circumstances. Some of the occasions for poetry were highly formalized. A person who was invited to a party would be expected to produce a poem in the same way that someone in the modern world is expected to play a parlor game the host might choose. One consequence of such uses of poetry was a vast quantity of second- and third-rate poetry. The pleasures of such poetry for the host and other guests were modest: the celebration of that moment, a fine turn of phrase, the way in which someone they knew expressed himself. These modest pleasures hold little allure for readers a thousand years later. However, some of the greatest poems of the dynasty can be found within that vast corpus of occasional poetry.

Partings and parting banquets were another important occasion for poetry. The friends and associates of the person leaving would often accompany the traveler a small distance on the journey. Then they would stop, set up a feast, and drink until late in the night. The next morning the bleary-eyed traveler would begin the serious part of the journey. This activity called for the composition of poems that would often be written out in a scroll and presented to the traveler on his final departure.

To drop in on a friend for a visit or, having dropped in, to find the person not at home were occasions that called for poems. Like banquet poems and other kinds of occasional poetry, such poetic "house gifts" might be modest verse, but they might also rise to the level of great art. "Visiting the Recluse on Mount Tai-t'ien and Not Finding Him In" is a famous poem by Li Po (701–762):

A dog barks amid the sound of waters,
Peach blossoms dark and heavy with dew.
Where trees are thickest I sometimes see a deer,
Noon in the ravine, but I hear no bell.
Bamboo of wilderness split through blue haze,
A cascade in flight, hung from an emerald peak.
No one knows where you've gone—
But I linger, disappointed, among these few pines.

It is worth our while to linger a while with this poem, to consider both how it functioned as a social act and how it transcended that immediate social purpose to become one of Li Po's best-known poems. On one level, the level most Western readers can see directly, Li Po is simply describing the scene around the recluse's dwelling and politely stating his disappointment that the man was not at home. But to be a good reader of the poem and of Li Po, to be the *chih-yin,* requires a special kind of attention on our part: we must follow the movement of Li Po's perception, and in that movement we must understand where the poet is and what he cares about. Learning to be a good reader of Chinese poetry is an art as fine as being a good poet.

Some of the things necessary to understand the poem are "lore." The good reader would associate peach blossoms with the story of "Peach Blossom Spring," in which a fisherman followed a trail of peach blossoms deep into the mountains where he found a village that had remained cut off from the outside world for centuries; the reader would know that Buddhist monasteries, located deep in the mountains, would ring the monastery bell at noon; and the reader would know that the pine was the emblem of moral integrity and the solitary life. But apart from these bits of lore, the art of reading requires only an intuitive sense of the way in which a description implies a particular "stance" and state of mind on the part of the person giving the description. If we learn this art of reading, we can easily understand why this poem was an appropriate "house gift" on this particular occasion, and why it became a very famous poem for future generations; we can also begin to see something of the immense appeal T'ang poetry held and still holds for Chinese readers.

The opening, "A dog barks amid the sound of waters," is a bold juxtaposition of sounds. The good reader knows at once that Li Po has been traveling through the mountains to find the recluse, hearing nothing but the sound of rushing waters. The intrusion of the dog's barking is a sign to the traveler of a human presence in the landscape; at the same time, to the person living hidden in the mountains, the barking announces the arrival of someone from the outside world. But beyond revealing the visitor to the recluse and the closeness of the recluse's dwelling to the visitor, this juxtaposition of sounds—the flowing waters and the dog's barking—is a structure of abrupt intrusion, the sensuous counterpart of the poet's intrusion into the quiet world of the recluse.

To notice the peach blossoms is an allusion to the story of "Peach Blossom Spring," explained earlier. As the dog's barking tells the poet that he has finally reached the dwelling of the recluse, the peach blossoms heavy with dew reveal to us how the poet knew the way there. We smile. The heavy peach blossoms fall into the water (whose sounds the poet heard in the first line) and are carried by the current down the mountain, forming a trail for an outsider to follow to reach the home of someone hiding away in the mountains.

The poem is a search; the poet is looking for someone who is "hidden away" but is only finding elusive traces of the recluse's presence, traces half appearing in the landscape. In the thickest part of the forest a deer briefly appears, a creature whose wariness of humans is like the wariness of the recluse toward outsiders. For Li Po, looking intently to find the man, that movement might have been him. But the very fact that the deer would let itself be seen is evidence that the recluse has been here: in this place the shy animal has little to fear from a human. Like the barking of the dog, its appearance is another mark that the recluse is nearby—somewhere.

The water rushing down the mountain forms a ravine, along which the poet climbs. The steep sides and the thick trees growing along them keep the ravine in shade through the morning and afternoon. There is only one moment of full light, at noon when the sun is directly overhead. As the poet climbs through the shadows and approaches the home of the recluse, suddenly the sun breaks into the ravine. He stops and listens, knowing that in a place as remote as this one there might be a monastery, whose presence he can know by the sound of the noontime bell, just as he knew the presence of the recluse by the sound of the dog's bark intruding on the sound of the waters. However, there is only silence; and in that silence he realizes just how far into the wilderness he has come.

The next two lines are very beautiful, fine examples of the T'ang art of the couplet and of the way in which the description of the natural world is a mirror for human concerns. He sees a blue haze, and within that haze are tall straight stalks of bamboo, green and barely defined against the background of mist. After the intrusive barking of the dog, which let the poet know how close he was to the recluse and let the recluse know an outsider had come, everything seems to elude Li Po: he looks intently for something or someone; a shape half appears, then recedes—a deer, the bamboo in haze. Then that solid vertical figure of bamboo in the fluid haze becomes the vertical figure of the fluid waterfall, set against the solid background of the cliff. This waterfall becomes the "sound of waters" that carries the peach blossoms down into the mortal world.

In the last couplet the poet reaches the recluse's dwelling (which fortunately has a servant present to tell him that his master is not there). All the figures that half appeared, then disappeared, are gone; what remains is only a stand of pine trees where the poet leans, disappointed at not finding the recluse. Here a bit of lore is necessary. Li Po and his readers all know that the pine tree is the emblem of the recluse. Li Po has found the recluse in finding the surroundings that make the recluse what he is. Finding the person is unnecessary. Like the sounds of the mountain landscape when the dog is not barking at an intruder, the recluse has merged perfectly with nature, has disappeared into it. Li Po pretends to be a "worldly" person who does not recognize that he has truly found the recluse by finding his surroundings.

Ch'iu Wei, a contemporary of Li Po, wrote a poem on a similar subject; Ch'iu Wei climbs the mountain to the dwelling of the recluse, discovers that the man is not at home, and at the end of the poem states the principle more obviously than Li Po:

Though we didn't assume the roles of guest and host,
I have found the pure truth of your life here:
My impulse finished, I go back down the mountain—
Why should I have to wait for your return.

On one level Li Po has written a polite occasional poem, praising the man for the beauty of his home in the wilderness and the perfect life he has found there. It is the sort of poem one is supposed to write when paying an unexpected visit on a friend and not finding him at home. On another level it is a deeper poem about human beings and nature. On this level Li Po's poem goes beyond its use in a social occasion to become a very famous work that has appealed to readers for a thousand years.

Occasional poetry was an important form of participation in the social world; it was the most common context for writing poetry. It was not, however, the only kind of poetry. As in Western poetry, there were poems on general topics; and although poets still preferred concrete occasions for composition, those occasions did not have to be social ones. In Li Po's poem, for the sake of a compliment he assumes the role of a worldly intruder into the pure world of the recluse. Elsewhere, in "Question and Answer in the Mountains," he assumes the role of the recluse who rejects the common world.

You ask me why I choose
  to lodge in emerald hills;
I laugh and do not answer you,
  my heart is calm and still.
Peach blossoms in flowing water
  disappear into the distance:
There is another universe
  apart from the human world.

Together with Li Po, Tu Fu (712–770) is considered the greatest poet of traditional China. Tu Fu was caught in the middle of the great rebellion of the northeastern armies under the leadership of their general An Lu-shan. His captivity behind rebel lines, his escape to the loyalist court, and his later wanderings through the western provinces of the crumbling T'ang state made him a witness to great political events; in that role he fulfilled perfectly the definition of poetry given in the Great Preface of the *Book of Songs:* he unified the personal and the public aspects of the age. Many of his poems comment directly on battles and imperial policy; but toward the end of his life, traveling down the Yangtze River, he wrote some of his finest work, integrating private experience with the T'ang vision of the universal order. The following poem, "Spending the Night in a Tower by the River," is from this period.

> The color of darkness extends on the mountain paths,
> As I lodge by the river gate, high in a study,
> A thin cloud spends the night on cliff's edge,
> The lonely moon topples in the wave.
> Storks and cranes fly calmly one after another,
> Wild dogs and wolves howl over their prey.
> I cannot sleep for worry over battles—
> I have no strength to right the universe.

As in Li Po's poem, description here is the movement of Tu Fu's attention, first watching the darkness as it rises up the paths through the mountains (when the sun sets, the mountaintops catch the last light, so darkness seems to rise "up" the mountain). Tu Fu is in K'uei-chou, built on a steep mountainside that slopes down to the Yangtze River. High in the tower by the river, he feels he is clinging to the very edge of the land; then looking out, he sees his counterpart in the cloud, hanging motionless on the cliff's edge, as if about to fall into the river. That precarious position directs his attention to something falling; he looks down into the river and there sees the moonlight tossed about in the turbulent waters, as if the moon itself had fallen. Darkness and danger seem to surround him.

Hanging at the edge of things, there are two possibilities, falling to destruction or flying free, the actual movement of the cloud that seems so precariously balanced on the cliff. Poems like this one by Tu Fu are built of parallel images and oppositions: every shape has counterparts and contrasts. The form of the cloud on the point of flight finds a parallel in the image of cranes and storks, birds associated with recluses and immortals, moving easily through the air. Below the cranes and storks in the darkness Tu Fu hears "wild dogs and wolves," associated with violent men, howling over some victim taken in the darkness. Images of fear and hope of escape surround him in his precarious perch. The sleeplessness follows naturally from these images but also from the sense of his own powerlessness; he has "no strength to right the universe."

The poem is a private statement, yet at the end it raises a public value, if only to confess the impossibility of realizing that value: Tu Fu would "right the universe" if he could; he cannot.

Rather than an art that is separate from the common world in which we live, Chinese poetry tried to be part of life, giving words to complex feelings. Even in a private poem like Tu Fu's, poetry was a means to make a public statement, even if the statement would have to take the place of action. The great poets are not figures apart but remain some of the most memorable figures in Chinese civilization: personalities like T'ao Ch'ien, Li Po, and Tu Fu remain a living part of that community across time.

THIRTEEN

□

The Distinctive Art of Chinese Fiction

Paul S. Ropp

Storytelling in China probably began in the cave, and it continues to flourish in the late twentieth century. For a civilization as old and continuous as China's, a complete history of fiction would fill many books. My purpose in this chapter is more modest: to suggest the uses and pleasures of reading Chinese fiction in English translation, to give a sense of the distinctive qualities of fiction (especially vernacular fiction) in China as compared with Western fiction, and to review some of the highlights of the Chinese tradition.

There are many ways to try to understand a civilization. No one way is necessarily superior to the others, but certainly one of the most enjoyable ways to explore the riches of Chinese civilization is through its fiction. As a very popular art form in China, fiction can tell us a great deal about the beliefs, values, and customs of ordinary people. In describing the details of daily life Chinese storytellers from at least the fifth century A.D. onward have given us our most extensive sources on the actual texture of Chinese life, what Lionel Trilling once called the "hum and buzz of implication" that we take for granted in our own lives but that gets lost in most formal or official records from the past.

Fiction naturally invites analysis from many different perspectives.[1]

Although I have not always been able to implement their suggestions, I am very grateful to the following people for very helpful criticisms of earlier drafts of this chapter: Sunhee Kim Gertz, C. T. Hsia, David L. Rolston, Yaohua Shi, Virginia Vaughan, and Judith Zeitlin.

1. Four useful introductory works illustrating different approaches to the study of fiction are René Wellek and Austin Warren, *Theory of Literature,* 3d ed. (New York: Harcourt, Brace & World, 1956); Wilbur Scott, ed., *Five Approaches of Literary Criticism* (New York: Collier-Macmillan, 1962); Elizabeth Burns and Tom Burns, eds., *Sociology of Literature and Drama* (Harmondsworth: Penguin, 1973); and Terry Eagleton, *Literary Theory: An Introduction* (Minneapolis: University of Minnesota Press, 1983).

Part of its perennial appeal is that it can be read and enjoyed on so many different levels. The highly trained literary theorist might probe a particular work with mind-boggling erudition, but a beginning student can read the same work at a less sophisticated level and still gain a great deal of pleasure and understanding.

Fiction can also be an illuminating vehicle for the comparison of two civilizations. Chinese fiction has not had much influence on Western literature, and until the late nineteenth century the West had little or no impact on Chinese fiction. In part, this separation is what makes Chinese and Western literatures interesting to compare. In such a comparison we see both universals of human storytelling and evidence that different civilizations with their particular conceptions of human life, social and political organization, moral and religious teachings, and modes of entertainment inevitably shape their fictions to meet their own needs and concerns.

The development of fiction in China and the West offers many striking parallels. In both China and the West fiction has generally been seen to have a dual mission: to entertain and to instruct; and in both cultures these two goals have frequently been in conflict. Until relatively recently (perhaps the eighteenth century in the West and the twentieth century in China) the social status of the practitioners of fiction has been relatively low. Fiction was frequently condemned by philosophers and moralists in both cultures for "leading people astray," "glorifying vile behavior," and "wasting valuable time" that would otherwise be spent, it was assumed, in more uplifting or productive pursuits. (These arguments alone have always assured fiction a ready audience in both cultures!)

Apart from moral attitudes toward fiction, there are also important parallels in the evolution of storytelling forms in China and the West. In both cultures there has been a general development from shorter to longer works, from an earlier emphasis on myths and folktales to a later emphasis on the individual experience and observations of particular authors. As fiction became more sophisticated and self-conscious in both cultures it also evolved from an earlier tendency to endorse wholeheartedly the society's common values and moved instead to a more ironic stance that questioned or criticized the dominant values of the civilization. Although fiction was to some extent more valued in the West than in China early on, the direction of change in both has been toward a growing appreciation of the serious importance of fiction not just as entertainment but as a way of exploring profound social, moral, philosophical and psychological questions.

To be slightly more specific and to anticipate the second half of this chapter, it is worth noting the parallel development of the novel in both China and the West. The extended prose narrative that realistically creates a believable world of its own evolved in China from the fourteenth through the eighteenth centuries, slightly anticipating but very closely paralleling the development of the novel in Europe. In both cultures these literary developments seem to accompany the rise of a money economy, urbanization, a growing entertainment industry, and the spread of printing, literacy, and education. In both China and the West the novel was also primarily the work of a highly educated elite writing for educated readers. Most striking are the parallels from the sixteenth through the early nineteenth centuries when the novel in both cultures became increasingly autobiographical and increasingly serious in the exploration of social, moral, and philosophical problems.[2]

In addition to these similarities, there are some important differences between Chinese and Western fiction. Several themes from the other chapters in this volume are especially important in the traditions of Chinese fiction. Among these I would emphasize the importance of history and historical-mindedness, the relative optimism of the Chinese worldview, the moral humanism of Confucian philosophy, and the relative emphasis from very early in Chinese history on collective behavior and the welfare of the group rather than the individual.

As I already noted, early fiction in China and in the West was assumed to have a moral purpose, but the moral emphasis has generally been stronger, or has survived longer, in the Chinese tradition. Michael Sullivan (see Chapter 11) has remarked on the Chinese tendency to assume that great art is by definition moral. The dominant stated purpose of Chinese storytellers has been to uplift their readers, to reassure them that the universe is friendly, that human life is meaningful, and that human morality above all makes it so. This moralistic humanistic optimism in traditional Chinese fiction (despite exceptions to be noted later) gives it a didactic quality that contemporary Westerners have sometimes criticized as trite at best and dishonest at worst.

It would be a great mistake, however, to assume that Chinese storytellers lacked courage or insight into society because they were optimistic and didactic. We should note that fiction writers had to attract readers somehow; unlike poets and philosophers, storytellers had no captive audience among aspiring scholar-officials. The need to attract and keep a reader's attention cut against the Confucian grain of moralistic optimism. As Tolstoy wrote at the beginning of *Anna Karenina,* "All happy families are alike; each unhappy family is unhappy in its own way." Virtue is unfortunately boring in its predictability, and evil is fascinating in its sheer variety. For these reasons Chinese storytellers have never stayed wholly within the bounds of respectability. The audience for tales of sex,

2. An excellent discussion of the development of the novel in China and the West is by Andrew H. Plaks, "Full-length *Hsiao-shuo* and the Western Novel: A Generic Reappraisal," *New Asia Academic Bulletin* 1 (1978): 163–76.

violence, intrigue, and adventure has been as vast and as eager in China as anywhere else.

The storyteller's most common solution to the conflicting demands of didacticism and attracting an audience was to put a moral gloss on every story and then (as often as not) ignore or contradict the self-proclaimed "message" while trying to make the story as exciting, as funny, or as believable as possible. This pattern is most obvious in traditional Chinese love stories. These stories, particularly the erotic or pornographic ones, invariably pose as moral tales warning readers of the dire consequences of romantic love and unbridled sexual indulgence. Yet the storytellers often take such graphic delight in the love scenes in these stories that they could not possibly have succeeded in their proclaimed goal of encouraging sexual abstinence and debunking romantic love.[3] The point here is not to question the honesty or virtue of the storyteller or his audience, but simply to note how fiction can illustrate the social and moral tensions of a civilization.

Among the important sources of optimism and moral didacticism in Chinese fiction were its origins in the writing of history and what David N. Keightley notes as the profound philosophical optimism of the early Chinese (see Chapter 2). If the universe is friendly, if it "makes sense" morally, and if human beings have the power to make collective improvements in their lives, the possibilities for a tragic view of life are greatly diminished. Needless to say, there have been tragedies in Chinese literature and more tragedies in Chinese life, but the relative Chinese disinterest in tragic stories is very striking in its contrast with Western traditions from ancient Greece onward. More than anything else, this profound philosophical optimism is what modern Western critics have found objectionable in the Chinese storytelling tradition. But a disinterest in tragedy does not mean that human ignorance, folly, greed, and misery are ignored or glossed over in Chinese fiction. On the contrary, these themes occupy a well-deserved place in Chinese, as in all human, fiction. The task of the Chinese fiction-writer (and the Chinese historian) was to redeem these dark themes from the abyss of despair by "making moral sense" of them.

In Chinese fiction the moralistic and optimistic emphasis of Confucianism was ironically reinforced by the spread of Buddhism and the concepts of reincarnation, karma, and moral retribution. Although Confucian scholars often criticized Buddhism, the religion flourished in

3. The triumph of the entertainer over the moralist among the writers of erotic fiction that poses as "avoidance" literature may be seen from the titles of two representative works in English translation: Li Yü, *The Prayer Mat of Flesh,* trans. by Richard Martin from a German version by Franz Kuhn (New York: Grove Press, 1963), and John Scott, trans., *The Lecherous Academician and Other Tales by Master Ling Mengchu* (London: Rapp & Whiting, 1973).

China, as T. H. Barrett describes (see Chapter 6), from the second century A.D. onward, and Buddhist views of reincarnation and moral retribution came to be embedded in the popular Chinese worldview. This belief could explain away the most horrible examples of apparent injustice, and thousands of Chinese short stories take as their theme the rewarding of good and punishment of evil in this life or the next (or the one after that).

As a part of their mutual faith in a moral universe, Confucians and Buddhists both saw the primary value of fiction in moral terms. One might even go so far as to suggest that Confucian historiography and Buddhist missionary efforts provided the first great impetus for the development of storytelling in China. Confucian historians developed narrative models that storytellers copied verbatim, and Buddhist missionaries discovered that a good exciting story was a far better lure to religion than the dry explication of a sacred text. Despite their radical disagreement on the meaning of life, Buddhists and Confucians agreed on the moral purpose of fiction, and each group affirmed an ethicoreligious order with little room for tragedy or despair.

Confucians and Taoists shared a faith in harmony, balance, and a cyclical view of reality that also worked against the development of tragedy. Confucians urged moderation in all things, and Taoists argued that all situations and qualities contain the seeds of their opposite. Extreme power leads to defeat, extreme wealth to poverty, and any one virtue, if carried to extremes, becomes a vice. In this view (shared by Confucians and Taoists alike) a hero is by definition moderate. Thus, in contrast to the typical Greek tragic hero, the Chinese hero is not likely to be destroyed by a noble impulse carried too far. A faith in the cyclical nature of life also helps to rob death of its sting. When the philosopher Chuang Tzu surprised his friends by singing cheerfully after the death of his wife, he responded by defining death as a natural part of life, not something to be feared or mourned. For Confucians death brings sadness—the sadness of parting—but not terror or pity, the stuff of Greek tragedy.

Another factor that worked against a tragic view of life in China was the emphasis Keightley notes (see Chapter 2) on the society or the collectivity rather than the individual. This collective emphasis with its bureaucratic overtones may seem inhibiting and confining to contemporary Westerners, but it was a source of great social strength and stability in traditional China. If an individual is defined solely in individual terms, the opportunities for tragedy are unlimited, but where individuals are defined by their social function and their ties to society, the possibility of tragedy quickly recedes. An individual might die a horrible death, but in the Chinese view an individual's death is understood less as the fate of an individual soul and more as an event in the ongoing stream of humanity. If a good person suffers injustice and dies for a lost cause, it is not to be seen as a terrible tragedy. The very praise of the storyteller or historian affirms and perpetuates the values of society and thus redeems the tragedy.

The greater emphasis on the group rather than the individual in early China is also evident in another way in Chinese fiction. In general (some exceptions are examined later) early Chinese storytellers were more interested in plot and incident than in psychological description. I should note that the "psychological novel" with its detailed exploration of individual consciousness is a relatively recent phenomenon even in the West. But placing Western and Chinese traditions side by side, we see more emphasis on individual psychology in the West, at least from the sixteenth century onward. Chinese storytellers tended to take a longer-range view than their Western counterparts and to focus on the broad canvas of human society (which of course has its own charms, as in a Chinese handscroll or a Brueghel painting).

The relative inattention to individual psychology in much Chinese fiction is partly a matter of perspective, for in the grand totality of the universe, the individual human psyche may not amount to much. Chinese thinkers (including storytellers) have generally viewed human nature as very malleable and as heavily influenced by the larger society. By contrast, Westerners have tended to view the individual as morally and socially autonomous, with the power to shape his or her own destiny. A traditional Chinese critic might well respond to the Western approach by saying that so much attention to individual psychology trivializes and distorts reality by ignoring the more important factors of social pressures and role expectations and by being too concerned with the "short run" rather than with the more significant long-term development of a whole society.

One final comparison of Chinese and Western approaches to literature illustrates another recurrent theme: what may appear to modern Westerners as defective Chinese literary technique often reflects deep differences in worldview. Western readers have sometimes criticized Chinese fiction for its lack of coherence in plot development, its highly episodic quality, and its general looseness in structure. Andrew Plaks has made two astute observations regarding these criticisms: first, the holistic and organismic Chinese worldview, which sees life in recurrent cyclical and interrelated patterns, does not encourage the development of the Western-style unilinear plot; second, the preferred plot structure in Chinese fiction is borrowed from drama, in which the climax or pivotal point in a work occurs not at the end but two-thirds or three-fourths of the way through the story. Whereas Western audiences may see the concluding, rather quiet, section of such a work as anticlimactic and therefore unsatisfying, Chinese appreciate in the final calming "afterglow" a sense of the completion of a cycle, the implicit assumption that "life goes on," and that the completion of one cycle is the prologue of another.[4] This insistence on seeing life as the ceaseless alternation and interplay of life and death, joy and sorrow, summer and winter, order and chaos, has been an awe-inspiring vision the Chinese have found deeply satisfying and meaningful. Such a worldview goes far to account for the relative absence of tragedy and unilinear plots in Chinese fiction.

I have described some of the main characteristics of Chinese fiction and have compared in very broad terms the traditions of storytelling in China and the West. In the remainder of this chapter I focus on Chinese fiction itself. After touching very briefly on the major categories of fiction in China and noting the development of different types of short stories from the tenth century onward, I conclude with a discussion of the most famous traditional Chinese novels written from the fourteenth to the nineteenth centuries.

Patrick Hanan has identified three distinct literatures in the Chinese tradition corresponding to three general audiences. The bulk of the population, illiterate and relatively poor, enjoyed an oral tradition, consisting of stories told in vernacular Chinese at marketplaces and in urban entertainment districts. For the highly educated literati class literature included the short tale in classical Chinese, the highly allusive written language of officialdom (little changed from the time of Confucius to the twentieth century) that required years of study to master. From at least the fourteenth century onward a written vernacular literature that drew on both oral and classical traditions also developed; it appealed especially to an urban "middle class" of semiliterate shopkeepers, merchants, artisans, clerks, bookkeepers, and low-level officials. Scholars once assumed that the written vernacular stories were composed primarily by urban storytellers themselves as promptbooks for their live performances. This may have happened in some cases, but we now know that many highly educated writers also borrowed the storytellers' conventions in writing these stories for a relatively well educated reading public.

These three literatures, Hanan is quick to point out, have always existed in close proximity, and there is a good deal of overlapping and mutual influence among them.[5] The written vernacular, as a kind of middle-level literature, is no doubt the most eclectic of the three and by far the most fertile in the development of the Chinese novel. Both written traditions borrowed heavily from oral storytelling conventions as well as from music, drama, and poetry. The vernacular authors com-

4. Andrew H. Plaks, "Towards a Critical Theory of Chinese Narrative," in *Chinese Narrative: Critical and Theoretical Essays,* ed. Andrew H. Plaks (Princeton: Princeton University Press, 1977), 334–39.

5. Patrick Hanan, "The Development of Fiction and Drama," in *The Legacy of China,* ed. Raymond Dawson (London: Oxford University Press, 1964), 115–43.

monly interspersed their narratives with verses (in classical Chinese), popular songs, sayings, and ballads, occasionally in such profusion as to overshadow the prose narration itself.

In general Chinese storytellers, novelists, and compilers of stories have been voracious borrowers of plots, dialogue, poems, and sayings from any and all available sources. As a result, a common stock of plot lines has been cycled and recycled through all the main types of literature. Some stories exist in dozens of different versions, ranging from classical tales to poetic ballads (*chantefables*) to dramas to vernacular tales, and even novels that might string together a number of preexisting stories. This profusion of recycled stories makes the history of Chinese fiction especially complex for scholars tracing the entangled webs of borrowed sources. What mattered most to a traditional Chinese audience was not an author's originality but the cleverness with which he could weave borrowed material into a believable pattern with no seams showing.

As in the West, fiction in China evolved from shorter to longer forms. The earliest written fiction in China (popular by the fourth century A.D.) consisted of very short notes, tales, observations, and anecdotes called *pi-chi,* or simply jottings, mostly a paragraph or two in length. In the T'ang period (seventh to tenth centuries) a somewhat longer and more precisely defined type of story evolved called *ch'uan-ch'i* (literally meaning "propagation of wonders"). Both *pi-chi* and *ch'uan-ch'i* authors delighted in the strange, the supernatural, and the bizarre, although the *ch'uan-ch'i* stories dealt with a broader range of fictional topics, including love, knight-errantry, and a variety of historical themes. In the seventeenth century the *ch'uan-ch'i* reached its greatest perfection in the work of P'u Sung-ling, who wrote a marvelous collection titled *Strange Stories from Liao-chai* (P'u's studio). P'u's tales are an eery blend of humor, satire, mild eroticism, reports of exotic or strange phenomena, and terrifyingly vivid descriptions of suffering and injustice.[6]

Two short story forms that particularly reflect the didactic emphasis of Chinese fiction are the *pien-wen,* Buddhist-inspired tales of moral retribution in parallel prose or alternating verse and prose, and the *kung-an,* or detective story. Partly spoken and partly sung or chanted, the *pien-wen* apparently flourished in the ninth and tenth centuries, but they were rediscovered only in the twentieth century in the caves of Tun-

6. Two translations of selected stories from P'u's work are P'u Sung-ling, *Strange Stories from a Chinese Studio,* trans. Herbert Giles (reprint, New York: Dover, 1969), P'u Sung-ling, *Selected Tales of Liaozhai,* trans. Hsien-yi Yang and Gladys Yang et al. (Peking: Panda Books, 1981). One can quickly gain a sense of P'u's narrative power from the elegant translations of his stories sprinkled throughout Jonathan Spence, *Death of Woman Wang* (New York: Knopf, 1978).

huang, after lying unnoticed for nearly a thousand years. Their emphasis on moral retribution came to be a main feature of most later Chinese short stories. The detective story has probably enjoyed a longer run in China than in any civilization (roughly from the eleventh century to the twentieth). In the *kung-an* (literally, "court case"), a crime is committed, often in full view of the reader. A magistrate then proceeds to solve the crime, usually through elaborate and clever stratagems. The suspense is not in discovering the criminal but in following the magistrate's thought and action to see *how* justice will be served.

The most important short stories in the Chinese tradition are the vernacular tales, *hua-pen* (usually called "promptbooks"), which became increasingly popular from the eleventh century onward. Originally thought to have been nothing more than the notes of oral storytellers, *hua-pen* are now recognized as a fully developed written genre in vernacular Chinese that borrowed the conventions of the storyteller but were written for and sold to the literate reading public. These stories cover a broader range of subjects than the literary tales, and they reflect the growth of cities and the spread of printing and literacy in China from the Sung period onward. They were especially popular in the late Ming period (sixteenth and seventeenth centuries) when they were first published by professional writers and compilers who signed their works and defended fiction as a worthwhile and even noble endeavor.[7]

When we consider the traditional Chinese novel, an almost universal consensus affirms six works as truly great. These books were created from the sixteenth through the eighteenth centuries. Although many other novels were written during these years, these six almost alone have been widely known, read, and loved by educated Chinese from the time they were first published (usually some years after their author's death) to the present. These novels are comparable in scope, ambition, and skill to the Western novel from the sixteenth through the nineteenth centuries.[8]

Given the strong influence of historical narrative on Chinese fiction, it is not surprising that the earliest great work of extended prose narrative is *Romance of the Three Kingdoms* (*San-kuo-chih yen-i*), a historical narrative

7. An excellent small collection of *hua-pen* stories is Cyril Birch, ed., *Stories from a Ming Collection* (New York: Grove Press, 1958). The most comprehensive sampling of all the major Chinese short story forms in English translation is Y. W. Ma and Joseph S. M. Lau, eds., *Traditional Chinese Stories: Themes and Variations* (New York: Columbia University Press, 1978). A fine critical history of *hua-pen* stories is Patrick Hanan, *The Chinese Vernacular Story* (Cambridge: Harvard University Press, 1981).

8. For a far more detailed introduction to these major Chinese novels, including numerous critical comparisons between Chinese and Western literature, see C. T. Hsia, *The Classic Chinese Novel* (New York: Columbia University Press, 1968). As will be clear to Hsia's readers, my assessment of these novels is deeply indebted to his work.

based on the dissolution of the Han Dynasty into three competing kingdoms after A.D. 220.[9] Although traditionally attributed to Lo Kuan-chung (1330–1400), the earliest extant version of *Romance of the Three Kingdoms* dates only from the early sixteenth century. It was probably compiled by a number of anonymous authors and editors over several generations. All the characters are historical, the general plot outline is based on historical fact, and the mode of narration is little different from that of official histories. The purpose of the work is also (ostensibly at least) the same as the historian's: to give meaning to the past through the preservation and presentation of a moral order in history.

The main characters in *Three Kingdoms* are heroic in stature. Three men, Liu Pei, Kuan Yü, and Chang Fei swear an oath of brotherhood at the beginning of the story, and much of the rest of the tale follows as a consequence of this act. This brotherhood celebrates the Confucian virtue that personal loyalty in a good cause assumes and even surpasses the force of blood ties. Liu Pei is the rightful heir of the Han throne; his chief foe is Ts'ao Ts'ao, a high Han official with his own dynastic ambitions. Ts'ao Ts'ao, perhaps the most famous "villain" in popular Chinese historiography, is one of Lo Kuan-chung's greatest triumphs in characterization. An ambitious man adept at manipulating Confucian symbols while violating Confucian virtue, Ts'ao Ts'ao is ruthless in his quest for fame and power. But he is also a sensitive poet and an impulsive man vulnerable to anxieties and violent swings of mood.

One of the chief virtues of Lo's *Three Kingdoms* is its level of complexity and irony in narrating the struggle for power in an era of dynastic collapse. With its vast canvas encompassing the length and breadth of China over a century of political and military turmoil, this novel shows the great generals and statesmen of that era as mortal men with very human passions (the chief ones being the desire for fame and power) and ultimately with little individual power to change the inexorable sweep of great historical events. The virtue of Liu Pei, in accord with orthodox Confucian theory, wins him loyal followers and retainers, but virtue alone is not enough to overcome bad decisions, bad strategy, and (perhaps) the workings of fate or Heaven.

Even more than in China's dynastic histories, *Three Kingdoms* reveals history to be a seamless web of closely interwoven factors. Morality and Heaven are important but no more so than courageous fighting, daring maneuvers, clever tactics, and sagacious strategies; and the ability of the evil general may even surpass that of the virtuous one in these areas.

9. English translations of this novel include C. H. Brewitt-Taylor, trans., *Romance of the Three Kingdoms,* 2 vols. (reprint, Rutland, Vt.: Tuttle, 1959), and an excellent one-volume abridgment by Moss Roberts, *Three Kingdoms: China's Epic Drama* (New York: Pantheon, 1977).

Blind luck and supernatural phenomena may occasionally intervene, but it is abundantly clear that treachery and deceit can at times pay handsome dividends. The only consolation seems to be that those short-term gains at the cost of virtue stand condemned forever in the cold and clear-eyed assessment of the chronicler.

Three Kingdoms approaches a tragic view of human life in its often pessimistic picture of dynastic collapse, but the view is ultimately too long-term and too morally confident to be defined as tragic. The assumption remains that human life goes on, and the narrator (and implicitly his audience) appreciates and affirms the good cause. The confident hope also remains, whatever the concrete evidence to the contrary, that the people will ultimately flock to support the virtuous ruler and allow him to re-establish a just order. It may take centuries, but China's experience is so long and the Chinese viewpoint so long-term that centuries of disorder, even a few in succession, are not enough to shake this confidence in the eventual return to virtue, peace, and harmony. In its complexity and irony, *Three Kingdoms* has given Chinese through the centuries a relatively sophisticated picture of politicomilitary history that is ultimately affirmative, even though focused on some of history's darker sides. The virtues and failings of its characters have also given the Chinese a rich short-hand vocabulary in the politics of intrigue, warfare, villainy, and statesmanship.

The next great novel in the Chinese tradition, *Water Margin* (*Shui-hu chuan,* also available in translations titled *All Men Are Brothers* and *Outlaws of the Marsh*)[10] also evolved over a long period and passed through the hands of numerous authors, editors, and compilers. *Water Margin* is the story of a band of outlaws, some of whom really existed, in the Northern Sung dynasty (1101–1125). But compared with *Three Kingdoms* it is far less rooted in historical events and far more indebted to the vernacular short story tradition. Its origins in the vernacular short story can be seen in its language, which is far more colloquial than that of *Three Kingdoms,* and in its style, which is far less dependent on historical narratives and

10. There are three complete English translations of this novel: J. H. Jackson, trans., *Water Margin,* 2 vols. (reprint, Boston: Cheng & Tsui, 1976); Pearl S. Buck, trans., *All Men Are Brothers,* 2 vols. (reprint, New York: Crowell, 1968); and Sidney Shapiro, trans., *Outlaws of the Marsh,* 2 vols. (Peking and Bloomington: Foreign Languages Press and Indiana University Press, 1981). The text of the *Water Margin* has had a messy history; countless different versions have been compiled and published by many different (usually anonymous) editors. Different versions have ranged from seventy to one hundred and twenty chapters. The shorter versions, especially a seventy-one-chapter edition published in the seventeenth century, have generally been more popular and critically praised than the longer versions. The Jackson and Buck translations are based on the popular seventy-one-chapter edition; the recent Shapiro translation is taken from an earlier one-hundred-chapter edition.

more indebted to the storyteller's conventions of stock phrases, poems, songs, and parallel prose interspersed throughout the narrative. In its theme *Water Margin* is also more potentially subversive than *Three Kingdoms* because its bandits are frequently the heroes of the story and government officials, right up to the emperor, are either ignored or portrayed as weak, misguided, venal, and corrupt.

In a sense *Water Margin* celebrates the virtues of righteousness, loyalty, and justice, which are quite respectable Confucian virtues. In Confucian terms the problem with the book is that these virtues seem to be the monopoly of outlaws, and they are often carried to such excess that they violate all sense of Confucian propriety and moderation. The impetuous righteousness of the heroes leads them to break the law and join the bandit brotherhood under the leadership of Sung Chiang in his mountain lair of Liang-shan-po (named for Mt. Liang and its marshy and conveniently inaccessible borders in Shantung province). Eventually, 108 of these heroes find their way to Liang-shan-po in a rambling series of discrete episodes (taking up much of the novel's one hundred chapters) that culminate when all the heroes celebrate a banquet on the mountain. From this high point the excitement tapers off as the heroes gradually disperse, die out, or surrender to the government.

There is a good deal of blood and gore in this novel, albeit in the name of justice and righteous vengeance. Some Chinese editors have attempted to impart the story with socially redeeming value by having the rebels finally surrender to the throne and begin to work for the state by turning their wrath on other presumably less virtuous rebels. *Water Margin* has frequently been condemned by modern critics for its brutality (the righteous rebels sometimes eat their defeated rivals), its misogyny (promiscuous women are brutally slain by the self-righteous and sexually puritanical bandits), and its gang morality (outlaws who join the Liang-shan group are often oppressed in turn by the strict but selective mores and social pressures of the outlaw band).

Andrew Plaks has recently argued that *Water Margin,* at least in one sixteenth-century version, is actually an ironic Neo-Confucian critique of its popular heroes; their brutality is exaggerated so as to undercut all the surface praise of their heroism.[11] Despite Plaks's ironic interpretation and despite the criticisms of other nonironic interpreters of the novel, *Water Margin* has always been a favorite of young Chinese readers who appreciate it for its vivid characterizations of brave exciting heroes who are larger than life, fun-loving, hard-drinking, loyal companions to the death. As a tale of adventure, it has been appreciated for its drama and not for its morality; in the service of excitement its brutality has been

11. Andrew H. Plaks, *The Four Masterworks of the Ming Novel* (Princeton: Princeton University Press, 1987), chap. 4.

accepted without many qualms. In a society where learning to read and write has been a tedious task inextricably bound up with submission to the authority of the past and to one's elders, *Water Margin* has afforded each new generation the vicarious thrill of rebellion and revenge.

The next great Chinese novel, *Journey to the West* (*Hsi-yu chi,* known as *Monkey* in Arthur Waley's abridged translation),[12] was also inspired by an actual historical event: the pilgrimage of Hsuan-tsang, a pious Buddhist monk, to India in the seventh century to bring important Buddhist scriptures back to China. Hsuan-tsang's courageous seventeen-year journey inspired many tales of adventure and religious devotion, particularly useful to Buddhist proselytizers in search of an audience. In the sixteenth century many of these popular stories and legends were woven together, perhaps (although we cannot say with certainty) by Wu Ch'eng-en, a witty poet and minor official. In any case, *Journey to the West* was first published in 1592, a decade after Wu's death.

In its form *Journey to the West* marks a significant advance in the Chinese novel. Far more than embellished history or loosely connected short stories, *Journey* is a coherent work of fantasy; it incorporates a far wider range of sources than its predecessors, and it also shows a much higher degree of control by an individual author. It is as interlaced with poetry as *Water Margin,* but most of the poetry in *Journey* is original and inventive, whereas *Water Margin* tends to rely heavily on popular songs, stock phrases, and preexisting poems that are little better than doggerel. The plot of *Journey* is also more unified than those of its predecessors. The personalities of its heroes (although not explored in great depth) are more consistent and complex than the generals and bandits of the more historical novels. Particularly striking is the comic interplay between the novel's main characters.

In *Journey* the serious moral story of a pious monk becomes intertwined with countless supernatural figures and fables and is transformed into a sprawling comic allegory full of gentle and humane satire. The vast stretches of desert and mountains in China's "wild west" had inspired a rich Chinese lore of monsters and perils, a lore deeply tapped by Wu Ch'eng-en. Hsuan-tsang is about the only "normal" human being in a world of gods, monsters, fallen angels, and wizards of all shapes and sizes; but unlike his historical model, the novelist's Hsuan-tsang is hopelessly incompetent and dull. He despairs over the slightest obstacle in his path and is successful in the end almost in spite of himself. The real heroes of *Journey* are Hsuan-tsang's assistants, protectors, and guides, Chu

12. Arthur Waley, trans., *Monkey* (New York: Grove Press, 1958), includes less than one-fourth of the entire novel, but it is remarkably true to the original spirit of the work. A masterful complete translation has recently been completed by Anthony C. Yu, trans., *Journey to the West,* 4 vols. (Chicago: University of Chicago Press, 1977–1984).

Pa-chieh and Sun Wu-k'ung, both "fallen angels" expelled from Heaven for misdeeds, and both trying (or at least willing to appear to try) to regain their heavenly status by assisting the poor lonely monk on his treacherous pilgrimage. Chu Pa-chieh is a pig (Pigsy in Arthur Waley's translation), embodying all the earthly appetites and inclinations associated with that animal. Sun Wu-k'ung (whose name, "Aware of Vacuity," ironically suggests enlightenment) is a magical monkey, as quick-witted, energetic, and anarchistic as Hsuan-tsang is slow, dull, and orderly.

Much of the comic content of this novel rests on the interplay of the hedonistic Pigsy, the irrepressible Monkey, and their "master," the helpless plodding monk. In the world of this journey all the gods, goddesses, demons, and devils who threaten the pilgrims are utterly self-seeking, lustful, petty, and corrupt; they mirror every imaginable human weakness. Hsuan-tsang finds his life or his purity constantly threatened; the female demons pose a particularly frightful threat for they believe having sexual intercourse with a human being will prolong their lives. The cumulative effect of the journey is to make of Hsuan-tsang a nervous wreck lacking the courage and imagination even to face each new day. Pigsy, utterly practical and unconcerned about purity, constantly looks out for the short run, ever hopeful of finding a good hot meal, a warm lover, and a soft bed.

Hsuan-tsang's timidity and Pigsy's laziness leave Monkey as the principal fighter and strategist against all comers. Fortunately, Monkey has innumerable powers of transformation, including the possession of a magical, toothpick-sized instrument that can be expanded into a great deadly cudgel when the need arises (giving Freudian interpreters much cause for fascination with "Monkey's rod"). Although Hsuan-tsang depends entirely on Monkey's powers for his own safety, Monkey's impulsive audacity poses threats of its own, for the little ape is so quick, so energetic, and so uninhibited that he is constantly on the verge of forgetting the religious purpose of the journey and seeking adventure purely for its own sake. What ultimately keeps Monkey in line is his slim metal headband controlled by Hsuan-tsang; the monk can tighten the band to produce such excruciating headaches that Monkey simply has to obey despite all his contrary instincts. The interplay of Hsuan-tsang, Pigsy, and Monkey is reminiscent of the dialogue between that great duo of Western literature, Don Quixote and Sancho Panza. Monkey's imagination and energy propel him beyond the wildest thoughts of Hsuan-tsang and Pigsy, yet their commonsense survival instincts are occasionally all that save Monkey from self-destruction.

Journey is a complex novel that can be read and enjoyed on many levels. Although technically a Buddhist novel on the quest for enlightenment, it pokes as much fun at Buddhism as at any other human institution. The entourage of the Buddha himself is as corrupt as any customs office in the underpaid Confucian bureaucracy. Yet for all its satiric barbs aimed at the Buddhists, the novel also lends itself to a Buddhist—or, more broadly, a Buddhist-Taoist-Confucian—allegorical interpretation. The journey of Hsuan-tsang and his companions is a religious quest, and each of the quest's participants faces a different kind of temptation. If Pigsy needs to overcome animal appetites and lust, Hsuan-tsang must try to conquer his own self-centered fears and anxieties, and Monkey has to learn the humility to accept limitations in his quest for power and knowledge. Through all the comedy and satire shine what we might call a Taoist amusement at human absurdities, a Buddhist critique of greed and materialism, and a Confucian appreciation for moderation in all things. In *Journey* Wu Ch'eng-en (and/or other anonymous authors) created a universal fable of human foibles in a unified work of inventive imagination, comic whimsy, and philosophical insight.

Another late-sixteenth-century work of a very different kind marks a similar advance in the art of the Chinese novel. *Chin P'ing Mei* (which is also translated under the title *The Golden Lotus*)[13] is the first great Chinese novel of morals and manners, a meticulously detailed portrait of the daily lives of a Chinese merchant, Hsi-men Ch'ing, and the many members of his household. Perhaps one should call *Chin P'ing Mei* the great Chinese novel of the absence of morals and (good) manners because it has long been recognized as one of the least inhibited works of erotic and pornographic literature in the relatively rich Chinese tradition.

As I noted earlier, didacticism has been one trademark of Chinese literature, and certainly many Chinese moralists (not to mention parents) have condemned *Chin P'ing Mei* for its most imaginative and unrelenting eroticism. However, the whole framework of the novel is a moral one; it shows the dire and unavoidable consequences of a life of sexual hedonism. What is more important in an artistic sense is the stark realism of the novel, which makes it a truly compelling multidimensional portrait of a rapidly changing, money- and status-crazed society.

Chin P'ing Mei is far more firmly rooted in everyday life than any of the other works thus far discussed. As Patrick Hanan astutely observes: "If one defines the novel as in some way concerned with depicting social change or conflict by the careful documentation of the texture of society, then the *Chin P'ing Mei* is the first true Chinese novel."[14] Not surpris-

13. This novel also exists in a one-volume abridgment, [Bernard Miall, trans.], *Chin P'ing Mei,* [translated from a German version by Franz Kuhn] (Toms River, N.J.: Capricorn, 1960), and a more complete but still abridged scholarly translation, Clement Egerton, trans., *The Golden Lotus,* 4 vols. (reprint, London: Routledge & Kegan Paul, 1972). A full new translation that will far surpass its predecessors is currently being undertaken by David Roy of the University of Chicago.

14. Hanan, "The Development of Fiction and Drama," 134. Hanan elaborates further on this theme in another essay, "A Landmark of the Chinese Novel," *University of Toronto Quarterly* 30, no. 3 (April 1961): 325–35.

ingly, this work appeared at the turn of the seventeenth century, a time of rapid economic expansion, the growth of cities, and the increased use of money. The seventeenth century was also a time of considerable philosophical ferment in China; the Confucian world was shaken by the growth of an iconoclastic, idealistic, and individualistic school of thought that attacked conservative orthodoxy; and the literary world witnessed similarly shocking changes as a movement sprang up to proclaim fiction as a valuable and worthwhile pursuit.

Such Western critics as Lionel Trilling and Ian Watt have noted the importance of economic growth, social mobility, and urbanization in the rise of the Western novel.[15] The anonymity of city life allows for the fascinating interaction of many different types of people; the decline of a stable rural society, together with the corresponding increase in social mobility (both upward and downward), provides authors with many new plot possibilities; the increasing pace of social and economic change gives authors and audiences alike a new and often intense fascination with questions of status, wealth, and power. Economic expansion and urbanization also stimulate the entertainment industry and the growth of publishing. In some ways these kinds of changes had already occurred in China in the Sung period (from the tenth century onward), but the sixteenth and seventeenth centuries marked an acceleration of long-term trends in economic growth and urbanization. The changes that occurred in the last century of the Ming dynasty (roughly 1540–1640) were as dramatic in literature and philosophy as in the economy and society. *Chin P'ing Mei,* with its unprecedented level of social realism, is in both form and content a vivid reminder of the rapid social and intellectual change that occurred in late Ming China.

The plot of *Chin P'ing Mei* is more unified and focused than any of China's earlier novels, even though the anonymous author seems deliberately to quote popular songs and to make references to other stories, dramas, and novels at every conceivable opportunity. As a result of such borrowing, the novel is a kind of encyclopedia of literary and dramatic quotation, an unprecedented eclectic creation that weaves disparate materials into a coherent story. *Chin P'ing Mei* is framed as a spin-off from the plot of the *Water Margin:* Wu Sung, one of the toughest heroes of Sung Chiang's band, avenges the murder of his brother by killing his brother's former wife and murderess, Pan Chin-lien (the Golden Lotus). But the incident involving Wu Sung is in fact only a tiny thread that appears at the beginning and the end of the *Chin P'ing Mei;* in between is a vast tapestry totally different from *Water Margin* in almost every way.

15. See, for example, Lionel Trilling, "Manners, Morals, and the Novel," in *The Liberal Imagination,* by Lionel Trilling (New York: Viking Press, 1951), and Ian Watt, *The Rise of the Novel* (Berkeley: University of California Press, 1972).

In some respects *Chin P'ing Mei* is a parody of *Water Margin*'s heroes. Like Sung Chiang, Hsi-men Ch'ing is also surrounded by a group of "sworn brothers," but in contrast to the courage and derring-do of the Liang-shan bandits, Hsi-men Ch'ing's entourage is made up entirely of weak ciphers, social-climbers, and hangers-on. There is nothing remotely heroic in this group. Hsi-men Ch'ing is not a malicious person, but he has his weaknesses: chief among them is an insatiable lust. Almost a tragicomic figure, Hsi-men Ch'ing is at the center of a whirlwind he cannot control. When he finally dies of sexual overexertion, his friends, who depended entirely on his largesse for their lives of ease and pleasure, are sorry chiefly for themselves. To express their deep respect, they jointly compose a eulogy for their benefactor that is notable primarily as a hymn of praise that describes him in unmistakably phallic terms.

Perhaps the most striking innovation of *Chin P'ing Mei* lies in its characterization of women. We might not think of an erotic and pornographic novel as the likeliest place to find psychological insights regarding women, but by focusing on domestic life in a well-to-do urban household the author of *Chin P'ing Mei* took a much closer look at the psychology of women than any earlier Chinese novelist. Hsi-men Ch'ing has six wives, all of them bound to serve him and, if possible, to produce strong, healthy male heirs. Their utter dependency on his favor produces a palpable air of lethal competition in the household, in large part because of the machinations of the fifth wife, Lotus (the same Golden Lotus Wu Sung eventually kills). As a former slave who has suffered much abuse, Lotus is driven by insecurity and insatiable desires for power and sexual pleasure. Because Lotus is a stronger personality than Hsi-men Ch'ing, he is unable to bring order to his household or to resist her manipulations even when his own interests are threatened. She finally drives him to sexual exhaustion and death in a chilling series of scenes where she keeps him sexually aroused with aphrodisiacs and ointments even after he falls into a coma.

Chin P'ing Mei contains some of the most sexually gruesome scenes in Chinese literature, but it also exhibits a great deal of lighter satire and comedy (often involving sex) before turning dark and ugly near the end of the work. Despite the heavy erotic and comic emphasis, however, the novel remains a serious work of literature that integrates its moral message convincingly into the fabric of the story. Buddhist reincarnation and moral retribution are central to the novel; the main sinners all come to a bad end, and eventually Hsi-men Ch'ing's son (who may or may not be his own reincarnated soul) becomes a monk in order to compensate for his father's misdeeds. The novel also lends itself to a Confucian interpretation: Hsi-men Ch'ing fails to cultivate virtue in his own person; failing that, he also fails to order his own household; and as a prominent merchant with good political connections, Hsi-men in his failure symbolizes a larger social and political failure in Ming China. By the end of the novel the entire state is near collapse, and the cause is clearly a moral one that ascends from the individual to the family to the bureaucracy and finally to the court. The eclectic author of *Chin P'ing Mei* assumes a compatibility between Buddhist and Confucian messages and an inseparable bond linking the individual, the society, and the state.[16]

In a tour de force of literary historical scholarship Andrew Plaks has analyzed the four novels discussed so far as serious works of Neo-Confucian commentary on sixteenth-century Chinese society. Drawing on all available critical scholarship in Chinese, Japanese, and Western languages, Plaks interprets these works with special attention to their sixteenth-century editors, authors, and commentators. He notes the many structural features the works have in common, including "their paradigmatic length of one hundred chapters [with one exception], narrative rhythms based on division into ten-chapter units, further subdivision into building blocks of three- or four-chapter episodes, contrived symmetries between the first and second halves of the texts, special exploitation of opening and closing sections, as well as certain other schemes of spatial and temporal ordering, notably the plotting of events on seasonal or geographical grids."[17]

In contrast to the earlier emphasis in much scholarship on the origins of these novels in popular storytelling, Plaks demonstrates how the sophisticated and highly literate authors and compilers of these works manipulated the conventions of popular storytelling in a variety of subtle ways so as to assume an ironic stance toward the surface meaning of the texts. Thus, *Three Kingdoms* contrasts the ideal of dynastic order with the realities of dynastic collapse and disorder; *Water Margin* deflates the heroic myths and stereotypes of the popular tradition; *Journey to the West,* in more comic ways, undercuts the proclaimed high seriousness of the religious quest; and *Chin P'ing Mei,* most clearly of all, satirizes the moral bankruptcy of society by juxtaposing pedestrian proclamations of conventional piety with the grossest immoral behavior.[18]

Plaks may not win universal assent on all points, but he has raised the level of criticism of the traditional Chinese novel to new heights of sophistication. His emphasis on the progressive development of irony is particularly useful and illuminating for my purposes in this discussion because irony reached its fullest development in the Chinese tradition in

16. An illuminating study of *Chin P'ing Mei* that highlights the Confucian interpretation of the novel is Katherine Carlitz, *The Rhetoric of "Chin p'ing mei"* (Bloomington: Indiana University Press, 1986).

17. Plaks, *Four Masterworks of the Ming Novel,* 497–98.

18. Plaks summarizes his closely reasoned book-length argument in *Four Masterworks of the Ming Novel,* chap. 6.

the two great works of the eighteenth century, *The Scholars* and *Dream of the Red Chamber.*

The Scholars was written nearly two centuries after *Chin P'ing Mei* and one full century after the tumultuous collapse of the Ming dynasty and the conquest of China by the Manchus.[19] A satirical novel above all else, *The Scholars* resembles *Chin P'ing Mei* in its focus on ordinary people and everyday life, its didactic assumptions, and its obsession with questions of money and status, but it differs from that erotic novel in most other ways. The author of *The Scholars,* Wu Ching-tzu (1701–1754), focuses not on the bedroom but rather on the public aspects of urban life, particularly the life of the literati class. Wu Ching-tzu borrowed jokes, anecdotes, and subplots from a variety of sources, but his borrowing was far less extensive than that of any earlier Chinese novelist. Poems and stock storyteller phrases still appear at chapter breaks in *The Scholars,* but they no longer bear much burden in carrying the story along. Instead, a relatively objective narrator sets scenes in which the characters reveal themselves entirely through their own words and deeds. Wu Ching-tzu's vernacular prose description and his heavy incorporation of autobiographical experience into the fabric of his work were major developments in the Chinese narrative tradition.

The Chinese title of this work is *Ju-lin wai-shih* (An informal history of the literati). *Ju-lin,* literally, "forest of Confucian scholars," was a category of orthodox Confucian historiography. The *ju-lin* section of official histories (following the example of the great Han historian, Ssu-ma Ch'ien) consisted of biographies of important scholars. *Wai-shih,* "outer history," denotes an informal history (often including gossip and hearsay) as opposed to the orthodox *cheng-shih,* or official history. Whereas the orthodox Chinese historian emphasizes the major events, offices, honors, and accomplishments of the great and near-great (as well as the evil deeds of great villains), Wu Ching-tzu in his informal history concentrates on the daily lives, the petty cares and concerns, and the pretensions and posturings of the literate and semiliterate aspirants to elite status.

In Wu Ching-tzu's novel, status is the most important thing in existence; it is a tangible commodity avidly sought through success in the civil service examinations and readily bought, sold, traded, or stolen in many ways. The biographies in *The Scholars* amount to a veritable catalogue of status-seekers. Examination success is of course the first and most assured route to high status, but failing that, one can ingratiate oneself with those who have won examination degrees, marry one's children into prominent families, impersonate famous poets and scholars,

19. Wu Ching-tzu, *The Scholars,* trans. Hsien-yi Yang and Gladys Yang (Peking: Foreign Languages Press, 1957).

or edit and publish selections of "successful" or "model" essays for the preparation of examination candidates. If one finds these strategies too demeaning, as Wu Ching-tzu himself clearly did, one could adopt the opposite position of the proud eccentric, hold in contempt all examination candidates and their feeble examination essays, sponsor poetry outings and drama contests with one's like-minded friends, lavish money on all "good causes" that come along, and generally thumb one's nose at the establishment. The middle part of *The Scholars* describes one such proud eccentric, Tu Shao-ch'ing (a self-portrait of Wu), who adopts this latter strategy so enthusiastically that he squanders his rather substantial family inheritance.

The satire of *The Scholars* is somewhat uneven and alternately mixed with slapstick comedy and heavy-handed invective. The plot is a loose and rambling affair that seems particularly unfocused in the last third of the story. Yet this work has long been cherished by Chinese readers for the purity of its vernacular prose, for its distinctive and self-assured authorial personality, and for its vivid gallery of unforgettable social types from the hurly-burly of an increasingly urban society "on the make" in eighteenth-century China. A civilization as old as China's invites, almost requires, a burdensome pedantry in its intellectuals, and Wu Ching-tzu provides a delightful pin prick in the balloon of intellectual pomposity. As China's first long work of sustained social satire, *The Scholars* has continued to inspire Chinese writers into the nineteenth and twentieth centuries.[20]

The greatest Chinese novel, all agree, is Ts'ao Hsueh-ch'in's *Dream of the Red Chamber* (*Hung-lou meng*), also known as *The Story of the Stone*.[21] First published in 1792, *Dream of the Red Chamber* is unparalleled by any other Chinese novel in its psychological depth, philosophical ambition, and multilayered complexity. Unfinished at the time of Ts'ao Hsueh-ch'in's death, *Dream of the Red Chamber* has provoked more textual and interpretive controversies than all other traditional Chinese novels combined. In the twentieth century research on this work has grown into a virtual industry called "Red Studies" (*hung-hsueh*) in which hundreds of

20. For a useful study of Wu Ching-tzu's satirical art see Timothy C. Wong, *Wu Ching-tzu* (Boston: Twayne, 1978). Social criticism in *The Scholars* is the subject of Paul S. Ropp, *Dissent in Early Modern China: "Ju-lin wai-shih" and Ch'ing Social Criticism* (Ann Arbor: University of Michigan Press, 1981).

21. The most elegant translation of Ts'ao Hsueh-ch'in's novel is David Hawkes and John Minford, trans., *The Story of the Stone,* 5 vols. (Harmondsworth: Penguin, 1973–1986). Another complete recent translation is Hsien-yi Yang and Gladys Yang, trans., *A Dream of Red Mansions,* 3 vols. (Peking: Foreign Languages Press, 1978–1980). The best one-volume abridgment is Florence McHugh and Isabel McHugh, trans., *Dream of the Red Chamber* (reprint, Westport, Conn.: Greenwood Press, 1975). A shorter one-volume abridgment is Chi-chen Wang, trans., *Dream of the Red Chamber* (New York: Anchor, 1958).

scholars and students have tried to resolve questions concerning its authorship, early commentators, different editions and manuscripts, and hidden meanings. The novel has been proclaimed, among other things, an autobiographical confession, a tragic triangular love story, an apolitical Buddhist allegory, an elaborate anti-Manchu tract in disguise, an encyclopedic summation of Chinese civilization, and a revolutionary attack on a decadent feudal culture.

The complexity of *Dream of the Red Chamber* begins with its language. The work is full of homonyms and homophones with double and triple meanings. The surname of the main family is Chia, a pun on "false"; there is also a Chen (which sounds like the Chinese word for "real") family that mirrors the Chia family in all details. The novelist delights in foreshadowing events and dropping everywhere hints of predestination and reincarnation. There is a running dialogue through 120 chapters on the alternation and confusion between illusion and reality. The possibilities for allegorical readings are almost endless, and the messy textual history of the novel insures against any one interpretation ever becoming definitive.

On one level *Dream of the Red Chamber* is a Buddhist work on the theme of the illusory and transitory nature of the material world. A stone, literally a discarded piece of Heaven, is curious about the human world of the "red dust" (Buddhism's term for the illusory world of material things and human attachments and entanglements) and so is incarnated in the human form of Chia Pao-yü, the young protagonist of the novel, whose name means Precious Jade to signify the magical piece of jade found in his mouth at birth. Pao-yü is plunged into this world of human attachments to experience all its suffering so that he may eventually attain enlightenment and detachment from the material and psychological world of the "red dust." As the stone is disillusioned, the whole story of its astonishing experience is carved out on the very piece of jade originally found in Pao-yü's mouth. The story of the stone is also the story on the stone.

On another level *Dream of the Red Chamber* is an exciting human story of a large complex family on the decline. The Chia family is prominent: a daughter serves as an imperial concubine, and the father is a respected official. Yet the future of the family is in doubt because none of the young males is responsible or capable. Befitting its high status, the family must keep up appearances—weddings and funerals, for example, must be lavish—but ample funds for such elaborate displays have long ago disappeared. As the family slips into financial trouble it also gradually loses favor at court. Eventually, the family's property is confiscated, its once-high position is destroyed, and the novel ends on a despairing note of disillusionment. Downward social mobility is a common theme in Chinese fiction, but nowhere else in the Chinese novel is its psychological pain spelled out in such vivid detail.

The main narrative of *Dream of the Red Chamber* focuses on the young people of the Chia family, particularly the youngest son, Chia Pao-yü, his maids, and his female relatives (sisters, cousins, aunts, mother, and grandmother). Pao-yü, patterned at least in part after Ts'ao Hsueh-ch'in himself, is a thoroughly irresponsible young man. He cares nothing for appearances (except in girls' faces and clothes), nor for success, fame, orthodoxy, respectability, or work. In these traits he is the exact opposite of his father, who cares precisely and exclusively for these things. Pao-yü is usually protected from his father's wrath by his mother and especially his grandmother, a fun-loving and compassionate old lady who is unspoiled by the artificiality of aristocratic and official life.

As a pampered young aristocrat, Chia Pao-yü lives in a magnificent garden compound along with several female cousins and their many solicitous serving maids. In intimate daily contact they enjoy feasts of the richest food, dramatic performances, parties, wine, and poetry-writing games and contests. Pao-yü is a sensitive friend of all the young women in the household. He prefers the company of girls over boys, but to the puzzlement (or disbelief) of his elders, he seems relatively indifferent to female sexual enticements. Except for a few elegant young men who excite him, all other males in the story appear to be vulgar bores to Pao-yü. Most of Pao-yü's male cousins seem obsessed with sex, an obsession he finds both strange and disgusting.

The novel's most popular subplot revolves around the important question of Pao-yü's marriage. He loves his beautiful hypersensitive cousin Lin Tai-yü above all others. Her name means Black Jade, after her own jade locket that matches Pao-yü's jade piece. In addition to their common stones these two share artistic temperaments that love true beauty and detest shallow superficiality in all forms and guises. Unfortunately, Tai-yü is too frail and neurotic to be judged an acceptable mate by the senior women in the Chia household. They conspire instead to arrange Pao-yü's marriage to another beautiful cousin, Hsueh Pao-ch'ai, who is much more conventional, sane, and healthy than the increasingly ill Tai-yü. As the marriage takes place, Tai-yü dies a pitiful death, feeling abandoned by Pao-yü and everyone else.

One of the many titles this novel has been given in its various stages is *The Twelve Beauties of Chin-ling,* after twelve of the main young women in the Chia household (located in Chin-ling, or Nanking). One by one these women come to a tragic end: maids and mistresses alike are forcibly married to undesirable mates; several take refuge in Buddhist nunneries; some are cruelly expelled from the idyllic life of the garden; others commit suicide in protest against unjust accusations of wrongdoing; and several die painful deaths as much from psychological as physical causes.

For all his sympathy for these women, Pao-yü is weak and incapable of doing anything to help them avoid their painful fates. The novel is especially revealing in its portrait of family dynamics and the psychological development of the Chia women. Details of dress, gestures, makeup, tone of voice, dreams, intimate conversations, and confessions are all used most effectively in creating vivid portraits of individual personalities. *Dream of the Red Chamber* is unique in the Chinese tradition in its apparent obsession with individual feelings and the smallest details of daily life.

By the end of the novel Pao-yü, who earlier detested all thought of examination competition, relents, studies, and passes the all-important examination that will admit him to the elite status of officialdom. But instead of returning home to enjoy his moment of glory as the savior of the Chia family, he abandons his wife and infant son and disappears with the Buddhist priest and Taoist monk who have wandered in and out of the story from the beginning proclaiming the vanity of the world of the red dust and the virtue of detachment and withdrawal.

The intense contradiction at the heart of *Dream of the Red Chamber,* between human passion and Buddhist detachment, is thus ultimately resolved in favor of enlightenment and withdrawal. Or is it? Ironically, this novel, which proclaims the illusory nature of the world of the red dust, has recreated that world so lovingly and artfully that it gives that world the permanence in art that it lacked in the painful experience of Ts'ao Hsueh-ch'in and his family. For all its proclamations of Buddhist meanings, this work remains the sharpest example of social realism in the Chinese tradition. No other Chinese novel creates such an entire world so believably. The real allegiance of Ts'ao in the final analysis would seem to be not to Confucian familial responsibility or Buddhist-Taoist detachment but to the truth of the novelist's art and to the magic of storytelling.[22]

The classic Chinese novel reached its apogee with *Dream of the Red Chamber* but did not end there. In the early nineteenth century two works in particular deserve mention: *Six Chapters of a Floating Life,* by Shen Fu, and *Flowers in the Mirror,* by Li Ju-chen.[23] *Six Chapters* (of which only four chapters survive) is more an autobiography than a novel, but its casual, simple, and straightforward style, its intensity of feeling, and

22. Two fine literary studies of *Dream of the Red Chamber* are Lucien Miller, *Masks of Fiction in "Dream of the Red Chamber": Myth, Mimesis, and Persona* (Tucson: University of Arizona Press, 1975), and Andrew H. Plaks, *Archetype and Allegory in "Dream of the Red Chamber"* (Princeton: Princeton University Press, 1976).

23. The most recent and accurate translation of Shen Fu's work is Leonard Pratt, trans., *Six Records of a Floating Life* (Harmondsworth: Penguin, 1983). An effective abridged translation of *Flowers in the Mirror* is by Dai-yi Lin (Berkeley: University of California Press, 1965).

its intimate description of married love make it a minor landmark in the Chinese narrative tradition. *Flowers in the Mirror* is a mixture of fantasy and satire that marks the culmination of the traditional scholarly Chinese novel. It is most famous in the modern West as a work sympathetic to women; a few of its chapters portray a Kingdom of Women where traditional Chinese sex roles are completely reversed, with predictable consequences for the male Chinese travelers who visit there hoping to make their fortune selling cosmetics. *Flowers in the Mirror* is a gentle satire of all kinds of human quirks and shortcomings and a clever vehicle for Li Ju-chen to show off his esoteric knowledge of everything from table games and poetry to phonetics and etymology. It combines the air of fantasy of *Journey to the West* and the social commentary of *The Scholars.*

Six Chapters of a Floating Life and *Flowers in the Mirror* are charming if minor works, and they mark a logical conclusion to this survey of traditional Chinese fiction. The genre of the Chinese novel seems in its conclusion to imitate the internal architecture of the novel itself. *Dream of the Red Chamber* marks the climax of the tradition, and the two later works form a kind of afterglow, a quiet and final recycling of earlier themes in a less ambitious and slightly minor key. When more Chinese novels were written in the late nineteenth century, followed by still more in the twentieth, they had begun to absorb Western influences.

As I noted earlier, the development of the Chinese novel offers many illuminating contrasts and parallels with the Western novel. In China, as in the West, from the sixteenth century to the nineteenth century the novel came to be recognized by some as a serious intellectual endeavor capable of addressing and illuminating the most important social, political, and philosophical issues of an entire civilization. Drawing on the tradition of classical commentaries, Chinese fiction critics and editors wrote detailed chapter-by-chapter or even line-by-line commentaries on all the major novels. They analyzed these works from many different perspectives including narrative structure and composition, style and pacing, artistic and philosophical strengths and weaknesses, and the relationship of each work to the major intellectual traditions of Confucianism, Buddhism, and Taoism. Although these commentators remained something of a minority within the Chinese intellectual elite, they articulated a kind of poetics of the novel that can be extremely valuable to the modern student hoping to understand these works and their original authors on their own terms.[24] The traditional Chinese commentators remained less secure and more defensive than their Western contemporaries in proclaiming the legitimacy of fiction, but their efforts clearly parallel

24. For an introduction to these traditional Chinese commentators, with full translations of important commentaries on the six "classic novels," see David L. Rolston, ed., *How to Read the Chinese Novel* (Princeton: Princeton University Press, 1989).

Western developments in the growing intellectual respectability of prose fiction.

One of the most striking differences between the novel in China and the West lies in the absence in China of anything approaching the great explosion of works of genius in the nineteenth-century West. There were notable works written in nineteenth-century China, but nothing to compare with the amazing production of the Western greats: Austen, Thackeray, Dickens, the Brontës, Eliot, and Hardy in England; Stendhal, Balzac, Dumas, Hugo, Sand, Baudelaire, and Zola in France; Gogol, Turgenev, Dostoevsky, and Tolstoy in Russia; Hawthorne, Melville, Twain, and James in the United States. The list could be longer, but one has only to hear the Western novelists' names to realize the enormous contrast with nineteenth-century China.

Instead of the geometrical growth of great works as the novel matured, the Chinese tradition seemed to leapfrog along at a leisurely pace, producing a couple of great novels every other century. Despite a far less spectacular flowering, however, in a rough way the changes in these two-century leaps parallel the Western experience: with increasing narrative sophistication came a deepening sense of irony toward society's mainstream values, a gradual decline in mythic and supernatural elements, and a corresponding increase in reliance on individual authorial experience and creativity.

What does not occur in China is an artistic declaration of independence or autonomy for literature. In one of the classics of Western literary criticism, *The Mirror and the Lamp,* M. H. Abrams sees in Western romanticism of the early nineteenth century a radical break with the previous two thousand years of Western critical thought. Whereas the Western poet had earlier been identified with the image of the mirror, passively reflecting external objects, the romantic movement identified the poet with the image of a lamp, an active illuminator that shines on reality and thus transforms it literally into something new. In the nineteenth-century Western romantic view the individual author thus assumed a role of tremendous power and importance. Although dealing explicitly with poetry rather than fiction, Abrams draws attention to the kind of revolutionary changes that occurred in European literary traditions only as recently as the nineteenth century.[25]

In China, by contrast, the novelist remained as much a peripheral figure in the nineteenth century as in the sixteenth. Despite the minority movement extolling the importance of fiction in the sixteenth century, the Chinese novelist was not prominent, powerful, or influential until the twentieth century, and even then prominence more often brought

25. M. H. Abrams, *The Mirror and the Lamp: Romantic Theory and the Critical Tradition* (Oxford: Oxford University Press, 1953).

persecution than power. Of the six major novels I discuss, only the last two—*The Scholars* and *Dream of the Red Chamber*—have clearly identifiable individual authors, and their identity was not known with certainty until the 1920s. In some ways Wu Ching-tzu and Ts'ao Hsueh-ch'in fit the stereotype of the modern Western alienated artist, but even in alienation the modern Western artist has had a powerful sense of importance, of widely shared artistic traditions and assumptions, and of artistic autonomy from political and economic forces. The traditional Chinese novelist did not enjoy such a sense of importance and autonomy. In the light of this difference the accomplishments of the Chinese novelists from the sixteenth to the nineteenth centuries are more striking than their shortcomings: their works are among the most accessible, enjoyable, illuminating, and inspiring documents from China's late imperial era.

APPENDIX 1

□

Maps

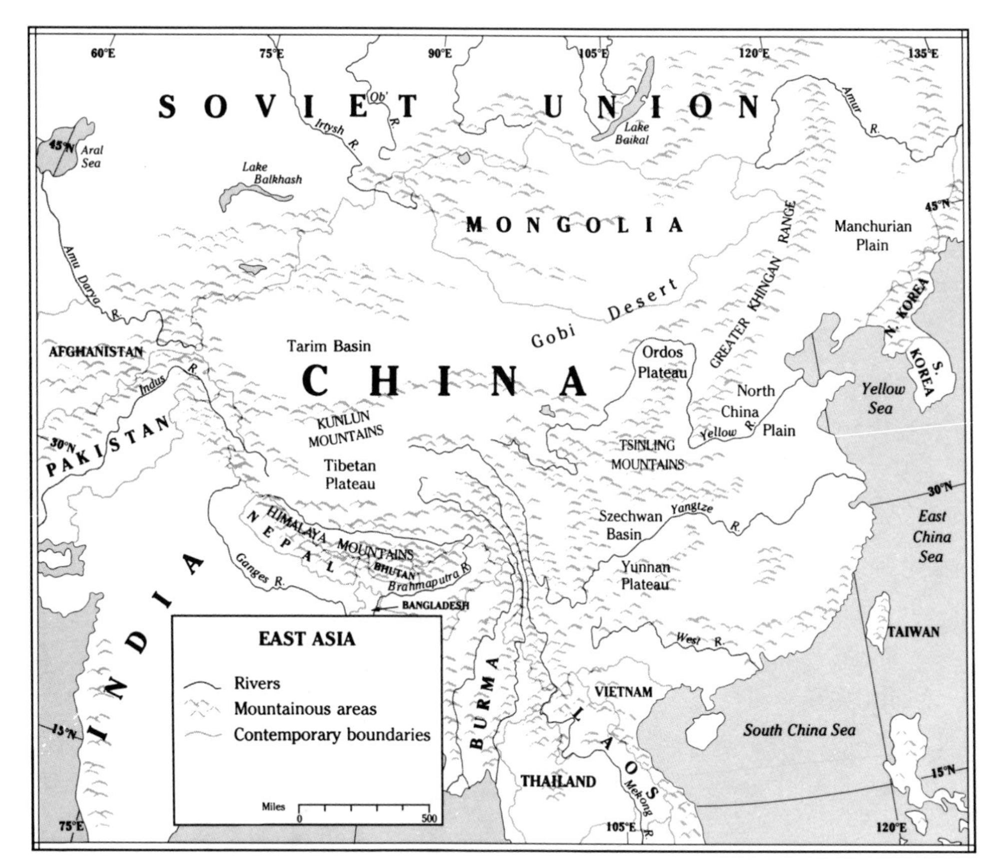

Map 1. The topography of East Asia.

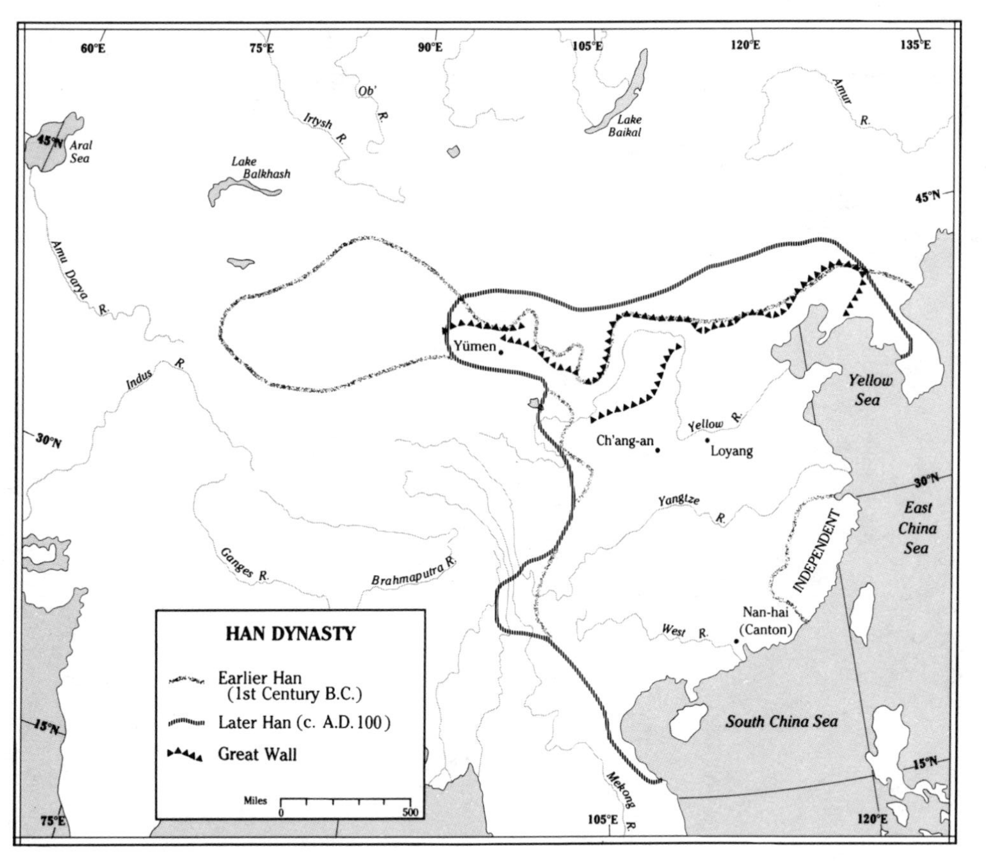

Map 2. Boundaries of the Han dynasty.

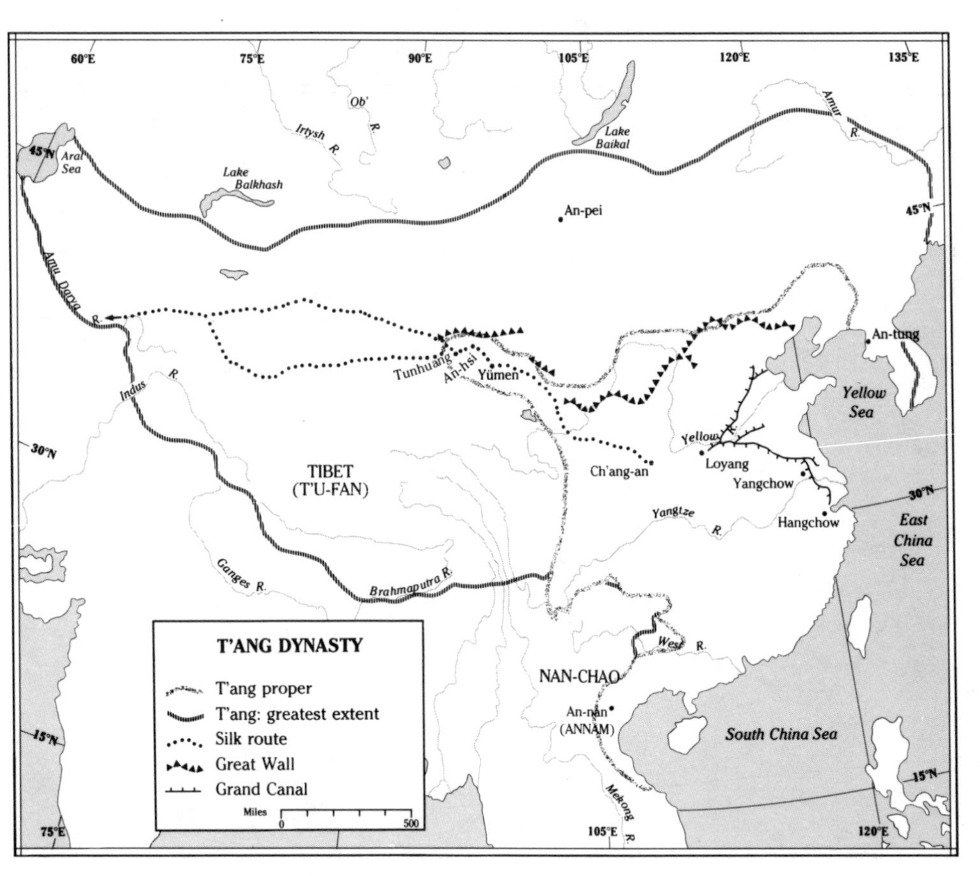

Map 3. Boundaries of the T'ang dynasty.

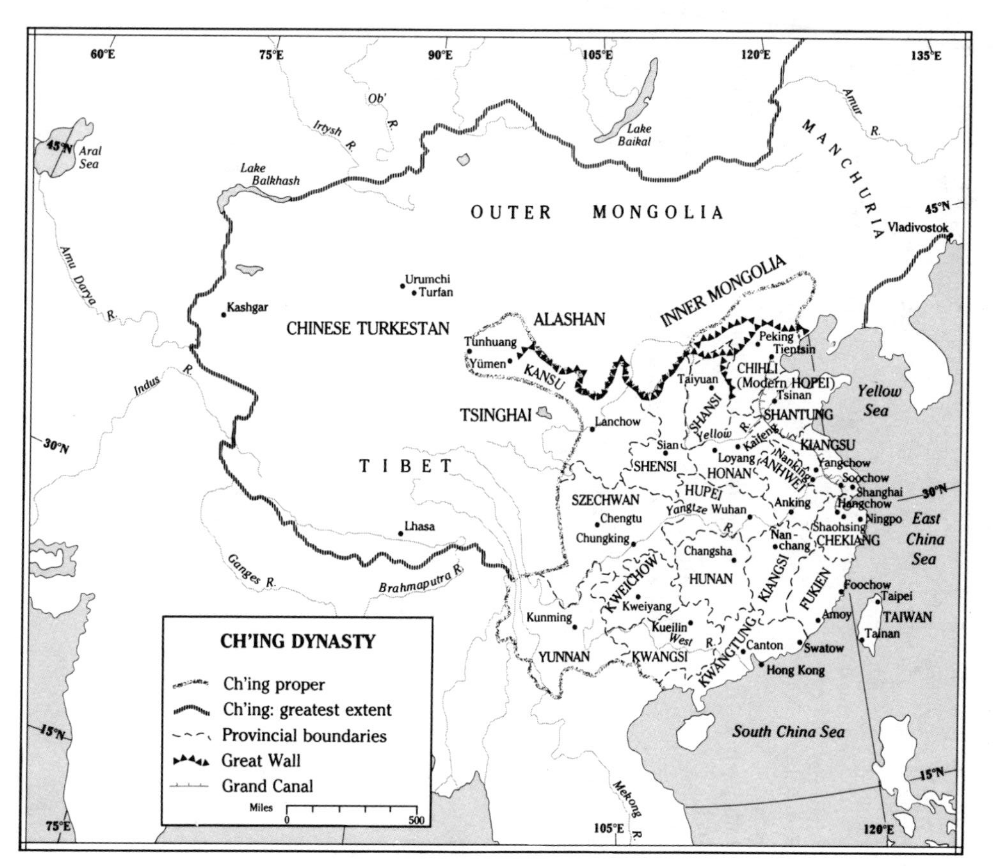

Map 4. Boundaries of the Ch'ing dynasty.

SOURCES CONSULTED IN PREPARING THE MAPS

Central Intelligence Agency. "China," Map number 800029 (545114). Washington, D.C.: Central Intelligence Agency, 1984.

———. "Soviet Union, East and South Asia, 1:46,000,000." Washington, D.C.: Central Intelligence Agency, 1987.

Fairbank, John K., Edwin O. Reischauer, and Albert M. Craig. *East Asia: Tradition and Transformation.* Boston: Houghton Mifflin, 1973.

Hermann, Albert. *An Historical Atlas of China.* Rev. ed. Edited by Norton Ginsburg. Chicago: Aldine, 1966.

Hsieh, Chiao-min. *Atlas of China.* Edited by Christopher L. Salter. New York: McGraw-Hill, 1973.

Hucker, Charles O. *China's Imperial Past.* Stanford: Stanford University Press, 1975.

Meskill, John T. *An Introduction to Chinese Civilization.* Lexington, Mass.: Heath, 1973.

New York Times. *The Times Atlas of China.* New York: Times Books, 1974.

Rand McNally. *Rand McNally Atlas of World History.* New York: Rand McNally, 1987.

Schirokauer, Conrad. *A Brief History of Chinese and Japanese Civilizations.* New York: Harcourt Brace Jovanovich, 1978.

APPENDIX 2

□

A Brief Chronology of Chinese History

ca. 5000–ca. 2000 B.C.	A variety of Neolithic cultures appear in north, central, and south China. Primitive agriculture, stone tools, and increasingly elegant pottery. Age of mythical sage emperors Yao, Shun, and Yü.
ca. 2205–ca. 1766 B.C.	*Hsia dynasty* (unverified).
ca. 1766–ca. 1045? B.C.	*Shang dynasty:* Earliest documented civilization. Hereditary monarchy, divination, earliest writing and bronze technology.
1045–256 B.C.	*Chou dynasty:* Patrimonial-bureaucratic government, formation of basic social and political ideals.
1122–771 B.C.	*Western Chou:* Relatively stable and strong Chou dynasty, the "Golden Age."
770–256 B.C.	*Eastern Chou:*
770–481 B.C.	Spring and Autumn period: Steady decline of Chou power and authority. Emergence of independent kingdoms.
403–221 B.C.	Warring States period: Development of iron weapons, crossbow, and cavalry in warfare. Total collapse of Chou power and authority.
551–479 B.C.	Confucius (K'ung Fu-tzu).
371–289 B.C.	Mencius (Meng Tzu).
369–286 B.C.	Chuang Tzu (traditional dates).
298–238 B.C.	Hsun Tzu.
ca. 280–233 B.C.	Han Fei Tzu.

221–206 B.C.	*Ch'in dynasty:* Ch'in state eliminates rival states, abolishes hereditary ranks, and unifies under direct imperial rule.
221–210 B.C.	Reign of Ch'in Shih Huang-ti (First Emperor of Ch'in).
215–214 B.C.	Earlier fortifications linked to form the Great Wall.
213 B.C.	Confucian classics burned and their private circulation banned.
209–206 B.C.	Ch'in collapse and civil war.
206 B.C.	Han dynasty established by Liu Pang (Han Kao-tsu).
206 B.C.–A.D. 220	*Han dynasty:* Formative Chinese dynasty. Legalist-inspired political institutions modified and rationalized with Confucian doctrines. Pre-Han aristocracy not restored, but powerful landed families begin to rise, especially in Later Han. The Han is noted for great historical writing, *fu* (rhyme-prose), Confucian thought, bronze mirrors and horses, clay figurines, and silk paintings.
206 B.C.–A.D. 9	Western or Former Han dynasty (capital at Ch'ang-an).
ca. 179 B.C.–ca. 104 B.C.	Tung Chung-shu, Han Confucian synthesizer.
141–87 B.C.	Reign of Emperor Wu (Han Wu-ti): Expands Han boundaries into central Asia; establishes Confucianism as state orthodoxy.
145–90 B.C.	Ssu-ma Ch'ien, author of *Shi-chi* (*Records of the Grand Historian*), which set standard for China's "dynastic histories."
A.D. 9–23	Wang Mang usurps throne and establishes short-lived Hsin dynasty.
25–220	Eastern or Later Han dynasty (capital at Loyang).
65	First documented case of Buddhism in China.
ca. 105	Paper invented.
184	Yellow Turban uprising in eastern China.
184–215	Five Pecks of Rice Rebellion in Szechwan.
220–589	*Era of division:* Several weak regimes in the south; domination by a succession of

non-Han rulers in the north. Steady rise of landed aristocratic families. Rapid growth of Buddhist and Taoist religions. Beginnings of landscape painting, Buddhist sculpture and grotto paintings.

220–285 *Three Kingdoms era* (Han, Wei, and Wu).

265–420 *Chin dynasty* (in south only after 316).

317–589 *Northern and southern dynasties*

386–534 *Northern Wei (T'o-pa Wei) dynasty:* Pacifies north China under strong central rule.

581–618 *Sui dynasty:* Military and political reunification of north and south China (Grand Canal connects north and south, ca. 610).

618 T'ang dynasty founded by Li Yuan (T'ang Kao-tsu)

618–907 *T'ang dynasty:* Strong, expansive, and cosmopolitan dynasty. Society and upper levels of government dominated by a few powerful landed aristocratic families. Great age of poetry, Buddhism, and beginnings of Confucian revival. Beginnings of great porcelain and landscape painting traditions, gold and silverworks, and silk stuffs.

626–649 Reign of Li Shih-min (T'ang T'ai-tsung): Era of military expansion, effective government, and intellectual eclecticism.

684–705 Empress Wu proclaims short-lived Chou dynasty (only female to assume direct control of throne in Chinese history).

ca. 700–850 "Great age of poetry": Wang Wei (d. 759), Li Po (d. 762), Tu Fu (d. 770), Han Yü (d. 824), Po Chü-i (d. 846).

713–756 Reign of T'ang Hsuan-tsung: Era of cultural brilliance and political ineptitude, ends in rebellion.

755–763 Rebellion of General An Lu-shan (leading to weakening of T'ang rule).

ca. 840–846 Suppression of Buddhism under Emperor Wu-tsung.

874–884 Huang Ch'ao Rebellion.

907 T'ang rule collapses.

907–960 *North-south division:* Five Dynasties in north; Ten Kingdoms in south.

916–1125	Liao Empire dominates Manchuria, Mongolia, and most of northern border areas.
960	Chao K'uang-yin (Sung T'ai-tsu) founds Sung dynasty.
960–1279	*Sung dynasty:* T'ang-style closed aristocratic elite disappears. Beginning of the social, economic, political, and cultural trends of "late imperial China": Maturation of civil service examination system and Confucian scholar-official government. Elite status becomes more dependent on education, examination success, and official government service, giving rise to the "literati ideal" of the refined gentleman-scholar. Era of commercial expansion and urbanization, spread of printing and foot-binding, growth of vernacular literature, great age of landscape painting, monochrome porcelain. Neo-Confucian revival.
960–1127	*Northern Sung dynasty* (capital at Kaifeng).
ca. 1000–1200	Rise of Neo-Confucianism: Fan Chung-yen (d. 1052), Chou Tun-i (d. 1073), Shao Yung (d. 1077), Chang Tsai (d. 1077), Ch'eng Hao (d. 1085), Ch'eng I (d. 1107), and Chu Hsi (d. 1200).
1012	First large-scale use of early-ripening rice.
1065	Civil service examinations fully institutionalized.
1069–1076	Wang An-shih as chief councillor implements reforms to strengthen central government.
1076	Wang An-shih resigns; policies reversed by conservatives Ssu-ma Kuang (d. 1086) and Su Tung-p'o (d. 1101).
1115–1234	Chin dynasty established in Manchuria and north China by Jurchen tribes.
1125–1127	Sung capital of Kaifeng falls to the Chin.
1127–1279	*Southern Sung dynasty* (capital at Hangchow).
1167–1227	Genghis Khan unifies Mongols and conquers most of Asia.
1234	Fall of Chin dynasty and establishment of Mongol power in north China.

1260	Khubilai becomes Great Khan of the Mongols.
1272–1368	*Yuan dynasty:* Mongol rule of China. Era noted for development of drama and continuity of Chinese cultural traditions.
1272–1279	Mongol conquest of south China.
1275–1291	Marco Polo serves in Khubilai's court.
1279	Last Sung emperor commits suicide.
1351–1368	Red Turban Rebellion.
1368	Chu Yuan-chang (Ming T'ai-tsu) founds Ming dynasty (with capital at Nanking; permanently moved to Peking in 1421).
1368–1644	*Ming dynasty:* Chinese control reestablished; maturation of authoritarian bureaucratized monarchy; further development of Neo-Confucianism. Noted for development of extended vernacular prose fiction (the "novel"), blue and white polychrome porcelain, and further development of poetic and painting traditions.
ca. 1400	Early versions of *Romance of the Three Kingdoms* and *Water Margin* first published.
1404–1433	Under court sponsorship the eunuch Cheng Ho (1371–1433) leads seven maritime expeditions to the Indian Ocean.
1472–1529	Wang Yang-ming, founder of the idealistic "learning of the mind" school of Neo-Confucianism.
ca. 1570–1600	First publications of *Journey to the West* and *Chin P'ing Mei.*
1559–1643	Nurhaci (1559–1626) and Abahai (1592–1643) establish Manchu state in northeast.
1582–1610	Jesuit missionary Matteo Ricci lives in China, eventually residing in Peking (1600–1610) with imperial sponsorship.
1620–1647	Peasant rebellions destroy Ming dynasty.
1644	Manchus conquer China and establish Ch'ing dynasty.
1644–1911	*Ch'ing dynasty:* Continuation of Ming culture and institutions. Further strengthening of monarchy; steady economic growth, commercial development and

	population expansion; era of "evidential scholarship," literary inquisition, and compilation of encyclopedias; further development of prose fiction, poetry, and painting.
1662–1796	"High Ch'ing": Three great emperors—K'ang-hsi (r. 1662–1722), Yung-cheng (r. 1723–1735), and Ch'ien-lung (r. 1736–1796)—preside over extended period of peace, prosperity, and stability.
ca. 1750	Satirical novel *The Scholars* completed.
1774–1789	Ch'ien-lung emperor's literary inquisition; compilation and cataloguing of all books in the empire (*Complete Library of the Four Treasuries*).
1792	The great novel *Dream of the Red Chamber* first published.
1796–1804	White Lotus Rebellion.
ca. 1800–	Arrival of competitive Western powers in China.
1839–1842	First Opium War between China and Britain.
1850–1864	Taiping Rebellion.
1856–1860	Second Opium War between China and Britain and France.
1894–1895	China defeated in Sino-Japanese War.
1898	Hundred Days' Reform defeated by conservatives.
1900–1901	Boxer Rebellion (Peking occupied by allied Western powers).
1905	Civil service examination system abolished.
1911	Ch'ing dynasty falls.
1912	Republic of China proclaimed.
1949	People's Republic of China established. Republic of China continues rule on Taiwan.

APPENDIX 3

□

A Guide to Further Reading

This brief annotated guide is intended to suggest general works particularly useful for the beginning student. Most of the works cited include more extensive bibliographies. Following the first two sections on bibliographies and general histories, the guide is arranged according to the topics of the preceding chapters. Most of the chapters include notes with more extensive listings of additional sources.

BIBLIOGRAPHIES

Association for Asian Studies. *Bibliography of Asian Studies.* Ann Arbor: Association for Asian Studies, 1965–. An annual listing of books and articles on Asia arranged by area and topic.

Chang, Ch'un-shu. *Premodern China: A Bibliographical Introduction.* Ann Arbor: University of Michigan, Center for Chinese Studies, 1971. An annotated guide to works on China from earliest times to the nineteenth century.

Gentzler, J. Mason. *A Syllabus of Chinese Civilization.* 2d ed. New York: Columbia University Press, 1972. A detailed course outline with suggested topics, readings, and discussion questions designed for a liberal arts college curriculum.

Hucker, Charles O. *China: A Critical Bibliography.* Tucson: University of Arizona Press, 1962. A detailed annotated listing of works on all aspects of Chinese civilization from earliest times through the mid twentieth century. This valuable bibliography is currently being updated by David M. Deal of Whitman College.

GENERAL HISTORIES OF CHINA

Gernet, Jacques. *A History of Chinese Civilization.* Translated by J. R. Foster. Cambridge: Cambridge University Press, 1982. A detailed history of China that blends social, political, economic, and cultural history and places China within the context of world history.

Hucker, Charles O. *China's Imperial Past: An Introduction to Chinese History and Culture.* Stanford: Stanford University Press, 1975. An authoritative history of China from earliest times to the nineteenth century with topical coverage of political history, social-economic history, religion and thought, and art and literature.

———. *China to 1850: A Short History.* Stanford: Stanford University Press, 1978. A distillation of *China's Imperial Past* into a very compact introduction.

Reischauer, Edwin O., and John K. Fairbank. *East Asia: The Great Tradition.* Boston: Houghton Mifflin, 1960. An authoritative survey text of traditional East Asia; it was later incorporated into a survey that includes the modern period: John K. Fairbank, Edwin O. Reischauer, and Albert M. Craig. *East Asia: Tradition and Transformation.* Boston: Houghton Mifflin, 1978. A revised edition on China alone, *China: Tradition and Transformation,* was also published (Houghton Mifflin) in 1989 under the authorship of Reischauer and Fairbank.

Schirokauer, Conrad. *A Brief History of Chinese and Japanese Civilizations.* New York: Harcourt Brace Jovanovich, 1978. A valuable and wide-ranging one-volume survey of Chinese and Japanese history from earliest times to 1977.

WESTERN PERCEPTIONS OF CHINA

Dawson, Raymond. *The Chinese Chameleon: An Analysis of European Conceptions of Chinese Civilization.* London: Oxford University Press, 1967. A study of Western reportage on China from Marco Polo in the fourteenth century to the "China-watchers" in the mid twentieth century.

Hudson, G. F. *Europe and China: A Survey of Their Relations from the Earliest Times to 1800.* 1931. Reprint. Boston: Beacon Press, 1961. A history of cultural and commercial contacts between China and Europe from the sixth and seventh centuries B.C. to 1800.

Isaacs, Harold. *Images of Asia.* New York: Harper Torchbooks, 1972. Originally published as *Scratches on Our Minds* in 1958, this book is a survey of American attitudes toward China and India, primarily in the modern era. It is based on interviews, opinion surveys, and wide reading in Western journalistic and scholarly writings.

EARLY CHINESE CIVILIZATION

Boltz, William G. "Early Chinese Writing." *World Archaeology* 17 (1986): 420–36. A relatively technical but fundamental analysis of the origin, nature, and development of Chinese characters; it examines the topic from a comparative perspective.

Chang, Kwang-chih. *Art, Myth, and Ritual: The Path to Political Authority in Ancient China.* Cambridge: Harvard University Press, 1983. A stimulating attempt to characterize the links between the political, religious, social, and artistic realms of the Chinese Bronze Age.

———. *The Archaeology of Ancient China.* 4th ed. New Haven: Yale University

Press, 1986. The most recent, quasi-encyclopedic survey of a rapidly changing field; it covers the period from early man to ca. 1000 B.C.

Creel, Herrlee Glessner. *The Birth of China: A Survey of the Formative Period of Chinese Civilization.* New York: Ungar, 1937. Although dated by new archaeological discoveries, this highly readable account of the Shang and Chou dynasties still provides an excellent introduction to early Chinese culture.

Keightley, David N. "The Religious Commitment: Shang Theology and the Genesis of Chinese Political Culture." *History of Religions* 17, no. 3–4 (1978): 211–25. An exploration of the mutually reinforcing values in Shang religion, administration, and art.

———. "Late Shang Divination: The Magico-Religious Legacy" in Henry Rosemont, Jr., ed., *Explorations in Early Chinese Cosmology* (First published in *Journal of the American Academy of Religious Thematic Studies* 50.2). Chico, Calif.: American Scholars Press, 1984: 11–34. The worldview revealed by oracle-bone inscriptions suggests how Shang religious views shaped the secular concerns of later ages.

Wang, C. H. "Towards Defining a Chinese Heroism." *Journal of the American Oriental Society* 95, no. 1 (1975): 25–35. The absence of martial heroism and the epic form in early Chinese literature permits the identification of a characteristically Chinese style of heroic action.

Wheatley, Paul. *The Pivot of the Four Quarters: A Preliminary Inquiry into the Origins and Character of the Ancient Chinese City.* Chicago: Aldine, 1971. The evolution of Chinese urbanism is placed in comparative perspective with particular emphasis on the role played by religious belief.

GOVERNMENT IN TRADITIONAL CHINA

The Cambridge History of China. Cambridge: Cambridge University Press, 1978–. A projected fifteen-volume comprehensive history of China; includes the most detailed and authoritative essays in English on Chinese political history.

Goodrich, L. Carrington, and Fang Chao-ying, eds. *Dictionary of Ming Biography.* New York: Columbia University Press, 1975. An indispensable reference work that includes detailed and authoritative biographies of major political, cultural, and intellectual figures of the Ming period.

Huang, Ray. *1587: A Year of No Significance.* New Haven: Yale University Press, 1981. A sensitive and detailed exploration of court politics, dynastic decline, and social, economic, and intellectual problems in the late-Ming period.

Hucker, Charles O. *A Dictionary of Official Titles in Imperial China.* Stanford: Stanford University Press, 1985. A masterful reference work that includes authoritative translations of political titles and institutions, a table of organization, and a brief historical essay for each dynasty.

Hummel, Arthur W., ed. *Eminent Chinese of the Ch'ing Period, 1644–1911.* Washington, D.C.: Government Printing Office, 1943–1944. An indispensable reference on major figures of the Ch'ing dynasty.

Spence, Jonathan. *Emperor of China: Self-Portrait of K'ang-hsi.* New York: Vintage, 1975. Illuminating translations from the imperial edicts and other writings of the great K'ang-hsi emperor, who ruled from 1662–1722.

LAW IN CHINESE HISTORY

Bodde, Dirk. *China's First Unifier: A Study of the Ch'in Dynasty as seen in the Life of Li Ssu.* Hong Kong: Hong Kong University Press, 1967. A clear overview of Legalist principles in action in the state of Ch'in.

Bodde, Dirk, and Clarence Morris. *Law in Imperial China.* Philadelphia: University of Pennsylvania Press, 1967. A classic work on later legal thought and practice; it includes 190 Ch'ing dynasty cases translated from the *Hsin-an hui-lan* ("Conspectus of Penal Cases").

Duyvendak, J. J. L., trans. and ed. *The Book of Lord Shang.* 1928. Reprint. Chicago: University of Chicago Press, 1963. Translations from the writings of the great Legalist statesman of the fourth century B.C. Shang Yang.

Hsu, Cho-yun. *Ancient China in Transition: An Analysis of Social Mobility, 772–222 B.C.* Stanford: Stanford University Press, 1965. A classic study of social, political, and intellectual change in the formative era of the Eastern Chou.

Hulsewe, A. F. P., trans. *Remnants of Han Law.* Leiden: Brill, 1955. An annotated translation of the chapter on "punishments" in Pan Ku's *Han-shu.*

———, trans. *Remnants of Ch'in Law.* Leiden: Brill, 1985. Illuminating translations of important Ch'in laws and administrative rules from the third century B.C. that were discovered in Hupei in 1975.

Watson, Burton, trans. *Records of the Grand Historian of China.* 2 vols. New York: Columbia University Press, 1961. Expert translations from the monumental history by the great Han dynasty historian Ssu-ma Ch'ien. It is also available in a one-volume paperback abridgment: *Records of the Historian.* New York: Columbia University Press, 1969.

———, trans. *Courtier and Commoner in Ancient China: Selections from the History of the Former Han by Pan Ku.* New York: Columbia University Press, 1974. Selections from Pan Ku, Ssu-ma Ch'ien's successor; it includes colorful biographies of Han emperors in action.

Yang, Gladys, and Hsien-yi Yang, trans. *Selections from the Records of the Historian.* Peking: Foreign Languages Press, 1977. Selected pre-Han biographies by Ssu-ma Ch'ien, including accounts of Lord Shang and the first emperor of Ch'in.

THE CONFUCIAN TRADITION

Chan, Wing-tsit. *A Source Book of Chinese Philosophy.* New York: Columbia University Press, 1969. Important selected translations from the major works of Confucianism, Taoism, and Buddhism.

De Bary, William Theodore, Wing-tsit Chan, and Burton Watson, comps. *Sources of Chinese Tradition.* 2 vols. New York: Columbia University Press, 1960. Selected translations from major Chinese works of philosophy, history, and religion.

Mote, F. W. *Intellectual Foundations of China.* 2d ed. New York: Knopf, 1988. A wise and succinct survey of early Chinese thought in comparative perspective.

Schwartz, Benjamin. *The World of Thought in Ancient China.* Cambridge: Harvard

University Press, 1985. A challenging exploration of early Chinese thought that is rich with comparative insights.

Tu, Wei-ming. *Humanity and Self-Cultivation: Essays in Confucian Thought.* Berkeley: Asian Humanities Press, 1979. Fifteen essays on the Confucian tradition with emphasis on its "inner dimensions" from classical to modern times.

CHINESE RELIGIONS

Ch'en, Kenneth. *Buddhism in China: A Historical Survey.* Princeton: Princeton University Press, 1964. A useful introduction to the topic.

De Bary, William Theodore, ed. *The Buddhist Tradition in India, China, and Japan.* New York: Vintage, 1972. Valuable translations from important Buddhist texts.

Jochim, Christian. *Chinese Religions: A Cultural Perspective.* Englewood Cliffs, N.J.: Prentice-Hall, 1986. A useful introductory survey.

Overmyer, Daniel L. *Religions of China: The World as a Living System.* San Francisco: Harper & Row, 1986. A very concise introductory survey that covers the practices and beliefs of both the elite and the popular traditions.

Thompson, Laurence G. *Chinese Religion: An Introduction.* 4th ed. Belmont, Calif.: Wadsworth, 1988. A recent updated version of a long-standard introduction to the structures and functions of Taoism, Buddhism, and what Thompson calls "literati religion."

Wright, Arthur R. *Buddhism in Chinese History.* Stanford: Stanford University Press, 1959. Reprint. New York: Atheneum, 1965. Brief but wide-ranging essays on the interaction of Buddhism with Chinese culture and society from the Han period into the twentieth century.

Yang, C. K. *Religion in Chinese Society.* Berkeley: University of California Press, 1961. A classic study of the sociology of Chinese popular religion.

CHINESE SCIENCE AND MEDICINE

China: Seven Thousand Years of Discovery: China's Ancient Technology. Peking: China Reconstructs Magazine, 1983. A brief history of Chinese technology that is well illustrated in color.

Chinese Academy of Sciences. Institute for the History of Natural Sciences. *Ancient China's Technology and Science.* Peking: Foreign Languages Press, 1983. A clearly written summary of Chinese inventions.

Needham, Joseph, et al. *Science and Civilisation in China.* 14 vols. to date. Cambridge: Cambridge University Press, 1954–. A monumental survey of the field with full bibliographies and lavish illustrations. Recent abridgments of this work do not fully convey some of Needham's most interesting ideas or the grace of his writing; they also do not revise obsolete parts of the earlier volumes in light of the later volumes and other recent scholarship.

Sivin, Nathan. "An Introductory Bibliography of Traditional Chinese Science: Books and Articles in Western Languages." In *Chinese Science: Explorations of an Ancient Tradition,* ed. by Shigeru Nakayama and Nathan Sivin, 279–310. Cambridge: MIT Press, 1973. A guide to further reading, which is brought up to date in Sivin's "A Supplementary Bibliography of Traditional Chinese Science." *Chinese Science* 7 (1986): 33–41.

———. "Science and Medicine in Imperial China—The State of the Field." *Journal of Asian Studies* 47, no. 1 (1988): 41–90. A survey of recent studies in Chinese, Japanese, and Western languages.

———. *Traditional Medicine in Contemporary China.* Ann Arbor: University of Michigan Center for Chinese Studies, 1988. Translations from part of a textbook of traditional Chinese medicine; translations include explanations and historical discussion.

WOMEN, MARRIAGE, AND THE FAMILY IN CHINA

Buxbaum, David C., ed. *Chinese Family Law and Social Change.* Seattle: University of Washington Press, 1978. Contains fifteen articles, some by leading Chinese and Japanese scholars.

Ebrey, Patricia Buckley. *Family and Property in Sung China: Yuan Ts'ai's Precepts for Social Life.* Princeton: Princeton University Press, 1984. Examines attitudes toward family relations and property management among the upper class.

Ebrey, Patricia Buckley, and James L. Watson, eds. *Kinship Organization in Late Imperial China, 1000–1940.* Berkeley: University of California Press, 1986. Nine studies of kinship activities outside the sphere of the domestic household.

Guisso, Richard W., and Stanley Johannesen, eds. *Women in China: Current Directions in Historical Scholarship.* Youngstown, Ohio: Philo Press, 1981. Thirteen studies of women in literature, art, and history; emphasizes the premodern period.

Hanley, Susan B., and Arthur P. Wolf, eds. *Population in East Asian History.* Stanford: Stanford University Press, 1985. Includes six studies of Chinese historical demography in comparative perspective.

CHINESE ECONOMIC HISTORY

Chao, Kang. *Man and Land in Chinese History: An Economic Analysis.* Stanford: Stanford University Press, 1986. An imaginative and wide-ranging survey using sparse and sometimes unreliable data.

Eastman, Lloyd E. *Family, Fields, and Ancestors: Constancy and Change in China's Social and Economic History, 1550–1949.* New York: Oxford University Press, 1988. A recent synthesis of Western scholarship on social and economic history with emphasis on the sixteenth through the nineteenth centuries.

Elvin, Mark. *The Pattern of the Chinese Past.* Stanford: Stanford University Press, 1973. An ambitious attempt to analyze the longevity of China's imperial system, its "precocious" economic productivity in the Sung period, and its "stagnation" in late imperial times.

Ho, Ping-ti. *Studies on the Population of China, 1368–1953.* Cambridge: Harvard University Press, 1959. Pioneering essays on tax registration data and rapid population growth, particularly in the Ming and Ch'ing eras.

Perkins, Dwight H. *Agricultural Development in China, 1368–1968.* Chicago: Aldine, 1969. A detailed economic study of expanding agricultural productivity in late imperial times within the constraints of traditional technology.

CHINESE SOCIAL HISTORY

Huang, Philip C. C. *The Peasant Economy and Social Change in North China.* Stanford: Stanford University Press, 1984. A rigorous and multifactored analysis of "what went wrong" with Chinese agriculture in the last several centuries. Difficult, but probably the best study of Chinese rural society available in English.

Meskill, Johanna M. *A Chinese Pioneer Family: The Lins of Wu-feng, Taiwan, 1792–1895.* Princeton: Princeton University Press, 1984. A vivid depiction of life on the frontier (in this case Taiwan) that shows the successive ways in which elites maintained their dominance over local society.

Naquin, Susan. *Shantung Rebellion: The Wang Lun Uprising of 1774.* New Haven: Yale University Press, 1981. A vivid narrative of a disastrously failed rebellion that analyzes the underside of late imperial society, that is, its sects and secret societies.

Naquin, Susan, and Evelyn S. Rawski. *Chinese Society in the Eighteenth Century.* New Haven: Yale University Press, 1987. The best overall introduction to late imperial Chinese society; it downplays change over time but correctly emphasizes regional diversity.

Rowe, William T. *Hankow: Commerce and Society in a Chinese City, 1796–1889.* Stanford: Stanford University Press, 1984. A structural analysis of trade and urban society before and after the Western "opening" of the city.

Spence, Jonathan. *The Death of Woman Wang.* New York: Viking, 1978. A remarkable and highly literary reconstruction of Ch'ing society as experienced by some of its least fortunate members.

CHINESE ART

Cahill, James. *Chinese Painting.* Cleveland: World, 1960. An excellent introduction to the history of Chinese painting, a subject Cahill has explored in many fine, more specialized studies.

Sickman, Laurence, and Alexander C. Soper. *The Art and Architecture of China.* Rev. ed. Baltimore: Penguin, 1971. An informative survey of sculpture, painting, and architecture with many black-and-white illustrations.

Siren, Osvald. *Chinese Painting: Leading Masters and Principles.* 7 vols. New York: Ronald Press, 1956–1958. A monumental history of Chinese painting with hundreds of illustrations and information on over fourteen hundred painters.

Sullivan, Michael. *The Meeting of Eastern and Western Art.* Greenwich, Conn.: New York Graphic Society, 1973. A study of the mutual artistic influences between China, Japan, and the West over the past four centuries.

———. *The Arts of China.* 3d ed. Berkeley: University of California Press, 1984. A concise, richly illustrated and authoritative survey from earliest times to the twentieth century.

CHINESE POETRY

Graham, A. C. *Poems of the Late T'ang.* Baltimore: Penguin, 1965. Translations of some of the most exciting poems in Chinese with an excellent introduction on translating Chinese poetry.

Liu, James J. Y. *The Art of Chinese Poetry.* Chicago: University of Chicago Press, 1962. A general introduction to the forms and values of Chinese poetry.

Liu, Wu-chi, and Irving Yucheng Lo. *The Sunflower Splendor: Three Thousand Years of Chinese Poetry.* New York: Anchor Books, 1975. A massive and comprehensive anthology of Chinese poetry by many hands; it contains a useful bibliography and notes on individual poets.

Owen, Stephen. *The Great Age of Chinese Poetry: The High T'ang.* New Haven: Yale University Press, 1982. A literary history of the period traditionally considered to be the high point of classical poetry.

———. *Traditional Chinese Poetry and Poetics: Omen of the World.* Madison: University of Wisconsin Press, 1985. Eight somewhat eccentric essays on the fundamental concerns of classical poetry and the role it played in traditional Chinese civilization.

Waley, Arthur, trans. *Translations from the Chinese.* New York: Knopf, 1941. More than two hundred poems, mostly reprinted from Waley's *Chinese Poems* (first published in 1918), which first created a taste for Chinese poetry in the West.

———. *The Life and Times of Po Chü-i.* New York: Macmillan, 1949. A very readable biography of a major poet of the early ninth century that gives a good sense of the role of poetry in public and private life.

CHINESE FICTION

Birch, Cyril, ed. *Anthology of Chinese Literature.* 2 vols. New York: Grove Press, 1965–1972. An excellent selection of translations by many hands from all genres, including poetry, prose essays, short stories, dramas, and novels from early times to the contemporary era.

———, ed. *Studies in Chinese Literary Genres.* Berkeley: University of California Press, 1974. Scholarly essays on major genres of poetry, drama, and fiction in the Chinese tradition.

Chang, H. C., comp. *Chinese Literature.* Vol. 1, *Popular Fiction and Drama.* Edinburgh: Edinburgh University Press, 1973. Highly readable and lively translations of brief sections from the major novels and two famous dramas.

Hsia, C. T. *The Classic Chinese Novel.* New York: Columbia University Press, 1968. A beautifully written introduction to the six great novels with an emphasis on comparisons with the best of Western fiction.

Liu, Wu-chi. *An Introduction to Chinese Literature.* Bloomington: Indiana University Press, 1966. A brief but comprehensive and reliable history of Chinese literature, including poetry, drama, and fiction.

Nienhauser, William, Jr., ed. and comp. *The Indiana Companion to Traditional Chinese Literature.* Bloomington: Indiana University Press, 1986. An extremely valuable reference work on all facets of traditional Chinese literature with authoritative entries and bibliographies by 170 contributors.

Plaks, Andrew H., ed. *Chinese Narrative: Critical and Theoretical Essays.* Princeton: Princeton University Press, 1977. Scholarly essays on Chinese narratives, mostly fiction, with emphasis on the Ming and Ch'ing periods.

———. *The Four Masterworks of the Ming Novel.* Princeton: Princeton University Press, 1987. A masterful analysis of the four "great Ming novels" with detailed discussion of their sixteenth-century social, intellectual, and cultural context.

CONTRIBUTORS

T. H. Barrett received his doctorate at Yale University. He is professor of East Asian history at the University of London's School of Oriental and African Studies, a post he assumed in 1986 after teaching eleven years in the Department of Chinese Studies at Cambridge University. A specialist in the religious history of China (especially of the T'ang period), he has written *Singular Listlessness: A Short History of Chinese Books and British Scholars* (1989) and the introduction to the English translation of H. Maspero, *Taoism and Chinese Religion* (1981). His book *Li Ao: Buddhist, Taoist or Neo-Confucian?* is due to appear soon.

Jack L. Dull received his Ph.D. from the University of Washington, where he is associate professor of history and director of the East Asian Language and Area Center. He was chair of Washington's Chinese Studies Program from 1975 to 1985. A specialist in the social and intellectual history of early imperial China, he has edited *Han Social Structure* by Ch'ü T'ung-tsu (1971), and *Han Agriculture* by Hsu Cho-yun (1980). He is currently researching Han dynasty law.

Patricia Ebrey received her doctorate from Columbia University. She is professor of East Asian studies and history at the University of Illinois. She has published several books including *The Aristocratic Families of Early Imperial China* (1978), *Chinese Civilization and Society: A Sourcebook* (1981), *Family and Property in Sung China: Yuan Ts'ai's Precepts for Social Life* (1984), and most recently, *Kinship Organization in Late Imperial China, 1000–1940* (1986), coedited with James Watson. She is currently engaged in research on Chinese family rituals (weddings, funerals, and ancestral rites), especially in the Sung dynasty.

Albert Feuerwerker holds a Harvard Ph.D. and is the A. M. and H. P. Bentley Professor of History at the University of Michigan, where he served as director of the Center for Chinese Studies, 1961–1967 and 1972–1983, and chair of the history department, 1984–1987. A specialist in the economic history of China, he has published articles and monographs on many aspects of modern Chinese social, economic, political, and intellectual history. His works include *China's Early Industrialization* (1958), *The Chinese Economy, 1912–1949* (1968), *The Chinese Economy, ca. 1870–1911* (1969), *Rebellion in Nineteenth-Century China* (1975), *State and Society in Eighteenth-Century China* (1976), and *Economic Trends in Republican China, 1912–1949* (1977). He has also edited and contributed to *History in Communist China* (1968), *Chinese Social and Economic History from the Song to 1900* (1982), and (with John King Fairbank) *The Cambridge History of China,* vol. 13 (1986).

David N. Keightley received his Ph.D. in East Asian history from Columbia University. Professor of history and chair of the Center for Chinese Studies (1988–1990) at the University of California at Berkeley, Keightley specializes in China's Neolithic and early Bronze Age cultures. The author of *Sources of Shang History: The Oracle-Bone Inscriptions of Bronze Age China* (1978) and the editor of *The Origins of Chinese Civilization* (1983), he has written a variety of articles on early Chinese archaeology, historiography, inscriptions, metaphysics, religion, and political culture. Keightley was one of the founders and has served as the editor of the journal *Early China.* He was named a MacArthur Fellow in 1986.

Stephen Owen holds a doctorate from Yale University and is presently professor of Chinese and comparative literature at Harvard. He is the author of five books on T'ang poetry and traditional Chinese poetics, including *The Poetry of the Early T'ang* (1977), *The Great Age of Chinese Poetry* (1981), *Traditional Chinese Poetry and Poetics: An Omen of the World* (1985), *Remembrances: The Experience of the Past in Classical Chinese Literature* (1986), and *Mi-lou: Poetry and the Labyrinth of Desire* (1989).

Paul S. Ropp received his doctorate from the University of Michigan and is currently associate professor and chair of history at Clark University. A specialist in Chinese social and intellectual history, he has written *Dissent in Early Modern China: "Ju-lin wai-shih" and Ch'ing Social Criticism* (1981) and several articles on women, literature, and society, primarily in the Ch'ing period (1644–1911). He is currently engaged in research on women in late imperial Chinese literature and society.

William T. Rowe received his doctorate from Columbia University and is currently professor of history at the Johns Hopkins University. Specializing in modern Chinese social and economic history, he has written *Han-*

kow: Commerce and Society in a Chinese City, 1796–1889 (1984), *Hankow: Conflict and Community in a Chinese City, 1796–1895* (1989), and numerous articles. He has also edited *Perspectives on a Changing China* (1979) with Joshua A. Fogel.

Nathan Sivin received his doctorate in the history of science from Harvard University. He is currently professor of Chinese culture and of the history of science at the University of Pennsylvania. His publications include *Chinese Alchemy: Preliminary Studies* (1968), *Cosmos and Computation in Early Chinese Mathematical Astronomy* (1969), and, with Joseph Needham, Lu Gwei-djen, and Ho Ping-yü, *Science and Civilisation in China,* vol. 5, part 4, *Chemical Discovery* (1980). He is the editor and publisher of the journal *Chinese Science,* and he has also edited and contributed essays to *Chinese Science: Explorations of an Ancient Tradition* (with Shigeru Nakayama, 1972), *Science and Technology in East Asia: Articles from ISIS, 1913–1975* (1977), and *Astronomy in Contemporary China: A Trip Report of the American Astronomy Delegation* (1979).

Jonathan Spence received his doctorate from Yale University, where he is currently the George Burton Adams Professor of History. A specialist in Chinese history and Chinese-Western relations from the sixteenth century to the present, he recently received a MacArthur Fellowship. His books include *Ts'ao Yin and the K'ang-hsi Emperor, Bondservant and Master* (1968), *To Change China: Western Advisors in China from 1620 to 1960* (1969), *Emperor of China: Self-Portrait of K'ang-hsi* (1974), *The Death of Woman Wang* (1978), *The Gate of Heavenly Peace* (1981), *The Memory Palace of Matteo Ricci* (1984), and *The Question of Hu* (1988).

Michael Sullivan received his doctorate from Harvard University. He is currently Fellow by Special Election of St. Catherine's College, Oxford University. His many books include *Chinese Art in the Twentieth Century* (1959), *An Introduction to Chinese Art* (1961), *The Birth of Landscape Painting in China* (1962), *Chinese and Japanese Art* (1965), *The Meeting of Eastern and Western Art* (1965, rev. ed., 1989), *Chinese Art: Recent Discoveries* (1973), *The Arts of China* (1973, 4th ed., 1984), *The Three Perfections: Chinese Poetry, Painting and Calligraphy* (1974), *Symbols of Eternity: The Art of Landscape Painting in China* (1979), and *Chinese Landscape Painting,* vol. 2, *The Sui and T'ang Dynasties* (1980).

Tu Wei-ming received his doctorate from Harvard University, where he is now professor of Chinese history and philosophy. A specialist in Confucian thought, he has written many books and articles, including *Neo-Confucian Thought in Action: Wang Yang-ming's Youth* (1976), *Centrality and Commonality: An Essay on Chung-yung* (1976), *Humanity and Self-Cultivation: Essays in Confucian Thought* (1980), *Confucian Ethics Today: The*

Singapore Challenge (1984), *Confucian Thought: Selfhood as Creative Transformation* (1985), and *The Way, Learning and Politics: Perspectives on the Confucian Intellectual* (1989).

Karen Turner received her doctorate in Chinese History at the University of Michigan. She is currently assistant professor of history at the College of the Holy Cross and a visiting scholar in the East Asian Legal Studies Program at Harvard University School of Law. A specialist in early Chinese legal thought, she studied at Beijing University under the auspices of the Committee on Scholarly Communication with the People's Republic of China in 1979 and has returned to China several times in the past decade to research the Ma-wang-tui documents on law. She has written on legal theory and is completing a book-length manuscript on monarchy and law in the early imperial period in China. She has been active in China exchange programs and is the author of *China Bound: A Guide to Academic Life and Work in the PRC* (1987).

INDEX

Compositor: G & S Typesetters, Inc.
Text: 10/12 Baskerville
Display: Baskerville
Printer: Maple-Vail
Binder: Maple-Vail